Forensic Pathoradiology of Virtual Autopsy

Virtual autopsy is a burgeoning field that employs imaging methods to find causes of death. This book critically analyses and compares different post-mortem features and their radiological appearance in diverse cases. It orients forensic doctors trained in traditional autopsy to understand the radiological appearance of their gross findings and radiologists to comprehend the pathology in an imaging study. Further, it provides the standard operating protocols to be followed in different cases. This can be an alternative to standard autopsies for broad and systemic examination of the whole body as it saves time, aids better diagnosis, and respects religious sentiments.

Key features:

- Provides the reader with an in-depth review of the value of a CT-directed virtual autopsy complementing a regular autopsy and how it can enhance the quality of medico-legal death investigation in a jurisdiction.
- Bridges the gap between the specialities of Forensic Medicine and Radiology and helps the readers co-relate and understand the concept of Virtual Autopsy.
- Features over 500 original autopsy photographs and CT images with over 100 case reports including a stepwise approach to each case along with comparative radiological images.

Forensic Pathoradiology of Virtual Autopsy

Dr Sudhir K Gupta
MBBS, MD, DNB, MNAMS, FICS (Chicago)
Professor and Head
Department of Forensic Medicine and Toxicology
All India Institute of Medical Sciences, New Delhi, India

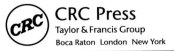

CRC Press
Taylor & Francis Group
Boca Raton London New York

CRC Press is an imprint of the
Taylor & Francis Group, an **informa** business

Designed cover image: Author

First edition published 2024
by CRC Press
6000 Broken Sound Parkway NW, Suite 300, Boca Raton, FL 33487-2742

and by CRC Press
4 Park Square, Milton Park, Abingdon, Oxon, OX14 4RN

CRC Press is an imprint of Taylor & Francis Group, LLC

© 2024 Sudhir K Gupta

ISBN: 978-1-032-46903-4 (hbk)
ISBN: 978-1-032-46902-7 (pbk)
ISBN: 978-1-003-38370-3 (ebk)

DOI: 10.1201/9781003383703

Typeset in Warnock Pro
by Deanta Global Publishing Services, Chennai, India

CONTENTS

Contents

PREFACE

Every human being wants a life of dignity, in life and death. Post-mortem dissection/cutting during autopsy of the deceased body is an unpleasant experience for the relatives of the deceased. It adds to the mental trauma at a time when the family is grieving/mourning. Virtual autopsy (VA) has come as a boon to forensic experts and the family of the deceased to avoid this painful experience. The concept of dignified management of the dead is the need of the hour as every person deserves dignity and respect. This concept also includes not only handling the deceased bodies with dignity, but also safe preservation in a cold cabinet, proper autopsy in medico-legal cases, surgical restoration of mutilated or dismembered body parts, embalming for preservation, and packaging and hygienic and safe transportation for the last ritual. In medico-legal cases, forensic autopsy or post-mortem examination is mandatory as per the provision of the law of countries across the globe. The conventional medico-legal autopsy techniques worldwide comprise of opening all the body cavities and the examination of the visceral organs by detailed dissection. Generally, a long incision is made from the chin to the pubic symphysis to open the body cavities. These long stitches and post-mortem alterations of the body give a very unpleasant visual appearance to the aggrieved relatives and well-wishers. We conducted a survey of a large number of aggrieved relatives of the deceased persons undergoing autopsy examination in the Department of Forensic Medicine and Toxicology, All India Institute of Medical Sciences (AIIMS), New Delhi. This survey concluded that 92% of the family members didn't want the practice of traditional dissection from chin to symphysis pubis dissection (Figure 0.1).

The mental agony of relatives caused by post-mortem dissection is a well-established fact. Studies have shown that society at large does not want the deceased body to undergo autopsy involving invasive dissection of the body. They will willingly opt for an alternative technique which involves zero to minimal cuts/dissection in the body of the deceased person. This has led to finding an alternate, non-invasive or minimally invasive technique without compromising the purpose of the conventional autopsy and also fulfilling the medico-legal queries for the legal purpose. The solution was found through virtual autopsy. Advancement in medical diagnostic technologies has given many tools for autopsy surgeons to conduct autopsy in a non-invasive or minimally invasive way. The cross-sectional imaging technique has further helped doctors to view the pathology and post-mortem findings in 2D and 3D imaging without dissecting the body. This concept of digital or virtual autopsy has already been adopted by autopsy centres in Switzerland, Australia, and England and has proven to be very useful to meet the needs of the legal system. And it has given relief to the concerned relatives in mourning from the unpleasant experience of their loved one's body being dissected. Most religious and cultural beliefs prevalent in Indian society are against the post-mortem dissection of corpses as per their religious faith. However, they are bound to follow the law of the land and the same has been in practice for decades. Even though the pace of modernization in the field of Forensic Pathology in developed/developing countries is well appreciated, the same has not been fully utilized in most developing countries. This is mainly due to the limited resources or under-rutilization of available radiological advancement in their respective hospitals by autopsy surgeons. This drawback has led to the scientific development and value of medico-legal work in developing countries decades behind when compared to that of developed countries. The multi-cultural and multi-religious population of India is an ideal beneficiary of concepts like computed tomography (CT) augmented autopsy, CT-guided minimal invasive autopsy, and interpretation of PMCT internal findings in the form of virtual autopsy as many cases will not at all require conventional autopsy. In light of advancements in radiological science and its use in post-mortem surgery to protect the dignity of the dead by minimum use of scalpel in the body, the Department of Forensic Medicine, AIIMS, New Delhi, submitted a proposal to the Indian Council of Medical Research headquarters to establish a Centre for Advanced Research and Excellence in Virtual Autopsy. The Indian Council of Medical Research (ICMR) approved the proposed study on 24 September 2018 in the Vide ICMR letter no. Coord/7(3)/CARE-VA/2018-NCD-II and the same research proposal was submitted to AIIMS institutional ethics committee which was approved after detailed scrutiny Vide Ref. No: IEC-575/02.11.2018, RP-28/2018 dated 30 November 2018, Vide Ref. No: IEC-577/02.11.2018, RP-29/2018 dated 30 November 2018, and Vide Ref. No: IEC-633/07.12.2018, RP-37/2018 dated 31 November 2018. This study was titled 'Centre for Advanced Research & Excellence in Virtual Autopsy' which played a vital role in the inception of India's first dedicated virtual autopsy centre. The primary objective of this study was to assess if we could incorporate modern imaging techniques including CT in autopsy so that the technique of minimal dissection of the corpse could be followed. CT scanning of the dead body will also be useful in two key areas of research and reference. First, it is used for age estimation by studying the ossification centres in various bones. Second, it will also be used before opening the body for analysing the internal findings of the organs which can be missed in conventional autopsy like internal neck findings in hanging and strangulation which are crucial aspects of forensic medicine. Conventional autopsy findings are documented by a subjective observer-dependent method which cannot

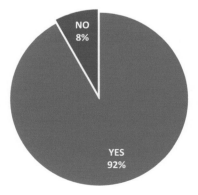

FIGURE 0.1 Result of a survey conducted at the AIIMS, New Delhi, mortuary.

be recreated or cross-examined. The findings and the ones that have not been documented are permanently lost especially if the body has been cremated. For decades, there has been a delay in applying imaging techniques in forensics and the medico-legal system, which provides objective, scientific, reliable, reproducible, and permanent documentation of relevant forensic findings. The rich radiological data obtained from virtual autopsy can also be very useful for research purposes. It can be used for various medical research like anatomical variations of skeletal/organs in the human body and age-related ossification studies in the Indian population. PMCT data in sudden death cases can be a good source to study the pathology of diseases and a form of feedback to the treating clinicians in clinical care. The ICMR is the first to introduce the concept of virtual autopsy in India at the Department of Forensic Medicine, AIIMS, New Delhi, which involves zero to minimal cuts to the body of the deceased person in medico-legal autopsy.

ABOUT THE AUTHOR

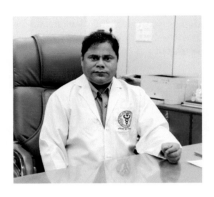

Dr Sudhir K Gupta is a Professor and Head of the Department of Forensic Medicine, AIIMS, New Delhi, India. He excelled right from his undergraduate times, securing a Gold Medal in the MBBS examination. He completed his post-grad at Banaras Hindu University, Varanasi, India and was awarded Diplomate by the National Board. He is a well-known teacher and researcher at AIIMS, New Delhi, for the past 28 years and has also been recognized by the Indian Association of Medico-legal Experts. He has worked towards the sensitization of doctors working in the mortuaries to handle the deceased in addition to inculcating an aura of respect and teaching the doctors how to treat their work with utmost dignity. Since taking the mantle of the Head of the Department of Forensic Medicine in 2013, he has been working towards converting the AIIMS mortuary into a Centre of Excellence for forensic studies. He remains a member of many state service commissions and union service commissions in confidential assignments. Dr Gupta is the pioneer of virtual autopsy in India by establishing the AIIMS and ICMR Centre of Advanced Research and Excellence in Virtual Autopsy, a first of its kind in India and South Asia. He has also been awarded a fellowship from Windsor University, Canada. His work has been internationally recognized across the globe from Australia to the United States of America.

Dr Gupta has been associated with AIIMS for more than a quarter of a century and has used the opportunity to promote progress in the field of Forensic Medicine. He has served the Nation and has helped bring justice through forensic investigations in various challenging cases in partnership with the CBI, NIA, NHRC, Delhi Police, various state police, and all the levels of the judiciary. He has served at AIIMS teaching MBBS, MD, and PhD students and providing specialized training to National and International doctors. Besides India, he has also received recognition for his work in the field of Forensic Medicine by the Coroners Association of Europe; American Academy of Forensic Science, Scotland Yard Police, UK; the FBI; and police services of countries including Australia and all Asian countries like Taiwan, Singapore, and Nepal. He has been recognized by the American Association of Surgeons and was invited to the United States for training in emergency and trauma care in 2005 with CME credit and was even made a member of the technical specification committee for initiating an AIIMS Trauma Centre, in 2005. The AIIMS Forensic Medicine Department has attained new horizons under his stewardship and has established various new facilities such as the 24-hour embalming facility, forensic radiology unit, virtual autopsy unit, DNA laboratory, and modern toxicology laboratory. He has promoted the establishment of a cadaver organ retrieval facility for therapeutic transplantation. Several other facilities like modular odourless autopsy suites are also in the process of being established. Recently the Delhi High Court expressed its gratitude and appreciated his efforts in preserving and conducting a third autopsy on an Indian citizen about 14 months after their death in Saudi Arabia. He has published more than 150 scientific papers in different National and International medical journals and has 6 chapters in books and textbooks on legal medicine. He has authored two books titled, *Forensic Medicine and Toxicology* and *Forensic Pathology of Asphyxial Deaths* with CRC Press, Boca Raton, Florida, United States. Under his leadership, a record number of cornea donations has taken place in the time period of 2013 to 2021 at AIIMS, New Delhi. He is working on a research project to assess the viability of different organs and tissues after death for transplantation purposes. As a doctor, one of his missions is to establish a breakthrough cadaver organ retrieval facility which would save countless lives. He has collaborated with an NGO to provide free hearse van services to help in the cremation of the deceased who belong to the poorer sections of society. Dr Gupta holds the record of being the first autopsy surgeon to be awarded a fellowship diploma by the International College of Surgeons, Chicago, Illinois, United States. He has developed an ultra-modern toxicology lab with analytical instruments like GCHS, HPLC, trace metal analyser, UV visible double beam spectro-photometry, TLC, biochemistry analyser, and microwave digestion unit. The laboratory is currently serving as a nodal centre for alcohol estimation in medico-legal cases in south and southeast Delhi. The lab is also a registered centre for the estimation of mercury in biological samples for the global mercury lab databank as per UNEP. He was awarded Medical Doctor of the Year by *E-Medinews* and *Indian Journal of Clinical Practice* in 2010.

Here is a list of the prominent cases of National and International repute handled by Dr Gupta for CBI and other investigating agencies: Virtual autopsy of veteran actor-comedian Raju Shrivastava, 2022; CBI Delhi/investigation in the death of Sh. Y.S. Vivekananda, brother of previous Chief Minister of Andhra Pradesh, 2022; CBI Chandigarh/investigation of the death of three children in a canal at Panipat, 2022; CBI Delhi/investigation to identify individuals in objectionable photo/videos, 2022; CBI Kolkata/investigation in the death of Sh. Niranjan Baishnab, an eye witness to a murder case, 2022; CBI Shimla/investigation on the death of Mr Parveen Sharma, 2022; Delhi police/facial reconstruction and skull superimposition of an unidentified dead body, 2022; investigation of the death of Mr Devendar Kumar on the directions of Hon'ble Tiz Hazari Court, Delhi, 2022; examination of mortal remains of Foreign Secretary Late. Jaswinder Singh, External Affairs Ministry, 2022; Delhi police/investigation of the death of Yogesh K Jude, 2022; NIA Jammu/forensic analysis of exhibits containing medicines, 2022; CBI Kolkata/investigation of post-poll violent deaths of Kolkata in 2021 and 2022; CBI Delhi/investigation of Bakoria encounter case, 2021; CBI Delhi/death investigation of Late Dheeraj Ahalawat, Vice President, Yes Bank, 2021; death investigation of Priyanka Sharma case, triple murder by Thallium poisoning, 2021; CBI Delhi/investigation of alleged medical negligence in death of Ms Rosy Sangma, 2021; CBI Vishakapatnam/investigation of death of Ms Ayesha Meera in Vijaywada, 2021; CBI Delhi/investigation of child sexual abuse in Goa and Bhiwandi Maharashtra, 2021; CBI Delhi/investigation of online child sexual abuse and exploitation (OCSAE) prevention, 2021; CBI Delhi/investigation of Chitrakoot child sexual abuse case – examination of the accused and 30 abused children, 2021; CBI Kolkata/investigation of a suspicious hanging death of a girl student in her school hostel in Manipur, which created public unrest in the state 2020; CBI Delhi online child sexual abuse and exploitation (OCSAE) prevention – investigation unit – cases of child pornography 2020; CBI Chandigarh case – murder case of Sukhamnpreet Singh at Sippy Siddhu, 2020; CBI Lucknow/death investigation of Mr Pravish Chman who died in a rock concert in Greater Noida, 2020; death investigation of Indian film star Sushant Singh Rajput 2020; Disha gang rape and murder case – appointed as chairman of the medical board to conduct the second autopsy of four accused that were killed in exchange of fire, 2019; homicide of Mr Rohit Shekhar Tiwari S/O veteran politician late Mr N D Tiwari, 2019; CBI/investigation of gang rape and custodial death of father of victim in Unnao 2018. Cases done prior to 2018 are CBI/death investigation of Finnish citizen Mr Felix Dahl Valdimar in Goa; the demise of Mrs Sunanda Pushkar, Supreme Court monitored CBI enquiry in more than 40 cases of extrajudicial killings in Manipur; death of Cabinet Minister Sh Gopi Nath Munde in an RTA by CBI, CBI/Sheena Bora murder case Mumbai, CBI/death investigation of IAS officer Anurag Tiwari in Lucknow; CBI/Investigation of Promila Gandhi mysterious death case Chennai, CBI/inquiry into Sara Singh murder case, Lucknow; CBI/Shimla gang rape and custodial death case, Kotkhai; CBI/investigation of the suicide of IAS officer DK Ravi, CBI investigation; reinvestigation by CBI in the death of Dr Y S Sachan, an accused in NHRM scam; Jessica Lal murder case, the High Court of Delhi; NIA investigation of Vidyacharan Shukla ex Union Minister bomb blast death; scribe Nirupma Pathak Case; Uphaar fire tragedy cases; Nitish Katara murder case; BMW Lodhi road accident case; Shivani Bhatnagar murder case; judicial inquiry into death of Ram Singh the main accused in Nirbhaya case; Tihar jail, CBI/invesigation of Dy SP Mangalore; M K Ganpathy death, Karnataka; deputed by the High Court of Madras to supervise the autopsy in custodial death of P Ramkumar, the accused in public hacking of a female Infosys employee; Deputed by the High Court of Madras for third autopsy of Ilavarsana, Chennai; CBI/Geetanjali Garg, wife of Chief Judicial Magistrate, Gurgaon death case; CBI/death of journalist Akshay Singh; VYAPAM scam in Madhya Pradesh; CBI/Puja Mishra death case; CBI/Denisye Carole Sweeney death investigation – British citizen found dead in Goa; death investigation of a teenage couple in a suspected rape/drowning in Jind and Kurukshetra which shocked the entire Haryana State; CBI/suicide of AIIMS student Rishikesh; CBI/suspected gang rape and murder of a minor girl in Haridwar.

ACKNOWLEDGEMENTS

This book, the first of its kind book in medical science, is based on more than 28 years of experience and research on forensic autopsy by the author. In his experience, he has seen many cases of sudden and suspicious deaths due to various manners/modes of death, and there has been unrest at national and international levels to know the cause and manner of death.

Several case studies have been added to help readers understand how the principles of forensic medicine are applied practically and to help the judiciary in judging crimes. Numerous colour photographs and illustrations have been added to support the text and help the readers to visualize concepts for better understanding. I dedicate this book to all the deceased whose contributions through photographs are highly educative. In this fast-paced era of technology, the field of forensic medicine is rapidly and constantly evolving. To this end, I have made every effort to fortify this book with updated and relevant knowledge, particularly with regard to medico-legal investigations and causes of death in medico-legal cases. The needs of medical students, autopsy surgeons, judicial officers, and forensic fraternity, medical practitioners, autopsy surgeons, criminal lawyers, and police officers have been taken into consideration to make this book a useful source of reference in forensic pathology radiology. Considering the extensive and highly scientific amount of work that went into bringing out this edition, I am most grateful to Dr Kulbhushan Prasad, Dr Abhishek Yadav, Dr Swati Tyagi, Dr Karthi Vignesh Raj K, Dr Jay Narayan Pandit, Dr Zahid Ali CH, Dr Balaji D, and I am especially grateful to Dr Abilash S, Assistant Professor from the Department of Forensic Medicine, AIIMS, New Delhi, without whose active and wholehearted contribution and direct participation this would not be possible.

I thank my wife Dr Madhu Gupta and son Keshav Karan whose active support helped make this endeavour successful. I dedicate this book to my loving father **Shri Kashi Nath Gupta** and mother **Kasthuri Devi**.

1 CONCEPT OF VIRTUAL AUTOPSY

In the modern era of medical care delivery system all over the world, the use of advanced radiological images in the form of digital X-ray, computed tomography, and magnetic resonance imaging are being used frequently and routinely, and the same needs to be adopted in the practice of forensic autopsy. Hence there is a requirement for clearly defining the role and application. The author in his experience has seen many cases, a few of which are mentioned in the last chapter indicating the potential areas of use of forensic radiology in trauma deaths, foreign body discovery, mass fatality, and body identification post-mortem computed tomography (PMCT) as a substitute for dissectional autopsy. The use of images from CT scanning is one possible way of reducing the number of unnecessary dissection in autopsy. Certain faith groups are particularly keen to avoid an autopsy dissection, and many others will be pleased if it's possible to avoid one.

The history of forensic medicine/pathology in India can be traced back as early as 1250–1000 B.C. where there is mention of medico-legal aspects like sexual offences and their punishments, intoxication and the loss of mental capacity, etc. Charaka Samhita is an ancient script that gave guidelines for the training of physicians in treating poisoning cases. Arthashastra of Kautilya outlines the application of medical knowledge in helping the Justice system. It also describes the examination of dead bodies in suspected unnatural death cases. 'Modi's Medical Jurisprudence' traces the evolution of medico-legal work in British India. The earliest incident of custodial death and its certification by medical practitioners was reported in Madras in 1678. A soldier, Thomas Savage, abused his superior officer in a drunken brawl. He was tied to a cot and died. Surgeons John Waldo and Bezaliel Sherman inspected the body and they were the first to issue a death certificate in British India. The first medico-legal autopsy was performed in India by Dr. Edward Bulkley in 1693. However, the first medico-legal case of injury was documented in the form of a medico-legal report by Dr. Bulkley in 1695 in British India.

The evolution of Forensic Medicine/Forensic Pathology/ Legal Medicine happened in various other places of the world in a sporadic fashion up to the late 16th century when many places had identified Forensic Medicine as a distinct specialty. During this phase of evolution of forensic medicine, one of the greatest medicolegists or a forensic physician was Paulus Zacchias (1584–1659) who was a papal physician and head of the medical system. His work which was published in three volumes known as the '*Quaestiones medico-legales*' was one of the most important pieces of literature which recorded and established legal medicine as a distinct topic of medicine and as an important specialty. The sporadic evolution of various other countries prior to the 16th century included:

Babylon: The Code of Hammurabi from Babylon, which dates back to about 2200 B.C., mentions medicine and its relation with the legal system.

Egypt: In Egypt, medical experts were required to give opinions at judicial hearings and were requested to carry out autopsy examinations. Imhotep, who was the personal physician of King Zoster, initially combined law and medicine. Worldwide, the inquest procedure was first done in the colony of New Plymouth, New England, in the year 1635 related to the death of John Deacon. The rule of exclusion was applied here, where the deceased John Deacon had no signs of external violence in the form of blows, wounds, or any other hurt and the conclusion related to the cause of death was given as bodily weakness due to long fasting and extreme climatic variations.

Greece: Hippocrates, who lived in Greece from 460–355 B.C., has given significant contributions to the matter of toxicology, medical ethics, and the prevention of abortion. The Hippocratic Oath is still an important pillar guiding physicians and also a signpost for doctors to avoid negligence in practice.

Rome: Numa Pompilius was a prominent figure in Rome who contributed significantly to medico-legal work. The Lex Aquillia, published in 572 B.C., is an article discussing the significance and lethality of wounds and also provides an expert medical opinion on wounds. After the death of Julius Caesar, the cadaver was examined in the forum of physicians and the examining physician. Antistius found that out of the 23 stab wounds on his body only one was found to be fatal. Pliny the Elder (23–79 A.D.) did significant work on topics like superfetation and suspended animation.

Jerusalem: Godfrey de Bouillon in 1100 A.D. made an important code of laws which introduced the principles of feudalism but took the help of physicians. This made provisions for the courts to order medical examinations by a physician if they felt the need. In cases of death by murder, the dead body was examined for injuries and to determine the possible weapons causing those injuries.

Italy: Autopsies and other medico-legal examinations were very common in Italy. Pope Innocent III, in 1209 A.D., initiated appointments of doctors in the courts of law for interpretation of the nature of wounds sustained. Pope Gregory IX, in 1234 A.D., initiated the *Nova Compilatio Decretalium* which is a collection of previous councils and Popes' decisions in medical matters relating to marriage, nullity, impotence, delivery, caesarean section, legitimacy, sexual offences, abortion, crimes against the person, and witchcraft.

China: The earliest mention of post-mortem examination in China was during the 1250s A.D. in the book named *His Yuan Lu*. The contents of the book were mainly related to autopsy techniques, post-mortem guidelines, injuries caused by blunt and sharp objects, and identification of death due to drowning and thermal burns.

France: In 1260 A.D. the book of common law of St. Louis highlighted the role of surgeons and medical experts in helping the law to come to a conclusion on medico-legal matters by taking the role of witness. In Paris, recognized medical experts were part of the preparation of injury reports and other medico-legal reports. Reports by these surgeons were founded on external inspection of the body and of any wounds on it, with at most superficial incisions. No autopsy was made.

Medical experts took the role of expert witnesses addressing the medico-legal matters in courts of law relating to injury reporting, weapons examination, toxicology cases, the examination of sexual offences, and pregnancy. The right of conducting an autopsy was granted to the Faculty of Montpellier by

DOI: 10.1201/9781003383703-1

the Pope in 1374 A.D. The Constitutio Criminalis Carolina in Germany (1532) and the ordinance of Francois I focused on bridging the gap between medicine and law which was later further strengthened by Henri IV and other kings.

Germany: In 1507 A.D., a systemized code of penal law and procedure was made under George, Prince Bishop of Bamberg. This code emphasized and required evidence from a medical expert in cases related to violent deaths. Under Emperor Charles V a similar code was adopted in almost all states of Germany. The Constitutio Criminalis Carolina came to being in 1532 A.D., and it was based on the *Codex Bambergensis*. It dealt with aspects like injuries, murder, suicide, infanticide, abortion, pregnancy, poisoning, etc. It also recognized the significance of medical examination in cases of insanity among the accused. It also showed the importance to the courts to consider medical evidence and understand its significance. It paved the way for the practice of medico-legal autopsies by allowing the opening of dead bodies for examination. Legal medicine which also included public health in those times with all these changes started emerging as a separate and important branch which was later recognized by prominent universities. In North America, the first autopsy was conducted by Champlain's surgeon, Estienne, near the initial periods of the 17th century.

Autopsy and its types

An autopsy or post-mortem examination is a systematic examination of a person's dead body, which is conducted by a doctor or by a medical board consisting of doctors to ascertain the cause, manner, and time of death for legal reasons, which is called a legal autopsy. Autopsies are also taught in medical school and used for various research purposes. Autopsies are of the following types:

i. Medico-legal: This refers to the post-mortem examination of a dead body performed by a doctor or by a medical board of doctors under the legal jurisdiction of the State. The consent of the deceased's relatives is not required in such cases.

ii. Academic/Anatomical: These are carried out by medical students to learn about the anatomy of the human body. This type of autopsy is done on human cadavers kept preserved in special chemicals specifically for this purpose.

iii. Pathological/Clinical: These are conducted by pathologists to diagnose or confirm the cause of a patient's death in cases where the physician is not certain of the same. However, this type of autopsy can only be done with the consent of the next of kin. These autopsies are not ordered by any legal authorities. Once the autopsy is done, the body is handed over to the deceased's relatives. Ancillary investigations such as microbiology, histology, etc., are routinely carried out by the pathologist conducting the autopsy.

The main objectives of a medico-legal autopsy include the determination of the cause and manner of death, confirmation of the identity of the dead person, and collection of all possible evidence needed for investigation or legal process in case of any expected foul play or future litigation. A medico-legal autopsy is being conducted under Sections 174 and 176 in Criminal Procedure Code 1973 as discussed extensively above. The law directs the investigating officer to take the body of the deceased to the concerned designated hospital/post-mortem centre. The nature and extent of the examination are not formulated or

described in these sections or any other law in Indian Penal Code or Criminal Procedure Code. The holistic procedure currently followed during any autopsy examination by most of the autopsy centres includes:

i. The receipt of the inquest papers from the police or magistrate.

ii. Detailed perusal history or the inquest findings as detailed by the legal authorities in the inquest papers.

iii. The witness statements related to the circumstances surrounding the death.

iv. Clarification of the queries raised by the autopsy surgeon with the authorities.

v. Identification of the deceased by the relatives (preferably two).

vi. Thorough External Examination of the deceased and documenting the findings like identification marks, clothes, etc.

vii. Detailed examination of the external injuries if any present over the body.

viii. Internal examination of the body by adhering to various techniques performing various dissection of cavities.

ix. Preservation of the samples like blood, urine, vitreous, and viscera for toxicology analysis on account of suspicion or samples from internal organs for histopathology examination if required.

x. Conclude the cause of death after receipt of preserved viscera analysis in cases where samples are preserved or directly conclude the cause of death on the account of non-preservation of samples.

In the author's experience almost 80–90% of the cases, the cause of death is known from the extensive inquest procedures undertaken by the legal authorities. The extensive dissection at autopsy examination in such cases is carried out only to confirm the findings concluded during the inquest or inquiry by the legal authorities. The remaining 10–20% of cases may require an extensive dissection where the history given by the relatives or the inquest procedure conclusion may be inconsistent with the external examination findings seen at the autopsy examination. Hence, the internal dissection could be curtailed and supplanted by Post-Mortem Computed Tomography (PMCT)–aided virtual autopsy examination in 80–90% of cases where the inquest findings including the circumstances surrounding the death, history given by the relatives, history given by the investigative authorities, external examinations observed at the autopsy procedure, and the findings observed at the PMCT-aided virtual autopsy procedure are consistent and coinciding.

Legal aspects of virtual autopsy in India

The main objectives of a medico-legal autopsy include the determination of the cause and manner of death, confirmation of the identity of the dead person, and collection of all possible evidence needed for investigation or legal process in case of any suspected foul play or future litigation. A medico-legal autopsy is conducted under Sections 174 and 176 of The Code of Criminal Procedure (CrPC), 1973. The law directs the investigating officer to take the body of the deceased to the concerned designated hospital/post-mortem centre for autopsy. The nature and extent of the post-mortem examination procedure are not formulated or described in these sections of the CrPC, the Indian Penal Code, or any other law in India.

Virtual autopsy (VA) reports are exactly the same as traditional autopsy reports with the only difference being that advanced radiological imaging techniques are used to examine the findings instead of invasive internal dissection of the body. The following legal sections of law in India support the admissibility of electronic documents or evidence in a court of law. It will also be applicable to VA documents or evidence. It is a well-settled fact that CT scans and X-ray reports have already been accepted as scientific evidence in a court of law in India.

- Section 3, Indian Evidence Act, 1872:

    It states that all documents including electronic records produced for the inspection of the court are called documentary evidence.
- Section 2 (1) (t), The Information Technology Act, (IT Act), 2000:

    It defines 'electronic record' which means data, record, or data generated, image or sound stored, received, or sent in an 'electronic form' or microfilms or computer-generated microfiche.
- Section 6, The Information Technology Act, (IT Act) 2000:

    It provides for the use of electronic records and electronic signatures in the Government and its agencies.
- Sections 65A and 65B, Indian Evidence Act, 1872:

    This details the admissibility of electronic records as evidence and states that the information contained in an electronic record that is printed on paper, stored, recorded, or copied in optical or magnetic media produced by a computer shall also be deemed to be a document and shall be admissible in any proceedings.
- National Human Rights Commission (NHRC) guidelines:

    The NHRC has issued guidelines for post-mortem examination in custodial deaths. In India, the post-mortem reports and procedures even in state medico-legal manuals are broadly based on these guidelines. The NHRC also issued an advisory for upholding the dignity and protecting the rights of the dead (14 May 2021), keeping in view the large number of deaths during the second wave of the COVID-19 Pandemic. National Human Rights Commission, India in its 'Advisory for Upholding the Dignity and Protecting the Rights of the Dead' at page 5, point 6: A-IV, it states that:

    The Government/National Medical Commission may consider adopting a partial autopsy method in cases where the complete autopsy is not necessary, arrangements of techniques, experts and training of the forensic experts shall be conducted to promote advanced methods of the autopsy

    It encourages the use of minimally invasive methods in autopsy using advanced techniques like VA.
- Kehar Singh & Ors vs. State (Delhi Admn.) on 3 August 1988. Hon'ble Supreme Court of India. 1988 AIR 1883, 1988 SCR Suppl. (2) 24 (Assassination of Mrs Indira Gandhi ex-Prime Minister of India case)

    The Honourable Supreme Court observed that:

    It is not always necessary to have a complete post-mortem in every case. Section 174 CrPC confers discretion to the Police Officer not to send the body for post-mortem examination if there is no doubt as to the cause of death. If the cause of death is certain and beyond the pale of doubt, or controversy, it is unnecessary to have the post-mortem done by Medical Officer. In the instant case, there was no controversy about the cause of death of Mrs. Gandhi. A complete post-mortem of the body was therefore uncalled for.

This statement supports the case to avoid unnecessary autopsy where the cause of death is very clear and fulfils the requirement of the law. In such cases, VA could be the right scientific option to document the findings by digital imaging techniques without opening the body and preserve the document for future reference in case any dispute arises.

Global outlook of virtual autopsy

Switzerland: Switzerland has a few pioneer institutes in the field of post-mortem imaging, i.e., the Institute of Forensic Medicine, the University of Zurich, the Institute of Forensic Medicine, the University of Bern, and the University Centre of Legal Medicine, Lausanne. All of these institutes have dedicated post-mortem CTs (PMCTs) scanners, and they utilize them for research as well as for medico-legal investigation purposes. An approach for a standard protocol in forensic radiology is given by the Institute of Forensic Medicine, the University of Zurich, the Institute of Forensic Medicine, the University of Bern in collaboration with the Institute of Diagnostic and Interventional Radiology, and the University of Zurich as 'imaging in forensic radiology: an illustrated guide for post-mortem computed tomography technique and protocols.' Further Swiss legal regulations introduced a criminal procedure stating 'imaging is a good method for screening and is a useful examination in combination with autopsy.' In practice, PMCT is performed along with autopsy as an adjunct method, i.e., when a responsible person has already decided that there is a need for an autopsy. In criminal trials in Switzerland, imaging has already been accepted as reliable and therefore admissible evidence in several forensic cases.

United Kingdom: In the United Kingdom, the University Hospital of Leicester has been providing post-mortem imaging services for forensic and coronial investigations for over two decades. Post-mortem imaging requests must always come from a coroner. This request is not free, as per the "Chief Coroner's Guidance No. 1 The use of Post-Mortem Imaging (Adults)" – the purpose of which is to provide a sound working procedure with minimum requirements where post-mortem imaging is used. Whenever an examination of the body is required, the coroner must decide in each case with the assistance of a pathologist (and where appropriate, a radiologist) what type of examination is appropriate. The coroner will bear in mind, among other things, the wishes of the deceased or the bereaved family. The guidance mentions the Royal College of Pathologists (RCPath) statement on the standards for medico-legal post-mortem cross-sectional imaging in adults in October 2012, from the largest study conducted by two UK centres in Manchester and Oxford between 2006 and 2008 in a study called: 'Postmortem imaging as an alternative to autopsy in the diagnosis of adult death: A validation study' which concluded that invasive autopsy was not needed in 48% of cases. In these cases, the major discrepancy rate compared with invasive autopsy was 16%. Apart from that Section 14 of the Coroners and Justice Act 2009 (in force from 25 July 2013) suggests that 'a post-mortem examination of a body' is not limited to an autopsy and may include CT (or MRI) imaging. This is achieved by Section 14(1) and (2) which provides that a senior coroner may 'specify the kind of examination to be made' and may request 'a suitable practitioner' to carry it out.

Japan: In 1985 Tsukuba Medical Center started to conduct PMCTs for the first time in Japan. In 2000, Dr. Hidefumi Ezawa, a pathologist at the Research Center Hospital for Charged Particle Therapy of the National Institute of Radiological Sciences in Japan, described the importance of Postmortem Imaging (PMI) examination before autopsy, and proposed a new type of PMI, that is, Ai. In Japan, PMI is generally referred to as 'autopsy imaging' and abbreviated as 'Ai.' In 2004, members with specialized expertise from the Tsukuba Medical Center and the National Institute of Radiological Science published the book 'Autopsy imaging (Ai).' Other pertinent publications include 'Guidebook for Interpretation of Ai,' 'Guidelines for Ai,' and 'Guidelines for Ai scanning technique.' In 2015, the 'Postmortem imaging interpretation guideline' was developed as a part of the Ministry of Health, Labour and Welfare (MHLW)'s grant-in-aid of the Scientific Research project, "Research for Implementation of Postmortem Imaging of Deaths Outside Medical Institutions" in collaboration with the Japan Radiological Society, the Japanese Society of Legal Medicine, and the Japan Society of Autopsy Imaging. The guideline was designed to provide a pathway for physicians who will keep it at hand when interpreting post-mortem images. There is a lot of literature present, however, as most of the documentation on Japanese PMI (Ai) is in the Japanese language, it remains relatively unknown to other countries. PMI data is collected data for the identification of individuals, for judicial matters, and for educational purposes.

Australia: The Victorian Institute of Forensic Medicine has a dedicated PMCT facility, and they work on medico-legal autopsy along with standard autopsy in forensic cases.

the Netherlands: In 2000, under the concept of Forensic Radiology, a collaboration between the Netherlands Forensic Institute, and the Department of Radiology in the Groene Hart Hospital (GHH) retrospectively studied around 1700 cases over a 15 years period, which included cases of blunt trauma, natural, fire, submersion, etc. All the cases were included in a database that comprises both deceased victims in which a forensic autopsy was designated and cases of living victims, for gathering forensic evidence for their case in court, e.g., after maltreatment or accidents. Apart from that, a thesis study 'Forensic radiology in the Netherlands: Results of a symbiotic collaboration in the pathological-radiological field,' by the University of Amsterdam, is published and is available for reference. Along with a Dutch guideline for clinical fetal-neonatal and paediatric post-mortem radiology, including a review of the literature.

China: Post-mortem forensic imaging started late in China, and the Institute of Forensic Science, the Ministry of Justice, PRC (IFS), is the first organization to systematically carry out research. The research team conducted a comparative study between post-mortem forensic imaging and autopsy findings in different cases like traffic accidents, falls from a height, occupational accidents,

intentional injury, drowning, burning, etc. Apart from PMCT, they are also working on the concept of Postmortem Magnetic Resonance Imaging (PMMRI) and Postmortem Computed Tomography Angiography (PMCTA). Apart from that the City University of Hong Kong started a course titled 'Forensic Imaging' with course code: CHEM3084 offered by the Department of Chemistry with complete course details

Sweden: VA procedures at the Center for Medical Image Science and Visualization (CMIV), Department of Radiology, Linköping University Hospital, Sweden, have been developed in collaboration with the Swedish National Board of Forensic Medicine and are now routinely used for forensic examinations. VA activities are added to the traditional workflow procedure and enable an interactive approach. This gives the investigators time to complete the crime scene investigation before the physical autopsy. The procedure is based on continuous interaction between the forensic pathologist, the radiologist, and the police. VA is currently used as a compliment to the standard autopsy procedure and can make the autopsy more efficient as the pathologist has prior knowledge of the case before conducting the standard autopsy.

France: PMCT in France is in a budding phase, growing as a collaboration of the Department of Forensic Medicine, Timone Hospital, and the Department of Medical Imaging. They have conducted a study to determine the diagnostic capabilities of unenhanced PMCT (UPMCT) in detecting traumatic abdominal injuries from November 2011 to October 2016 in a single institution. Inclusion criteria were traumatic deaths that underwent both UPMCT and standard autopsy. And concluded that the low sensitivity and low negative predictive value (NPV) do not support the use of UPMCT as an alternative to conventional autopsy to diagnose and/or rule out traumatic abdominal injuries. Nevertheless, UPMCT remains a helpful tool as it helps detect hemoperitoneum and virtually excludes the presence of perihepatic haematomas.

Malaysia: In Malaysia, at the National Institute of Forensic Medicine (NIFM) Hospital Kuala Lumpur, there is a dedicated CT machine to scan forensic cases sent to NIFM, whereby since 2010 all cases sent to the institute have a whole-body CT scan prior to a standard autopsy. The use of PMCT at the institute has been a valuable adjunct to conventional autopsy procedures as it allows the pathologist to plan aspects of the procedure in advance by identifying potential hazards, such as tuberculosis or sharp metallic object.

Mexico: In Mexico, the Office of the Medical Investigator (OMI) is a centralized medical examiner office, where the deceased (found dead, sudden death, cause of death unknown) come for autopsy. The Centre for Forensic imaging (CFI) was built by the State of New Mexico at the OMI and contains a CT scanner. From 2010 to 2017, because of projects related to post-mortem computed tomography a database and a website were created, called the New Mexico Decedent Image Database (NMDID).

Africa: In the African continent, the University of Cape Town, South Africa, the University of Uyo and Lagos State University, Nigeria, and Egypt have taken the idea of PMCT and initiated the procedure with the collaboration of respective radiology departments and published a few studies and case reports.

Apart from the previously mentioned, Germany, Russia, Poland, and Denmark are also working in the same direction to uplift the research work in the field of PMCT in collaboration with radiology units.

Establishment of a Centre for Advanced Research and Excellence (CARE) in virtual autopsy at the All India Institute of Medical Science (AIIMS), New Delhi, India

Forensic medicine/Pathology is the application of the principles and knowledge of medical science along with circumstantial evidence, for legal investigation and proceedings of the court of law, to help in the administration of justice. An autopsy is a systematic examination of a person's dead body, which is conducted by a doctor or by a medical board consisting of doctors to ascertain the cause, manner, and time of death and for other medical, legal, and research purposes. For decades, the traditional autopsy techniques have remained the same without many notable changes. Even with the introduction of newer techniques in different fields of medicine, still, in forensic medicine, post-mortem examination has been limited mainly to invasive autopsy and conventional photography. This is an observer-dependent method and in case of any missed finding, it will be lost when the deceased's body is cremated. The application of imaging technologies to visualize internal findings in the field of medico-legal post-mortem examination started to be noticed in the early 1990s. Multi-slice computed tomography (MSCT) is identified as the most promising tool among them and is already an established method in many Western countries. The use of imaging techniques like CT and magnetic resonance imaging (MRI) and optical surface scanning of the exterior was postulated as an alternative method to internal dissection in the 1980s. This technique was first started by the Institute of Forensic Medicine, University of Bern, Switzerland, in the mid-1990s. In 2018, the Indian Council of Medical Research (ICMR) headquarters introduced a scheme to establish ten centres to encourage in-depth research on an identified research area with the aim to generate new knowledge and have a better understanding of a particular disease or a health condition. These centres were named 'Centres for Advanced Research and Excellence.' Forensic medicine was one of the specialities among the ten in which applications were sought. Dr. Sudhir Kumar Gupta, Professor and Head of Department of Forensic Medicine, AIIMS, New Delhi, submitted a proposal to the ICMR headquarters to establish a CARE in virtual autopsy.

On 24 September 2018 the 'Centre for Advanced Research and Excellence in Virtual Autopsy' was selected as one of the CAREs by the ICMR. As a part of the project, three research proposals were submitted to AIIMS institutional ethics committee which were approved after detailed scrutiny.

Validation of virtual autopsy by the Honourable Union Health Minister, of India

In a sitting of the Rajya Sabha held on Tuesday, 3 December 2019, the Honourable Member of Parliament (Rajya Sabha) Shri. Rewati Raman Singh put up a starred question (No: 152) on the topic of a new technique for the post-mortem of the body, that asked:

(a) Whether it is a fact that the AIIMS and the ICMR are working together on a technique that would allow post-mortem without incising the body; and
(b) If so, by when this technique would be implemented?

To this question, the Honourable Health Minister replied that AIIMS and ICMR (Figure 1.1) have put forth a project after studying and researching this topic around the world wherever this technique has been implemented and emphasized that virtual autopsy would strengthen the humanitarian approach and thereby facilitate dignified management of the dead. In continuation, he explained that the virtual autopsy project in India is the first of its kind in the South Asian Association for Regional Cooperation (SAARC) nations. In response to another question, 'Will the records of the deceased be available in digital format?' from the same member, he replied that the records/data of the virtual autopsy would be digitalized and preserved, which would be helpful if a need for an expert review of the case arises.

Honourable Member of Parliament (Rajya Sabha) Shri K. T. S Tulsi congratulated AIIMS for the path-breaking research in the virtual autopsy. He also enquired:

About the total number of CT machines required in the country and financial allocation to ICMR for procuring the same.

The Honourable Health Minister, in his reply, stated that INR50 million (~US$600,000) had been allocated and the procurement process was in its final stages. He stated that it will be initiated by AIIMS at first and that the institute will later provide training to other institutions in the country to facilitate the same in other centres across the country.

Conflict over the practice of 'integrative medicine'

*151. DR. SANTANU SEN: Will the Minister of AYURVEDA, YOGA & NATUROPATHY, UNANI, SIDDHA AND HOMOEOPATHY be pleased to state:

(a) whether the Minister is aware of the growing differences between Ministry of AYUSH and Ministry of Health and Family Welfare's National Health Authority (NHA) over the practice of 'integrative medicine'; and

(b) if so, the details of alternative treatments that the AYUSH Ministry has talked about?

New technique for postmortem of body

†*152. SHRI REWATI RAMAN SINGH: Will the Minister of HEALTH AND FAMILY WELFARE be pleased to state:

(a) whether it is a fact that the All India Institute of Medical Sciences (AIIMS) and Indian Council of Medical Research (ICMR) are working together on a technique that would allow postmortem without incising the body; and

(b) if so, by when this technique would be implemented?

Losses incurred by Power DISCOMs

*153. SHRI B. K. HARIPRASAD: Will the Minister of POWER be pleased to state whether the Power DISCOMs are running under huge losses, if so, the details of losses and separate consolidated loss details of other distribution and power generation companies?

Finance sector and climate change risk

*154. SHRI PARTAP SINGH BAJWA: Will the Minister of FINANCE be pleased to state:

(a) whether the Ministry has studied the

AIIMS and ICMR working on developing 'virtual autopsy' technique, Harsh Vardhan says

PTI 3 December, 2019 05:49 pm IST

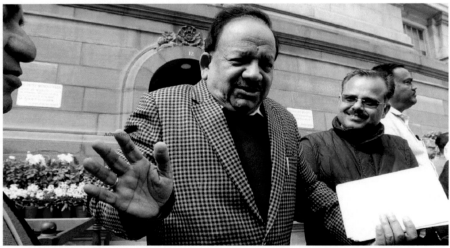

File photo of Union Health Minister Harsh Vardhan at Parliament House | Photo: Praveen Jain | ThePrint

New Delhi: Delhi's AIIMS and Indian Council of Medical Research are jointly working on a technique for postmortem without dissecting the body and it is likely to be functional within the next six months, Health Minister Harsh Vardhan said in Rajya Sabha Tuesday.

FIGURE 1.1:   Honourable Health Minister's media briefing on AIIMS ICMR Virtual Autopsy project.

Inauguration of the centre

On 20 March 2021, the Centre for Advanced Research and Excellence in Virtual Autopsy was inaugurated by Prof. Balram Bhargava, then Director General of the Indian Council of Medical Research, and Head of Department, Dr. Sudhir K. Gupta, the author of this book and principal investigator of virtual autopsy (Figure 1.2).

Need and rationale for a virtual autopsy in the Indian medico-legal system

VA is a joint collaboration of two premiere institutes, i.e., the Department of Forensic Medicine and Toxicology, AIIMS, New Delhi, and the ICMR headquarters with a global vision in order to achieve the concept of humanitarian forensics and dignified management of the dead. The need and rationale for VA in the Indian medico-legal system are as follows:

1. Dignified management of the dead: VA brings a more humanitarian approach to the post-mortem examination by preserving the dignity of the deceased using non-invasive or minimally invasive methods. It decreases the mental trauma of relatives and friends by reducing avoidable/unnecessary internal dissection and respecting religious beliefs.
2. Credible and scientific reports: VA using PMCT will help in a detailed study of minute internal findings that are not visible to the naked eye, which makes the report more scientific and credible. Forensic findings are currently documented in an observer-dependent subjective way. Findings that have not been documented are destroyed if the body has been cremated. With the application of VA, digital documentation of relevant forensic findings helps to reduce inter-observer variation and assists in reviewing the findings if required.
3. Reproducibility: VA reports have digital data archiving which can be reproduced for any legal forum or investigative agencies. The data can be reviewed by other forensic radiology experts at the request of higher investigative agencies like the Central Bureau of Investigation (CBI), National Investigation Agency (NIA), judicial enquires, etc., if required for second or third opinions.
4. Time-saving procedure: VA takes much less time compared to conventional autopsy which allows the early handing of the body to the relatives for cremation and reduces emotional stress.
5. Human resource utilization: As VA uses non-invasive/minimal invasive methods it requires less manpower compared to traditional autopsies which require more assistants during internal dissection.
6. Digitization of records: VA data can be stored for years in digital format utilizing very little space and can be studied, analysed, and reviewed anytime as per the requirement for medico-legal and research purposes.
7. Infection control: VA has a very significant role in high-risk cases like HIV, Hepatitis B and C, Tuberculosis, Rabies, COVID-19, etc. It provides an alternative to conventional autopsy and has an important advantage in minimizing the transmission of infection in the mortuary among autopsy surgeons and their post-mortem assistants. The ICMR and AIIMS, New Delhi formed the standard guidelines for medico-legal autopsy for COVID-19 deaths in India in 2020. It mentions that proactive steps should be taken to avoid invasive autopsy to prevent the spread of infection from biological fluids. It could be done using the method of verbal autopsy, circumstantial evidence, external examination/inspection of the body, photography recording, complete digital X-ray of the whole body, and criteria of elimination and exclusion method. Virtual autopsy using an X-ray and PMCT is a very good option in cases of high-risk infection. The Department of Forensic Medicine, AIIMS, New Delhi has done many cases of medico-legal autopsy using

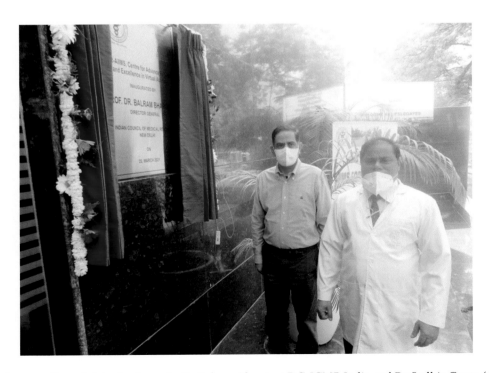

FIGURE 1.2:   Inauguration of virtual autopsy by Dr Balram Bhargava DG-ICMR India and Dr Sudhir Gupta (Author).

non-invasive virtual autopsy techniques in cases with positive COVID-19 and there have been no medico-legal complications/objections in the investigation and the court of law.

8. Database for age estimation: Estimation of age is important for various medico-legal purposes like determination of juvenility, age determination of sexual assault survivors, unknown dead bodies, and in disputed age categories referred by the sports authority of India. VA provides a large amount of data for preparing a database for age estimation in the Indian population by studying the ossification centres of different bones and joints.

9. Research: In VA whole-body CT is taken where the detailed data can be used for even clinical research.

10. Teaching tool: VA has shown an important potential for teaching both undergraduate and postgraduate medical education and in super specialities. Through 3D virtual imaging technology, coloured 3D images like real human anatomical structures can be constructed for understanding pathological disorders. VA digital images supplemented with other case details provide vivid and real-life learning material for medical students and postgraduate trainees.

Infrastructure

The Centre for Advanced Research and Excellence (CARE) in virtual autopsy (Figure 1.3) has been established by the joint collaboration of two premiere institutes AIIMS, New Delhi and ICMR headquarters. The centre has a dedicated research facility in an area of about 2400 square feet and a PMCT set-up in an area of about 800 square feet. The facility along with its PMCT set-up is interconnected with the odourless modular autopsy suite (Figure 1.4) and post-mortem embalming wing. The scanning room (Figure 1.5) of the PMCT is equipped with a Canon Medical Systems', Aquilion Lighting, 16-slice MSCT scanner (TSX-035A). The console room (Figure 1.6) of the PMCT set-up has dedicated workstations (Vitrea 6.9. and Vitrea 7.10), viewing stations, and a RAD storage system. All existing radiation safety regulations in the PMCT set-up are in accordance with the current regulation of the Atomic Energy Regulatory Board (AERB) of India and the Bhabha Atomic Research Centre (BARC).

The centre has a dedicated board room (Figure 1.7) and an advanced research section (Figure 1.8) with an HD video conferencing facility, internet facility, multiple desktops/laptops, a digital podium, and an audio system, all connected to a touch interactive display for smooth conduction of intra/inter-departmental and institutional academic activities. Local Area Network (LAN) connectivity is used to connect the board room with the console. There is also a waiting lobby (Figure 1.9), reception area (Figure 1.10), pantry room, and three restrooms.

Technical aspects of virtual autopsy

PMCT refers to a computerized X-ray imaging procedure that was first introduced by Godfrey Hounsfield of EMI Laboratories in 1972. It uses a narrow beam of X-rays around the body, which is processed by a computer to generate cross-sectional images or slices of the body.

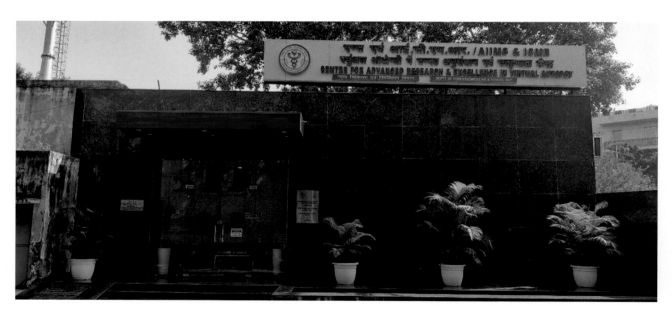

FIGURE 1.3: Virtual autopsy centre AIIMS, New Delhi, India.

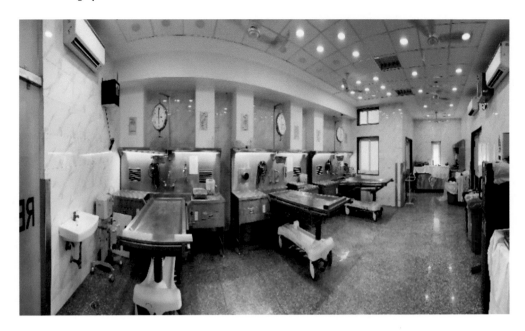

FIGURE 1.4: Odourless modular autopsy suite of AIIMS New Delhi, the Author's Centre.

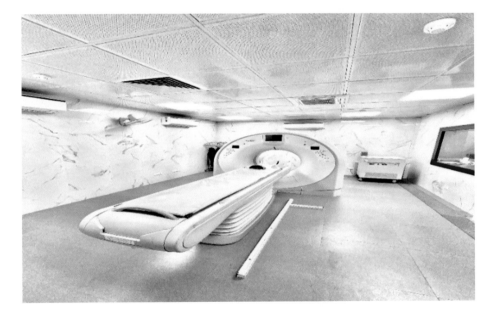

FIGURE 1.5: Scanning room (gantry and couch) of Virtual Autopsy Centre AIIMS New Delhi.

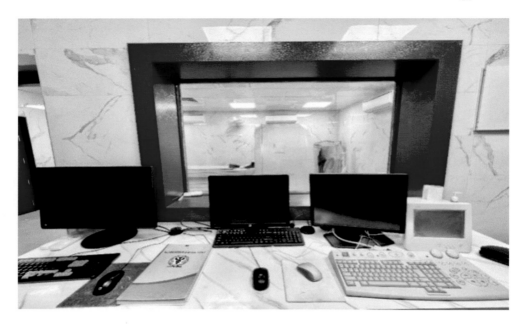

FIGURE 1.6:   Console room of PMCT of Virtual Autopsy Centre AIIMS New Delhi.

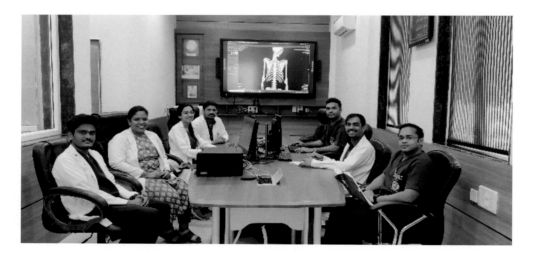

FIGURE 1.7:   Virtual autopsy reporting/ board room with the researcher resident doctors of AIIMS New Delhi.

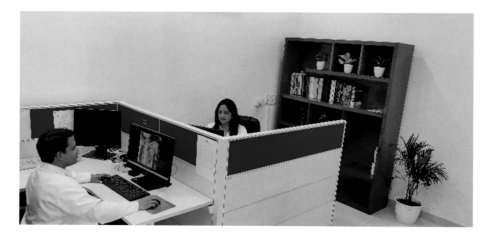

FIGURE 1.8:   Dr Abilash S (Asst. Prof.) and Dr Swati Tyagi (Asst. Prof.) of Department of Forensic Medicine & Toxicology, AIIMS New Delhi at the Advanced research section of Virtual Autopsy Centre.

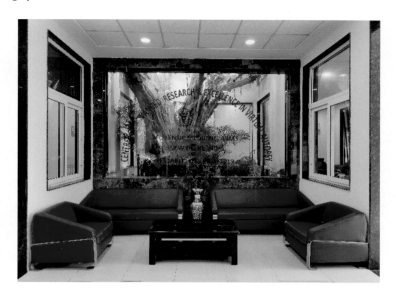

FIGURE 1.9: Waiting lobby of the Virtual Autopsy Centre, AIIMS New Delhi.

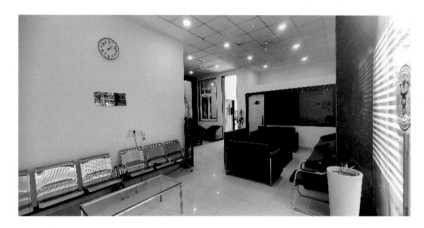

FIGURE 1.10: Reception area of the Virtual Autopsy Centre, AIIMS New Delhi.

Gantry

The gantry of the helical CT scanner contains the X-ray tube, pre-patient filter, and beam collimator on the same side as a unit (Figure 1.11). Post-patient filter and detector arrays are present on the diagonally opposite aspect. These two units rotate inside the gantry at the same speed to achieve simultaneous signal capturing and transmission. The deceased is placed at the iso-centre of the gantry over the couch which passes through the aperture of the gantry at a pre-fixed speed.

Parts of Gantry

1. X-ray source:

| Produces the monochromatic X ray beam. | ⇒ | Electricity passed heats up tungsten filament (cathode) | ⇒ | starts discharging electrons by thermionic emission. | ⇒ | Electrons are attracted towards the positively charged anode-target (tungsten) | ⇒ | This produces heat and X ray photons which is directed to the detector through a window. |

2. Filters: Filters are layers made of metals like aluminium that filter low-energy X-rays. These low-energy X-rays otherwise increase the total dose to the patient and do not contribute to image formation. The filters are placed in front of the X-ray tube across the pathway of the X-ray photon beam. Post-patient filters, between the patient and the detector arrays, are also used to filter distracting photons.
3. Collimator: Between the filter and the patient the X-ray beam is narrowed by calculated pre-set commands to determine the width of the X-ray beam collimation. The narrow beam collimation of the Canon Aquilion 16-slice scanner at our centre exposes the 16 central (0.5 mm) detector elements, i.e., beam collimation is 8 mm.
4. Detector array: 16-slice CT scanners have 16 functional rows of detectors (Figure 1.12). Each row will have 1000–2000 detectors. The Canon Aquilion Lighting has 16 0.5 mm and 24 1 mm detector rows.

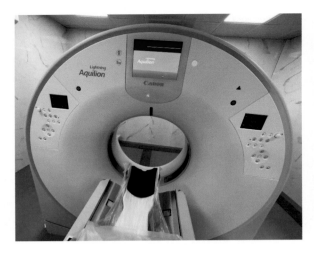

FIGURE 1.11:   Gantry exterior.

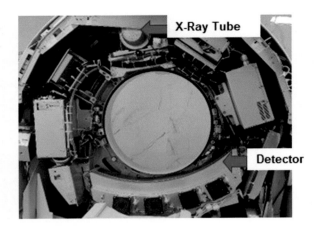

FIGURE 1.12:   Gantry interior.

Technical terms used in PMCT

1. Pitch: It gives the overlap between slices. It's calculated as 'couch travel increments per rotation inside gantry/ total width of acquired slices.'
2. Attenuation: In CT, a slice during acquisition is divided into multiple small blocks called voxels. Each block is assigned a number according to the attenuation that happened to the corresponding portion of the X-ray beam. The linear attenuation coefficient is the quantification of attenuation, generally expressed as a CT number or Hounsfield units. The linear attenuation coefficient is a property of a tissue depending on its composition, atomic number, and density. High-density tissues (such as bone) absorb or reflect the radiation to a greater degree, and a reduced amount is detected by the scanner on the opposite side of the body. Similarly, low-density tissue (such as the lungs), absorbs the radiation to a lesser degree, and there is a greater signal detected by the scanner. The CT number of water is considered as zero (0), that of cortical bone is about +1000 and that of air is about −1000.
3. Projection data/ raw data: Projection data is a raw set of data which is generally not visualized as images. This data set further undergoes post-processing to make the axial slices and further reformations. In the case of a medico-legal set-up for virtual autopsy, permanent storage of raw data is recommended.
4. Windowing: CT grayscale spread across attenuation coefficients of air, i.e., −1000 to those of metallic objects in the range of thousands. CT numbers of soft tissues and body fluids are in a narrow range. To distinguish these tissues visually, smaller ranges can be fixed for the grey scale by increasing the lower limit and by decreasing the upper limit. This narrowed grey scale represents the window width. Any value lower than the window width/range will be shown as black and any values above the range will be shown as white, giving a better vivid representation of the tissues that fall under the range. Although many pre-set named window levels and widths (like lung window, bone window, or soft tissue windows) are being supplied with various workstations, these settings can be later changed while viewing the reconstructed images in any plane.

Virtual autopsy data processing (Figure 1.13)

1. Data acquisition: The deceased body should be placed exactly at the iso-centre of the gantry whenever possible

to obtain better image quality. Usage of 120 kVp would be ideal for routine PMCT scans. High tube voltage scans with 140 kVp are advisable for cases with metallic foreign bodies like firearm bullets, and metallic implants inside the body which can be set immediately after screening the topogram. Low kVp is advisable for contrast-enhanced studies as suggested by several studies (Figure 1.13).

2. Data reconstruction: Projection data is first processed into axial data, also known as primary reconstruction. This can be made into different section thicknesses. Thin (0.5–1 mm) sections are desirable for better spatial resolution and for MPR and 3D reconstructions:

   i.   Multi-planar reconstruction or reformation (MPR): The data of axial images after primary reconstruction can be processed into volumetric data which is used to make 2D images of any plane of the body (secondary reconstruction). This post-processing technique is called MPR. It can be done in any plane including sagittal, coronal, and oblique planes.

   ii.   Curved planar reformation (CPR): This is a type of secondary reconstruction where the imaging plane is aligned along with the course of a structure or organ. Generally, the curved planes need to be manually derived which is a time-consuming process. CPR is especially useful in visualizing hollow tubular structures like arteries, veins, bile ducts, ureters, etc.

   iii.   Maximum intensity projection (MIP): MIP is a post-processing technique that displays the elements which show maximum attenuation in the linear path of the photons in the observer's view orientation. MIP is commonly used for better visualization of elements with high CT numbers like contrast materials and calcifications.

   iv.   Minimum intensity projection (MinIP): MinIP is a post-processing technique that displays the elements which show minimum attenuation in the linear path of the photons in the observer's view orientation.

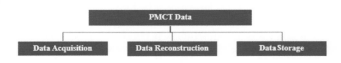

FIGURE 1.13:   Stages of data processing.

MinIP is commonly used for better visualization of elements with low CT numbers like airways, lungs, and any gas-filled regions of interest.

v. Volume rendering technique (VRT): VRT is one of the most advanced post-processing techniques for CT data. Volume rendering assigns a value for each voxel in a transparency spectrum ranging from 0% (totally transparent) to 100% (totally opaque). Here soft tissues, bones, cartilage, air, etc., can be visually interpreted as a representation with different colours.

3. Data storage: Scan data should be archived electronically as per the existing norms for medico-legal documentation. A picture archiving and communication system (PACS) is ideal for PMCT data storage over longer durations. Other modalities like network attached storage (NAS), dedicated external mass storage devices, or individual drives for each case can be used as per the volume of workload in the centre, available space, and financial considerations.

It is worth mentioning that the NMC professional conduct, etiquette, and ethics regulations, 2002, states that efforts should be made to computerize medical records for quick retrieval. The Ministry of Health and Family Welfare in the year 2016 has framed guidelines for Electronic Health Standards for India emphasizing the importance of e-health records.

Radiation safety measures

1. As per the Atomic Energy Regulatory Board (AERB) of India guidelines, an adequately shielded CT room needs to be ensured at the time of designing the infrastructure.
2. A radiation safety officer (RSO) with knowledge and training in ionizing radiation measurement and evaluation of safety techniques and the ability to advise the executive management regarding the radiation protection needs of the facility is required.
3. Protective accessories like lead aprons, protective glass eyewear, thyroid and gonadal shields, mobile protective barriers, hand gloves, etc.
4. Monitoring devices like thermo-luminescent dosimeter (TLD) badges, pocket dosimeters, etc., should be available.
5. Periodic maintenance, modification, and up-gradation of facilities and equipment, as and when required.
6. Periodic quality assurance for mechanical tests of the CT machine alignment and positioning accuracy, collimation, and other parametric tests like radiation dose test of the computed tomography dose index (CTDI), use of test phantoms for calibration and evaluation of the performance of CT scanners and examination of radiation leakage levels and a radiological protection survey.

Standard operating procedure of virtual autopsy

Case selection for virtual autopsy

This is one of the first and most important steps of the whole procedure. There are many cases in which a non-invasive/minimal invasive autopsy can be a very good alternative to the conventional autopsy upholding the humanitarian aspect of dignified management of the dead without compromising on the scientific medico-legal purpose of conducting an autopsy. The assessment of the suitability of the case for virtual autopsy

will vary from case to case keeping in view all the relevant circumstantial evidence, medical records and investigative findings. The autopsy surgeon has to look into all the relevant scientific facts and circumstantial evidence of the case while selecting the suitability of the case for virtual autopsy. The following case criteria needs to be taken into consideration while selecting cases for virtual autopsy:

1. Hospital admitted and treated cases of natural/accident/suicide deaths with complete history and treatment records.
2. Sudden natural death cases with a history of long-term illness with medical records and clear PMCT findings corresponding to the history and eye witness, for example – cases with a history of headache with evident intracranial haemorrhage in PMCT, chest pain with evident heart wall rupture in PMCT, or chest pain with evident coronary calcifications and occlusion.
3. Accidental deaths with eyewitness and clear PMCT findings corresponding to the history/eye witness, for example – road traffic accidents with polytrauma, falls from a height, choking while eating, etc.
4. Suicidal/homicidal/unnatural death cases examination can be done using PMCT if the conclusion can be drawn as for the law.

Apart from the above-mentioned case criteria, the following points also need to be considered:

i. Explain the procedure of non-invasive VA to the relatives.
ii. Assessment of foul play after perusal of initial investigative findings.
iii. Biological samples/evidence requested by the investigating officer (IO) that requires invasive procedure/internal dissection of the body.
iv. Is it a medical negligence case?
v. The perusal of all treatment records.
vi. Is external examination consistent with the alleged history, treatment records, and internal findings of PMCT?
vii. Whether PMCT is showing clear demonstrable internal injuries that are sufficient to conclude the cause of death and answer medico-legal queries for investigation and the court of law.

Flow chart showing methodology of virtual autopsy procedure (Figure 1.14)

Virtual autopsy is based on four aspects:

A) Verbal autopsy.
B) Visual autopsy.
C) PMCT with digital X-ray.
D) Miscellaneous procedures.

A) Verbal Autopsy:
1. A detailed perusal of inquest papers.
2. Interaction with relatives and IO regarding the case.

Step 1: A detailed perusal of inquest papers:
The IO submits a written requisition along with other inquest papers that need to be perused thoroughly:
- Police Form 25/35 A, B, and C, are filled up as per the type of case.
- Statements of the relevant witnesses and relatives.
- Hospital treatment records.
- Death summary in hospital death cases.

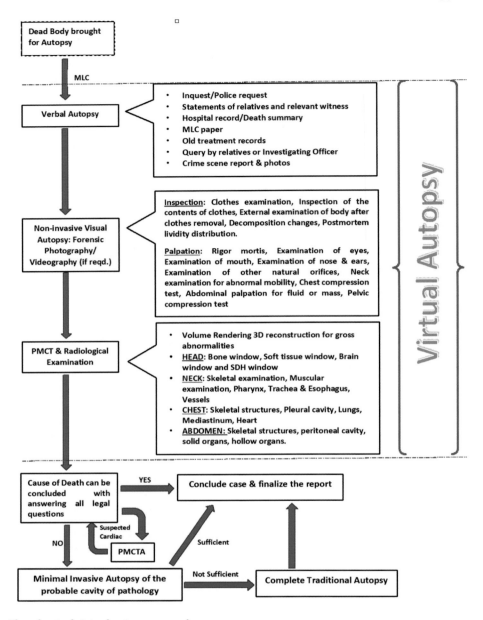

FIGURE 1.14: Flowchart of virtual autopsy procedure.

- Medico-legal report (MLR).
- Brought dead declaration report.
- Photographs/videography/CCTV footage of the scene of occurrence.
- Police hue and cry notice for identification in case of an unclaimed dead body.
- Seizure memo (items seized at the scene of occurrence).
- Any other relevant documents that are required for the case.

Step 2: Interaction with relatives and IO regarding the case: The autopsy surgeon will interact with the relatives and the IO also to understand their version of events regarding circumstances of death like recovery of the body, place of death, last seen alive, a witness account and preliminary investigation findings to rule out any foul play. After the perusal of inquest papers and other evidence as mentioned

in Step 1, a case assessment for non-invasive VA criteria will be done. Then relatives and IOs are to be informed and have the VA procedure explained (refer to Annexure I)

B) Visual Autopsy:
1. External examination (clothes, belongings, ligatures, foreign particles, etc.).
2. External injury examination.
3. Post-mortem photography.
4. Collection of biological samples/evidence by minimally invasive/non-invasive approaches.

Step 1: External examination (clothes, belongings, ligatures, foreign particles, etc.)
A detailed scientific external examination of the deceased's body is done in the following sequence:

- Body cover/bag.

- Length of body.
- Clothes worn and their condition.
- Personal belongings.
- Ligature material.
- Foreign particles.

After the removal of all the clothes and belongings, a systematic head-to-toe examination must be conducted in systematic and preformatted order:

Post-mortem changes are to be examined as follows: Rigor mortis, post-mortem lividity, and decomposition changes.

- The external appearance of the deceased.
- Scalp/scalp hairs/skull: For any palpable deformity.
- Eyes: Eyelids, conjunctivas, corneas, and pupils are to be examined.
- Nasal cavity: Nostrils, alae of the nose, and nasal bridge.
- Mouth; Lips, oral mucosa, teeth, gums, frenula, and tongue.
- Ears: Pinna of ears and external auditory meatus.
- Nails: Shape of nails, nail beds, and colour.
- Condition of body orifices: For any discharge.
- The neck.
- Ribs and chest wall: For any palpable deformity.
- Abdominal wall.
- Groin and genitals.
- Upper limb.
- Lower limb.

Step 2: External injury examination

It must be recorded systematically in the prescribed format in a head-to-toe manner. Any visible injury or palpable deformity is mentioned in a way that the injury description must include the following points:

- Type of injury.
- Site of injury.
- Colour of injury.
- Size of injury.
- Distance from prominent bony landmarks.
- Additional findings, e.g., surrounding area, margins, the base of wound, or foreign body (if found).

Step 3: Post-mortem photography

Forensic photography has become an important tool in the medico-legal system, as it gives a documented picture in an easy and effective way to capture and appreciate important evidentiary findings. The steps to be followed for photography in VA procedure are:

1. Verify date/time in-camera settings.
2. The photograph should contain the date and time.
3. Photography should be carried out in a systematic and clockwise manner. An overall view, mid-range, and close-up should be taken in every case.
   - Overall view: For seeing the relationship of the body with injury/other objects.
   - Mid-range: Relate the photograph with another immediate body part.
   - Close-up: For injury details or items in view.
4. During an external post-mortem examination (PE) the following photographs must be taken:
   PE1-Full front view of the body with clothing as the case is brought to the centre.

PE2-Full back view of the body with clothing.
PE3-Right side of the body.
PE4-Left side of the body.
PE5-Face, front view, and both sides.
PE6-Full front view of the body without clothing.
PE7-Full back view of the body without clothing.
From the anterior aspect:
PE8-Head and neck.
PE9-From shoulders, chest, and abdomen with upper limbs on sides.
PE10-From pelvis to the upper part of thighs.
PE11-From the lower part of thighs, legs, and feet dorsum.
PE12-Close-up of soles.
From the posterior aspect:
PE13-Head and neck.
PE14-From shoulders, chest, and abdomen with upper limbs on sides.
PE15-From pelvis to the upper part of thighs.
PE16-From the lower part of thighs and legs.
PE17-Right-hand front and back, left-hand front and back, both with fingers spread out.

Step 4: Collection of biological samples/evidence by minimally invasive/non-invasive approach

Biological sample collection during a virtual autopsy can be done with minimally invasive and non-invasive techniques. The samples are handed over to the IO after proper sealing, labelling and receipt to maintain the proper chain of custody. These samples may include:

- Femoral blood samples.
- Urine samples by suprapubic aspiration.
- Vitreous fluid.
- Air-dried blood in gauze or over FTA paper.
- Vaginal swabs.
- Hair samples.
- Nail clippings.
- Swab for gunpowder, etc.
- Seminal/saliva swabs.
- Subcutaneous bullet fragment/foreign object retrieved by minimal subcutaneous dissection.
- Samples collected for histopathology may be preserved by needle biopsy or other minimally invasive procedure.

C) PMCT with digital X-ray:
   1. Identification of the deceased body.
   2. PMCT and digital X-Ray examination.
   3. Assessment of the virtual autopsy findings.

Step 1: Identification of the deceased body

Deceased identification is an important step in the proceedings of medico-legal autopsy. It must be done by:

- Two relatives, whose names and signatures are mentioned on the requisition form.
- The IO.
- By the hospital tags/label pasted over the deceased body cover.

Step 2: PMCT and digital X-ray examination

Virtual autopsy involves a PMCT scan/digital X-ray of the deceased body and interpreting the findings for the medico-legal diagnosis.

Deceased bodies should always be covered/packed with water-impermeable/proof and artefact-free body bags. Scanning the body without breaking the rigor is the recommended method to avoid post-mortem artefacts. A second scan after repositioning is advisable if any body parts are missed out.

Metallic personal belongings need to be removed after screening the topogram or after the first scanning on a case-to-case basis.

After the PMCT scanning, the reconstruction of images is done automatically into different planes in the console system. Data is visualized through Vitrea software installed on a workstation (Figure 1.15). After opening the software, the deceased post-mortem details are to be selected for further proceedings.

Subsequently, 4-frame windows will be opened with sagittal, coronal, axial, and VRT images (Figure 1.16). Then all the planes are simultaneously set in the proper orientation for anatomical and pathological interpretation.

The brightness and contrast of CT images are optimized to view specific types of tissue. Each of these tissue-specific brightness/contrast settings is called a CT window.

The most used windows are:
- Bone window: Bone fractures and bone marrow are clearly visualized (Figure 1.17).
- Lung window: Pleura, lung parenchyma, airway, and pulmonary vessels (Figure 1.18).
- Soft tissue window: Muscles, vessels, and solid organs (Figure 1.19).

Before proceeding for virtual internal examination, the whole body is examined in VRT to note any apparent fractures or skeletal deformities in long bones and vertebrae, or any foreign bodies.

Examination of the layers of skin for any injuries and related pathology.

Normal post-mortem changes, e.g., post-mortem lividity with effusion (Figure 1.20), decomposition gases with pneumothorax/pneumoperitoneum/pneumocephalus, sedimentation of blood, etc. are

to be identified and differentiated (Figures 1.21 and 1.22).

Every body cavity is to be examined in a specific window as per pathological findings (Figure 1.23).

A. Head and neck: In the head and neck cavity (Figure 1.24), the PMCT is to be examined in three main windows along with a VRT image as described below:
    i.   VRT image: Fractures and foreign bodies can be identified (see Figure 1.25 A–F).
    ii. Bone window: Pineal gland, choroid, and other calcification, foreign body along with fracture (see Figure 1.26A, B) can be visualized.
    iii. Brain window: In the brain window (70–100 HU) the findings to be observed are soft tissue swelling, scalp laceration and hematoma, extra-axial haemorrhage, parenchymal lesions (Figure 1.27A), interventricular haemorrhage (Figure 1.27B), and pneumocephalus.
    iv. Subdural window: In some cases, a thin layer of subdural haemorrhage may not be visible, and then the window is changed to the subdural window (150–200 HU) for better visualization of subdural haematoma.

B. Chest cavity:
    Sudden death causes are often related to the cardiothoracic organs which makes its proper examination important, as it contains the vital organs, i.e., heart and lungs along with major blood vessels, i.e., aorta and inferior vena cava. The thorax part of the body anatomically contains the mediastinum and the lungs. Like the head CT, the chest PMCT is also visualized in three different windows, i.e., bone, soft tissue, and lung to examine bones, mediastinum, and lungs respectively (Figure 1.28).

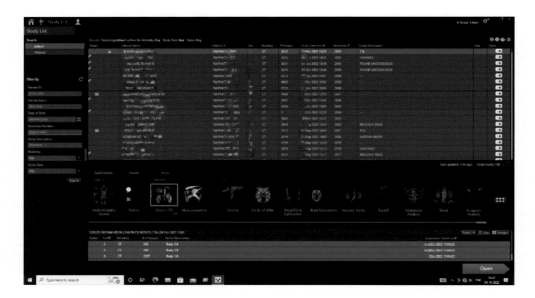

FIGURE 1.15:   Vitrea software home page.

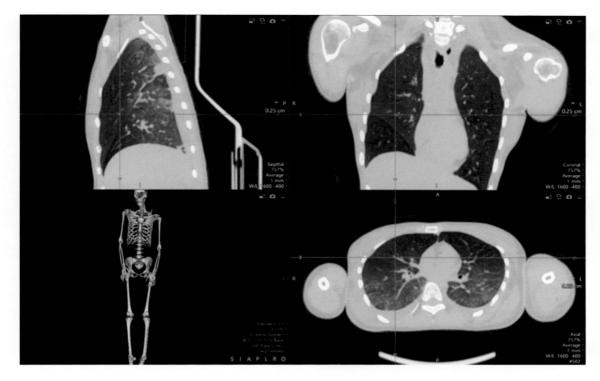

FIGURE 1.16: Sagittal, coronal, and axial along with VRT (volume reconstructed) image on a single screen.

i. Bone window: In this window, the bones of the chest cavity, i.e., rib, sternum, clavicle, and thoracic vertebra are better appreciated (Figures 1.29 and 1.30), and any fracture or age-related abnormality can be seen here. The thoracic level can be ascertained by rib attachment during scrolling of the axial plane. The exact location of the fracture can be confirmed by viewing three planes (axial, coronal, and sagittal) simultaneously with the help of a full crosshair.

ii. Soft tissue window: This window is primarily used in the chest region to visualize the mediastinum which includes the aorta and its branches, the inferior vena cava and its tributaries, the pulmonary trunk, the heart, trachea oesophagus, and lymph nodes. Calcifications of arteries (Figure 1.31 A, B), pericardial effusion, cardiomegaly, etc. are easily seen in this window.

iii. Lung window: In this window, lung parenchyma is seen along with bronchioles and vessels. The haziness of parenchyma, dilatation of bronchioles, dilatation of vessels, the collapse of the lung, etc. (Figure 1.32 A, B). can easily be appreciated. Further clarity can be assessed by using technical tools and parameters.

C. Abdomen and pelvis:
The abdomen is divided into retroperitoneal and peritoneal areas which should be delineated for

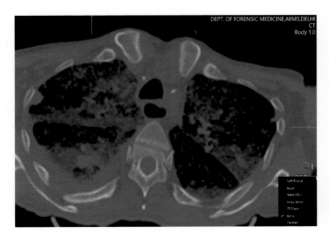

FIGURE 1.17: Bone window.

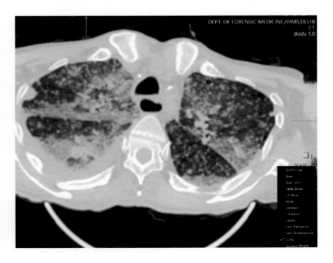

FIGURE 1.18: Lung window.

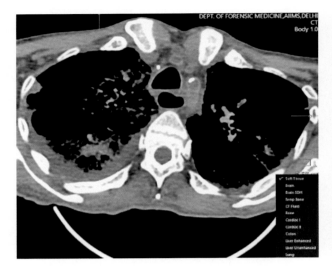

FIGURE 1.19:   Soft tissue window.

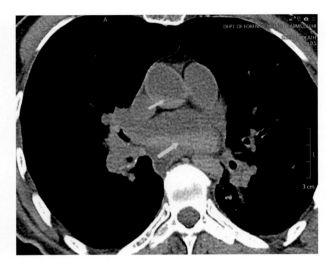

FIGURE 1.22:   Sedimentation of blood in great vessels (yellow arrow).

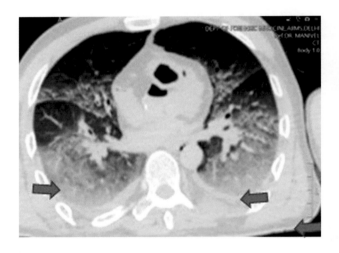

FIGURE 1.20:   PM lividity at the dependent area.

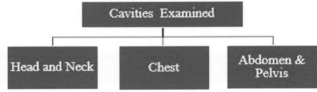

FIGURE 1.23:   Flowchart of PMCT cavity examination.

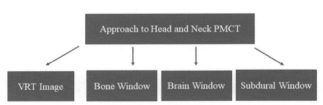

FIGURE 1.24:   Flowchart of PMCT head and neck examination.

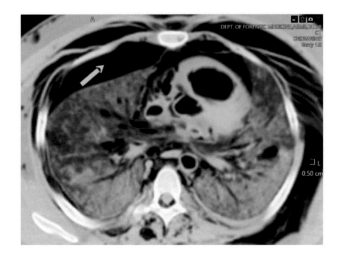

FIGURE 1.21:   Decomposition gas (yellow arrow).

the exact location of the deceased organ. PMCT abdomen is visualized in three different windows, i.e., bone, soft tissue, and lung to examine bones, solid organs, and air in the peritoneum along with gases in the intestines respectively (Figure 1.33).

i.   VRT image: Fracture's location and extension can be easily appreciated in volume reconstructed images (Figure 1.34).

ii. Bone window: In this window, the lumbar and sacral vertebra along with the pelvis bone are observed for any fracture or dislocation. The exact location of the fracture can be confirmed by viewing three planes (axial, coronal, and sagittal) simultaneously with the help of a full crosshair

iii. Soft tissue window: This window is primarily used for solid organs like the liver,

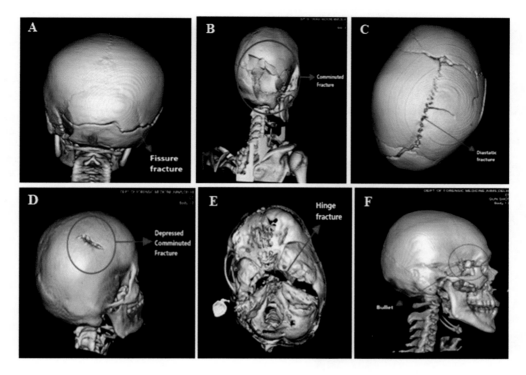

FIGURE 1.25: VRT image of the skull showing. (A) Fissure fracture on the occipital bone. (B) Comminuted fracture over the occipital and right temporal region. (C) A diastatic fracture involving the sagittal suture and partly the coronal suture and lambdoid suture. (D) Depressed comminuted fracture. (E) Type I hinge fracture seen placed coronally extending from one middle cranial fossa to the other running through the sella turcica. (F) The exact position of the bullet in the right temporal region.

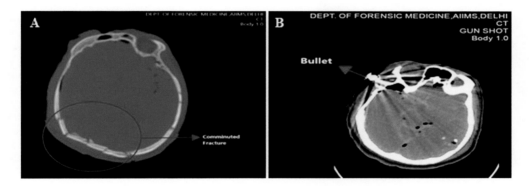

FIGURE 1.26: Axial section of brain showing. (A) Comminuted fracture over the occipital and right temporal region. (B) Foreign body in the right temporal region with streak artefact.

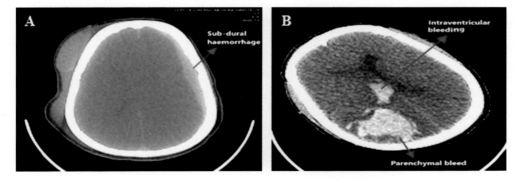

FIGURE 1.27: Axial plane showing. (A) Right side Subgaleal haematoma and left side subdural haemorrhage (red arrow). (B) Intraventricular bleeding and parenchymal bleeding.

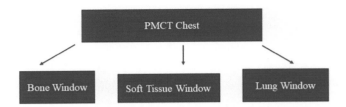

FIGURE 1.28: Flowchart of PMCT chest examination.

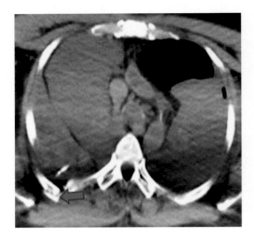

FIGURE 1.29: Axial image showing rib fracture.

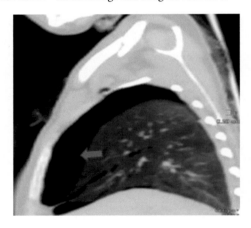

FIGURE 1.30: Sagittal image: Clavicle fracture and pneumothorax.

kidney, pancreas, adrenal, and spleen. Any nodularity of the surface of a solid organ, or any injury to the organ, can be interpreted in this window

iv. Lung window: The pneumoperitoneum can easily be assessed (Figure 1.35).

Step 3: Assessment of the virtual autopsy findings

Holistic assessment of the case will be done after the detailed consideration of the following examination findings and deliberation, so as to reach a scientific conclusion for cause/manner of death and other medicolegal queries:

- The perusal of all relevant Inquest paper findings.
- Interaction with relatives and the IO.
- PMCT/X-ray findings.
- External examination findings including injuries.

D) Miscellaneous procedures:
1. Proper cleaning, packing, and handing over the body to relatives through the IO.
2. Report writing and framing scientific opinion.
3. Maintaining proper autopsy records (hard copy/digital).
a. Step 1: Proper cleaning, packing, and handing over the body to relatives through the IO

The body is cleaned, properly packed in a waterproof bag and handed over to the relatives in a proper dignified manner through the police personnel in-charge/the IO.

b. Step 2: Report writing and framing scientific opinion

The virtual autopsy report is to be prepared in the same format as the conventional autopsy reports. In AIIMS, New Delhi, it is being done in the department's post-mortem report drafting software Medulla. The report begins with a detailed preamble, followed by the body of the report, and then the opinion portion. External examination findings including external injuries should be properly mentioned. The corresponding internal findings should be mentioned as per PMCT findings. The scientific opinion on the case will be framed after thorough deliberations of findings as per Step 3 (PMCT with digital X-ray: Assessment of the virtual autopsy findings).

c. Step 3: Record keeping

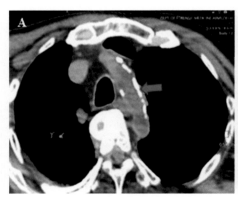
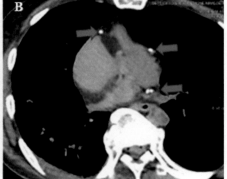

FIGURE 1.31: Axial section of PMCT chest showing. (A) Calcification of the arch of the aorta. (B) Calcification of all three coronaries.

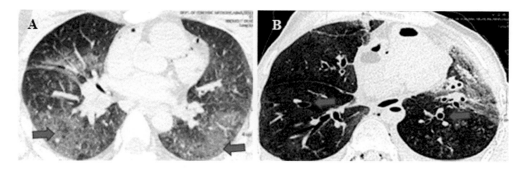

FIGURE 1.32: Axial plane of PMCT chest showing. (A) Bilateral ground glass opacity. (B) Bilateral dilated bronchioles and pleural effusion.

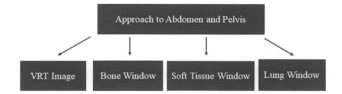

FIGURE 1.33: Flowchart of PMCT abdomen and pelvis examination.

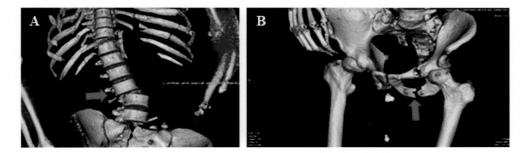

FIGURE 1.34: VRT image showing. (A) fracture of the lumbar and sacral vertebra. (B) Fracture of the pelvis.

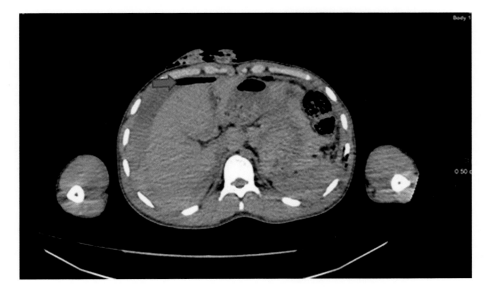

FIGURE 1.35: Axial section of PMCT showing pneumoperitoneum.

Photographs of external examination findings and PMCT data are to be stored in the department's medical records along with the detailed post-mortem report in digital form for easy retrieval and perusal. The medical record should be maintained in a safe and systematic way to ensure easy reproducibility and prevent manipulation.

Virtual autopsy conducted at CARE, AIIMS, New Delhi

Case 1: Treated natural death case

The deceased was brought to AIIMS, New Delhi's emergency centre in an unconscious state after collapsing at a gym in South Delhi on 10 August 2022. A medico-legal case was registered as he was brought to casualty in an unconscious state with unclear history. After resuscitation, he was shifted to the cardiac ICU. On Day 42 of his admission, he expired during his treatment on 21 September 2022. The body was then shifted to AIIMS mortuary. Since a medico-legal case was registered, the police requested for autopsy as a standard protocol. A virtual autopsy was conducted by a medical board, following the standard protocol.

Why was this case considered for virtual autopsy?

1. The case was registered as a medico-legal case (MLC), in AIIMS, New Delhi, as the history was unclear regarding the cause of the unconscious state. After the patient expired, the police requested for autopsy as per the standard protocol.
2. There was no allegation of foul play neither from police nor from the side of the relatives.
3. The deceased was treated in hospital for 42 days and the death was an in-hospital death.
4. A Medical Certification of Cause of Death (MCCD) and death report were already issued in standard Govt. of National Capital Territory of Delhi format mentioning preexisting morbid disease conditions directly leading to death
5. The deceased had a known case of Type 2 diabetes mellitus, hypertension, and coronary artery disease. There was a previous history of three percutaneous coronary interventions (PCIs).
6. The virtual autopsy centre in AIIMS, New Delhi provided an alternative non-invasive autopsy technique.
7. Considering the circumstantial facts, medical history, and medical records of the deceased case, the medical board decided it to be a fit case for virtual autopsy.

Assessment of the virtual autopsy findings

Findings in PMCT (Figures 1.36–1.42)

Collection of biological samples by minimally invasive/non-invasive approach

No samples were required in this case

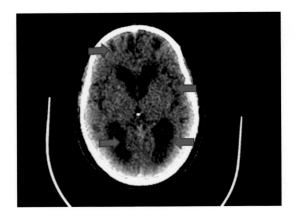

FIGURE 1.36: PMCT head showing generalized atrophic changes of the brain with dilated ventricles and prominent sulci and fissures.

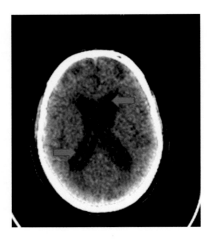

FIGURE 1.37: PMCT head showing generalized atrophic changes of the brain with dilated ventricles and prominent sulci and fissures.

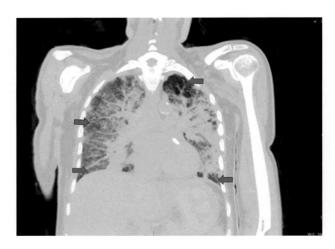

FIGURE 1.38: PMCT chest showing diffuse ground glass opacity and septal thickening.

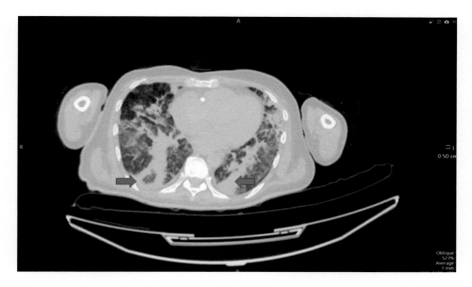

FIGURE 1.39: PMCT chest showing consolidation in bilateral lower lobes (blue arrows).

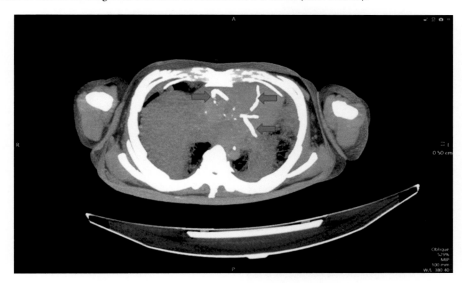

FIGURE 1.40A: PMCT chest with MIP showing multiple cardiac stents (blue arrows) suggestive of PCI.

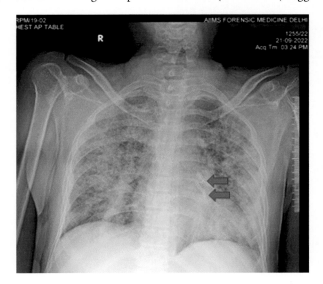

FIGURE 1.40B: Chest X-ray AP View showing multiple cardiac stents (blue arrows) suggestive of PCI.

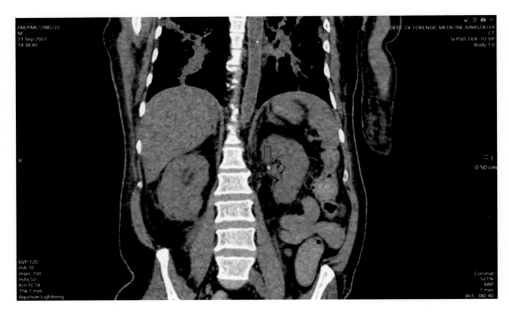

FIGURE 1.41:   PMCT abdomen showing calculi in the left renal pelvis.

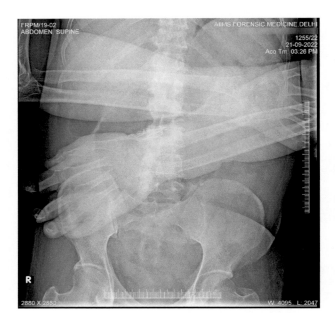

FIGURE 1.42:   X-ray of abdomen.

Case 1: Treated Natural Death Case...

शरीरमाद्यं खलु धर्मसाधनम्

POSTMORTEM REPORT
न्याय चिकित्सा एवं विषविज्ञान विभाग
Department of Forensic Medicine and Toxicology
अखिल भारतीय आयुर्विज्ञान संस्थान, नई दिल्ली - 110029
All India Institute of Medical Sciences, New Delhi -110029

Post-Mortem Report No.:   **Total Pages: 4**
FIR/DD Number:
FIR/DD Date:
Police Station:

Doctor/Autopsy Board Members

On the Body of {

Name:...
Father's Name:...
or
Husbands Name:.......................................
Sex:..
Age:...

Religion:..
Address:..

Body Brought and Identified By I.O
1
2

Body Identified By
1
2

Date & Hour of Receipt of dead body:.. *21/9/2022 2:30 pm*
Date & Hour of Receipt of Inquest Papers:................................ *21/9/2022 2:35 pm*
Date & Hour of Starting Autopsy:... *21/9/2022 2:35 pm*
Date & Hour of Concluding Autopsy:.. *21/9/2022 2:55 pm*

BRIEF HISTORY (as per Inquest Report):....................... *Alleged H/o deceased went to a gym in South Ex-2, New Delhi where while running in treadmill he suddenly collapsed due to an heart attack. The gym staff brought him to AIIMS Hospital Emergency immediately where he was admitted in ICU and was under treatment. During treatment he expired on 21.09.2022 at 10.07 AM and dead body was shifted to mortuary for postmortem examination. (Vide MLC no.   )*

In case of Hospital Death (Particulars as per Hospital Records) :
Name of Hospital... *AIIMS*
Date of Admission in Hospital:... *10/8/2022*
Date and Time of Death in Hospital:... *21/9/2022 10:07 am*
Central Registration Number of Hospital:................................. *UHID-*

न्याय चिकित्सा एवं विषविज्ञान विभाग, अखिल भारतीय आयुर्विज्ञान संस्थान, नई दिल्ली - 110029
Department of Forensic Medicine and Toxicology, All India Institute of Medical Sciences, New Delhi -110029

POST-MORTEM REPORT No.   Page 2 of 4

___

(A) GENERAL DESCRIPTION

Length of Body:.. *170 cm*

Clothes worn & their condition:.................................... *Wrapped in white hospital sheet. Blue full shirt, and blue and white checked pyjama. Clothes intact.*

Post-Mortem changes:

1. Rigor Mortis:.. *Upper limbs passed away, present over the lower limbs.*
2. Lividity:.. *Present over the back in the dependent regions in supine position no fixed, except for contact regions.*
3. Decomposition Changes:.................................... *NIL*
4. External appearance:... *Moderately built male. Generalized swelling present over the face and both hands. Cotton was present stuffed in the nostrils, mouth and tracheostomy stoma.*
a. Eyes:... *Closed, cornea hazy and conjunctivae pale.*
b. Mouth:... *NAD*
c. Nostrils.. *NAD*
d. Ears....:.. *NAD*
e. Nails:... *Pale nailbeds.*
f. Condition of orifices:... *Dark brownish serosanguinous fluid oozing from both nostrils and mouth.*

5. Injuries(Type,size,shape,location and direction etc.)
1) A brownish black scabbed abrasion of size 2 cm X 0.5 cm present over the anterior aspect of left leg over the shin 15 cm above the ankle with scab partially fallen off.

Iatrogenic wounds:
1) Bed sore of size 7.5 cm X 4.5 cm X skin deep present over the right infra-scapular region, with pale base and skin peeling.
2) Bed sore of 4 cm X 6 cm X soft tissue deep present over the upper part of the gluteal cleft and adjoining medial surface of both buttocks, pale base with unhealthy granulation tissue.
3) Partially healed, brownish scabbed, abrasion of size 0.3 cm X 0.3 cm X soft tissue deep present over the helix of left ear.
4) Tracheostomy stoma of size 2 cm X 0.5 cm X trachea lumen deep present over the anterior aspect of midline of neck, 2.5 cm above the supra-sternal notch. The surrounding margins have unhealthy granulation tissue with dark brownish sero-sanguinous fluid oozing out of the stoma.
5) Injection marks present over bilateral neck, dorsumm of both hands, bilateral cubital fossa and right inguinal region

(B) HEAD & NECK

1. Scalp & Sub Scalp:.. *NAD*
2. Skull:.. *INTACT*
3. Brain, Meninges and Cerebral Vessels:.......................... *Meninges unremarkable, cerebral vessels and sinuses intact. Generalized atrophic changes of brain seen with dialted ventricles and prominent sulci and fissures.*
4. Orbital, Nasal and Aural Cavities:
   (Examine if special indications present)........................... *NAD*
5. Mouth, Tongue:.. *Intact with pale mucosa and sero-sanguinous fluid oozing out.*
6. Neck, Larynx Thyroid and Other Neck Structures:........... *Tracheastomy stoma as described above. Congested mucosa, filled with dark brown sero-sanguinous fluid.*

(C) CHEST (THORAX)

1. Ribs and Chest Wall:... *Intact*
2. Diaphragm:.. *NAD*
3. Oesophagus:.. *NAD*
4. Trachea and Bronchi:... *NAD*
5. Pleural cavities:... *Bilateral minimal pleural effusion present.*
6. Lungs
   a. Right:.. *Diffuse ground glass opacity and septal thickening present with lower lobe consolidation.*
   b. Left:.. *Diffuse ground glass opacity and septal thickening present with lower lobe consolidation.*
7. Heart and Pericardial Sac:... *Pericardial sac intact. No pericardial effusion. Coronary stents present in the Left anterior descending artery, Left circumflex and Right Coronary artery.*
8. Large Blood Vessels:.. *Calcification present in the wall of ascending aorta, arch of aorta, descending thoracic aorta, descending abdominal aorta and bilateral common iliac artery.*

(D) ABDOMEN

1. Abdominal Wall:... *NAD*

न्याय चिकित्सा एवं विषविज्ञान विभाग, अखिल भारतीय आयुर्विज्ञान संस्थान, नई दिल्ली - 110029

Department of Forensic Medicine and Toxicology, All India Institute of Medical Sciences, New Delhi -110029

POST-MORTEM REPORT No.

Page 3 of 4

2. Peritoneal cavity:... *NAD*
3. Stomach
    A. Contents:... *Contains contents with heterogenous opacity, fluid and gas.*
    B. Mucosa:.. *NAD*
    C. Presence of any Abnormal Smell:............................. *NAD*
4. Small Intestine:.. *Has air-fluid levels and lumen is distended with gas.*
5. Large Intestine, vermiform appendix, Mesentery
   and pancreas... *Has air-fluid levels and lumen is distended with gas.*
6. Liver, gall bladder, biliary passage.................................... *Normal in size, smooth surface, parenchyma shows normal density.*
7. Spleen:... *NAD*
8. Kidney, renal pelvis, ureters
   a. Right:.. *Size 8.5 cm X 5.5 cm. Renal pelvis is unremarkable.*
   b. Left:... *Size 116 cm X 6 cm. Calculi of 3.5 mm diameter present in the renal pelvis.*
9. Pelvic Wall.. *NAD*
10. Urinary Bladder and Urethra:.. *Urinary bladder not distended and contains minimal residual urine.*
11 Genital organs:.. *NAD*
12. Uterus (Females):... *Not applicable*

(E) SPINAL COLUMN AND SPINAL CORD
(Note: The spinal cord need to be opened and examined if special indications present.)

1. Spinal Column and Spinal Cord:....................................... *No bony fractures, osteolytic or osteoblastic lesions.*

(F) ADDITIONAL REMARKS

Additional Remarks:... *On the request of near relative, virtual autopsy was conducted (External examination, Digital x-ray and PMCT). As per hospital records the deceased was diagnosed with Sepsis, Ventilator associated pneumonia with positive bacterial culture, Hypoxic ischemic encephalopathy, Dysautonomia, Stress induced upper gastrointestinal bleed and Malena. Type 2 diabetes mellitus, hypertension, coronary artery disease post PCI in 2006, 2013 and 2015. ACS- lateral wall myocardial infarction, post coronary angiography on 10.08.2022 showed left main (distal) 50% disease, LAD (ostium) 50-60% disease, (proximal) stent ISR 40 % diffuse stenosis, LCX (ostio-proximal)- ISR 95% disease, RI (ostium) - cut off, RCA (ostium) -50% stent patent, distal mild plaquing , post primary PCI 2 LM/LCX (RI 3.5 X 15) and LCX (distal) with RI 3 X 15, cardiogenic shock, improved LVEF 20-25% to 50-55%, paroxysmal AF.*

---END OF BODY OF REPORT---

न्याय चिकित्सा एवं विषविज्ञान विभाग, अखिल भारतीय आयुर्विज्ञान संस्थान, नई दिल्ली - 110029
Department of Forensic Medicine and Toxicology, All India Institute of Medical Sciences, New Delhi -110029

POST-MORTEM REPORT No.

(G) SPECIMEN COLLECTED FOR TOXICOLOGICAL ANALYSIS

(H) NATURE OF SPECIMEN PRESERVED
    Stomach with contents
    Small Intestine and contents
    Liver
    Kidney (one half of each)
    Spleen
    Sample of blood
    Other Viscera
    Preservative used

 Any other sample:

Received above marked material.

(Signature of Police official)

Name:
Belt No.:
Rank:

(I) ITEMS HANDED OVER TO POLICE
✓Dead Body
✓Post-Mortem Report No.
✓Inquest papers. Total number: 17
    Photograph/X-Ray, if any.
    Viscera, clothes & articles. if any.

Investigating Officer
Name:
Rank:
Police Station:

(J) TIME SINCE DEATH

Around 4-6 hours (Consistent with hospital records)

(K) OPINION

The cause of death to the best of my knowledge and belief is
Myocardial infarction and its subsequent medical complications

Signature of the Doctor / Autopsy Board Conducting Autopsy

Signature

Signature

Signature

Case 2: Treated Traumatic Death

POSTMORTEM REPORT

न्याय चिकित्सा एवं विषविज्ञान विभाग

Department of Forensic Medicine and Toxicology

अखिल भारतीय आयुर्विज्ञान संस्थान, नई दिल्ली - 110029

All India Institute of Medical Sciences, New Delhi -110029

Post-Mortem Report No.:   **Total Pages: 4**
FIR/DD Number:
FIR/DD Date:
Police Station:

Doctor/Autopsy Board Members

On the Body of
{
Name:...
Father's Name:...
or
Husbands Name:...
Sex:...
Age:...
Religion:...
Address:...

Body Brought and Identified By I.O
1
2

Body Identified By
1 Name:
2 Name:

Date & Hour of Receipt of dead body:.. *15/2/2023   2:00 pm*
Date & Hour of Receipt of Inquest Papers:................................. *15/2/2023   2:26 pm*
Date & Hour of Starting Autopsy:... *15/2/2023   2:55 pm*
Date & Hour of Concluding Autopsy:.. *15/2/2023   3:49 pm*

BRIEF HISTORY (as per Inquest Report):........................ *Allged history of deceased had a road traffic accident where pedestrain was hit by an auto rikshaw on 11/02/2023 at MB road,near railway under pass,Pul prahladpur. She was taken to Batra hospital and medical research centre where she expired during the course of treatment on 14/02/2023 at 7.16 PM vide MLC No. 16717/2023.*

In case of Hospital Death (Particulars as per Hospital Records) :
Name of Hospital:.. *Batra hospital and medical research centre*
Date of Admission in Hospital:... *11/2/2023*
Date and Time of Death in Hospital:... *14/2/2023   7:16 pm*
Central Registration Number of Hospital:..................................

(A) GENERAL DESCRIPTION

Length of Body:.. *5 feet cm*

Clothes worn & their condition:....................................... *Wrapped in white sheets.*

Post-Mortem changes:

1. Rigor Mortis:.. *Present over the lower limbs of the body*

2. Lividity:.. *Present over dependent parts of the body in supine position except pressure areas and it is fixed.*

3. Decomposition Changes:.. *Peeling of skin are present over bilateral wrist.*

4. External appearance:.. *Moderately built and nourished. Surgical adhesive tapes are present over bilateral wrist and right ankle. Multiple needle puncture marks are present over the bilateral dorsum of hands.*

a. Eyes:.. *Closed. On opening conjunctivae are pale and cornea are hazy.*

b. Mouth:... *Closed. On opening frenulae and gums are intact.*

c. Nostrils:... *Ala of nose are intact*

d. Ears....: .... *No abrnormality detected.*

e. Nails.. *Nail beds are pale bilaterally.*

f. Condition of orifices:... *No abrnormality detected.*

5. Injuries(Type,size,shape,location and direction etc.)

On external examination

1. A diffuse bluish black contusion of size 4 cm x 3 cm is present over the lateral aspect of left arm ,7 cm below the shoulder tip.

2. An obliquely placed reddish brown abrasion of size 3 cm x 1 cm is present over the lateral aspect of the left forearm,12 cm below the left elbow.

3. A diffuse bluish black contusion of size 7 cm x 6 cm is present over the left buttocks, 14 cm from the midline.

4. A horizontally placed reddish brown grazed abrasion of size 10 cm x 4 cm is present over the medial aspect of lower third of left leg,1 cm above the medial malleolus.

5. A sutured wound of length 8 cm is present over the heel of the right leg. On opening the sutures margins are crushed and contused.

(B) HEAD & NECK

1. Scalp & Sub Scalp:... *Soft boggy swelling on palpation is present over left temporal region with hyperdensity showing in the left temporal region on PMCT.*

2. Skull:.. *A fissure fracture involving the right occipital bone on the vault extending into the base of skull involving the right squamous and petrous part of temporal bone, right greater wing of sphenoid , pituitary fossa and ending at left greater wing of sphenoid.*

3. Brain, Meninges and Cerebral Vessels:....................... *Diffuse area of hyperdensity due to Subdural haemorrhage and area of hyperdensity into the sulci due to Subarachnoid haemorrhage are present over left fronto-parieto-temporal lobes. Area of hyperdensity surrounded by area of hypodensity due to contusion is present over the base of left frontal lobe which measures 1.7 cm x 1.5 cm. Left ventricle are compressed along with midline shift to the right side. Hyperdense area in the region of midbrain and pons due to brain stem haemorrhage is present.*

4. Orbital, Nasal and Aural Cavities:
   (Examine if special indications present)........................... *Hemosinus is present in bilateral maxillary sinus. Fracture of vomer bone is present in PMCT examination.*

5. Mouth, Tongue:... *No abnormality detected.*

6. Neck, Larynx Thyroid and Other Neck Structures:............ *No abnormality detected.*

(C) CHEST (THORAX)

1. Ribs and Chest Wall:... *A fracture of lateral third of clavicle is present on the left side.*

2. Diaphragm: .... *No abnormality detected.*

3. Oesophagus:.. *No abnormality detected.*

4. Trachea and Bronchi:... *Tracheal lumen is filled with fluid towards the distal end.*

5. Pleural cavities:.. *No fluid collection.*

न्याय चिकित्सा एवं विषविज्ञान विभाग, अखिल भारतीय आयुर्विज्ञान संस्थान, नई दिल्ली - 110029
Department of Forensic Medicine and Toxicology, All India Institute of Medical Sciences, New Delhi -110029

POST-MORTEM REPORT No.   Page 3 of 4

6. Lungs
    a. Right:.. *Ground glass opacities present along with patchy areas of consolidation over all the lobes.*
    b. Left:... *Ground glass opacities are present over all the lobes.*
7. Heart and Pericardial Sac... *Pericardium is intact, All four chambers are intact. No calcification noted in the coronary vessels.*
8. Large Blood Vessels:... *No abnormality detected.*

(D) ABDOMEN

1. Abdominal Wall:... *No abnormality detected.*
2. Peritoneal cavity:.. *No fluid collection.*
3. Stomach
    A. Contents:.. *Distended and contains contents with heterogenous opacities, fluid and gas along with multiple hyperdense material.*
    B. Mucosa:... *No abnormality detected.*
    C. Presence of any Abnormal Smell:............................ *NA*
4. Small Intestine:.. *Contains contents with heterogenous opacities, fluid and gas.*
5. Large Intestine, vermiform appendix, Mesentery
    and pancreas... *Contains contents with heterogenous opacities, fluid and gas along with multiple hyperdense material.*
6. Liver, gall bladder, biliary passage:................................. *No abnormality detected.*
7. Spleen:... *No abnormality detected.*
8. Kidney, renal pelvis, ureters
    a. Right:... *No abnormality detected.*
    b. Left:.. *No abrnormality detected.*
9. Pelvic Wall... *No abnormality detected.*
10. Urinary Bladder and Urethra:.. *Distended.*
11. Genital organs:.. *No abnormality detected.*
12. Uterus (Females):.. *No abnormality detected.*

(E) SPINAL COLUMN AND SPINAL CORD
(Note: The spinal cord need to be opened and examined if special indications present.)

1. Spinal Column and Spinal Cord:..................................... *Subarachnoid haemorrhage is present over the upper part of spinal cord. No fracture of spinal column is present.*

(F) ADDITIONAL REMARKS

Additional Remarks:.. *1) According to inquest paper no 14-16, NCCT head showed left frontoparietal subdural heamorrhage, diffuse subarachnoid haemorrhage in bilateral hemispheres with midline shift.*

--END OF BODY OF REPORT--

न्याय चिकित्सा एवं विषविज्ञान विभाग, अखिल भारतीय आयुर्विज्ञान संस्थान, नई दिल्ली - 110029

Department of Forensic Medicine and Toxicology, All India Institute of Medical Sciences, New Delhi -110029

POST-MORTEM REPORT No.   Page 4 of 4

(G) SPECIMEN COLLECTED FOR TOXICOLOGICAL ANALYSIS

(H) NATURE OF SPECIMEN PRESERVED
- Stomach with contents
- Small Intestine and contents
- Liver
- Kidney (one half of each)
- Spleen
- Sample of blood
- Other Viscera
- Preservative used

Any other sample:

Received above marked material.

(Signature of Police official)

Name:
Belt No.:
Rank:

(I) ITEMS HANDED OVER TO POLICE
- ✓ Dead Body
- ✓ Post-Mortem Report No.
- ✓ Inquest papers. Total number: 16
  Photograph/X-Ray, if any. -NIL
  Viscera, clothes & articles. if any. NIL

Investigating Officer
Name:
Rank:

(J) TIME SINCE DEATH

Consistent with hospital records(12 -18 hours before conducting autopsy)

(K) OPINION

The cause of death to the best of my knowledge and belief is
Head injury consequent upon blunt force or surface impact consistent with alleged history. All injuries are antemortem in nature.

Signature of the Doctor / Autopsy Board Conducting Autopsy

Signature

Signature

PROFORMA VERBAL AUTOPSY

Instructions for interviewer

- Conduct the interview in an enabling environment having in mind that they have lost their loved ones.
- Be polite and listen to what the relatives are saying rather than being judgemental.
- Choosing a respondent who has been the primary caregiver at the time of the terminal illness episode and death will be helpful both in getting a proper history thereby helping to narrow down to the exact cause of death.
- While interviewing, if the respondent or a family member expresses his/her grief by crying stop the interview for a while to comfort him/her.
- Do not be in a hurry to collect the information. Let them take their time.
- Look into the medical records after the entire interview is complete to prevent bias in concluding the cause of death.
- Seek all medical records after the interview and if possible, soft or hard copies may also be collected.
- You may add your comments after reviewing the records as supplementary information.
- Keep the information confidential.

Part 1: Identification Details

State_____ District_____Village_____

Verbal Autopsy Number
Name of the Deceased
Father/Husband's Name
Age in completed years
Sex: Male/Female
Date of Death:
Date of Interview:
Respondent Name:
Relationship with the Deceased:
Place of Death:
How long have you been living with the deceased before his/her death? (Months or years)
What is the cause of death as known to you?
If the deceased was a woman in the reproductive age group, was she amenorrhea or pregnant?
If yes, duration (in weeks)
Was the deceased in the habit of tobacco consumption?
Was the deceased in the habit of alcohol consumption?

How long was the person ill before his/her death?

Part 2: Narration by the Respondent

Describe the events in the patient's life just before his/her death as recalled by the relatives of the deceased. Write verbatim. Probe if necessary.

_____

_____

_____

_____

_____

_____

_____

_____

_____

_____

_____

_____

_____

_____
_____
_____
_____
_____
_____
_____
_____
_____
_____
_____
_____
_____
_____

Part 3: Past History

Was the deceased earlier taken to a doctor/hospital for any illness?
Tick those positive

Chronic Respiratory Illness	☐
Tuberculosis	☐
Heart Disease	☐
Heart Attack	☐
High Blood Pressure	☐
Diabetes	☐
Paralysis	☐
Cancer	☐
HIV/ AIDS	☐

Any other, specify:
Elaborate on the past history:

_____
_____
_____
_____
_____
_____
_____
_____
_____
_____

Part 4: Specific Symptoms:

Ask for the presence or absence of the following symptoms at the time of death and enquire about their duration. Ask about all the symptoms irrespective of the suggestive cause.

- Symptom:
- Duration:
- Weight loss:
- Unconsciousness:
- Swelling on any part of the body:
- Fits/convulsions:
- Decreased appetite:
- Vision disturbances:
- Voice disturbances:
- Disturbances while swallowing:
- Bleeding from any site:
- Ulcer/wound:
- Breathlessness:
- Sounds from chest:
- Headache:
- Urinary disturbances:
- Problems related to passing stools:
- Vomiting:
- Swelling of Abdomen:
- Fever (duration, grade, chills and rigors):
- Rash (duration, itching, place of spread):
- Swelling (duration, site, size, place, stationary, growing):
- Chest pain (site, type, onset, duration, associated with exertion):
- Cough (duration, dryness, expectoration, blood in sputum):
- Paralysis (duration, onset, dizziness, limbs involved, speech disturbance):
- Injury (duration, nature, site affected):

Part 5: Treatment History

Was the deceased taken to any doctor (any system of medicine/ traditional healer /hospital in his/her last days? (Probe for multiple diagnoses)
If yes, was the diagnosis told to the patient? If surgery was performed, details thereof (if the records are available please verify)

_____

_____

_____

_____

_____

_____

_____

To be filled by physician after reviewing the questionnaire

Probable diagnosis (cause of death) by the physician

Immediate cause

Underlying cause 1.

ICD 10 Code for cause of death

Other conditions related to death but not causal

Name and signature of physician with date

Medical records collected, please list ……………………………………..

List of abbreviations

1. AIIMS: All India Institute of Medical Sciences
2. VA: Virtual autopsy
3. CT: Computed tomography
4. PMCT: Post-mortem computed tomography
5. ICMR: Indian Council of Medical Research
6. CrPC: Code of Criminal Procedure
7. NHRC: National Human Rights Commission
8. MSCT: Multi-slice computed tomography
9. MRI: Magnetic resonance imaging
10. CARE: Centre for Advanced Research and Excellence
11. AERB: Atomic Energy Regulatory Board
12. BARC: Bhabha Atomic Research Centre
13. LAN: Local area network
14. MPR: Multi-planar reconstruction or reformation
15. CPR: Curved planar reformation
16. MIP: Maximum intensity projection
17. MinIP: Minimum intensity projection
18. VRT: Volume rendering technique
19. NAS: Network attached storage
20. PACS: Picture archiving and communication system
21. RSO: Radiation safety officer
22. TLD: Thermo-luminescent dosimeter
23. CTDI: Computed tomography dose index
24. MLR: Medico-legal report
25. PCI: Percutaneous coronary intervention
26. MCCD: Medical certification of cause of death

Bibliography

Abe K, Higuchi, K, Ino K. *Guideline for Ai scanning technique.* First edition. Vectorcore, Tokyo, 2009 (in Japanese).

Advisory for upholding the dignity and protecting the rights of the dead. National Human Rights Commission, India. 2021: 5. Available from: https://nhrc.nic.in/sites/default/files/NHRC%20Advisory%20for%20Upholding%20Dignity%20%26%20Protecting%20the%20Rights%20of%20Dead.pdf

Amadasi A, Merusi N,Cattaneo C. How reliable is apparent age at death on cadavers? *Int J Legal Med.* 2015;129:913–918. https://doi.org/10.1007/s00414-014-1042-9

Baccino E, Cunha E, Cattaneo C. Aging the dead and the living. In: Siegel JA, Saukko PJ, Houck MM (eds.), *Encyclopedia of forensic sciences.* Waltham: Academic Press, 2013, pp. 42–48.

Baccino E, Sinfield L, Colomb S, Baum TP, Martrille L. Technical note: The two step procedure (TSP) for the determination of age at death of adult human remains in forensic cases. *Forensic Sci Int.* 2014;244:247–251. https://doi.org/10.1016/j.forsciint.2014.09.005

Chief Coroner, Guidance No.1, The Use of Post-Mortem Imaging (Adults). Available from: https://www.judiciary.uk/wp-content/uploads/2013/09/guidance-no-1-use-of-port-mortem-imaging.pdf

Cunha E, Baccino E, Martrille L, Ramsthaler F, Prieto J, Schuliar Y, Lynnerup N, Cattaneo C. The problem of aging human remains and living individuals: A review. *Forensic Sci Int.* 2009;193:1–13. https://doi.org/10.1016/j.forsciint.2009.09.00825

Demirjian A. Dental development: Index of physiologic maturation. *Med Hyg. (Geneve)* 1978;36:3154–3159.

Demirjian A, Goldstein H. New systems for dental maturity based on seven and four teeth. *Ann Hum Biol.* 1976;3:411–421.

Ezawa H, Shiotani S. *Autopsy imaging (Ai).* First edition, Bunkodo, Tokyo, 2004 (in Japanese).

Flecker H. Roentgenographic observations of the times of appearance of epiphyses and their fusion with the diaphyses. *J Anat.* 1932;67:118–164.

Gakhar GK, Gupta V, Jasuja OP, Khandelwal N. Determining the ossification status of sternal end of the clavicle using CT and digital X-ray: A comparative study. *J Forensic Sci.* 2014 Mar 1;5(2):1.

Greulich WW, Pyle SI. *Radiographic atlas of skeletal development of the hand and wrist,* Second ed. Stanford, CA: Stanford University Press, 1959.

Japan Radiological Society and Study Group of Japan Health and Labor Sciences Research. Postmortem imaging interpretation guideline 2015 in Japan. Available from: https://cdicenter2016.med.hokudai.ac.jp/en/wp-content/uploads/2017/09/postmortem-Image-Interpretation-Guideline-2015.pdf

Jit I, Kulkarni M. Times of appearance and fusion of epiphysis at the medial end of the clavicle. *Indian J Med Res.* 1976;64:773–782.

Mincer HH, Harris EF, Berryman HE. The A.B.F.O. study of third molar development and its use as an estimator of chronological age. *J Forensic Sci.* 1993;38:379–390.

Mohanty A, Singh K and Others v State (Delhi Administration). Jus Corpus LJ. Available from: https://indiankanoon.org/doc/667073/#:~:text=Indian%20Penal%20Code%2C%201860%20Sections,upheld%2D%2DBalbir%20Singh%20acquitted.

Mughal AM, Hassan N, Ahmed A. Bone age assessment methods: A critical review. *Pak J Med Sci.* 2014 January;30(1):211.

Schmeling A, Dettmeyer R, Rudolf E, Vieth V, Geserick G. Forensic age estimation. *Dtsch Arztebl Int.* 2016;113:44–50. https://doi.org/10.3238/arztebl.2016.0044

Schmeling A, Olze A, Reisinger W, Geserick G. Forensic age diagnostics of living people undergoing criminal proceedings. *Forensic Sci Int.* 2004;144:243–245. https://doi.org/10.1016/j.forsciint.2004.04.059

Schmeling A, Schulz R, Reisinger W, Mühler M, Wernecke KD, et al. Studies on the time frame for ossification of the medial clavicular epiphyseal cartilage in conventional radiography. *Int J Legal Med.* 2004;118:5–8.

Schulz R, Mühler M, Reisinger W, Schmidt S, Schmeling A. Radiographic staging of ossification of the medial clavicular epiphysis. *Int J Legal Med.* 2008;122:55–58.

Shiotani S, Yamamoto S. *Guidebook for interpretation of Ai.* First edition. Bunkodo, Tokyo, 2008 (in Japanese).

The Japanese College of Radiology. *The Japan Association of Radiological Technologists, Guideline for Ai.* First edition. Vector-core, Tokyo, 2009 (in Japanese).

2   HEAD – ANATOMY, TRAUMA, AND PATHOLOGY

The head of the human body is a specialized globular cranial end region containing vital structures compacted into a small, complex area which is covered by a protective bone called a skull along with appendages like skin and hair, which protect the vital internal structures. In the animal kingdom, humans are placed at a higher level due to their brain, which is comparatively well-developed and large. This large brain is accommodated by a proportionally increased cranium size. This large brain also gives them the advantage of rational thinking, using judgment based on this rational thinking and also reasoning and analyzing every situation or problem encountered. The head has structures which are in close interrelation, including the sinuses, blood vessels, nerves, muscles, a ventricular system containing the cerebrospinal fluid, etc. This chapter has been written by the author from a regional point of view to give readers a better understanding. The gross and CT comparison is done in all possible places for easy understanding and also to act as a possible ready guide when readers encounter similar findings in cases.

The complex bony skull houses the brain, which is the control centre of all functions of the human body. The brain, along with many special sense organs like the eyes, ears, nose, and tongue, have very important functions. Human supremacy without this well-developed specialized region is questionable. Apart from the special senses, it also acts as the start of important tracts of human anatomy, which include the respiratory tract and digestive tract. Structurally and functionally, the head region is divided into:

1. Cranium.
2. Face.

Cross-sectional anatomy of the skull

Skull: The skull is the most complex human bone. It is formed by intramembranous ossification. It is symmetric along the median line and has mostly paired bone on either side or a single bone in the midline placed symmetrically such that the median line divides then into two similar halves. The head has 28 bones which include **8 cranial bones, 14 facial bones, and 6 auditory (ear) bones.**

The eight cranial bones
- **Two parietal bones:** (Figures 2.1A, 2.1B, 2.2A, and 2.2B)
  The parietal bones are paired bones which articulate with each other in the midline forming a sagittal suture. They also articulate with the frontal bone and the occipital bone anteriorly and posteriorly, respectively, forming the coronal suture in the junction with the frontal bone and lambdoid suture in its junction with the occipital bone. The common point where the two parietal bones and frontal bone meets and also the meeting point of the sagittal suture with the coronal suture is called the 'bregma'. Posteriorly, the common point where the two parietal bones and the occipital bone meet along with the meeting of the sagittal suture with the lambdoid suture is called 'lambda'. Laterally, the squamous suture is formed by parietal bones articulating with the squamous temporal bone.

- **Two temporal bones:** (Figures 2.3A, 2.3B, and 2.4)
  Temporal bones are paired bones which are situated on the sides of the skull. Temporal bones consist of the petrous part, which is seen in the base of the skull at the junction of the middle and posterior cranial fossa; it consists of the internal acoustic meatus and inner ear structures, and the middle ear with its ossicles. The tympanic part of the temporal bone forms the bony aspect of the external acoustic meatus. The mastoid process part houses the mastoid air cells. The squamous portion of the temporal bone is the largest of all its parts, and is also the thinnest bone of the cranium, making it the weakest and is prone to fractures. The spinous process and the zygomatic arch are two projections from the temporal bone. The temporal bone articulates the mandible below by a special and only mobile joint of the skull called the temporomandibular joint.

- **One frontal bone:** (Figures 2.1A, 2.1B, 2.2A, 2.2B, 2.3A, and 2.3B)
  The frontal bone is an anteriorly placed single cranial bone which forms the entire anterior part of the calvaria and also the upper third segment of the face, where it forms the boundary between the cranial and facial bones. This bone contains the frontal air sinuses found just above the orbits. This bone also forms the roof of the orbit, which in turn constitutes the anterior third of the base of the skull.

- **One occipital bone:** (Figure 2.2A, 2.2B, and 2.4)
  The occipital bone is a single trapezoidal-shaped bone and forms the major part of the posterior aspect of the cranium and the posterior cranial fossa of the base of the skull. It is the thickest of all the cranial bones. Fractures of this bone usually infer that the force transmitted to the skull is usually sufficient to be fatal. The most projecting part of this bone externally is termed external occipital protuberance, and on the inner aspect is an internal occipital protuberance. It also entirely supports the cerebellum and articulates with the cervical vertebra below and the sphenoid and parietal bone anteriorly. The occipital bone is divided into the basilar part, the condylar part, and the squamous part.

- **One ethmoid bone:** (Figure 2.4)
  The ethmoid bone is a single median pneumatic bone that is located in the anterior cranial fossa. It harbours the ethmoidal air sinuses, which drain into the nasal meatus. This bone forms the median wall of the orbits, which is called the lamina papyracea, and its cribriform plate has a perforated surface through which the filaments of olfactory nerves pass. Crista galli is the portion of the ethmoid bone which gives a bony projection in the anterior cranial fossa and acts as the anchor for attachment of falx cerebri.

- **One sphenoid bone:** (Figure 2.4)
  The sphenoid bone is a single median bone located in the central part of the base of the skull in the middle cranial fossa. It has an appearance of a butterfly along with its body, lesser wing, greater wing, and paired medial and lateral pterygoid plates. This complex-shaped bone articulates with all other bones of the cranium, which

DOI: 10.1201/9781003383703-2

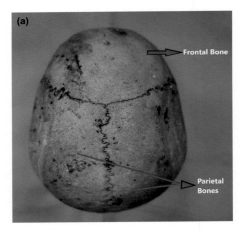

FIGURE 2.1A: Superior view of the skull shows frontal bone and parietal bones.

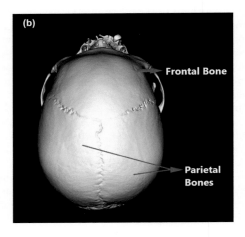

FIGURE 2.1B: Volume rendering CT image of the superior view of the skull showing frontal bone and parietal bones.

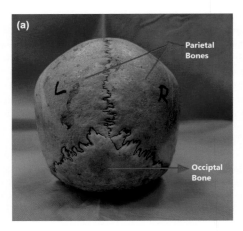

FIGURE 2.2A: Posterior view of skull shows occipital bone and parietal bones.

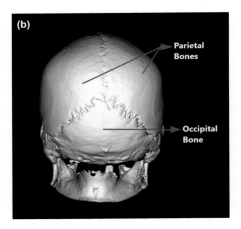

FIGURE 2.2B: Volume rendering CT image of a posterior view of the skull showing frontal bone and parietal bones.

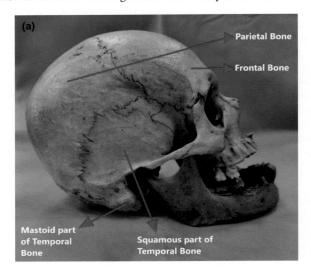

FIGURE 2.3A: Lateral view of the skull showing frontal bone, parietal bone, squamous part & mastoid part of the temporal bone.

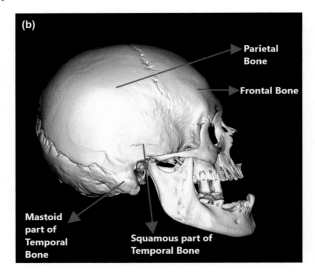

FIGURE 2.3B: Volume rendering CT image lateral view of the skull showing frontal bone, parietal bone, squamous part & mastoid part of the temporal bone.

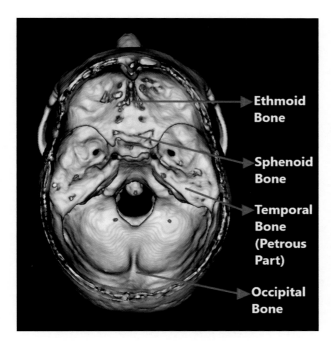

FIGURE 2.4: Volume rendering CT image of the base of the skull showing ethmoid bone, sphenoid bone, petrous part of the temporal bone and occipital bone.

include the frontal, parietal, temporal, and occipital bones.

The sphenoid bone also articulates with the following facial bones, the ethmoid, vomer, zygoma, palatine bones, and maxilla. It also acts as the channel through which the optic, oculomotor, trochlear, maxillary, mandibular, and abducens cranial nerves pass. It also hosts the sphenoidal air sinus and also the pituitary fossa (also called sella turcica or hypophysial fossa).

The 14 facial bones

- **Two nasal bones:** (Figures 2.5A and 2.5B)

   Nasal bones are paired rectangular-shaped bones, which form the nasal bridge. They are thicker in the upper part and as they come down they become thinner. They articulate superiorly with the frontal bone, medially with each other, and laterally with the frontal process of the maxilla. Inferiorly it articulates with the maxilla.

- **Two maxillary bones:** (Figures 2.5A and 2.5B)

   Maxillary bones are paired bones which form the upper jaw and the anterior part of the hard palate. It also forms part of the lateral wall of the nasal cavity and the inferior wall of the orbit. Maxillary bones are hollow pneumatic bones and contain the largest of the paranasal sinuses maxillary sinus. The maxillary bone has four processes, namely the frontal, alveolar, zygomatic, and palatine processes.

- **Two lacrimal bones:**

   The lacrimal bone is a paired bone. They are also the smallest and most fragile bones of the face. They are located on the medial wall anterior aspect of the orbit. The lacrimal bone articulates anteriorly and inferiorly with the maxillary bone, above with the frontal bone and posteriorly with the ethmoid. The bone is named due to

its close proximity to the lacrimal gland and associated structures. The lacrimal groove corresponds to the position of the nasolacrimal duct and is towards the orbital surface.

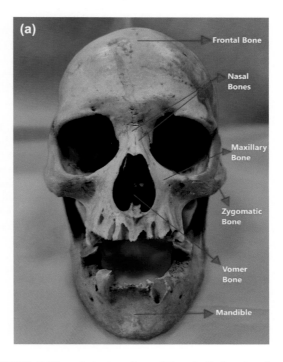

FIGURE 2.5A: Anterior view of the skull showing frontal bone, nasal bones, maxillary bones, vomer bone and mandible.

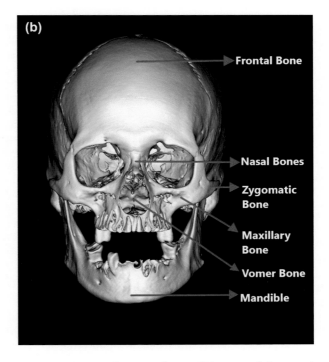

FIGURE 2.5B: Volume rendering CT image of the anterior view of the skull showing frontal bone, nasal bones, maxillary bones, vomer bone and mandible.

- **Two zygomatic bones:** (Figures 2.5A and 2.5B)

  The zygomatic bone is a paired bone which forms the anterolateral projection of the middle of the face forming the cheek prominence. This bone has four processes which include the frontal process, which forms the frontozygomatic suture with the frontal bone and also forms the lateral orbital wall. The temporal process is the most prominent one which forms the zygomatic arch after articulating with the corresponding process of the temporal bone. The maxillary process forms part of the floor of the orbit and articulates with the maxilla. The fourth process also joins with the maxilla bone giving the zygomatic eminence.

- **Two palatine bones:**

  Palatine bone is a paired bone, with a horizontal portion and vertical perpendicular plates. The horizontal plate of both sides together forms the posterior aspect of the hard palate. The vertical plates form a small part of the floor of the orbit and also articulate with the lateral pterygoid plate of the sphenoid bone. It has two foramina called the greater and lesser palatine foramina which transmit nerves and vessels of similar nomenclature.

- **Two inferior nasal conchae:**

  The inferior nasal concha is a paired bone, which is the skeletal support of the inferior turbinate in the nasal cavity. It helps in the formation of the meatuses of the nasal cavity to provide necessary channels and space for the air to get humidified as it travels.

- **One vomer bone:** (Figures 2.5A and 2.5B)

  The vomer is a single median bone located in the nasal cavity, and it forms the important support structure of the nasal septum in the posterior portion. It articulates with surrounding bones which include the palatine, maxillary, and ethmoid bones.

- **One mandible:** (Figure 2.5A and 2.5B)

  The mandible is an unpaired bone. It is the largest and strongest among the facial bones. The mandible structure consists of a body and two rami. The body has alveolar sockets which bear the dentition. The ramus has two processes which namely the anterior coronoid process and the posterior condyloid process, both of which are separated by a notch called the mandibular notch. The condyloid process is involved in the formation of the temporomandibular joint, which is the only mobile joint of the head. The mandible has two foramina namely the mental foramina, located on the outer surface of the body of the mandible, through which the mental nerve traverses and also the mandibular foramina, located on the inner surface of the ramus of the mandible and through which the inferior alveolar nerves and vessels traverse. The mandible also has a depression on the inner surface of the body called the submandibular fossa, which hosts the submandibular salivary gland.

The six auditory (ear) bones

- **Two malleus:** (Figure 2.6)

  The malleus is a paired bone with the outermost ear ossicle placed in the middle ear. It is the largest of the ear ossicles and is situated between the tympanic membrane and the incus. Due to being shaped like a hammer, it is called the malleus (Latin for hammer). It is held in position in the middle ear by ligaments, is the outermost bone of the middle ear, and is an important part of the

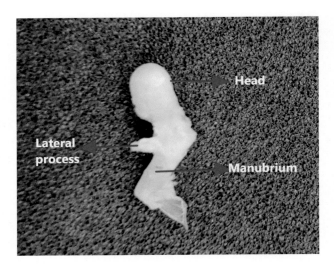

FIGURE 2.6: Malleus bone, the outermost ossicle of the middle ear, with a head, manubrium and lateral process.

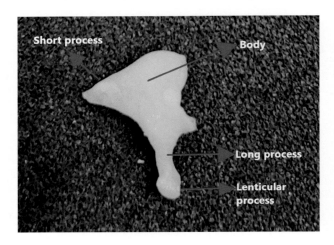

FIGURE 2.7: Incus bone, the middle ossicle of the chain located in the middle ear, shows the body, short process, long process, and lenticular process.

auditory system. The parts of the malleus include the head, manubrium (also called the handle of the malleus), anterior process, and lateral process. It has the role of transmitting sound from outside to the inner ear, and also, when loud sounds are encountered, they protect by reducing the transmission of such dangerous sounds.

- **Two incus:** (Figure 2.7)

  The incus is a paired bone and the middle of the ear ossicles. Its name, in Latin, means "anvil" due to its shape. It is held in position by the ligaments in the middle ear and also due to its articulation with the malleus and stapes. The ossicle is held in its appropriate place in the middle ear by ligaments. The incus structure consists of the body, the short process, the long process, and the lenticular process. The short process projects backwards, and the long process projects inferiorly and anteromedially. At the lower end of the long process, the bone bends at a 90° angle to form a lenticular process.

- **Two stapes:**

  The stapes is a paired bone with each bone presenting in the middle ear on both sides. It derives its name due to its shape resembling a stirrup, hence the name stapes, which means stirrup in Latin. Stapes bone is essential to the function of hearing, and it sets the oval window in vibration, which in turn transmits waves in the fluids of the cochlea. This moves the basilar membrane, which in turn triggers the sensory cells of the organ of corti. These sensory cells send nerve impulses to the brain, thereby converting the mechanical sound waves into electrical impulses. The stapes bone has a head, anterior limb, posterior limb, and footplate.

Cranial Sutures

Cranial sutures are fibrous joints which connect the different bones of the skull. This fibrous joint is made of connective tissue, which is mostly collagen. The process of the formation of this immobile fixed joint between these cranial bones is called synarthroses. The mandible is the only exception which forms a synovial joint which is mobile and is called the temporomandibular joint. There are many cranial sutures, namely:

Norma frontalis (**Anterior view of the skull**) (Figures 2.8a and 2.8b)	**Frontonasal suture:** This suture is located between the frontal and nasal bones. The midpoint of this suture, where both the nasal bones meet the frontal bone, is called a 'nasion'.
	Frontozygomatic suture: This suture is located between the zygomatic bone and the frontal bone. The articulation occurs between the zygomatic process (part of the frontal bone) and the frontal process (part of the zygomatic bone).
	Frontomaxillary suture: This suture is located between the frontal process (part of the maxilla) and the frontal bone. It is located in the nasal region lateral to the nasal bone.
	Zygomaticomaxillary suture: This suture is located between the maxillary process (part of the zygomatic bone) and the zygomatic process (part of the maxilla).
	Intermaxillary suture: This suture is located between the two maxillary bones, which form the two halves of the upper jaw.
	Metopic suture: The median cranial suture in the frontal bone, it is found in children but may be present in adults in 3–8% of cases. This suture shows the development of the frontal bone from two separate centres of ossification, which fuse in the midline.
Norma occipitalis (**Posterior view of the skull**) (Figures 2.9a and 2.9b)	**Sagittal suture:** This median cranial suture is located between two parietal bones. It is one of the most commonly studied sutures for determining age from the skull.
	Lambdoid suture: This suture is located between the parietal bone and the occipital bone. The junction of the two parietal bones with the occipital bone, also the point where the sagittal and lambdoid suture converge, is called 'lambda'.
Norma verticalis (**Superior view of the skull**) (Figures 2.10a and 2.10b)	**Coronal suture:** The suture's name is derived from its position in the skull, resembling a crown. It is present between the frontal bone and the parietal bones. The junction of the two parietal bones with the frontal bone, and also the point where the sagittal and coronal suture converge, is called 'bregma'.
Norma lateralis (**Lateral view of the skull**) (Figures 2.11a and 2.11b)	**Squamous suture:** This suture is located between the parietal bone and the squamous part of the temporal bone. It starts from the pterion anteriorly and posteriorly extends as the parietomastoid suture.
	Sphenofrontal suture: This suture is located between the frontal bone and sphenoid bone, near the pterion and, from an anterior view, located near the roof of the orbit.
	Sphenoparietal suture: This suture is located between the sphenoid bone and parietal bone, forming the horizontal 'H' line of the pterion.
	Occipitomastoid suture: This suture is located between the occipital bone and the mastoid process (part of the temporal bone). It is the downward continuation of the lambdoid suture.
	Temporozygomatic suture: This suture is located between the temporal bone and zygomatic bone on the lateral surface of the zygomatic arch.
Norma basalis (**Inferior view of the skull**) (Figure 2.12)	**Median palatine suture:** This suture is located between the horizontal plates of the palatine bone, on the posterior part of the hard palate.
	Transverse palatine suture: This suture is located between the palatine bone and the palatine process (part of the maxillary bone), on the hard palate.
	Petro-occipital suture: This suture is located between the occipital bone and the temporal bone's petrous part.
	Spheno-occipital suture: This suture is located between the sphenoid bone and the occipital bone.
	Petrosquamous suture: This suture is located between the temporal bone's petrous and squamous parts.
	Petrotympanic suture: This cranial suture is located between the temporomandibular joint and the tympanic cavity.

Premature fusion of the sutures poses a problem to the normal development of the skull bones also fails to properly accommodate the growing brain. This disorder is a common problem encountered in paediatric age groups and may be related to genetic mutations. This condition is called **craniosynostosis**.

Paranasal Sinuses

The paranasal sinuses are the hollow air-filled spaces present in the skull and facial skeleton and are connected to the nasal cavity. They are outgrowth pouches from the nasal cavity and are lined by the same continuous mucosa which lines the nasal cavity. The four paranasal sinuses include:

1. Frontal sinus.
2. Ethmoidal sinus.
3. Sphenoidal sinus.
4. Maxillary sinus.

The paranasal sinuses function by humidifying and heating the inhaled air before it enters the lower respiratory tract trapping dust particles and preventing them from entering, lightening the weight of the skull, and also acting to reduce the transmission of an impact's force to the vital structures in the case of facial trauma. Most of the paranasal sinuses are rudimentary or absent in newborns; they slowly increase in size and reach their mature size in the early 20s, but their shape greatly differs between individuals, and after that, they continue to enlarge

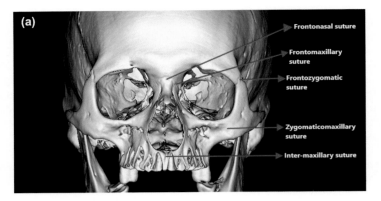

FIGURE 2.8A: Volume rendering CT image of the anterior view of the skull showing frontonasal, frontomaxillary, frontozygomatic, zygomaticomaxillary, and inter-maxillary suture.

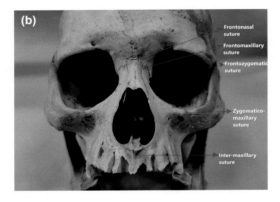

FIGURE 2.8B: Anterior view of the skull showing frontonasal, frontomaxillary, frontozygomatic, zygomaticomaxillary, and inter-maxillary suture.

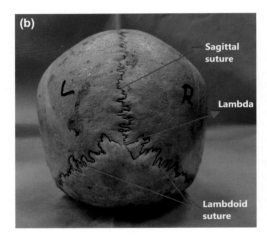

FIGURE 2.9B: Posterior view of the skull showing sagittal and lambdoid suture along with lambda.

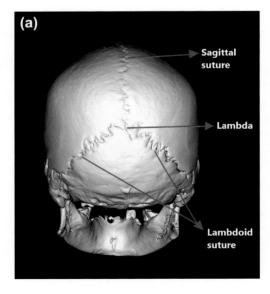

FIGURE 2.9A: Volume rendering CT image of a posterior view of the skull showing sagittal and lambdoid suture along with lambda.

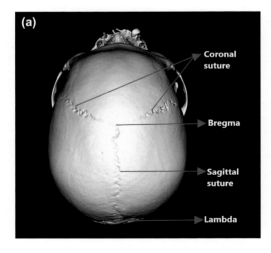

FIGURE 2.10A: Volume rendering CT image of the superior view of the skull showing coronal and sagittal suture along with bregma.

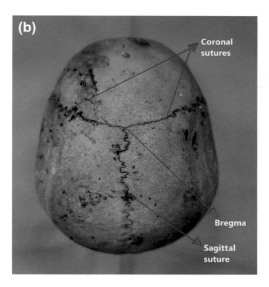

FIGURE 2.10B: Superior view of the skull showing coronal and sagittal suture along with bregma.

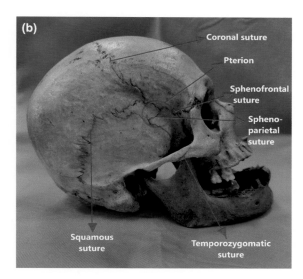

FIGURE 2.11B: Lateral view of the skull showing coronal, squamous, sphenofrontal, sphenoparietal, and temporozygomatic suture along with pterion.

slowly until death. The ethmoidal sinus is usually the first sinus to be pneumatized in a newborn child, followed by the usual pneumatization of the maxillary and sphenoid sinus. The frontal sinus is the last to pneumatize, and it gets completely pneumatized by the age of 14–15 years.

Frontal sinus: (Figures 2.13 and 2.15)

The frontal sinuses are paranasal sinuses which are present in the frontal bone. They are usually triangular in shape and are located above the inner end of the supraorbital crest and extend back into the medial part of the orbit. The two frontal sinuses present on either side of the midline are separated by a thin bony lamella. The frontal sinuses drain via the infundibulum into the middle meatus.

Ethmoidal sinus: (Figures 2.13, 2.14, and 2.16)

Ethmoidal sinus is a collection of air cells, usually 3–18 in number, which are separated by bony septa within the single

median ethmoid bone. The ethmoidal sinus is divided into the anterior and posterior groups, which are separated by the basal lamella. Previously, the ethmoid sinus was subdivided into three groups which were: the anterior, middle, and posterior ethmoidal air cells. However, in the current classification, the middle group are now incorporated into the anterior group. The anterior group drains via the ethmoid bulla into the hiatus semilunaris and middle meatus. The posterior group, via the sphenoethmoidal recess, drains into the superior meatus. A few of the named ethmoidal cells due to their clinical importance related to pathologies or surgical procedures include:

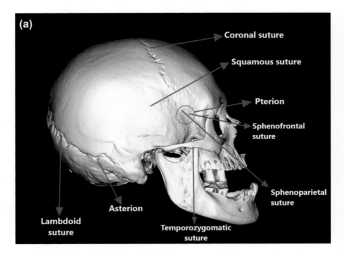

FIGURE 2.11A: Volume rendering CT image of the lateral view of the skull showing coronal, squamous, lambdoid, sphenofrontal, sphenoparietal, and temporozygomatic suture along with pterion and asterion.

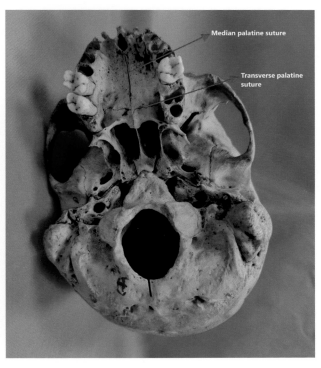

FIGURE 2.12: Inferior view of the skull showing median palatine and transverse palatine suture.

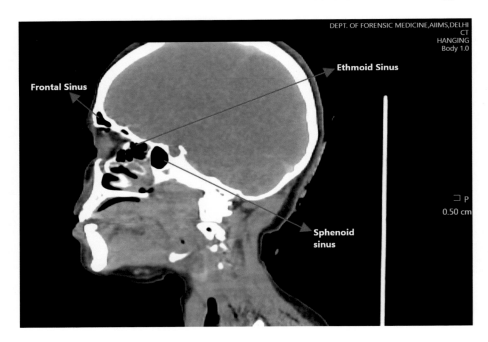

FIGURE 2.13: CT Sagittal section in the median plane showing the frontal sinus, ethmoid sinus, and sphenoid sinus.

1. Frontal recess cells, including the agger nasi cells.
2. Ethmoid bulla.
3. Haller cells.
4. Onodi cells.

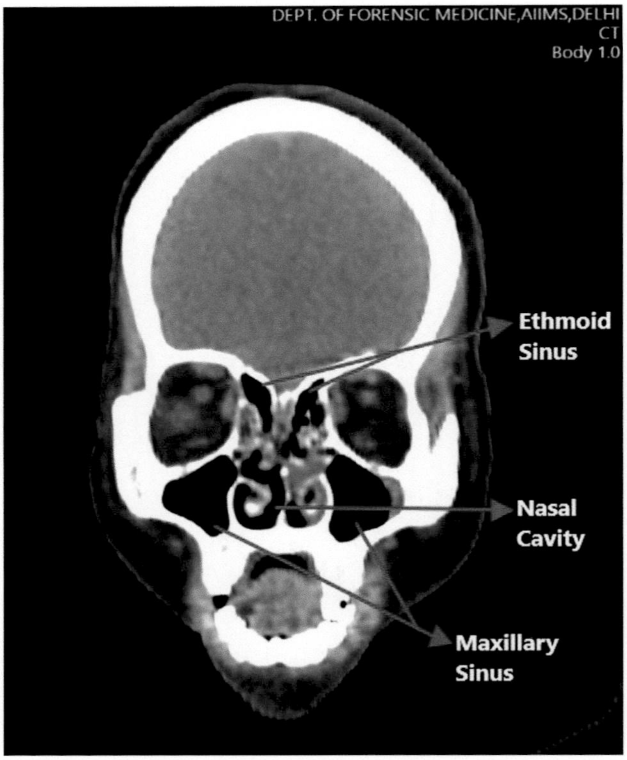

Sphenoidal sinus: (Figures 2.13, 2.16, and 2.17)

The sphenoidal sinuses are situated on the back of the nose in the sphenoidal bone and are the most posterior paranasal sinus. It contains a depression/fossa which hosts the pituitary gland. The sphenoidal sinuses are separated from each other by thin bony septae. The sinus drains above the superior concha into the sphenoethmoidal recess.

Maxillary sinus: (Figures 2.14 and 2.18)

Maxillary sinuses are paired pyramid-shaped sinuses located in the body of the maxillary bone. The apex of the pyramid

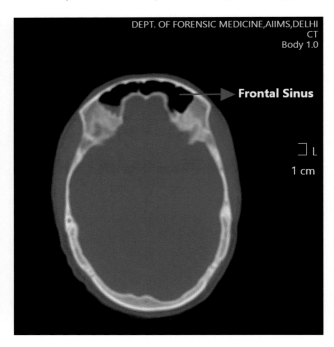

FIGURE 2.14: CT coronal section showing the ethmoid sinus and maxillary sinus. Air-filled nasal cavities with turbinates can also be appreciated in the view.

FIGURE 2.15: CT axial section showing both the frontal sinuses separated by a thin bony lamella.

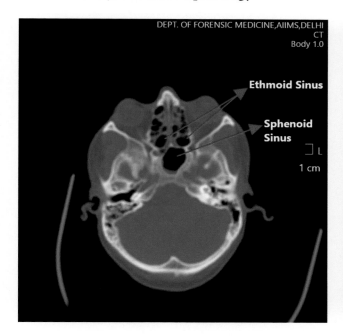

FIGURE 2.16: CT axial section shows the ethmoid sinus and sphenoid sinus.

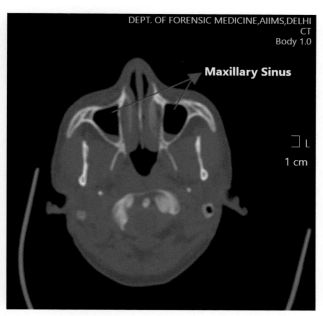

FIGURE 2.18: CT axial section shows the bilateral maxillary sinus.

Brain

The central nervous system (CNS) embryological origin is from a neural tube which has a central cavity that persists even after development. During development, the brain differentiates into the forebrain, midbrain, and hindbrain. The forebrain is comprised of the cerebrum and diencephalon. The cerebrum encloses its cavity, which includes the right and left lateral ventricles, and the diencephalon encloses its cavity, which is the third ventricle. The midbrain is a relatively smaller region which connects the forebrain and hindbrain. The cavity enclosed by the midbrain is the cerebral aqueduct of Sylvius. The hindbrain is comprised of the pons, medulla oblongata, and cerebellum. The hindbrain encloses the central cavity called the fourth ventricle. The adult human brain weighs about 1/50th, or 2%, of total body weight and roughly measures around 1180–1620 g in males and around 1030–1400 g in females. It is the receiving centre and receives all the information from the outside world with the help of the sense organs, including the five senses, which are smell, vision, hearing, taste, and various types of touch. The brain processes this information and stores them for short-term or long-term retrieval in the form of memory. It also controls the motor outcome in the form of speech, actions, functions, or emotions.

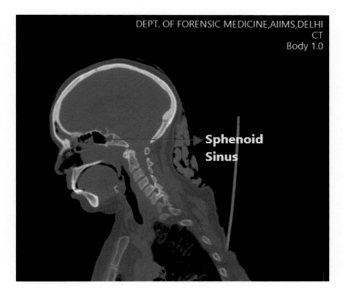

FIGURE 2.17: CT sagittal section in the midline, which shows the sphenoid sinus present below and in front of the pituitary fossa.

Cerebrum

The cerebrum is the largest and most prominent part of the brain. It is a part of the forebrain and consists of the right and left hemispheres which are in the anterior and middle cranial fossa, along with the supra-tentorial part of the posterior cranial fossa. The cerebrum is constituted by an outer grey matter, which is called the cerebral cortex, and below it is the white matter which forms the major core of the cerebral cortex. In the deeper aspect of the white matter, there are masses of grey matter known as the deep cerebral nuclei or basal nuclei/ganglia. The surface of the cerebrum is convoluted with surface elevations called the gyri and depressions called sulci. There are a few deep groves which are called fissures.

extends into the zygomatic process of the maxilla, while the base of the pyramid is formed over the lateral wall of the nose. The maxillary sinus roof is formed by the floor of the orbit, and the floor of the sinus is formed by the alveolar process of the maxillary bone. These sinuses are located above the first and second premolars and of the third molar and sometimes near the root of the canine, bilaterally. It drains via the hiatus semilunaris into the middle meatus of the nose. Fluid accumulates easily in this sinus due to the high position of the drainage point located high on the medial wall of the sinus.

The two cerebral hemispheres are separated by a deep central longitudinal fissure called the longitudinal cerebral fissure. In the floor of this fissure lies the corpus callosum, which is the largest commissure connecting the two cerebral hemispheres and contains the white matter connecting the corresponding areas of both cerebral hemispheres. The absence of corpus callosum is seen in genetic syndromes like Andermann, Aicardi, Shapiro, Acrocallosal, Menkes, or Mowat–Wilson. It could also be seen in cases of prenatal infection with the Rubella virus or brain malformations like hydrocephalus or Arnold-Chiari malformation.

The cerebral hemispheres (Figures 2.19–2.21) are divided into four lobes and are named corresponding to the overlying skull bone. The four lobes are:

1. **Frontal lobe:** Located above the lateral sulcus and in front of the central sulcus. It is the main centre for voluntary motor functions, awareness, motivation, aggression, and emotions.
2. **Parietal lobe:** Located behind the central sulcus and in front of the parieto-occipital sulcus, and above the lateral sulcus. It is the receiving and processing station for all sensory inputs except the special senses like taste, smell, and hearing.
3. **Temporal lobe:** Located below the lateral sulcus and in front of the pre-occipital notch. It is the receiving and processing place for smell and hearing and also plays a vital role in memory pathways.
4. **Occipital lobe:** Located behind the line that joins the parieto-occipital sulcus and the pre-occipital notch. It is the receiving and processing place for vision.

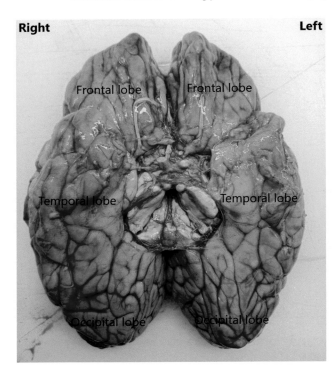

FIGURE 2.20: Inferior view of the cerebrum showing bilateral frontal, temporal, and occipital lobes.

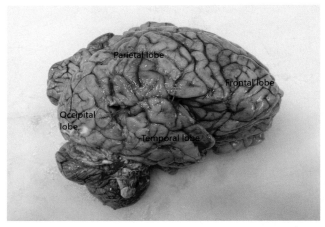

FIGURE 2.21: Right lateral view of the brain showing right frontal, parietal, temporal, and occipital lobes.

Basal ganglia/basal nuclei

The basal ganglia/basal nuclei are a grouping of grey matter located deep within the core of the cerebrum inside the white matter at the junction between the forebrain and midbrain (Figure 2.22). They are located symmetrically in both cerebral hemispheres. The basal ganglia play a vital role in functions like the control of voluntary motor movements, learning, cognition, eye movements, and emotion. Anatomically, the term basal ganglia include:

1. Corpus striatum.
2. Claustrum.
3. Amygdaloid body.

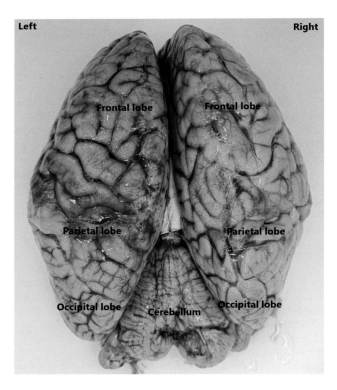

FIGURE 2.19: Superior view of the brain showing bilateral frontal, parietal and occipital lobes. Cerebellum is also appreciated in the posteroinferior aspect of the cerebrum.

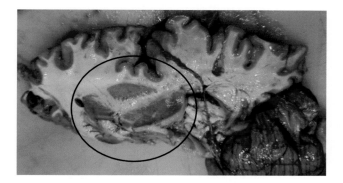

FIGURE 2.22: Deep nuclei present in the core of the cerebrum.

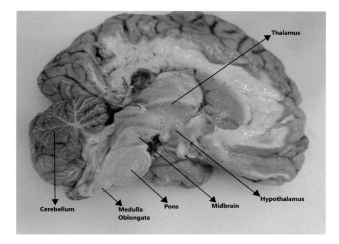

FIGURE 2.23: Mid-sagittal section of the brain showing thalamus, hypothalamus, and brainstem structures.

Functionally, the basal ganglia also include the substantia nigra, red nucleus, and subthalamus.

The fibres of the white matter converge near the subcortical masses form the internal capsule, which divides the corpus striatum into a medial caudate nucleus and a lateral lentiform nucleus. The lentiform nucleus has a paler medial part called globus pallidus and a darker outer part called the putamen.

Diencephalon

The second section of the forebrain after the cerebrum is the diencephalon which is part of the brain between the cerebrum and the brainstem. The main parts of the diencephalon include:

1. Thalamus.
2. Hypothalamus.
3. Metathalamus.
4. Epithalamus.
5. Subthalamus.
   - **Thalamus:** The thalamus is formed by two thalamic nuclei and forms the largest part of the diencephalon. The two nuclei are separated by a median slit-like third ventricle. The two thalamic nuclei are attached to each other by inter-thalamic adhesion. It forms the main relay station for all the sensory impulses like pain and touch but does not relay the special sensations. It also relays and integrates motor functions.

- **Hypothalamus:** Among all the parts of the diencephalon, the hypothalamus is the most inferiorly located portion having multiple small nuclei, of which the most conspicuous one is the mammillary bodies (Figure 2.23). This mammillary body is identified as rounded prominences on inspection of the base of the brain in the interpeduncular fossa. The hypothalamus has a stalk-like extension which forms the pituitary gland or also called hypophysis cerebri. The posterior lobe of the hypophysis cerebri is the direct neuronal continuation of the hypothalamus. Hypothalamus also regulates the body's homeostasis through its control over the autonomic nervous system and also the master endocrine gland, which is the pituitary.
- **Metathalamus:** It is mainly constituted by lateral and medial geniculate bodies and is located postero-inferior to the thalamus. The lateral geniculate body and medial geniculate body function as important relay stations for special sensory information of vision and hearing, respectively.
- **Epithalamus:** Located posterosuperior to the thalamus. It constitutes conspicuous structures called pineal gland and habenular nuclei. The pineal gland (Figure 2.24) is sometimes described as the 'third eye' or even as the 'seat of the soul'. It receives the sensory information of light and darkness and regulates the production of melatonin hormone, and holds a pivotal role in the sleep–wake cycle. It has an important role in regulating the onset of puberty. The habenular nuclei play a role in the olfactory sensation and also functionally are connected to the limbic system.
- **Subthalamus:** It is a part of the diencephalon that lies, as its name indicates, below the thalamus between the thalamus and the midbrain. It forms an important functional part of the basal ganglia and is involved in regulating and controlling motor functions.

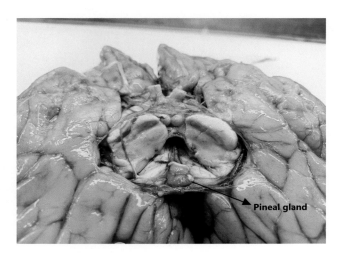

FIGURE 2.24: Inferior view of the brain after the removal of the brain stem shows the median structure of the diencephalon, which is the pineal gland.

Brainstem (Figure 2.25)

The brainstem is the posterior stalk-like part of the brain which connects the cerebrum with the spinal cord. It is the main relay station for all the sensory and motor tracts. It also has many regulatory centres which control vital systems of the human body like the respiratory and the cardiovascular system. The brainstem consists of the upper midbrain, middle pons, and lower medulla oblongata. These three parts of the brainstem are also connected to the cerebellum by the superior, middle, and inferior cerebellar peduncles. The fourth ventricle floor is made by the posterior aspect of the pons and upper medulla oblongata.

Midbrain (Figure 2.26)

The midbrain is a part of the brainstem and also the small connecting part between the forebrain and hindbrain. It is the uppermost segment of the brainstem, just above the pons. It hosts the nuclei of the third, fourth, and fifth cranial nerves, which are oculomotor, trochlear, and trigeminal cranial nerves, respectively. The midbrain also hosts the cerebral aqueduct of the Sylvius part of the ventricular system of the brain. The segment of the midbrain posterior to the cerebral aqueduct is termed the 'tectum'. The part in front of the cerebral aqueduct is divided into two equal cerebral peduncles with a central portion called the 'tegmentum'. Further anterior to it is the pigmented mass termed substantia nigra, which forms a functional part of the basal ganglia. Anterior to the substantia nigra lies the 'crus cerebri', which contains the nerve tracts and is the direct continuation of the internal capsule. The gap between these two cerebral peduncles forms the area termed the 'interpeduncular fossa'. The tectum part of the midbrain has four prominences called the colliculi. These colliculi are divided into two superior and two inferior colliculi. The

superior colliculi act as the relaying station for visual impulses, and the inferior colliculi act as the relay station for auditory impulses. The tegmentum part of the midbrain, on the other hand, hosts two large nuclei, which resemble the shape of a cigar and it is termed the red nuclei. These red nuclei help in regulating motor activity.

Pons (Figure 2.27)

The pons is the mid portion of the brainstem with the midbrain above and the medulla oblongata below. The term pons means bridge in Latin, and it is termed so due to its appearance with transverse fibres and its position between the two cerebellar hemispheres, giving it the appearance of a connecting bridge. The posterior aspect of the pons is triangular in shape, and it forms the floor of the fourth ventricle, which is present between the cerebellum and the pons. The anterior portion has a vertical median sulcus which lodges the basilar artery, and hence it is called the basilar sulcus. The pons has a small posterior region called the tegmentum and a large anterior portion which consists of descending fibres of the pyramidal tract and many pontine nuclei. The tegmentum portion holds the pontine sleep and respiratory centres, which are the vital centres. The respiratory centres regulate respiratory movements. The pons hosts the nuclei for the sixth, seventh, and eighth cranial nerves, which are abducens, facial and vestibulocochlear nerves, respectively.

Medulla oblongata (Figure 2.28)

The medulla oblongata is the lower region of the brainstem, below the pons. It continues below the spinal cord near the foramen magnum. The posterior aspect of the medulla oblongata forms the lower floor of the fourth ventricle. The anterior aspect of the medulla has two pyramidal-shaped elevations

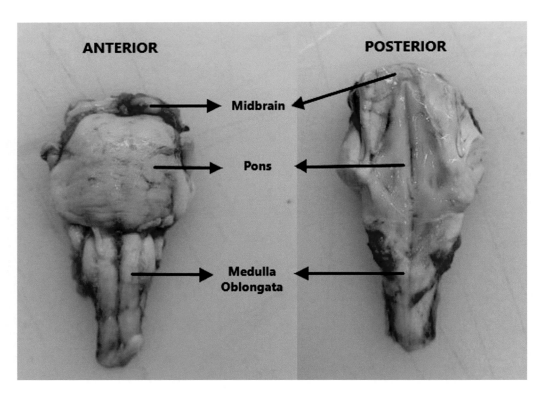

FIGURE 2.25: Anterior and posterior view of the brainstem shows the three structures forming the brainstem, which include the midbrain, pons, and medulla oblongata.

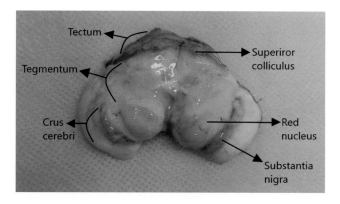

FIGURE 2.26: Section of the midbrain at the level of the superior colliculus shows the tectum, tegmentum, and the crus cerebri. The other prominent structures identified in the section include the superior colliculus, red nucleus, and substantia nigra.

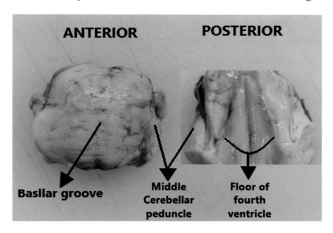

FIGURE 2.27: Anterior and posterior view of the pons shows the anterior median basilar groove, the middle cerebellar peduncle, and the posterior view shows the floor of the fourth ventricle.

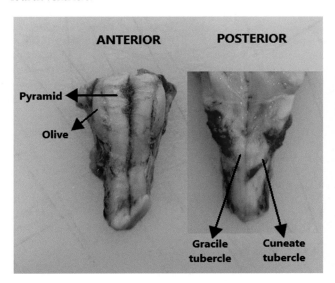

FIGURE 2.28: Anterior and posterior view of the medulla oblongata shows the pyramid and olive elevation on the anterior view, gracile tubercle, and cuneate tubercle on the posterior view.

called the pyramids, which mainly contain the corticospinal tracts. To the lateral aspects of these pyramids, there are elevations called the olives, which contain the olivary nuclei. The posterior aspect in the lower part medulla has four elevations, two on either side of the midline, which are called tubercles. The median two tubercles are the gracile tubercles, and the lateral tubercles are the cuneate tubercles. Medulla hosts most of the vital centres which regulate important functions like heart rate, breathing, and deglutition. It also regulates many reflexes by acting as the autonomic centre and also controls a few of the protective reflexes like coughing and sneezing. The medulla also hosts the nuclei for the ninth, tenth, eleventh, and twelfth nerves, which are the glossopharyngeal, vagus, accessory, and hypoglossal nerves, respectively.

Cerebellum (Figures 2.29 and 2.30)

The cerebellum, also called the little brain, is located in the posterior cranial fossa's infra-tentorial aspect. It is positioned posterior to the pons and medulla, with the diamond-shaped fourth ventricle intervening between these structures. The cerebellum consists of two cerebellar hemispheres with a median stalk called the vermis (called so due to its worm-like appearance), which connects the two cerebellar hemispheres. The cerebellum is connected to the midbrain, pons, and medulla by the superior, middle, and inferior cerebellar peduncles, respectively. The cerebellar surface has numerous slits called fissures and between these fissures there are folds of the cerebellum called folia (called so as they resemble leaves). The cerebellum regulates and controls motor activities, equilibrium, muscle tone, posture, proprioception, and coordinated movements. The cerebellum in each of its hemispheres hosts four nuclei, namely:

1. Dentate nucleus.
2. Emboliform nucleus.
3. Fastigial nucleus.
4. Globose nucleus.

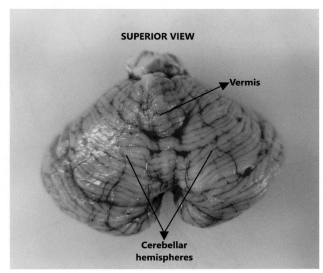

FIGURE 2.29: Superior view of the cerebellum shows the vermis and the two cerebellar hemispheres.

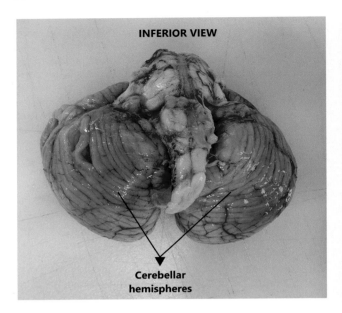

FIGURE 2.30: Superior view of the cerebellum shows two cerebellar hemispheres.

CT of the brain (Figures 2.31 and 2.32)

A brain CT examination is used to identify the anatomy and important landmarks of the brain and involves locating a few identifiable fissures which separate different lobes of the brain. The Sylvian fissure is an easily identifiable fissure separating the frontal and the temporal lobe, which is even appreciable on the axial sections. The central sulcus, which separates the frontal lobe from the parietal lobe, is usually less appreciable

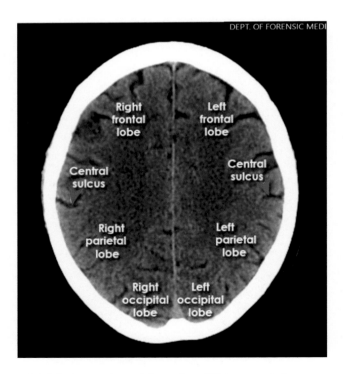

FIGURE 2.31: An axial section CT image of the upper level of the brain showing various regions of the brain, which include bilateral frontal, parietal, and occipital lobes/regions.

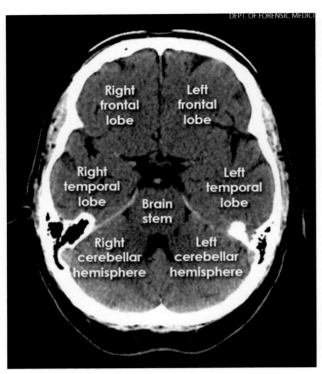

FIGURE 2.32: An axial section CT image of the lower level of the brain showing various regions of the brain, which include bilateral frontal, temporal, and occipital lobes/regions.

in the axial section of CT. However, it lies just posterior to the anterior limit of the lateral ventricle when the CT image is obtained parallel to the canthomeatal line. The parieto-occipital sulcus, which is appreciable in the medial surface of the cerebral hemisphere, can also be appreciated with difficulty at the level of the lateral ventricles on the mid-sagittal section. With CT scans, identification of anatomical landmarks, like the sulcus, are difficult; hence in practice, based on the approximate position of the lesion or finding, the term 'region' is used, for example, frontal region, parietal region, temporal region and occipital region. If the particular finding involves more than one region then terms like temporoparietal region or parieto-occipital region are used, combining the terms of the two regions.

Trauma to the head

Head Injury

Head injury is a broad term that describes a variety of injuries/damages that occur to the scalp, skull, brain, underlying tissue, and/or blood vessels in the head due to an external force. The term traumatic brain injury (TBI) is sometimes used as a synonym for the term head injury, but the actual meaning of traumatic brain injury does not represent the entire spectrum of head injury. The Brain Injury Association of America (2011) defines TBI as 'an alteration in brain function, or other evidence of brain pathology, caused by an external force'. This definition clearly shows that the term traumatic brain injury represents that part of the spectrum which involves damage to the brain and resultant dysfunction.

Head injuries can be classified in multiple different ways based on the below parameters:

Based on the mechanism causing the head injury, it is classified into:

- **Impact injuries:** The resultant injuries are due to head contact with an object, and are due to the local effects of contact with the head.
- **Acceleration/deceleration injuries:** These injuries occur when an unrestricted and sudden head movement causes compressive, tensile, and shear strains.

Based on the intact nature of the dura mater, head injuries are classified into:

- **Closed head injury:** This is a head injury where the dura mater remains intact, even when there is a skull fracture.
- **Open head injury:** This is a head injury in which the object causing the head injury is piercing the skull as well as breaching the underlying dura mater. This type of injury is referred to as a penetrating head injury.

Based on the morphology of the injury, it is classified into:

- **Scalp injury:** The scalp, being the outermost layer, is one of the common structures of the head to be injured. The injury to the scalp could be in the form of an abrasion, contusion or laceration.
- **Fractures of the skull:** This includes a variety of fractures like fissure fracture, comminuted fracture, depressed comminuted fracture, gutter fracture, pond fracture, hinge fracture, diastatic fracture, ring fracture, etc.
- **Contusion of the brain:** These injuries are to the part of the brain called the parenchyma; if the brain retains its shape though with vascular or parenchymal injury, it is a cerebral contusion, but if the disrupting force is large enough to cause the brain to lose its shape it is termed brain laceration.
- **Intracranial haemorrhages:** These are haemorrhages occurring in the parenchyma or the layers of the meninges, which also sometimes organize into haematomas. These include extradural haemorrhage, subdural haemorrhage, subarachnoid haemorrhage, and parenchymal haemorrhage.

Traumatic brain injury

During autopsy in cases of TBI, one of the fundamental duties of the autopsy surgeon is to assess the injury biomechanics. The primary impact surface or object should be matched with the injury pattern on the scalp. Identify the nature of the striking object, possible velocity, weight, contact surface, any projecting part, any specific pattern of surface, a possible position of the head, if the head was supported or freely mobile, etc. Consideration of all these factors helps predict the possible pattern of injury seen over the scalp, brain, and fracture of the skull. The autopsy surgeon should consider the overall picture in a case by understanding possible impact forces being linear or an acceleration/deceleration force. In contrast to the linear impacting forces, which cause the majority of localized injuries, acceleration/deceleration forces, though they cause localized scalp, meninges, and brain injuries, also produce a generalized injury to the entire head. The autopsy surgeon should always consider the dynamic nature of any injury, and most invariably involve a component of acceleration/deceleration forces

throwing the entire head separate from the impact site at equal risk of sustaining an injury. Biomechanics is the 'study of tissue failure (manifest as injury) when exposed to a given loading event, after which it ceases, either structurally or functionally, to perform normally'. This injury to the head may occur due to a direct crushing effect by impacting force or due to the displacement/deformation of the intracranial contents. This displacement/deformation of the intracranial contents occurs due to the differential motion between the skull/dura mater and the brain. This differential motion is due to the fact that the brain lags behind the skull/dura mater during acceleration of the head due to inertial or impulsive phenomenon. The injury to the head and intracranial contents also depends on the type of impacting force, like non-missile or missile, closed, or penetrating. In closed and non-missile injuries, usually, the impacting force causes acceleration/deceleration and also momentum, rotational, and linear forces. In cases of penetrating and missile injuries, a high kinetic energy but a low momentum is transmitted to the head. All these types of impact forces produce contact injuries like scalp laceration, skull fracture, intracranial haemorrhages, or brain contusion/laceration at the point of contact. However, the absence of any contact injury does not imply the absence of a head injury. In cases where the head is free to move, or the nature of impact force produces more acceleration/deceleration or rotational force on the head, this causes injury to the neurons of the brain, which sometimes could be microscopic without any gross changes. The combination of linear and angular force, usually termed curvilinear motion is the most common type of impacting force observed in practical situations. The cerebral hemispheres, in comparison with the brainstem, are more vulnerable to injury with curvilinear motion. Head injuries due to the impacting force can manifest as:

Primary outcome:

- Scalp injuries.
- Skull injuries.
- Intracranial haemorrhages/haematomas.
- Brain parenchymal injuries.
- Miscellaneous injuries.

Secondary outcome:

- Vascular injury.
- Cerebral oedema.
- Cerebral ischaemia.
- Herniation of the brain.
- Seizures.
- Hydrocephalus.

Assessment in cases of head injury

Head injury cases have a wide spectrum of appearances and manifestations. The external appearance and fatality do not always coincide and can be deceptive; hence complete assessment in every case is essential. Cases of head injury need the following assessments:

1. To confirm the presence of a head injury.
2. Approximate time of occurrence.
3. The possible mechanism causing head injury.
4. Nature of the injury and its distribution.
5. Pre-existing pathologies which could have an effect on the present finding.

6. The possible effect of post-mortem changes on the findings, especially the brain.
7. Possible artefacts which could mimic head injury, like an intracranial bleed.

Scalp injuries

It is the outer covering of the skull, protecting the skull and its contents from external forces mainly by dampening/reducing the transmission of force onto the brain and other vital structures. The scalp has its limit when the external force is beyond the limit of elasticity of the scalp, resulting in injury to the scalp. The scalp has five different layers, with each layer having its own limit of stretchability or elasticity. The layers are:

1. **Skin layer:** It consists of thick skin with dense hair follicles, sweat glands, and sebaceous glands.
2. **Subcutaneous tissue layer:** This layer is made of dense fibrous tissue, which forms fibrous septa which hold the skin layer and the aponeurotic layer firmly together. These outer three layers are firmly adherent to each other and cannot be separated and are together referred to as the 'surgical layers of the scalp'.
3. **Aponeurotic layer/galea aponeurotic:** It is the layer formed by the occipitofrontalis muscle along with the sheet of its aponeurotic layer. This layer is mainly responsible for the wrinkling of the forehead and the raising of the eyebrows.
4. **Loose areolar tissue layer:** This is the layer made of loose areolar tissue and is the layer on which the surgical layer moves under pressure. It is also considered the 'dangerous layer of the scalp' as blood or pus can easily accumulate in this layer. In blunt trauma to the scalp, haemorrhage and haematoma easily occur in this layer. It is the layer of scalp reflection in the autopsy (Figure 2.33).
5. **Pericranium layer:** It is the periosteal layer of the bones of the skull vault and is loosely attached over the bone and firmly attached near the sutures.

Scalp haematoma/contusion

The scalp is the outer layer of protection after head impact and protects underlying vital structures by absorbing, dispersing, and dampening some of the effects of trauma. The scalp is vascular, and it bleeds profusely after injury; if the skin is intact it results in scalp haematoma/contusion and if the overlying skin breaks causing a laceration, it results in profuse external bleeding.

A contusion or haematoma of the scalp can occur in different layers based on the characteristic of the external force and multiple external factors causing the injury. The most commonly encountered scalp contusion types are:

1. Subcutaneous haematoma.
2. Subgaleal haematoma.
3. Cephalhaematoma.

Subcutaneous haematoma: (Figure 2.34) Is a scalp haemorrhage occurring within the surgical layer of the scalp, in the subcutaneous layer. This is appreciated as a swelling of the scalp with a haemorrhage and it is difficult to differentiate the layer of the haemorrhage.

Subgaleal haematoma: (Figures 2.35 and 2.36) Is a haemorrhage which occurs below the aponeurotic layer of the scalp. This is the loose areolar tissue layer which lies below the tight surgical layer of the scalp. This haemorrhage is well appreciated in the CT scan by a bulge and haemorrhage in the layer of the scalp, and it crosses the sutures as it is in the layer that is not restricted by sutural lines. This haemorrhage/haematoma

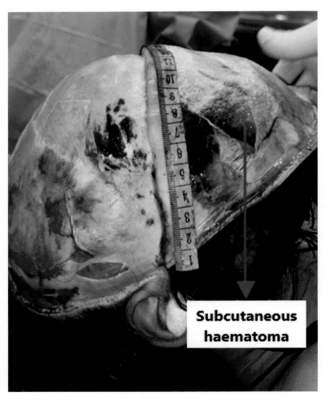

FIGURE 2.34: Blunt trauma to the head sustained by fall, causing haematoma in the subcutaneous layer of the scalp. On reflection of the scalp, the haematoma is appreciated in the surgeon's layer in the scalp reflected.

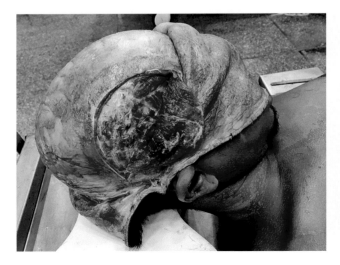

FIGURE 2.33: Layers of the scalp seen on dissection, red arrow showing separation of the scalp at loose areolar tissue layer on scalp reflection. Blue star shows temporalis muscle.

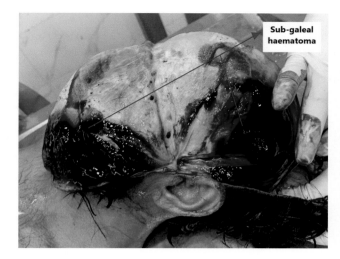

FIGURE 2.35: Subgaleal haematoma seen on reflection of the scalp, which is diffused and in the layer of scalp reflection during autopsy.

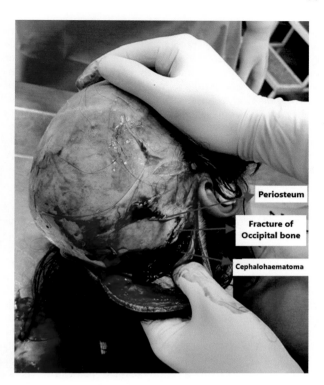

FIGURE 2.37: Cephalohaematoma is seen on removing the periosteal layer of the scalp; underlying fracture of the occipital bone is seen.

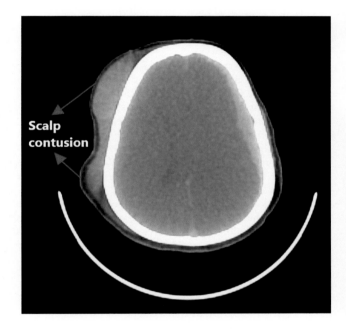

FIGURE 2.36: CT scan of the axial section shows a scalp contusion over the right frontoparietal region. The layer of scalp haemorrhage is not well appreciated in CT.

is well appreciated in autopsy as it is in the layer of reflection of the scalp where the haemorrhage is seen clearly.

Cephalohaematoma: (Figures 2.37 and 2.38) Is a scalp haemorrhage that occurs in the periosteal layer of the scalp and is usually associated with fractures of the underlying bone. It is seen in cases with instrumental deliveries. This haemorrhage usually does not cross the sutural lines due to the tight binding of fibrous tissue in the sutures.

Skull injuries

Skull fractures are an important indicator of severe craniocerebral trauma or head injury. Though they are an important indicator, in about 20% of cases of severe head injury, no

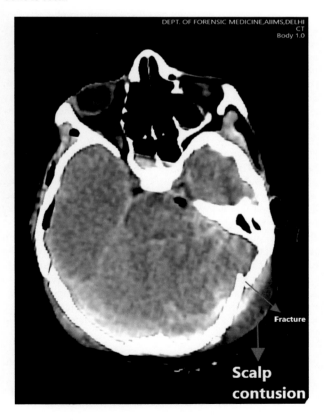

FIGURE 2.38: CT scan of the axial section shows cephalohaematoma as scalp contusion with difficulty in appreciating the layer of haemorrhage, underlying bone fracture is well appreciated.

fractures may be seen. Hence skull fractures, though, helpful in predicting severe head trauma are not a necessity to conclude fatal head trauma cases. Fractures of the skull can also occur in mild head injury cases; hence they are also not always predictive of severe head injury. Fractures are usually appreciated with radiological techniques and a CT scan in a bone window along with 3D surface-shaded volume rendering images help to obtain a complete picture of the fracture, including the shape and direction of the fracture. Small fissure fractures, especially in the base of the skull, may be difficult to identify in traditional autopsies.

Biomechanics of skull fracture

Skull fractures are the result of different external forces affecting the skull, causing disruption of its bony component. The skull bone is made of collagen fibres which are responsible for its strength, elasticity, and flexibility. The bone also consists of hydroxyapatite crystals which are the inorganic components, and they provide hardness, rigidity, and strength to the bone along with the ability of brittleness on compression. The major component of the bone is the organic element made of calcium and phosphate, along with collagen; this constitutes approximately 60–70% of the bone tissue. Water is the second most abundant component constituting approximately 25–30% of the total bone tissue weight.

Bone is known to be a highly adaptive connective tissue, which is influenced by multiple factors like heavy use, disuse, external forces, and even immobilization. Bone is a connective tissue which adapts to the demand placed on it and responds to the stress it is subjected to; for example, the same bone tissue differs in its internal architecture based on the physical activity of an individual like a sportsperson and a sedentary worker. Wolff's law which was proposed by a German anatomist and surgeon Julius Wolff in the 19th century, explains this phenomenon according to which 'Each change in the form and function of a bone or only its function is followed by certain definitive changes in its internal architecture, and secondary changes equally definitive in its external compliance, in accordance to the mathematics law'.

One should know that individual skulls will have a different range of tolerance to head injuries depending on multiple factors like skull thickness, age and gender, physical activity, and nutritional state of the individual, as all of these, along with many other factors, affect the architecture of the bone. The external forces involved in impact also play a major role, including factors like the duration of application of the force, the angle, area of distribution, direction, etc. Depending on the external force applied and the internal architecture of the bone to withstand the stress along with its elastic properties, the bone first absorbs the external energy exerted upon it up to a point called its elastic limit. After crossing this point, microbreaks in the internal architecture of the bone are observed, which is called the deformation point. This deformation is of two types:

1. **Plastic deformation:** This is where there is a permanent change in the shape of the bone.
2. **Elastic deformation:** This is where the bone regains its original shape when the external deforming force is removed.

The external deforming force applied upon the skull bone has generally termed the load or strain. This external force, as discussed above, has a number of factors based on which it determines the outcome on the bone; velocity/speed is one important factor based on which the load or strain is classified as:

1. **Slow load:** This includes cases of external deforming forces like road traffic accidents, assault, falls from a height, etc. The end result of such an external force on the skull bone could be either the bone returning to its original shape after the external force is removed (elastic deformation), permanent deformity in its shape (plastic deformation), or fracture.
2. **Rapid load:** This type of external deforming force is seen in ballistic injuries, which include firearm injuries, explosive injuries, etc. The bone, in such cases, acts more rigid and firm and also offers greater tolerance, finally resulting in shattering or fracture.

The difference in outcome in both types of loading forces is due to the time factor. In slow-loading forces, bone is under stress for a longer time and is subjected to elastic and plastic phases prior to failure. In cases of rapid-loading forces, bone can resist up to a certain point and beyond that, shatters or fractures, and there is negligible or no plastic deformation. Bone is a connective tissue due to its internal architecture and composition; it is a poor absorber of shock waves and rapid loads in comparison to surrounding tissue.

The specific pattern of fracture is produced by a specific type of external force which includes the direction of force, area transmitting the force and velocity of the external force. The pattern of fracture also depends on the specific region of the skull coming in contact with external force, the area of the surface, and whether the skull was free moving or supported when it was struck by an external force. The localized application of a certain amount of force is more dangerous than the same force applied over a larger area. The curve part of the bone, though based on internal architecture, is stronger than the flat surfaces of the skull; still, injuries in the curved regions are more serious than the flat regions as the curved regions have less contact area and more external force gets transmitted to this smaller area. Shape, size, weight, surface, and kinetic energy of the object transmitting the external force on the skull also determines the pattern of fracture that is possible. The overall practical picture which is to be considered in a case is, however, a dynamic one with usually moving head or object or both; hence a static theoretical explanation and expectation of fracture pattern in a scenario may sometimes be wrong or lead to misinterpretation. Even reproducing static models of the possible scenario may also not explain the complete picture in a case.

Fissure fracture (Figures 2.39 and 2.40)

It is a full-thickness fracture of the skull involving both the outer and inner table of the skull with no displacement. It is commonly seen over the calvaria but also seen over the base of the skull and other parts. This usually accounts for about 70 % of the fractures reported.

Mechanism: Fissure fractures are produced by:

1. Low external force impacts.
2. A force that is transmitted to the skull over a broad area.
3. Blows to a free-moving head have a higher chance of receiving a fissure fracture than when it is supported against a surface.

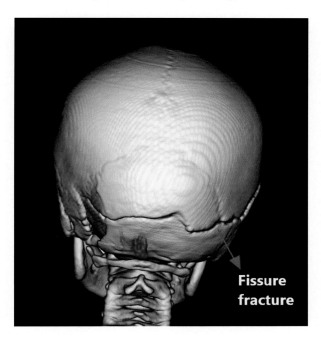

FIGURE 2.39: Volume rendering CT image showing fissure fracture involving the right temporal-occipital bone. Here the fracture line is seen crossing the lambdoid suture. The gaping of the fracture line is seen to reduce from right to left and tapers before ending near the left lambdoid suture.

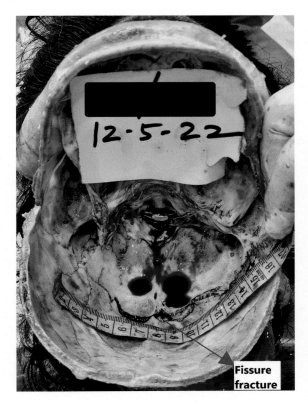

FIGURE 2.40: Fissure fracture in the same case seen on opening the skull during the autopsy, the fracture line is seen extending from the right temporal bone and crossing the right lambdoid suture traverses the occipital bone to end at the left lambdoid suture. The thickness of the gaping fracture is seen to decrease as it ends over the left side of the occipital bone.

4. When a blow strikes the skull, and if it is at an angle rather than perpendicular to the surface.

Fissure fractures usually end in the sutures or in other fracture lines, but if the force is sufficient enough, they can continue beyond the sutures or even as a diastatic fracture along the sutures. They are usually thicker with a little more gaping at the point of impact, and as the fracture line continues, it becomes thinner; this also helps in identifying the possible position of the impact. They also occur as terminal fractures extending from a comminuted or depressed fracture as the force reduces from the centre to the periphery.

Diastatic fracture (Figures 2.41 and 2.42)
This is a fracture of the skull involving sutures of the skull causing their widening. Sutures are fibrous joints which connect the bones of the skull.

Mechanism: This type of fracture is more common among infants and young people as their sutures are not yet fused, but they are also seen in adults. They can occur due to a fissure fracture entering the suture and extending along the suture. A diastatic fracture involving only the suture without any surrounding fracture may be difficult to identify in a CT scan alone, and careful inspection is needed to differentiate non-fusion from diastatic fracture.

Comminuted fracture (Figures 2.43–2.47)
This is a fracture in which the skull bone is broken into three or more fragments or pieces. The fracture is similar to a fissure fracture where both the outer and inner tables are fractured along with multiple fragments; the underlying dura mater may or may not be involved.

Mechanism: The head is struck or strikes a broad flat surface, especially when it is supported rather than free moving; the part of the skull coming in contact with the surface flattens to

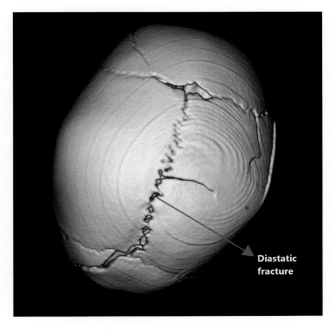

FIGURE 2.41: Volume rendering CT image of skull showing diastatic fracture involving the sagittal suture and partly the coronal suture and lambdoid suture. The fracture line extends into the occipital bone as a fissure fracture, and also few fissure fractures are seen over the right parietal bone and frontal bone.

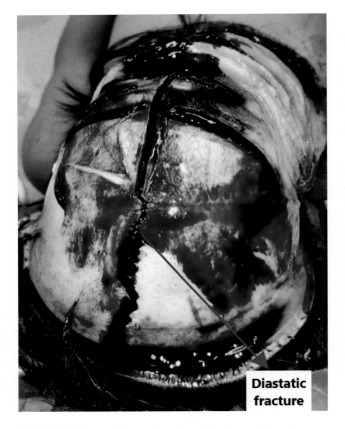

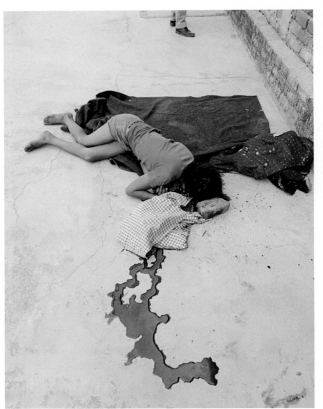

FIGURE 2.42: A fissure fracture of the frontal bone is causing a diastatic fracture involving the sagittal suture; the primary impact can be identified by seeing the contusion over the scalp present in the reflected flap of the frontal region.

FIGURE 2.43: A case of a 35-year-old male who was assaulted on the head with a brick when he was sleeping on the floor. Here the impacting surface of the brick is broad and flat, and the velocity involved is low. The head of the deceased was supported by the hard floor; hence the likely fracture pattern to occur in this case is comminuted fracture.

conform to the shape of the impacting surface. This results in plastic deformation when the external impacting force crosses the elastic limit. Berryman and Symes described a four-stage mechanism for this fracture:

1. A low-velocity impact by a flat surface causes initial in-bending at the point of contact and peripheral out-bending; if the contact area is small, the point of impact skull bone may get displaced inwards, causing a depressed comminuted fracture.
2. Radiating fractures start at the place of out-bending at one or multiple places which extend inwards towards the impact site or outwards.
3. Radiating fractures usually stop when they reach a skull suture.
4. Concentric fractures may form perpendicular to the radiating fractures.

This theory of Berryman and Symes has been accepted and proved by many forensic pathologists' experiments; however, a Kroman et al. study gave a contradictory result to this theory. Their experiment showed that the fractures started at the point of impact and radiated peripherally instead of coming from periphery to centre.

Depressed comminuted fracture
(Figures 2.48–2.53)

Depressed comminuted skull fractures are due to a more focal impact, and such fracture patterns have a higher

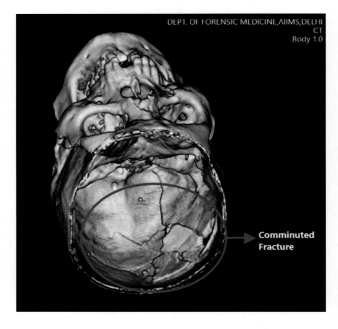

FIGURE 2.44: Volume rendering CT image of the skull in the above case showing comminuted fracture over the occipital and right temporal region.

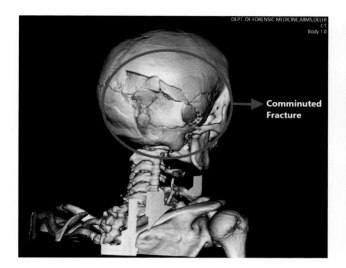

FIGURE 2.45:   Volume rendering CT image of the skull in the above case showing comminuted fracture over the occipital and right temporal region.

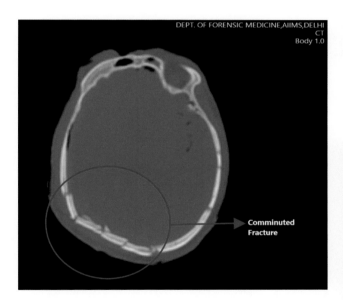

FIGURE 2.46:   Axial section CT image of the skull in the above case showing comminuted fracture over the occipital and right temporal region.

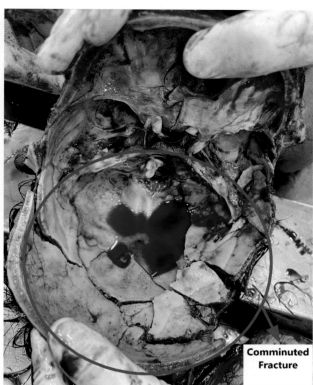

FIGURE 2.47:   Autopsy showing comminuted fracture over the occipital and right temporal region in the same case.

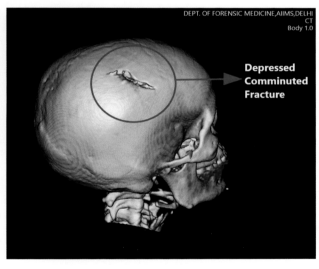

FIGURE 2.48:   Volume rendering CT image of the skull showing depressed comminuted fracture of the right parietal bone.

likelihood of causing intracranial injury than non-depressed fractures. These fracture patterns usually involve the bone fragment or pieces getting displaced inwards at the point of contact with the impacting force. This inward-displaced fragment has the probability of causing more brain injury than non-depressed similar fractures. When the object used to cause the injury makes a fracture whose dimensions are similar and the overall fracture pattern resembles the object used for causing the injury, it is called a 'fracture ala signature' or 'signature fracture'.

Hinge fracture
This is a type of fracture involving the base of the skull, where it is separated into two halves. This is commonly referred to as

motorcyclist fracture, as it is common among motorcyclists in road traffic accidents. There are three types of hinge fracture (Figure 2.54):

1. Type I (posterior transverse): (Figure 2.55) It is coronal in position extending from one middle cranial fossa to the other of the base of the skull through the sella turcica.

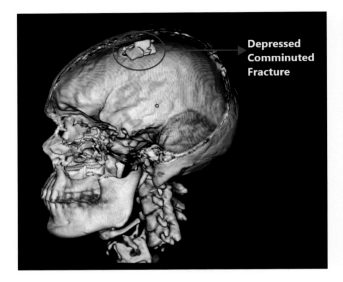

FIGURE 2.49: Volume rendering CT image of the skull showing depressed comminuted fracture of the right parietal bone with multiple bone fragments.

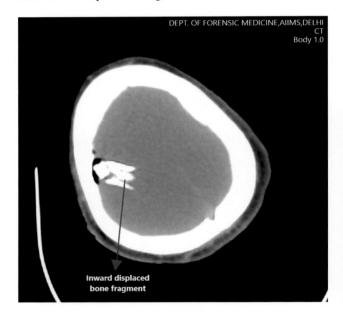

FIGURE 2.50: Axial CT image of skull showing the inward displaced bony fragment in the depressed comminuted fracture.

2. Type II (lateral frontal diagonal): Extends from the anterior cranial fossa to the opposite side, middle, or posterior cranial fossa of the base of the skull passing through the sella turcica.

3. Type III (anterior transverse): It is coronal in position, usually extending from the junction or one middle/anterior cranial fossa to the other but not through the sella turcica.

Mechanism: There are two possible mechanisms for hinge fracture-

1. Heavy impact on the side or top of the head extending into the base of the skull, separating into two halves.

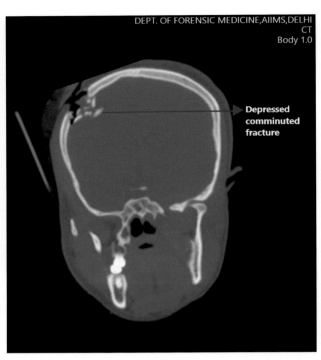

FIGURE 2.51: Coronal section CT image of a skull in the bone window showing the depressed comminuted fracture of the right parietal bone with inward displaced bone fragments.

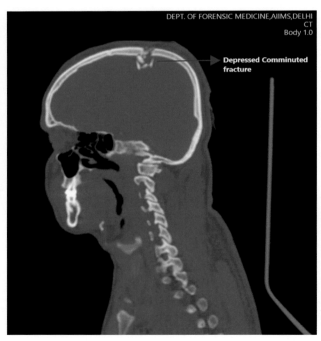

FIGURE 2.52: Sagittal section CT image of a skull in the bone window showing the depressed comminuted fracture of the right parietal bone with inward displaced bone fragments.

2. Impact on the chin or jaw, which transmits the impact force to the mandibular fossa causing fracture of the base of the skull. This mechanism usually shows injury like a contusion, abrasion, laceration, or fracture of the mandible (Figure 2.56), which is the primary impact point.

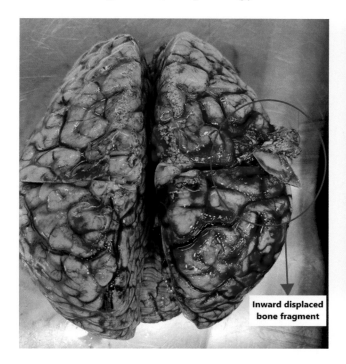

FIGURE 2.53: Autopsy in the above case showed a fragment of bone which was displaced inwards due to a depressed comminuted fracture attached to the brain over the right parietal region.

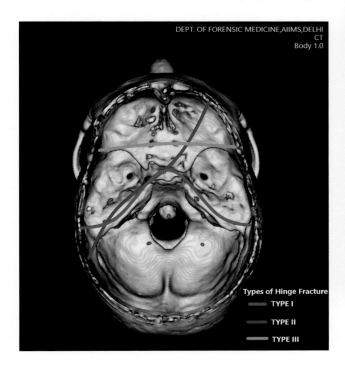

FIGURE 2.54: Three types of hinge fractures over the base of the skull. Type I (Red), Type II (Blue), and Type III (Green) hinge fractures.

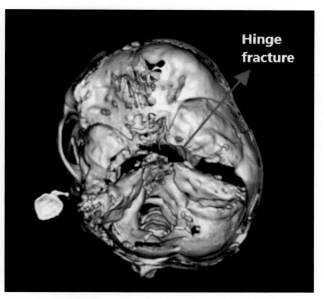

FIGURE 2.55: Volume rendering CT image showing Type I hinge fracture seen placed coronally extending from one middle cranial fossa to the other running through the sella turcica.

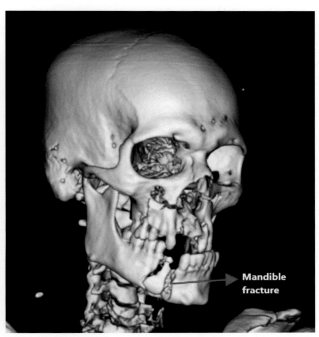

FIGURE 2.56: Volume rendering CT image showing mandible fracture in the above case, which was the primary point of impact finally causing the hinge fracture substantiating the second mechanism for the hinge fracture.

Fractures of the skull by firearm/gunshot injury

Firearm injuries by high-velocity bullets produce a perforating injury due to high kinetic energy; this includes entry and exit wounds from the bullet. In cases of low-velocity bullets, usually, a penetrating injury is produced; this involves an entry wound along with the projectile/bullet lodged in the opposite side skull bone or soft tissue; or in the brain parenchyma or other tissues after internal ricocheting. The entry wounds of the firearm are usually smaller than the exit wounds, with some exceptions like shored exit wounds or fragmentation of the projectiles.

Entry wound

The entry wound is usually round or ovoid in shape, with some exceptions like loose contact shots causing stellate entry wounds. The entry wound in the cranial bone, due to its architecture of outer and inner tables, produces two fractures. The fracture on the outer table is usually smaller than the fracture on the inner table, causing a cone-shaped appearance which is termed internal beveling (Figure 2.57). Along with the circular or ovoid bone defect at the entry, many fissure fractures radiate from the defect and rarely other fractures far from the defect may also be appreciated (Figure 2.58). There is the inward displacement of the bone fragments into the cranial vault (Figure 2.59) along the direction of entry of the projectile along with haemorrhage (Figure 2.60) and sometimes blackening or dispersion of brain parenchyma.

Exit wound

When the gunshot has high velocity, the projectile leaves the cranial vault through an exit wound which, again, due to the architecture of the cranial bone, has an inner and outer table. This exit wound involves two fractures, one each of the inner and outer tables (Figure 2.61). The inner table fracture is small, and the outer table fracture is bigger, giving a conical shape called external beveling (Figure 2.62). Sometimes the exit wound is more irregular in comparison with the entry wound. The bleeding is more compared with the entry wound, and also, the expulsion of brain parenchyma is sometimes appreciated.

Cerebral oedema

Cerebral oedema following a head injury can occur due to the following mechanisms:

1. Vascular engorgement in the brain passively due to venous obstruction or actively due to arterial dilatation.
2. The increased amount of water content in the brain cells.

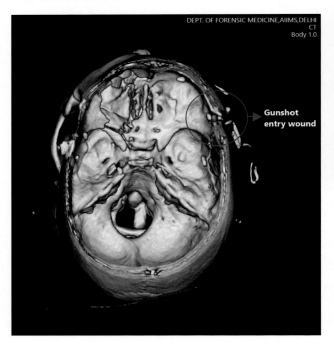

FIGURE 2.57: Volume rendering CT image of skull showing gunshot entry wound causing a cone-shaped defect with a small fracture in the outer table and a bigger fracture in an inner table called internal beveling.

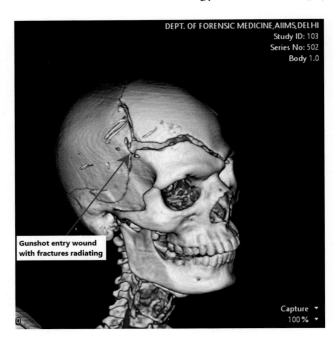

FIGURE 2.58: Volume rendering CT image of skull showing gunshot entry wound with a defect from which multiple fractures are radiating.

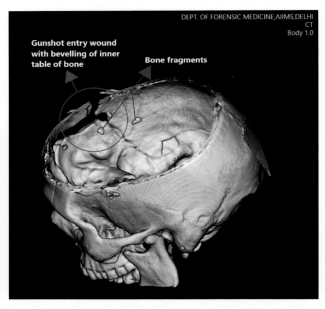

FIGURE 2.59: Volume rendering CT image of skull showing gunshot entry wound with bone fragments displaced inwards.

These mechanisms can cause cerebral oedema rapidly after the trauma or in a delayed manner, depending on the nature of the impacting force and the structures affected by the trauma. As cerebral oedema sets in the brain, the white matter becomes softer than normal, and also, the sharp distinction which exits between the grey matter and white matter becomes obscured. Severe cerebral oedema causes flattening of the gyri and narrowing of the sulcus. In cases where oedema occurs due to the breakdown of the blood–brain barrier causing vasogenic oedema with extravasation of protein-rich fluid, this gross examination shows some greenish discolouration of the white matter. Microscopic examination of swelling of pericapillary

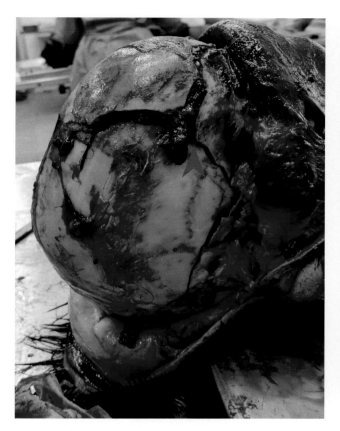

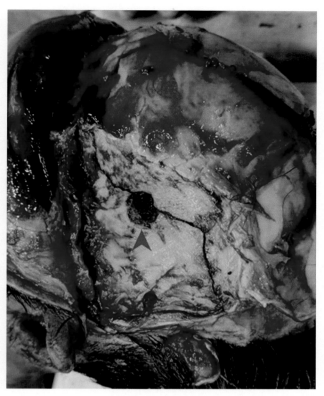

FIGURE 2.60: Autopsy image of skull showing gunshot entry wound with haemorrhage and multiple fractures radiating from the bullet entry defect.

FIGURE 2.62: Autopsy image of a skull with an exit wound in the left temporal region; the outer table fracture is bigger than the inner table fracture, causing a cone-shaped defect called external beveling. Multiple fracture lines are seen radiating from the defect.

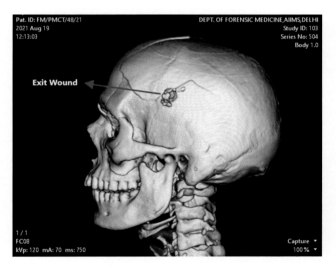

FIGURE 2.61: Volume rendering CT image of skull showing gunshot exit wound over the left temporal region.

astrocytic foot processes and oligodendroglial cytoplasm along with fluid extravasated in the extracellular space of white matter. In cases where there is trauma or haemorrhage to one cerebral hemisphere, there is unilateral cerebral oedema causing the shift of the midline and asymmetry. The intracranial pressure, when it increases, creates a pressure difference across the foramen magnum, and the vermis of the cerebellum gets displaced distally, causing herniation through the foramen

magnum called the cerebellar coning or herniation of the cerebellar tonsils called as tonsillar herniation. The increased intracranial pressure can also cause herniation of other parts of the brain like subfalcine herniation, uncal herniation, transtentorial herniation, etc.

Intracranial haemorrhages/haematomas
Extradural haemorrhage

Epidural (extradural) haemorrhage occurs between the inner table of the skull bone and the dura mater of the meninges. This is a potential space, and hence any collection to happen in this space needs more pressure than an existing space to have a haemorrhage or haematoma; hence extradural haemorrhage is mostly arterial in origin. Extradural haemorrhage usually occurs due to direct trauma to the skull, which damages the blood vessels causing the haemorrhage. As it is mostly arterial in origin, the most common artery injured is the middle meningeal artery (90% of cases) and in 10% of cases it is venous in origin due to damage to the dural venous sinuses. Extradural haemorrhages are less common in children and the elderly; it is more common in adults. The lucid interval is a period of consciousness between the initial prior loss of consciousness due to trauma and later loss of consciousness due to coma or neurological deficit following head trauma.

Extradural haemorrhages appear as a biconvex haematoma which causes flattening of the adjacent brain parenchyma and is usually adjacent to the fracture of the skull. Extradural haemorrhages are mostly supra-tentorial in location, and squamous temporal bone is the commonest site of occurrence.

CT findings

Extradural haemorrhages appear as a biconvex haematoma (Figures 2.63 and 2.64) with an adjacent fracture of the skull. 'Swirl sign' is a CT finding in the extradural haemorrhage showing a small hypodense region within the hyperdense haematoma; this indicates the area of a fresh bleed within the haematoma.

Subdural haemorrhage (SDH)

Subdural haemorrhage/haematoma is an intracranial haemorrhage where blood accumulates in the meninges between the dura mater and the arachnoid layer (Figures 2.65–2.70). It is one of the most common haemorrhages encountered in trauma cases. SDH can occur due to direct trauma to the head and also non-impact injuries. SDH is usually venous in origin and occurs due to the rupture or tear of the bridging veins, which cross the subdural space to enter the venous sinuses. This tear of the bridging veins can occur due to local blunt trauma force or acceleration/deceleration forces, shear strain due to rotational forces caused by brain rotation (Figures 2.66–2.69). Rarely cases of spontaneous arterial SDH have been seen to occur due to aneurysm rupture (Figure 2.70), tumours, or bleeding disorders. SDH can occur in all ranges of ages, from infancy to the elderly.

CT findings

Subdural haemorrhage is a crescent-shaped haemorrhage placed between the meningeal layers, and it displaces the brain medially (Figure 2.65). They usually are not restricted to sutural lines, crossing them but restricted by the venous sinuses, which they do not cross. Solid haematoma is appreciated in CT as a hyperdense crescent-shaped haemorrhage. A swirl sign may be seen for fresh bleeding inside the haematoma.

Subarachnoid haemorrhage (SAH)

Subarachnoid haemorrhage is the most common trauma-related intracranial haemorrhage (Figures 2.71–2.73). SAH also occurs in non-traumatic cases due to aneurysm rupture. Minor SAHs may be difficult to differentiate from artefacts of autopsy due to the rupture of blood vessels in the subarachnoid space. SAH, after occurring at the place of blood vessel damage, also spreads to other places; it appears to be more prominent at the leak site than at the place where it has spread. In cases of non-traumatic SAH, the circle of Willis is to be examined in detail to identify the leak site. The most common place of an aneurysm that ruptures is the junction between the anterior communicating artery and the anterior cerebral artery. In most cases of non-traumatic SAH, there is a history of headaches which is usually described as the 'worst headache of their life' or thunderclap headache.

CT findings

In cases of aneurysm rupture, the basal cistern is usually filled with blood, but the SAH depends on the site of rupture of the aneurysm. In cases of traumatic SAH, it is less widely

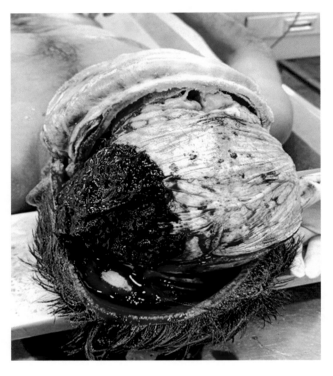

FIGURE 2.63: EDH present over left parietal and occipital region seen on removing skull vault.

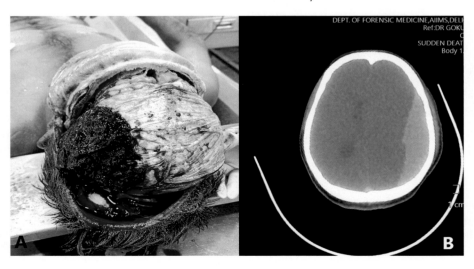

FIGURE 2.64: EDH present over left parietal and occipital region in PMCT axial section.

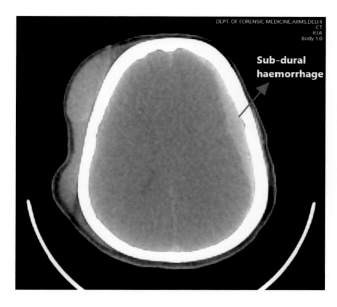

FIGURE 2.65: Crescent-shaped subdural haemorrhage present over the left frontoparietal region.

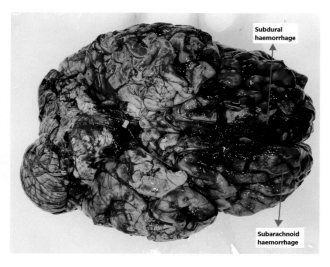

FIGURE 2.67: Diffuse subdural haemorrhage present over bilateral cerebral hemispheres along with subarachnoid haemorrhages at places over the base of the brain.

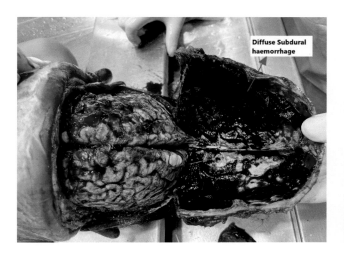

FIGURE 2.66: Diffuse subdural haemorrhage present over bilateral cerebral hemispheres seen stuck to the reflect skull vault with dura mater.

spread compared to aneurysm SAH, and it is located near the brain contusion or laceration (Figure 2.71).

Intraparenchymal haemorrhage

Intraparenchymal haemorrhage is proper bleeding in the brain parenchyma. There are many causes of such haemorrhage which include:

- Trauma.
- Hypertension.
- Eclampsia.
- Arteriovenous malformation.
- Amyloid angiopathy.
- Aneurysm rupture.
- Tumour.
- Coagulopathy.
- Infection.
- Vasculitis.

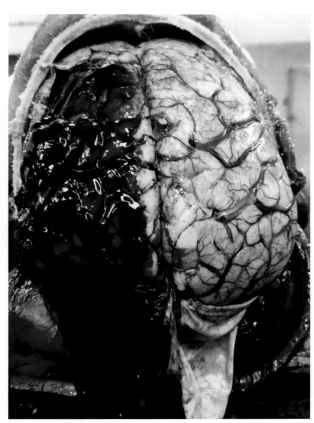

FIGURE 2.68: Subdural haemorrhage present over the entire left cerebral hemisphere.

Such haemorrhages push the brain parenchyma and also lead to increased intracranial pressure. The haemorrhage and raised intracranial pressure may also cause herniation of the brain. Intraparenchymal bleeds are usually presented as neurological deficits or strokes on presentation or even in cases of sudden death. A seizure episode before sudden death could also be the presentation. When such parenchymal bleeds happen close to

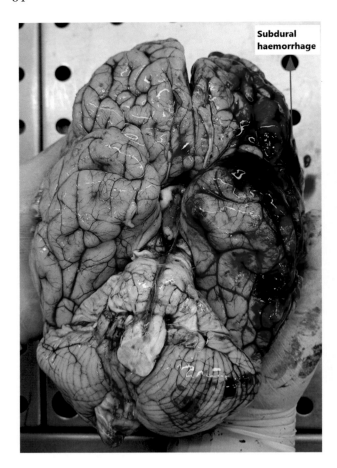

FIGURE 2.69: Subdural haemorrhage present over the left frontotemporal region.

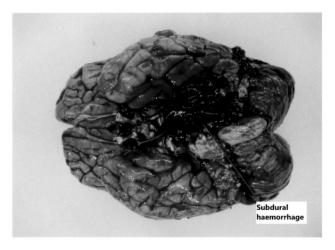

FIGURE 2.70: Subdural haemorrhage present over the base of the brain extending into the basal cisterns region.

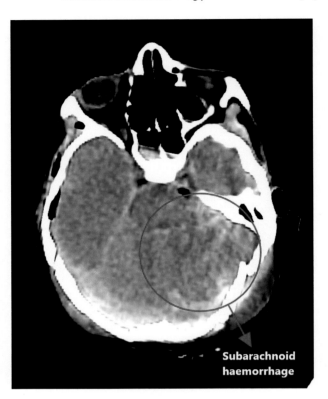

FIGURE 2.71: Axial section of CT shows a traumatic SAH is seen over the left temporal lobe of the brain with an adjacent fracture of the skull and scalp contusion.

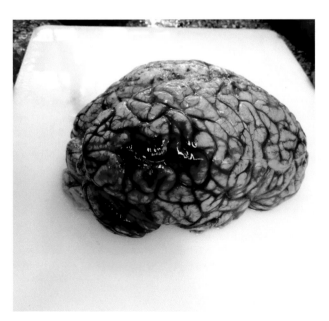

FIGURE 2.72: Subarachnoid haemorrhage present over the right parieto-occipital lobe and the right cerebellar hemisphere.

the ventricles of the brain, there may be an extension into the ventricles (Figure 2.74).

Ventricles of the brain

The ventricles of the brain are filled with cerebrospinal fluid and are interconnected cavities within the brain parenchyma. They are composed of two lateral ventricles, one-third ventricle and one-fourth ventricle. The two lateral ventricles communicate with the third ventricle by the interventricular foramen of Monro. The third ventricle communicates with the fourth ventricle by the cerebral aqueduct of Sylvius (Figure 2.75). The ventricles continue into the spinal cord as the central canal.

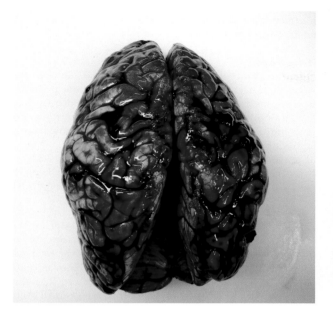

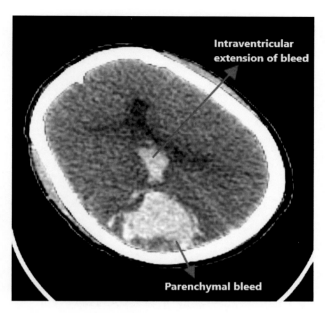

FIGURE 2.73: Diffuse SAH is present over both cerebral hemispheres with SDH present at places over bilateral parietal lobes.

FIGURE 2.74: Axial section of CT shows intraparenchymal bleed in the right parieto-occipital region extending into the right lateral ventricle.

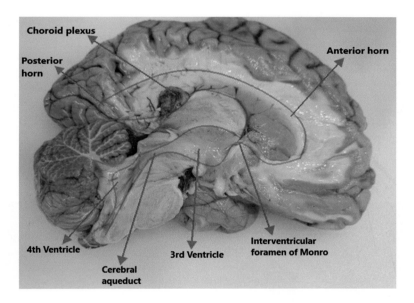

FIGURE 2.75: Rough outline of ventricles of the brain on sagittal section showing the lateral ventricle, third ventricle, and fourth ventricle along with the interventricular foramen of Monro and cerebral aqueduct.

Intraventricular haemorrhage

Intraventricular haemorrhage is a common complication of traumatic brain injury when a heavy impacting external force is involved. This intraventricular haemorrhage could also be non-traumatic and extension of the parenchymal bleed into the ventricles. One of the most commonly encountered cases is hypertensive bleeding and haemorrhagic stroke cases. Intraventricular haemorrhage could be present sometimes in all components of the ventricular system like lateral ventricles (Figures 2.76–2.80), third ventricle and fourth ventricle (Figures 2.77–2.79). In certain cases, the haemorrhage could be

only a specific part of the ventricular system or sometimes may extend to the surrounding cisterns (Figure 2.81).

Bullet injury to brain parenchyma

Bullets or projectiles can damage the brain by many mechanisms. As the bullet travels, it causes shock waves due to its motion, and this can damage the brain tissue. As the bullet physically travels through the brain parenchyma, it creates a permanent track (Figures 2.82–2.87), which usually contains blood and sometimes even blackening, depending on the distance of the firearm shot. Sometimes the bone fragments

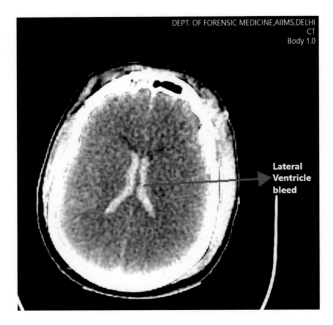

FIGURE 2.76: Axial CT scan image of the brain showing bilateral lateral ventricle haemorrhage in a case of traumatic brain injury.

which enter along with the bullet from the entry wound can also create multiple different tracks. In cases of shotgun injury, multiple tracks are formed by the pellets, and the length of each of these tracks depends on the kinetic energy possessed by the individual pellets. As the projectile penetrates the brain parenchyma, it causes tissue destruction in the permanent track (Figures 2.82 and 2.87) and stretching and elongation of the adjacent tissues mainly due to the formation of the temporary track, which is due to the kinetic energy of the projectile transferred in radial direction once the projectile strikes the brain parenchyma. This temporary track forms a large temporary cavity which is responsible for major damage to the neurons.

This temporary cavity depends on the velocity of the projectile and the issue density at which it penetrates.

CT findings

Identification of bullet tracks (Figure 2.82): CT scan images show haemorrhage along the track and bone fragments dispersed inwards or outwards, which helps to identify entry and exit wounds. There are metal fragments or projectile fragments in the track of the bullet. Beveling of the bone helps in identifying entry and exit wounds.

Localization of projectile/bullet: CT scan (Figure 2.83) and 3D reconstruction by volume rendering help in localizing the position of the bullet and its fragments (Figures 2.84 and 2.85).

Brainstem haemorrhage

The brainstem is the location where most of the vital centres of the respiratory and cardiovascular systems are present, and any haemorrhage in this part is considered the fatal subtype among intracranial haemorrhages. It is the relay centre for many long tracks traversing from the brain to the spinal centres; hence, in a compact place like this, even a small haemorrhage can lead to a major neurological deficit or death. The mortality rate is about 30–90% in brainstem haemorrhages. Among the brainstem haemorrhages, pontine haemorrhage is the most frequent (Figure 2.88). The reasons for brainstem haemorrhages are both traumatic and non-traumatic. Non-traumatic hypertension is the most common risk factor, along with other risk factors like anticoagulation therapy, coagulopathies, amyloid angiopathy, etc.

Cerebellar haemorrhage

Cerebellar haemorrhage is bleeding that occurs in the cerebellum, which accounts for about 9–10% of intracranial haemorrhage. Cerebellar haemorrhage occurs due to traumatic and non-traumatic haemorrhage. Hypertension is an important risk factor for spontaneous cerebellar haemorrhage (Figures 2.89–2.92). Tumours and trauma also contribute to the incidence of cerebellar haemorrhage.

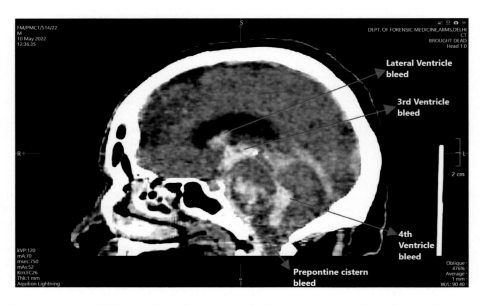

FIGURE 2.77: Sagittal section of CT brain shows Intraventricular haemorrhage involving the lateral ventricle, third ventricle, fourth ventricle and also in the interventricular foramen and cerebral aqueduct. The bleeding is also extending to the prepontine cistern.

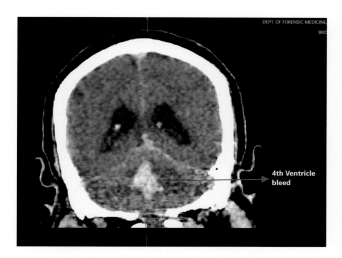

FIGURE 2.78: Coronal section of the CT brain shows an intraventricular haemorrhage in the fourth ventricle; the haemorrhage is seen taking the shape of the fourth ventricle, which resembles a diamond or rhomboid.

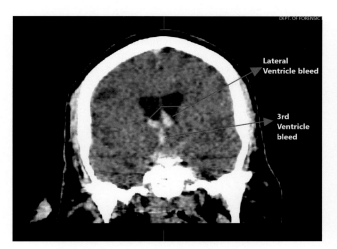

FIGURE 2.79: Coronal section of CT brain showing intraventricular haemorrhage in the lateral ventricles and the third ventricle.

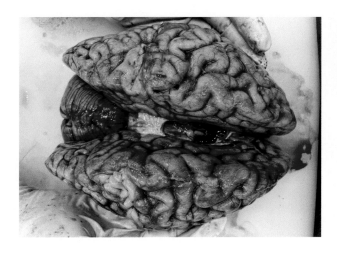

FIGURE 2.80: Superior view of the brain after dissection of the corpus callosum showing lateral ventricular bleed.

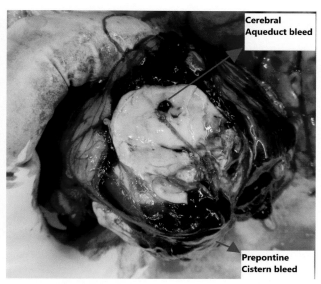

FIGURE 2.81: Cross section at the level of the brain stem shows haemorrhage in the cerebral aqueduct and also prepontine cistern haemorrhage.

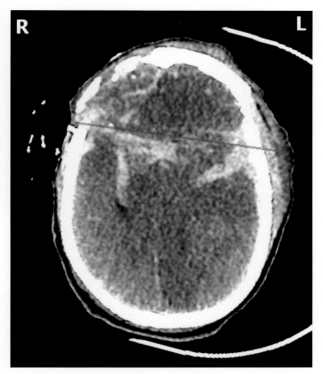

FIGURE 2.82: Red arrow showing the track of bullet piercing the brain parenchyma running horizontally backwards from right to left along with surrounding haemorrhage extending into the left lateral ventricle and surrounding parenchyma.

Brain Contusion

Brain contusions are focal surface bruises of the brain parenchyma. They are not mandatory for describing a case of fatal traumatic brain injury; however, their presence can depict the level of trauma that occurred. They are the result of damage to small cerebral blood vessels or the parenchyma. They are

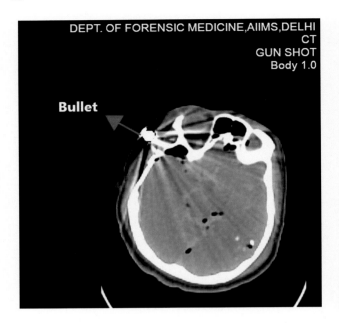

FIGURE 2.83: Bullet is lodged in the right temporal region after just exiting the skull. The metal artefact can also be appreciated.

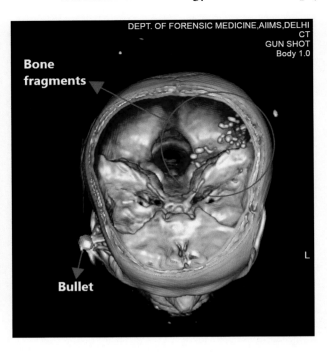

FIGURE 2.85: The volume rendering 3D image in the above case shows the bullet in the right temporal region and also inwards displaced bone fragments from the entry wound, helping in determining the track and direction of the bullet.

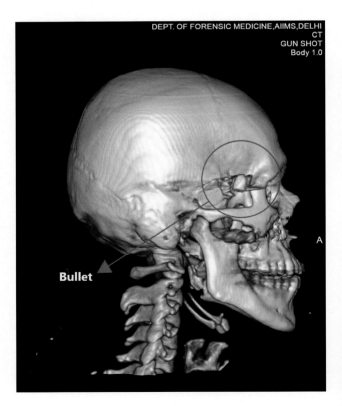

FIGURE 2.84: Volume rendering 3D reconstruction in the above-mentioned case showing the exact position of the bullet in the right temporal region.

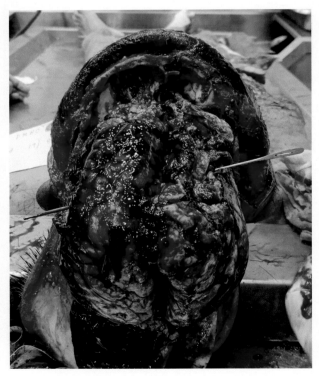

FIGURE 2.86: Autopsy of a case of bullet injury to the brain; the probe is placed along the permanent track of the brain created by the bullet entering from the right frontal lobe and is directed backwards and slightly upwards towards the left frontal lobe, where it exits the brain. Surrounding haemorrhage and necrosis can be identified.

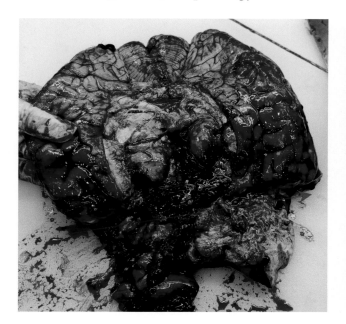

FIGURE 2.87: In this case, on dissection of the brain the permanent track of the bullet can be seen from the right frontal lobe to the left frontal lobe with damage to the brain parenchyma and haemorrhage. Haemorrhage is seen extending into the ventricles. SAH can also be observed in the brain parenchyma adjacent to the entry and exit points.

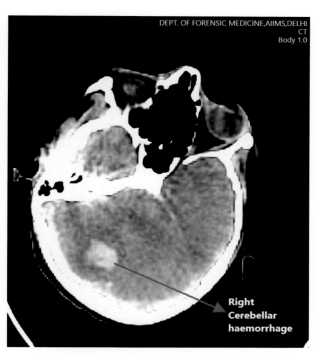

FIGURE 2.89: Axial section of CT brain showing right cerebellar bleed of non-traumatic origin in a case of sudden death.

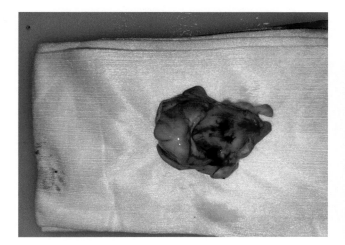

FIGURE 2.88: Multiple pontine haemorrhages appreciated over the pons.

identified by petechial haemorrhages present over the gyri. A contusion can be classified in multiple ways; one of the classifications is:

1. **Contusion haemorrhages** (Figures 2.93–2.94): They are a type of brain contusion which involves a vascular injury as the predominant feature.
2. **Contusion necrosis:** This is another type of brain contusion which may or may not contain haemorrhage; parenchymal injury is the main feature.

Contusion of the brain in practical scenarios rarely belongs purely to a single group and is usually in a

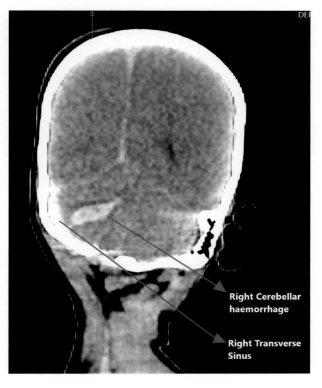

FIGURE 2.90: Coronal section of CT brain showing right cerebellar hemisphere, which has to be differentiated from the normal transverse sinus.

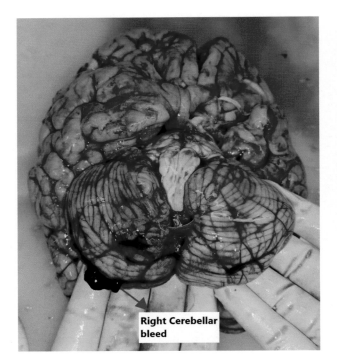

FIGURE 2.91:   The autopsy showed a blood clot oozing out of the right cerebellar hemisphere.

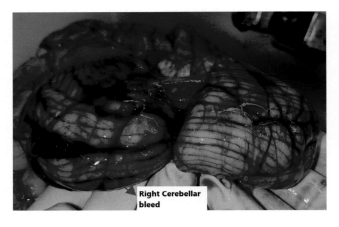

FIGURE 2.92:   The autopsy showed a blood clot oozing out of the right cerebellar hemisphere.

spectrum between these two extremes. Contusions are generally wedge-shaped on a cross-section of the brain surface having the broad base of the wedge, and they end in varying depths in the brain parenchyma, either grey matter or subcortical white matter. Contusions are generally associated with subarachnoid haemorrhage (SAH) due to the damage of blood vessels and their exposure to the subarachnoid space.

Based on the mechanism of occurrence of the contusion of the brain, they are classified into:

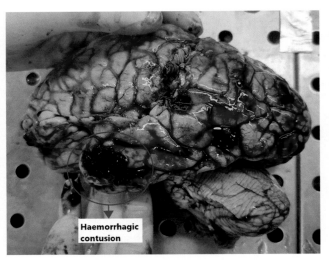

FIGURE 2.93:   Haemorrhagic contusion seen over the lateral surface of the left temporal lobe; the vascular injury is predominant with haemorrhage.

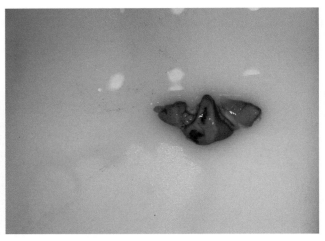

FIGURE 2.94:   Brain contusion is seen with petechial haemorrhages present over the gyri.

1. **Coup contusion:** It is the contusion of the brain occurring at the point of impact due to the direct impacting force.
2. **Contrecoup contusion:** It is the contusion of the brain occurring at the point opposite to the point of impact due to negative force or cavitation force.
3. **Intermediary contusion:** It is the contusion of the brain occurring in the deep brain in line of coup and contrecoup or along the line of impact.
4. **Fracture contusion:** It is the contusion of the brain occurring due to a fracture of the skull, usually different from the coup point.
5. **Gliding contusion:** It is the contusion of the brain occurring due to the displacement of the brain parenchyma during acceleration/deceleration caused by stretching of the neural tissue and resistance from more fixed structures like meninges.
6. **Herniation contusion:** It is the contusion of the brain occurring due to the herniation of part of the brain

either through bony passages like the foramen magnum or through meningeal structures like the falx cerebri or tentorium cerebelli.

Brain laceration

These are damage to the brain parenchyma where the neural tissues are stretched beyond the elastic limit of the neural tissue causing the disruption of the parenchymal surface (Figure 2.95). They are usually associated with high-impact injuries are have surrounding brain contusions and haemorrhages. They are also seen in ballistic injury cases due to the disrupting force of the projectile along with the shock waves which stretch the neural tissue beyond its limits.

Pneumocephalus

Pneumocephalus, also referred to by other terms like pneumatocele or intracranial aerocele, is a condition characterized by the presence of air inside the cranial cavity, which could be in between the meningeal layers (Figure 2.96) or brain parenchyma or the ventricles of the brain. There are various causes

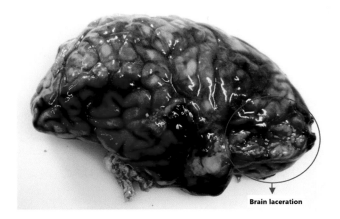

FIGURE 2.95: Brain laceration appreciated at the right frontal lobe; the tissue disruption along with surrounding haemorrhage and contusion is seen.

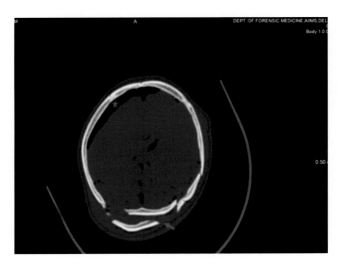

FIGURE 2.96: Pneumocephalus (red star) in an RTA case with fracture skull (red arrow).

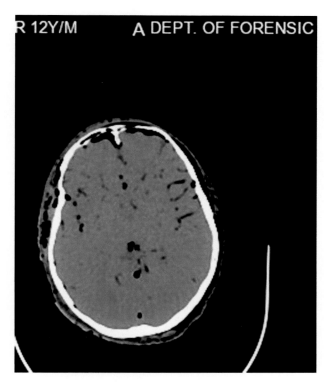

FIGURE 2.97: Air in the cranial cavity due to decomposition gases. The diffuse distribution of the gases is appreciable in the brain parenchyma and the subcutaneous tissues.

due to which air can enter the cranial cavity, which includes trauma causing fracture of the skull, laceration of the meninges, fracture of the paranasal sinuses, and base of skull fracture. Though trauma is a major cause of pneumocephalus, there are many other causes like iatrogenic causes, trans-cranial surgeries, trans-sphenoidal surgeries, lumbar punctures, ventriculoperitoneal shunts, etc. Infections like meningitis, sinusitis, or chronic otitis media due to gas-forming organisms can also cause pneumocephalus. In traditional autopsy, it is difficult to identify pneumocephalus; however, the use of radiological tools like digital X-ray and PMCT can help localize and also quantify the pneumocephalus. PMCT in the lung window helps in delineating the pneumocephalus and also identifies the aetiology for it, like any fracture of the skull or skull base or of any paranasal sinuses. It is important to differentiate from the air due to decomposition gases; here, we need to check the overall decomposition state of the case and also appreciate the diffuse distribution of air (Figure 2.97) in comparison with the localized distribution in pneumocephalus.

Bibliography

Adams JH. Brain damage in fatal non-missile head injury in man. In: Braakman R (ed.), *Handbook of clinical neurology*. Amsterdam, Netherlands: Elsevier, 1990. pp. 43–63.

Adams JH. Head injury. In: Adams JH, Duchen LM (eds.). *Greenfield's neuropathology*. London: Edward Arnold, 1992.

Adams JH, Graham DL, Scott G, et al. Brain damage in fatal non-missile head injury. *J Clin Pathol*. 1980;33:1132–1145.

Adams JH, Scott G, Parker LS, et al. The contusion index: A quantitative approach to cerebral contusions in head injury. *Neuropathol Appl Neurobiol*. 1980;6:319–324.

Adams RD, Sidman RL. *Introduction to neuropathology.* New York: McGraw-Hill, 1968.

Albrechtsen R. The incidence of so-called acute selective necrosis of the granular layer of cerebellum in 1000 autopsied patients. *Acta Pathol Microbiol Scand A.* 1977;85:193–202.

Ali TT. The role of white blood cells in postmortem wounds. *Med Sci Law.* 1988;28:100–106.

Alpers BJ, Forster EM. The reparative process in subarachnoid haemorrhage. *J Neuropathol Exp Neurol.* 1945;4:262–268.

Anderson R, McLean J. Biomechanics of closed head injury. In: Reilly PL, Bullock R (eds.), *Head injury: Pathophysiology and management.* London: Hodder Arnold, 2005. pp. 26–31.

Anderson RMcD, Opeskin K. Timing of early changes in brain trauma. *Am J Forensic Med Pathol.* 1998;19:1–9.

Auer RN, Dunn JF, Sutherland CR. Hypoxia and related conditions. In: Louis DN, Love S, Ellison DW (eds.), *Greenfield's neuropathology.* London, Arnold; 2008. pp. 233–280.

Beirowski B, Nogradi A, Babetto E, et al. Mechanisms of axonal spheroid formation in central nervous system Wallerian degeneration. *J Neuropathol Exp Neurol.* 2010;69:455–472.

Blumbergs PC. Pathology. In: Reilly PL, Bullock R (eds.), *Head injury: Pathophysiology and management.* London: Hodder Arnold, 2005.

Blumbergs PC, Jones NR, North JB. Diffuse axonal injury in head trauma. *J Neurol Neurosurg Psychiatr.* 1989;52:838–841.

Blumbergs PC, Scott G, Manavis J, et al. Staining of amyloid precursor protein to study axonal damage in mild head injury. *Lancet.* 1994;344:1055–1056.

Blumbergs PC, Scott G, Manavis J, et al. Topography of axonal injury as defined by amyloid precursor protein and the sector scoring method in mild and severe closed head injury. *J Neurotrauma.* 1995;12:565–572.

Brown AW. Structural abnormalities in neurons. *J Clin Pathol Suppl.* 1977;11:155–169.

Bryantseva SA, Zhapparova ON. Bidirectional transport of organelles: Unity and struggle of opposing motors. *Cell Biol Int.* 2012;36:1–6.

Cammermeyer J. The importance of avoiding "dark" neurons in experimental neuropathology. *Acta Neuropathol.* 1961;1:345–352.

Carey ME. Experimental missile wounding to the brain. *J Neurosurg.* 1989;71:754–764.

Carey ME. Experimental missile wounding of the brain. *Neurosurgery Clinics of North America.* 1995 Oct 1;6(4):629–642.

Chesnut RM, Marshall LF, Klauber MR, et al. The role of secondary brain injury in determining outcome from severe head injury. *J Trauma.* 1993;34:216–222.

Christman CW, Grady MS, Walker SA, et al. Ultrastructural studies of diffuse axonal injury in humans. *J Neurotrauma.* 1994;11:173–186.

Clark RSB, Kochanek P. *Brain injury.* Boston, MA: Kluwer Academic, 2001.

Dabbs DJ. *Diagnostic Immunohistochemistry.* Philadelphia, PA: Saunders Elsevier, 2010.

Denny-Brown D, Russell WR. Experimental cerebral concussion. *Brain.* 1941;64:93–164.

Dewey C, Downs M, Aron D, et al. Acute traumatic intracranial haemorrhage in dogs and cats. *Vet Comp Orthop Traumatol.* 1993;6:153–158.

DiMaio VJ, Di Maio D. *Forensic pathology.* Boca Raton, FL: CRC Press, 2001.

DiMaio VJM. *Gunshot wounds: Practical aspects of firearms, ballistics, and forensic techniques.* Boca Raton, FL: CRC Press, 1999.

Fackler ML. Civilian gunshot wounds and ballistics: Dispelling the myths. *Emerg Med Clin North Am.* 1998;16:17–28.

Fackler ML. Gunshot wound review. *Ann Emerg Med.* 1996;28:194–203.

Fackler ML, Bellamy RF, Malinowski JA. The wound profile: Illustration of the missile-tissue interaction. *J Trauma.* 1988;28 Supplement:S21–S29.

Fackler ML, Peters CE. The "shock wave" myth. *Wound Ballistics Rev.* 1991;1:38–40.

Finnie JW, Blumbergs PC, Manavis J, et al. Evaluation of brain damage resulting from penetrating and non-penetrating captive bolt stunning using lambs. *Aust Vet J.* 2000;78:775–778.

Finnie JW, Manavis J, Summersides GE, et al. Brain damage in pigs produced by impact with a non-penetrating captive bolt pistol. *Aust Vet J.* 2003;81:153–155.

Finnie JW. Neuroinflammation: Beneficial and detrimental effects after traumatic brain injury. *Inflammopharmacol.* 2013;21:309–320.

Finnie JW. Pathology of experimental traumatic craniocerebral missile injury. *J Comp Pathol.* 1993;108:93–101.

Finnie JW. Pathology of traumatic brain injury. *Vet Res Commun.* 2014;38:297–305.

Finnie JW. Animal models of traumatic brain injury: A review. *Aust Vet J.* 2001;79:628–633.

Finnie JW, Blumbergs PC. Animal models: Traumatic brain injury. *Vet Pathol.* 2002;39:679–689.

Finnie JW. Traumatic head injury in ruminant livestock. *Aust Vet J.* 1997;75:204–208.

Finnie JW. Brain damage caused by a captive bolt pistol. *J Comp Pathol.* 1993;109:253–258.

Finnie JW, Van den Heuvel C, Gebski V, et al. Effect of impact on different regions of the head of lambs. *J Comp Pathol.* 2001;124:159–164.

Freytag E. Autopsy findings in head injuries from firearms; statistical evaluation of 254 cases. *Arch Pathol.* 1963;76:215–225.

Kroman A, Kress T, Porta D. Fracture propagation in the human cranium: a re-testing of popular theories. *Clinical Anatomy.* 2011 Apr;24(3):309–18.

LeRoux PD, Haglund MM, Newell DW, et al. Intraventricular haemorrhage in blunt head trauma: An analysis of 43 cases. *J Neurosurg.* 1992;31:678–685.

Lewis SB, Finnie JW, Blumbergs PC, et al. A head impact model of early axonal injury in the sheep. *J Neurotrauma.* 1996;13:505–514.

Lindenberg R, Freytag E. The mechanism of cerebral contusions. *Arch Pathol.* 1960;69:440–469.

Loberg EM, Torvik A. Brain contusions: The time sequence of the histological changes. *Med Sci Law.* 1989;29:109–115.

MacKay RJ. Brain injury after head trauma: Pathophysiology, diagnosis, and treatment. *Vet Clin Equine.* 2004;20:199–216.

Oehmichen M, Auer RN, Konig HG. *Forensic neuropathology and associated neurology.* Springer-Verlag: Berlin Heidelberg, 2006. pp. 116–117.

Pillay VV. *Textbook of forensic medicine & toxicology,* 16th ed. Hyderabad: Paras Publisher, 2011, pp. 205–216.

Reddy KSN. *The essentials of forensic medicine and toxicology,* 29th ed. Hyderabad: K. Suguna Devi, 2010. pp. 218–238.

Russel RCG, Williams NS, Bulstrode CJK (eds.) *Bailey & love's short practice of surgery,* Twenty-third ed. London: Arnold, 2003, pp. 548–549.

Saukko P. Knight B. *Knight's forensic pathology,* 3rd ed. London: Arnold Publisher, 2004, pp. 174–221 (1, 20).

Vij K. *Textbook of forensic medicine and toxicology,* 4th ed. Noida: Elsevier, 2009, pp. 351–370.

3 THORAX – ANATOMY, TRAUMA, AND PATHOLOGY

The thorax is an important part of the trunk of the human body and also hosts some of the most vital organs. Diseases of the cardiovascular and respiratory systems are the leading causes of sudden death; the thorax is that part of the human body which contains the heart; great vessels like aorta, vena cavae, pulmonary arteries, and veins; and the lungs and their respiratory trees. Owing to these factors, examination of this anatomical region is crucial. The thorax contains the mediastinum, and the pleural sacs contain the lungs. Mediastinum is the central part of the thoracic cavity, and pleural sacs form the lateral aspect. The thoracic cage's roof is formed by the suprapleural membrane, and the floor is formed by the diaphragm. The walls are made of the skeleton (ribs, thoracic vertebra, and sternum), and these are interconnected by muscles.

The skeleton of the thoracic cage includes the anteriorly placed sternum, laterally placed 12 pairs of ribs on left and right sides and posteriorly placed 12 thoracic vertebrae (Figure 3.1).

Sternum

The sternum is the anterior midline skeleton of the thoracic cage; etymologically, the word 'sternum' is derived from the Greek word 'steron', which means chest. The sternum is commonly referred to as the breastbone too, due to its location. It is an anteroposteriorly flattened bone consisting of three parts: The manubrium, body, and xiphoid process (Figures 3.2 and 3.3). This bone articulates with the clavicle above and with the upper seven ribs directly, which are hence referred to as the true ribs, and the eighth to tenth ribs indirectly through the costal cartilage and hence they are referred to as false ribs, which gives direct or indirect anterior attachment to the upper 10 ribs through the costal cartilage. It is one of the bones whose ossification centres appear very early in the gestational period and helps in the age estimation of the foetus. The body of the sternum develops from left and right cartilaginous plates, which unite in the midline, and the manubrium and the xiphoid parts of the sternum develop from single separate ossification centres, which unite with the body late in adulthood.

- **Manubrium** (Figure 3.4): The manubrium is the upper, quadrangular-shaped part of the sternum bone, which articulates with the clavicles super-laterally, forming the sternoclavicular joint and laterally with the upper one and half costal cartilage of the ribs. The upper border of this quadrangular bone is a slight depression called the jugular notch and is between the articular facets of the sternoclavicular joint. The manubrium tapers below, and the lower part articulates with the body of the sternum where it forms the sternal angle or also referred to as the 'Angle of Louis', which is an important bony landmark which lies opposite T4/5 disc space and divides the mediastinum into the superior and inferior mediastinum.
- **Body:** The body of the sternum is also referred to by the name 'gladiolus'. This part of the sternum is anteroposteriorly compressed and flat, with a slight convex curve to the anterior and a slight concave curve to the posterior. The lateral surfaces have articular facets for the third to seventh ribs, along with a small lower portion of the second costal cartilage. The body of the sternum tapers

in the lower part, where it articulates with the xiphoid process.
- **Xiphoid process:** It is the lowest part and the tiniest part of the sternum bone and is also referred to as xiphisternum. It is highly variable in its shape and articulates with the lower part of the body of the sternum. It is cartilaginous and ossifies in the fourth decade of life. In certain cases, it may also articulate with the seventh rib.

Ribs

The ribs form the thoracic cage by articulating anteriorly with the sternum through costal cartilage and posteriorly with the thoracic vertebrae. A total of 12 pairs of ribs are present, which include 7 pairs of true ribs (as they are directly articulating with the sternum), 3 pairs of false ribs (as they articulate indirectly with the sternum), and 2 floating ribs (which do not have an anterior articulation). Another method of classification of the ribs is as typical and atypical ribs. The first, second, tenth, eleventh, and twelfth are atypical ribs (they have variations in comparison to generalized rib structure), and the rest are typical ones (they have a generalized structure) (Figure 3.5). The intercostal space between the ribs is covered by the muscles which consist of the external, internal, and innermost intercostal muscles which along with the lungs have a role in ventilation.

Typical ribs
The generalized structure of a typical rib includes a head, neck, and body. The head is usually wedge-shaped with two articular facets for the vertebrae. One facet articulates with the numerically corresponding vertebra and the other articulates with the vertebra above. The neck part bridges the head with the body. The junction of the neck and body has a roughed tubercle which contains an articulation facet for the corresponding vertebra's transverse process. The body is flattened and curves, and there is a groove on the inner side near the lower end for the neurovascular bundle.

Atypical ribs
Atypical ribs include the first, second, tenth, eleventh, and twelfth ribs, and they are referred to as 'atypical' as they have certain features that are different from the generalized structure of most ribs.

- **Rib 1:** It is short and wider compared to all other ribs. It only has a single facet on its head for articulation with its corresponding vertebra in contrast to two facets. The rib is flattened above-downwards and has grooves for the subclavian vessels on the upper surface.
- **Rib 2:** It is thinner and longer in comparison to the first rib and has a roughened area on its upper surface for the serratus anterior muscle.
- **Rib 10:** It has only one facet in the head for articulation with its numerically corresponding vertebra.
- **Ribs 11 and 12:** They have a head part with only one articular facet, they have no neck portion, and they don't articulate anteriorly, hence they are also referred to as floating ribs.

DOI: 10.1201/9781003383703-3

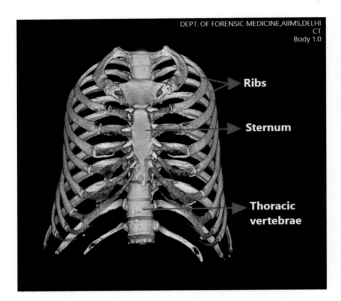

FIGURE 3.1: Volume rendering 3D CT image of the thoracic cage with the anteriorly placed sternum (blue), laterally placed ribs, and posteriorly placed thoracic vertebra (pink).

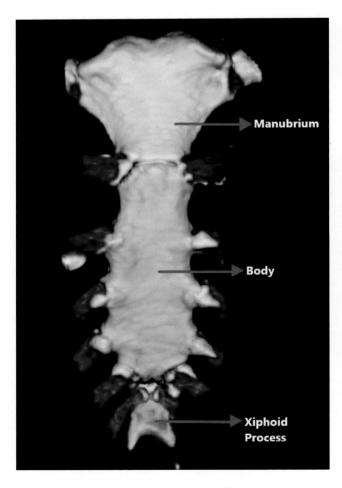

FIGURE 3.2: Volume rendering 3D CT image of the sternum consisting of three parts: Manubrium (pink), body (blue), and xiphoid process (green).

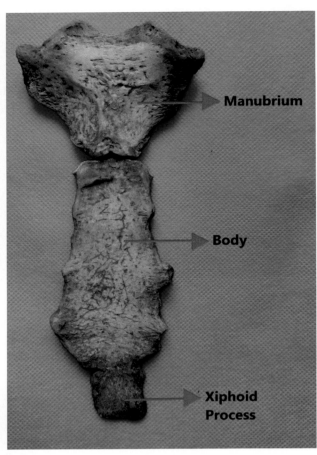

FIGURE 3.3: Gross photo of the sternum bone showing the manubrium, body, and xiphoid process.

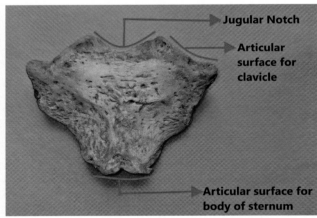

FIGURE 3.4: The gross image of the manubrium sternum showing the jugular notch and articular surfaces for the clavicle and body of the sternum.

Thoracic vertebrae

The thoracic vertebrae are 12 in number and form an important support structure for the thoracic cage. These 12 vertebrae are separated from each other by intervertebral discs. The thoracic vertebrae have a few generalized features, which include:

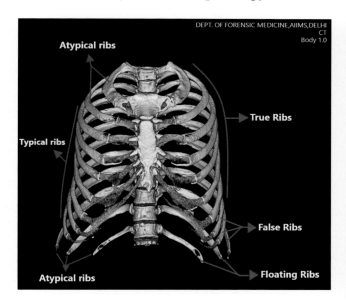

FIGURE 3.5: Volume rendering 3D CT image of the thoracic cage showing different types of ribs according to two methods of classification which are demarcated by colour coding for each method.

- Heart-shaped vertebral body.
- Demi-facets of the vertebral body on both sides for articulation with the heads of ribs.
- Costal facets on the transverse process for articulation with the tubercle of ribs.
- Long and inferiorly slanting spinous processes (Figures 3.6 and 3.7).

Mediastinum

The thorax's central compartment is the mediastinum, located between the two pleural sacs (Figure 3.8). It hosts most of the thoracic organs, and it also acts as a channel through which structures reach the abdomen through the thorax traverse.

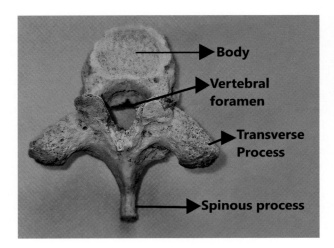

FIGURE 3.6: Thoracic vertebra gross examination shows a heart-shaped body long and inferiorly slanting spinous process.

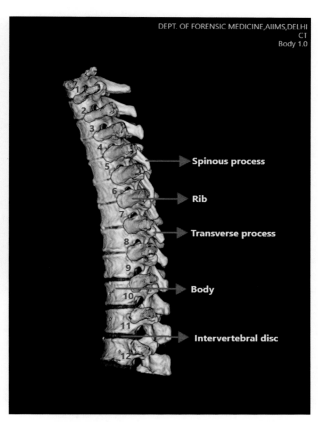

FIGURE 3.7: Volume rendering 3D CT image of the entire thoracic vertebrae showing the attachment of ribs and inferiorly slanting spinous process.

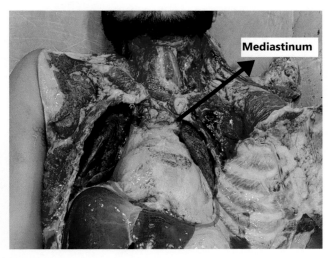

FIGURE 3.8: Mediastinum the central compartment of the thorax between the two pleural sacs.

It is marginated on each side by the mediastinal pleura, anteriorly by the chest wall and sternum, and posteriorly by the spine and chest wall. The mediastinum is divided into two parts, i.e., superior and inferior, by an imaginary line (plane of Louis) that runs from the **sternal angle to the T4 vertebrae** (Figures 3.9 and 3.10). Further anatomical structures present in a particular division are as follows:

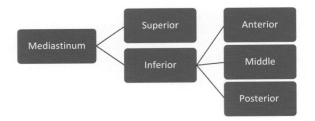

FIGURE 3.9: Classification of the mediastinum.

Superior mediastinum

The superior mediastinum (Figure 3.10) is an intrapleural space bounded superiorly by the thoracic inlet, anteriorly by the manubrium, posteriorly by vertebral bodies of T1–T4, laterally by pleura of both lungs, and inferiorly by an imaginary plane known as the plane of Louis, i.e., the transverse thoracic plane that runs from the **sternal angle** to the T4 vertebrae. The content of the area is as follows:

- **Major great vessels:** Superior vena cava and arch of the aorta with its three major branches, which are the brachiocephalic artery, left common carotid artery, and left subclavian artery.
- **Nerves:** Vagus, phrenic, and sympathetic nerves.
- **Other structures:** Trachea, oesophagus, thymus gland, thoracic duct and muscles, i.e., sternohyoid/sternothyroid muscles/inferior aspect of the longus coli muscle.

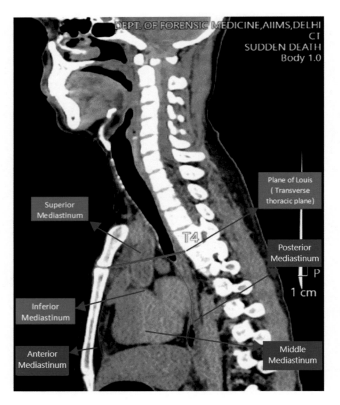

FIGURE 3.10: Sagittal section of the thorax showing various divisions of the mediastinum, i.e., superior, inferior, anterior, middle, and posterior mediastinum.

Inferior mediastinum

The inferior mediastinum (Figure 3.10) extends from T5–T12 and is further subdivided into the anterior, middle, and posterior parts as follows:

- The anterior mediastinum contains no major structures. It is located anteriorly by the sternum and posteriorly by the anterior margin of the pericardium. It accommodates fat, lymph nodes, loose connective tissue (including the sternopericardial ligaments, which tether the pericardium to the sternum), and branches of the internal thoracic vessels. The thymus extends inferiorly into the anterior mediastinum in the case of infants and children. However, it recedes during puberty and is mostly replaced by adipose tissue in adults.
- The posterior mediastinum is bound anteriorly by the pericardium and posteriorly by the T5–T12 vertebra. It accommodates the thoracic aorta (descending), oesophagus, thoracic duct, azygous, hemiazygous vein and sympathetic trunk.
- The middle mediastinum is bound anteriorly by the anterior margin of the pericardium and posteriorly by the posterior border of the pericardium. It contains the heart and its pericardium, along with the tracheal bifurcation and the left and right main bronchus. It is the main site of origin of all the great vessels running from or into the heart, i.e., the ascending aorta, superior vena cava, and pulmonary trunk.

Structures of the thorax

The major organs in the thorax are the heart and lungs; injury to these is highly fatal. The following are the major structures seen in the thorax:

Pericardium
The normal pericardium, i.e., the visceral and parietal pericardium along with pericardial contents, is visible as a 1- to 2-mm stripe of soft-tissue attenuation parallel to the heart and outlined by epicardial fat. The pericardium is best seen near the diaphragm, along the anterior and lateral aspects of the heart, where the fat layers are thickest.

Heart
The heart is a pyramidal shape structure that lies obliquely in the chest cavity. Its base points towards the posterior side, and the elongated apex is to the left and inferiorly. The left atrium forms the base or posterior part, receiving blood from superior and inferior pulmonary veins. The left ventricle forms the left border and the apex. The right atrium forms the right border, with superior and inferior vena cava draining into it. The right ventricle forms the anterior part. The inferior (diaphragmatic) part of the heart is formed by both ventricles anteriorly and a small part of the right atrium posteriorly (Figure 3.11). The oblique orientation of the heart causes the ventricles to lie anterior and inferior to the atria. The right atrium and ventricle are at a slightly higher level than their left counterparts, as the heart is also rotated in a clockwise fashion about its axis. The tricuspid and mitral valves, which separate the right and left atria and ventricles, respectively, are roughly vertically oriented. The plane of the valves is also inclined inferiorly and to the left. The aortic valves and the mitral valves are the most important to recognize, as they are most often affected by the

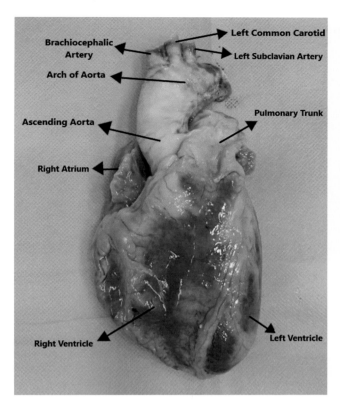

FIGURE 3.11: A gross examination of the heart showing the chambers along with the great vessels.

disease. The right and the left coronary arteries arise from the respective coronary sinus. The examination of this four-chambered organ, even in CT, is important. In the absence of a contrast medium, only a modest amount of the anatomy of the heart on CT can be appreciated (Figures 3.12 and 3.13) as compared to the anatomy with a contrast medium.

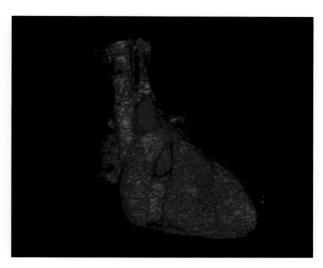

FIGURE 3.13: Volume rendering 3D reconstruction of the heart.

Aorta

It is the largest blood vessel of the human body, and its course in the thoracic region is divided into the ascending part, the arch of the aorta, and the descending part (Figures 3.14–3.16). The ascending aorta begins at the aortic valve at the level of the third costal cartilage's lower border; the first few centimetres of the ascending aorta, along with the pulmonary trunk, are enclosed in a common sheath of the pericardium. It then ascends to the right and arches over the pulmonary trunk to lie behind the upper border of the second right costal carti-lage, after which it continues as the descending aorta. During this course, the aorta gives certain branches, and the ascending aorta gives the right and left coronary arteries. The branches of the arch of the aorta are the brachiocephalic, the left com-mon carotid, and the left subclavian arteries (Figure 3.11). The

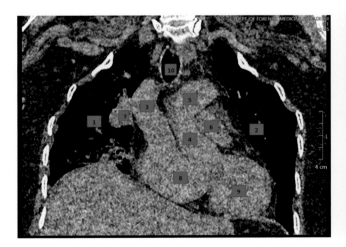

FIGURE 3.12: Coronal section of thorax showing in soft tis-sue window shows 1. The right lung, 2. The left lung, 3. Superior vena cava, 4. The ascending aorta 5. The arch of the aorta, 6. The main pulmonary trunk, 7. The right pulmonary artery, 8. The right ventricle, 9. The left ventricle, 10. The trachea. Red star: Pericardium.

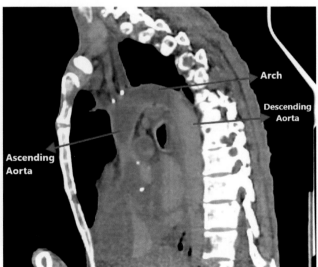

FIGURE 3.14: Sagittal section of thorax PMCT in soft tissue window showing the ascending, arch, and descending aorta. Post-mortem clot formation in the descending aorta due to the dependent position and pooling of blood is appreciated with the higher attenuation of the post-mortem clots.

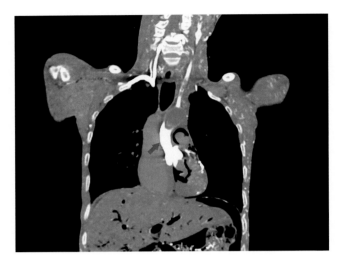

FIGURE 3.15: Coronal section of thorax PMCT with contrast, with the contrast seen in ascending aorta.

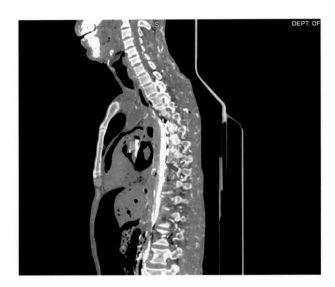

FIGURE 3.16: Sagittal section of thorax and abdomen PMCT with contrast, with the contrast seen in descending aorta.

brachiocephalic and left common carotid arteries ascend on either side of the trachea in a V shape to come to lie behind the sternoclavicular joints, at which point the brachiocephalic bifurcates into the major divisions, which are the right common carotid artery and right subclavian artery. The aortic isthmus is the junction of the arch and the descending aorta. This area is relatively fixed and is thus prone to injury with the shearing forces of blunt trauma; this is the most frequent site of aortic mural tear and transsection. The descending aorta passes inferiorly through the posterior mediastinum up to the diaphragm at the level of T12. The descending aorta then lies behind the oesophagus. The branches of the descending aorta are as follows: posterior intercostal arteries, bronchial arteries, oesophagal branches, mediastinal branches, phrenic branches, and pericardial branches to the posterior pericardium. As posterior intercostal arteries are the direct branch from descending aorta, so in cases of multiple rib fracture (4–5 ribs), blood

loss of about 1–2 litre is possible, and also it is considered sufficient to cause the death of the elderly patient or children.

Esophagus

Esophagus is the food passage connecting the pharynx with the stomach. It begins at the level of C5/C6 or the lower border of the cricoid cartilage as the continuation of the pharynx. It is subdivided into three parts, namely, the cervical, thoracic, and abdominal. The cervical part descends behind the trachea and thyroid and in front of the cervical vertebrae. The thoracic segment extends from the suprasternal notch till its exit through the diaphragm; the superior mediastinum is behind the trachea and then passes behind the arch of the aorta. As the oesophagus extends down, it passes into the posterior mediastinum to lie near the thoracic vertebrae. It enters the abdomen through the right crus of the diaphragm at the level of the tenth thoracic vertebra, and the final abdominal segment is the shortest, extends from the diaphragm to the cardia of the stomach (Figure 3.17) at the level of the eleventh thoracic vertebra.

Thymus

This organ is part of the lymphatic system, and it lies retrosternal in the superior mediastinum. It continues to grow after birth and reaches its maximum size at puberty. During infancy, the size of the thymus gland may extend down as far as the fourth costal cartilage (Figure 3.18). The normal thymus can be seen on CT long after it is no longer visible on a radiograph. On CT, it is homogeneous, with a density similar to that of muscle.

Pleura

The pleura is a serous membrane that not only covers the lung (i.e., the visceral pleura) but also lines the thoracic cavity and mediastinum (i.e., the parietal pleura). The visceral pleura

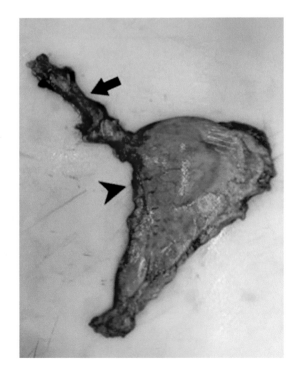

FIGURE 3.17: Traditional autopsy examination image showing Esophagus (black arrow) along with it continuing as stomach (black arrowhead).

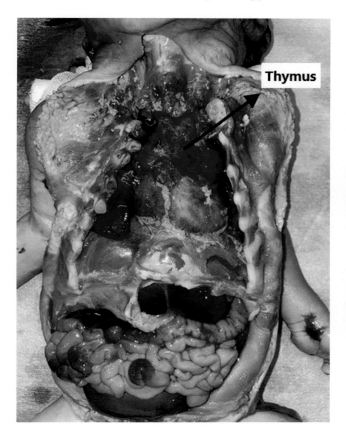

FIGURE 3.18: Thymus seen in the superior mediastinum extending into the inferior mediastinum up to the level of third costal cartilage.

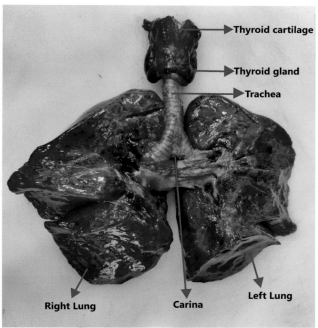

FIGURE 3.19: Gross anatomy of the lungs showing thyroid cartilage, thyroid gland, trachea, carina, right lung, and left lung.

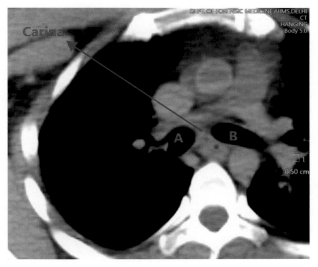

FIGURE 3.20: Axial section of the chest showing carina at the junction of main bronchi, right main bronchus (A), and left main bronchus (B).

spreads out to the interlobar and accessory fissures. Pleural parts are named according to the site, for example, costal, diaphragmatic, mediastinal, and apical.

Trachea

The trachea, also commonly referred to as the windpipe, is the passage for air from the atmosphere to enter the lungs during inspiration and for the expulsion of air from the lungs back to the atmosphere during expiration. Trachea starts at the lower border of the cricoid cartilage at the level of the sixth cervical vertebra and extends to the carina at the level of the sternal angle (T5 level), where it divides into the right and left primary bronchus (Figures 3.19 and 3.20). The trachea's length is 15 cm, and the diameter is 2 cm; it is made up of 15–20 incomplete cartilage rings which are bridged by the trachealis muscle posteriorly. The right bronchus is wider, shorter, and more vertical than the left main bronchus. Primary bronchus, after entering into the hilum, further divides multiple times, forming the bronchopulmonary tree. Carina is an anteroposterior ridge at the junction of the main bronchi, and it lies at the level of the sternal angle. The carinal angle measures approximately 60° +/−10. Enlargement of the left atrium on a PA chest radiograph causes widening of the carinal angle, which commonly occurs due to mitral valve dysfunction like stenosis or incompetence.

Lungs

The lungs are the organs responsible for respiration, where the exchange of oxygen and carbon dioxide occurs. The costal, mediastinal, apical, and diaphragmatic surfaces are the external surfaces of the lungs. The right lung comprises three lobes, while the left comprises two lobes. The lingula of the left upper lobe corresponds to the right middle lobe. Interlobar fissures, which are the oblique and horizontal fissures which run across the parenchyma, divide the lungs into the upper, middle, and lower lobes. On CT examination of the lungs in the axial section under the lung window, the oblique fissure appears as a thin hyperdense line extending from the periphery to the hilar region. This can be examined by checking the serial axial sections following the hyperdense line. This oblique fissure separates the middle lobe from the lower lobe in the right lung, while in the left lung, it separates the upper lobe from the lower lobe. On further examination of the axial sections, a horizontal/minor fissure can be appreciated, which separates the upper lobe from the middle lobe of the right lung. Each lobe is organized into several bronchopulmonary segments, which are supplied by a segmental bronchus, artery and vein. The two fissures (Figures 3.21–3.23) mentioned above are:

- The oblique (major) fissure is similar in both the right and left lungs. It extends from T4/T5 posteriorly to the diaphragm anteroinferior.
- The horizontal (minor) fissure in the right lung separates the upper and middle lobes. At the fourth costal cartilage level, it traverses horizontally from the hilum to the anterolateral surface of the right lung.

Lymph nodes

Lymph nodes are secondary lymphoid organs which are an integral part of the lymphatic system and are distributed throughout the body. Normal mediastinal lymph nodes typically measure less than 10 mm on the short axis; anything bigger than 10 mm is an indication of the need for evaluation. Thoracic lymph nodes form a major bulk of the lymph nodes of the body and are subdivided into 14 stations. These 14 stations are grouped into the following 7 zones (Figure 3.24) for a better understanding of their distribution and drainage.

1. **Supraclavicular zone:** It includes low cervical, supraclavicular, and sternal notch lymph nodes.
2. **Upper zone (superior mediastinal nodes):** It includes upper paratracheal, pre-tracheal (Figure 3.25), retro tracheal, and lower paratracheal lymph nodes.
3. **Aortopulmonary zone:** It includes subaortic and para-aortic lymph nodes.
4. **Subcarinal zone** (Figure 3.26): It is located between the right and left main bronchi and below the carina.
5. **Lower zone (inferior mediastinal nodes):** it includes para-oesophagal lymph nodes, i.e., below the carina (Figure 3.26).

6. **Hilar and interlobar zone (pulmonary nodes):** These are the proximal nodes adjacent to the bronchi near the hilar region of the lung.
7. **Peripheral zone (pulmonary nodes):** These are adjacent to distal lobar or segmental bronchi.

Examination of the lymph nodes is an important part of the gross examination, even though this is a difficult task owing to its size and variation on case to case basis. Anatomical orientation to the lymph node's location and morphology can help identify an abnormality in the gross appearance and is an important part of the complete autopsy examination. PMCT makes this task easier by helping locate and even measure these lymph nodes and check for any pathological pattern. The ability of PMCT to take thin sections and examine them in detail helps to locate and assess these lymph nodes. Calcification of the lymph nodes can also be well appreciated. Lymph nodes enlarged or calcified at certain times can be just an incidental finding but, in certain cases, could be part of the pathology leading to death.

Chest cross-sectional anatomy

Identifying and studying an organ or structure on only a single section of a CT scan is difficult, and it requires the examination of multiple sections above and below. This multi-level examination will help locate the structure and also identify its anatomical neighbours, and in certain scenarios, understand the pathway of a structure. Bony landmark assessment is an easy method for reading a CT scan and understanding the location. Vertebral bodies, which extend all along the thorax, are an important reference bony structure to determine the level of the axial section which is being examined. PMCT assessment is a little different from ante-mortem as the deceased body alignment can't be changed due to rigor mortis, and positioning with inspiration or expiration cannot be done. So due to these factors of body positioning, slight variation occurs in the level study. Important landmarks in the thorax anatomy considering superior and inferior mediastinum are as follows.

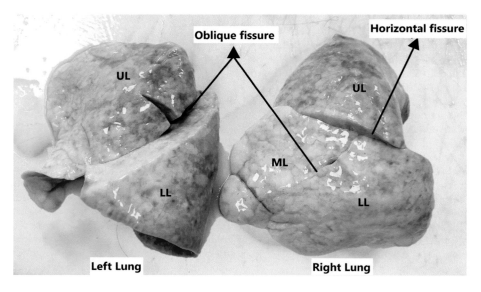

FIGURE 3.21: Coastal surface of both lungs examined shows the upper lobe (UL), the lower lobe (LL) in both lungs, and the middle lobe (ML) in the right lung. Oblique fissure is seen in both lungs, and a horizontal fissure is seen in the right lung.

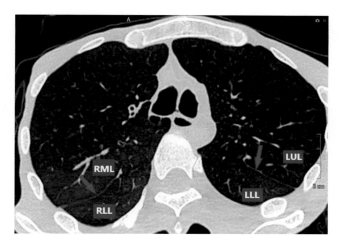

FIGURE 3.22: Axial section of chest CT in the lung window shows the oblique fissures in both lungs marked by red arrows. On the right side it separates the middle lobe (RML) from the lower lobe, and on the left side it separates the upper lobe (LUL) from the lower lobe (LLB).

Superior mediastinum

- **At the T2 level** (Figure 3.27)

    The trachea is the midline structure, in front of which are the strap muscles of the neck and posterior to which is the collapsed oesophagus. The apex of both lungs is present at this level, along with a portion of the first rib and clavicle, along with the vertebral attachment of the second rib, which is also appreciated. The head of the humerus, along with the glenoid cavity, is also

appreciated in this section. On the posterior aspect, a portion of the spine of the scapula is appreciated.

- **At the T3 level** (Figure 3.28)

    The trachea is seen in the midline, with the great vessels anteriorly and the oesophagus behind. The brachiocephalic veins are anterior and lateral to the arteries and unite to form the superior vena cava at about this level. The left brachiocephalic vein is seen passing anteriorly to the branches of the aortic arch. The three aortic branches, i.e., right brachiocephalic trunk, left common carotid, and left subclavian, are seen at this level. The third rib can be appreciated corresponding to its vertebra, and the complete spine of the scapula can be seen on both sides. The bulky para-vertebral muscles, which include the trapezius and erector spinae muscles, can be clearly appreciated.

- **At the T4 level** (Figure 3.29)

    This is an important level as the plane from the lower border of T4 and anteriorly ending at the sternal angle demarcates the superior and inferior mediastinum. It is also referred to as the plane of Louis or the transverse thoracic plane. At this level, to the left of the trachea is the lower part of the aortic arch, and the arch of the azygos vein is to the right. Superior vena cava formed by the right and left brachiocephalic veins can be seen at this level. The fourth rib corresponding to the vertebra level and upper border of the sternum can be seen.

Inferior mediastinum

- **At the T5 level** (Figure 3.30)

    This plane is at the level where the main pulmonary artery is seen dividing into the right and left pulmonary arteries. The right pulmonary artery is also seen running anterior to the right bronchus, whereas the left

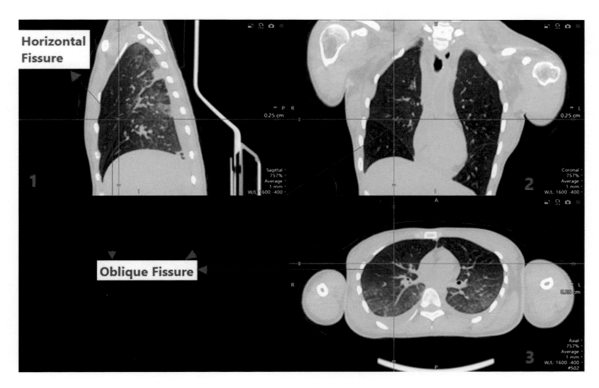

FIGURE 3.23: CT Lung in lung window of sagittal (1), coronal (2), and axial (3) section showing the oblique fissure and horizontal fissure in the right lung.

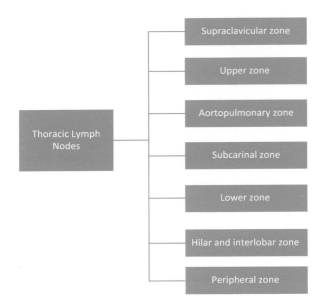

FIGURE 3.24:   Grouping of the thoracic lymph nodes into seven zones.

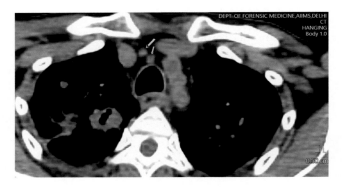

FIGURE 3.25:   Incidental finding of enlarged pre-tracheal lymph nodes (yellow arrows) in a case of hanging seen on an axial section of chest PMCT in soft tissue window.

pulmonary artery arches superiorly out of the plane to pass over the left bronchus. The ascending aorta is seen in a cross-section, lying in a more posterior plane than the origin of the main pulmonary artery. The oesophagus, azygos veins, and descending aorta are seen in the posterior mediastinum.

- **At the T6 level** (Figures 3.31 and 3.32)

  This section passes through the upper part of the heart. The right atrial appendage may be seen overlapping the origin of the aorta at this level. At this level, the coronary arteries, i.e., the left coronary artery, are divided into the circumflex and the left anterior descending artery (LAD) after originating from the aorta. On taking a section at a lower level of T6 right coronary artery is also visible along with the further path of the left circumflex and left anterior descending artery. The right ventricular outflow tract is seen anterior to the origin of the aorta.

- **At the T8 level** (Figure 3.33)

  This section passes through the chambers of the heart and shows the relationship of the chambers to each other. The left ventricular inflow and outflow tracts are separated from each other by the anterior leaflet of the mitral valve. The interatrial septum is also appreciated in this section. It can be noted in this section that the right atrium and right ventricle form the right border of the heart, the right ventricle also forms the anterior border, the left ventricle forms the left border, and the left atrium forms the posterior border.

Pathology of thorax

The biomechanics of thoracic pathologies are broadly classified into traumatic and non-traumatic patholiges (Figure 3.34).

Traumatic thorax pathologies

Thoracic trauma is a common cause of death, especially in the first three decades of life. Mortality rates from thoracic injuries are considered to be about 10%. Among the types of external forces causing thoracic injuries, blunt force accounts for about 96.3%, and due to sharp forces accounts for around the remaining 3.7%. The common causes of traumatic pathologies include RTAs, assault, homicide, sports injuries, and falls

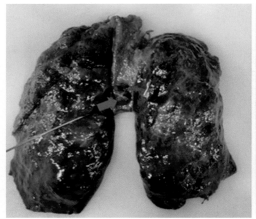

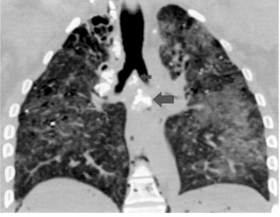

FIGURE 3.26:   Calcified enlarged subcarinal lymph nodes (red arrow) and inferior mediastinal lymph nodes (blue arrow) seen in the gross autopsy examination and coronal section of chest PMCT in lung window.

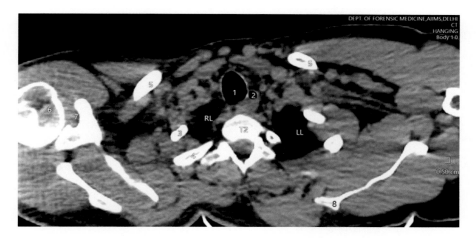

FIGURE 3.27: Axial section of the chest PMCT in soft tissue window at level T2 depicting the following: trachea, esophagus, first rib, second rib, clavicle, head of humerus, glenoid cavity, spine of scapula, RL: right lung, LL: left lung.

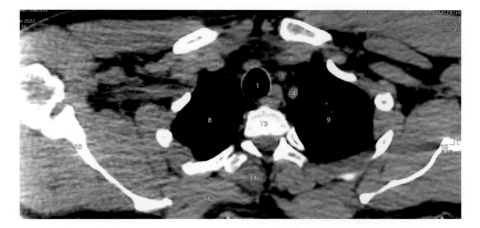

FIGURE 3.28: Axial section of the chest PMCT in soft tissue window at level T3 depicting the following: 1. Trachea, 2. Right brachiocephalic trunk, 3. Left common carotid, 4. Left subclavian, 5. Right brachiocephalic vein, 6. Left brachiocephalic vein, 7. Esophagus, 8. Right lung, 9. Left lung, 10. Spine of scapula, 11. Erector spinae muscle, 12. Trapezius.

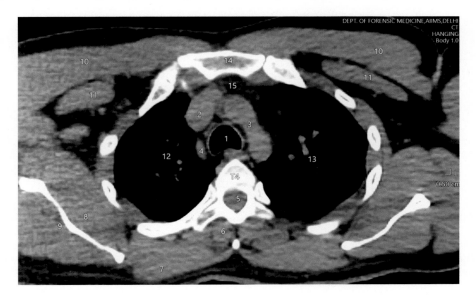

FIGURE 3.29: Axial section of the chest CT in soft tissue window at the level of T4 vertebra depicting the following: 1. Trachea, 2. Superior vena cava, 3. Arch of aorta, 4. Azygous vein, 5. Spinal cord, 6. Erector spinae, 7. Trapezius, 8. Subscapularis muscle, 9. Infraspinatus muscle, 10. Pectoralis major, 11. Pectoralis minor, 12. Right lung, 13. Left lung, 14. Sternum, 15. Retrosternal fat.

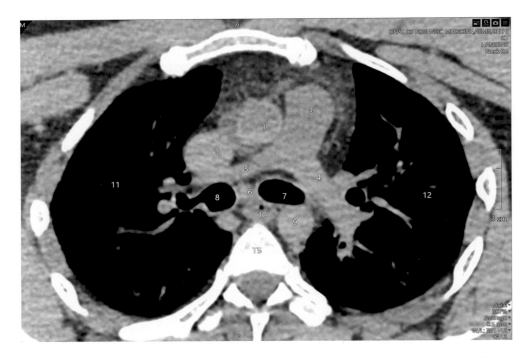

FIGURE 3.30: Axial section of the chest CT in soft tissue window at the level of T5 depicting the following structures as labelled: 1. Ascending aorta, 2. Superior vena cava, 3. Pulmonary trunk, 4. Left pulmonary artery, 5. Right pulmonary artery, 6. Carina, 7. Left main bronchus, 8. Right main bronchus, 9. Descending aorta, 10. Esophagus, 11. Right lung, 12. Left lung.

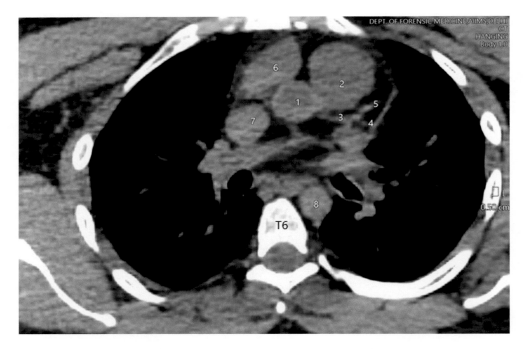

FIGURE 3.31: Axial section of the chest PMCT in soft tissue window at level T6 depicting the following: 1. Aorta, 2. Right ventricle, 3. Left coronary artery, 4. Left circumflex artery, 5. Left anterior descending artery, 6. Right atrium , 7. Superior vena cava, 8. Descending aorta.

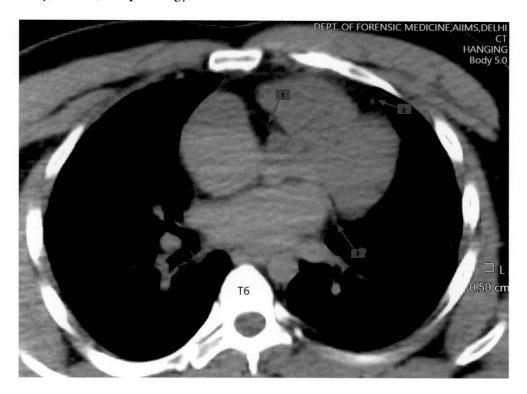

FIGURE 3.32: Axial section of the chest PMCT in soft tissue window at the lower level of T6 depicting coronary arteries, 1. Right coronary artery, 2. Left anterior descending artery, and 3. Left circumflex artery.

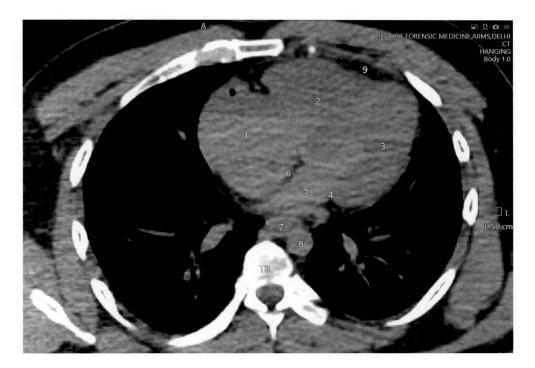

FIGURE 3.33: Axial section of the chest PMCT in soft tissue window at level T8 depicting the following: 1. Right atrium, 2. Right ventricle, 3. Left ventricle, 4. Mitral valve, 5. Left atrium, 6. Interatrial septum, 7. Esophagus, 8. Descending aorta, 9. Pericardial fat.

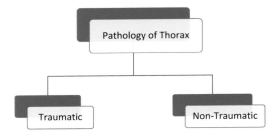

FIGURE 3.34: The pathology of thorax classification based on biomechanics.

from a height. There are various methods of classification of these thoracic injuries.

Injuries to the chest may be classified into:

1. **Closed injuries:** Closed injuries can occur as a result of blunt force or compressive force to the chest. Contusion or concussion to the internal organs can occur even without any external injury marks. In compressive force, as in accidents, rupture of the different organs occur between the sternum, rib cage, and spine.
2. **Open injuries:** Stab wounds and gunshots are the most common open injuries to the chest. Lacerations to internal organs also occur as a result of a fractured rib piercing the underlying organs and also the overlying skin.

Thoracic injuries can present as rib fractures, clavicle fractures, sternal fractures, thoracic vertebra fractures, pneumothorax, haemothorax, haemopneumothorax, cardiac tamponade, etc.

- Rib fractures

Rib fractures are the most common form of blunt trauma to the chest accounting for about 67.3% of trauma. It is common both among adults and children. Apart from autopsy examination, radiological examination helps to detect these fractures in an easier way (Figures 3.35 and 3.36), and PMCT helps in understanding the 3D distribution of the fracture and also the extent of the fracture, which is difficult with only autopsy examination. Ribs can fracture at any point, but they have a tendency to fracture at the point of maximum curvature or the place where force is applied. The rib fractures mechanism can be due to primary impact at the injury site or due to the compression of the thoracic cage. The best way to differentiate these mechanisms of rib fractures is to assess the pattern of distribution of these fractures and also examine the injury to the underlying viscera or mediastinal structures. In cases of fracture due to direct primary impact, the underlying viscera will also show features of local trauma, and the pattern of distribution of rib fracture will be more localized. Cardiopulmonary resuscitation (CPR) is also one of the most common causes for getting fractures in autopsy cases, which could be peri-mortem or post-mortem in origin, and the pattern is usually due to compression of the thoracic cage. The other mechanisms of rib fracture, apart from blunt trauma, could be due to penetrating instruments or objects/foreign bodies, like in the cases of stab or gunshot injury. The most common ribs fractured in trauma are usually the middle ribs, mostly from

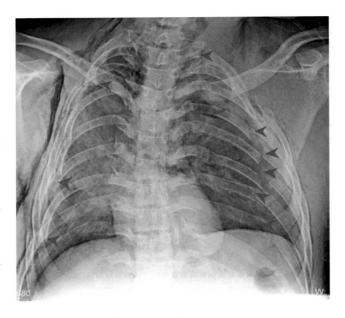

FIGURE 3.35: Chest X-ray AP view showing multiple rib fractures over bilateral ribs.

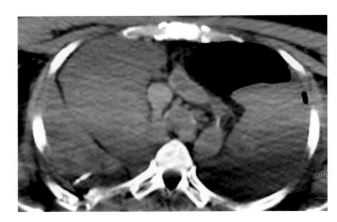

FIGURE 3.36: Axial section of PMCT thorax showing fractured rib on the right side in a case of fall from height.

the fourth to eighth ribs. Fractures of the first and second ribs are usually associated with injury to the neurovascular bundles closely associated with them. These broken ribs can cause secondary findings and injuries like pneumothorax, haemothorax, haemo-pneumothorax, lung contusion or puncture, and thoracic and even thoracic instability (flail chest). As rib fractures are very painful in ante-mortem conditions, they may result in shallow breathing and also retention of secretions. Flial chest or thoracic instability occurs due to heavy blunt force and is defined as 'two or more contiguous rib fractures with two or more breaks per rib' (Figure 3.37). This injury creates a mobile segment in the thoracic wall which moves paradoxically with the rest of the uninjured chest wall during respiration. Flail chest is associated with a high percentage of morbidity and mortality.

- Clavicle fractures

The clavicle is one of the most commonly fractured bones. The clavicle acts as a bridge between

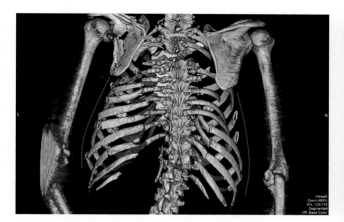

FIGURE 3.37: Volume rendering 3D image of the skeleton showing multiple contiguous rib fractures with two or more breaks per rib indicating a flial chest in a case of RTA.

the axial skeleton and the upper limb; hence any undue external force can cause a fracture, which is easily noted in the mechanism of injury causing such fractures. The clavicle is the first bone of the human body to develop, which by intramembranous ossification, starts ossifying in the fifth week of fetal life. Similar to all long bones, except for the fact it is placed horizontally, the clavicle has a medial and lateral epiphysis, but it lacks a well-defined medullary cavity. The mechanisms of clavicle fracture include a direct blow to the shoulder or blunt force on the shoulder due to a fall on the shoulder. The other common mechanism is the transmission of force which happens when a person falls with an outstretched hand; here, the force is transmitted from the periphery to the axial skeleton, and when this deforming force crosses the threshold of elasticity and plasticity of the bone it results in a fracture. In cases where the individual has osteoporosis, the strength and durability of the bone are less and hence fractures happen at even trivial forces. Radiological techniques like X-ray and CT scans (Figures 3.38 and 3.39) help for easier examination of the clavicle fracture compared to an autopsy examination. The fractures of the clavicle are classified into three types based on the position of the fracture:

i. Type I: Fracture occurring in the middle third of the clavicle (Figure 3.38).

ii. Type II: Fracture occurring in the lateral third of the clavicle.

iii. Type III: Fracture occurring in the medial third of the clavicle.

• Sternal fractures

The sternum, also referred to as the breast bone, is the central anterior bone of the rib cage. Fractures of the sternum usually occur due to RTAs, assault, sports injuries, falls from a height, etc. The mechanism of injury that is usually associated with sternal fracture can be categorized into direct or indirect trauma. The direct traumatic mechanism for sternal fractures includes deceleration injuries and blunt trauma to the anterior chest wall in RTA cases due to the striking of the steering wheel or dashboard or any other part of the vehicle to the anterior chest and

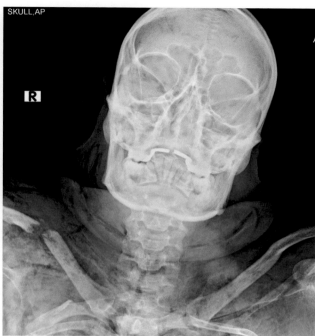

FIGURE 3.38: X-ray anteroposterior view showing fracture-dislocation in the middle one-third of the right clavicle, which is the commonest type (Type I).

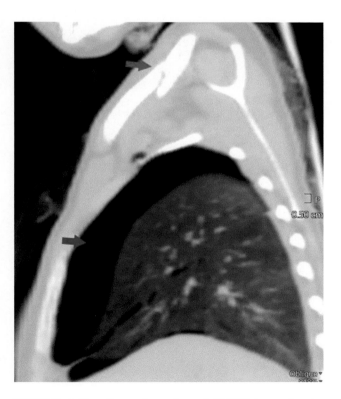

FIGURE 3.39: Coronal section of PMCT lung showing fractured clavicle (red arrow) along with pneumothorax (blue arrow).

in cases of falls from height (Figure 3.40) or assault. Seatbelt use, which protects the occupant from ejection, also restricts the anterior chest and shoulder, which results in direct transfer of force to the sternum, which can cause a fracture. Contact sports also include direct, blunt force trauma to the sternum resulting in fracture. Direct force by sharp force is rarely encountered and may be seen in cases of stabbing to the chest (Figure 3.41) or penetration by a sharp object. The indirect force transfer mechanism of sternal fractures includes cases of insufficiency fractures, stress fractures, and pathological fractures. Insufficiency fractures are those where the fracture occurs spontaneously in patients with anatomical defects or disorders of the ribcage or vertebra, like in severe thoracic kyphosis. Pathological fractures mostly occur due to the pathology of the bone, like osteoporosis seen in elderly patients, post-menopausal

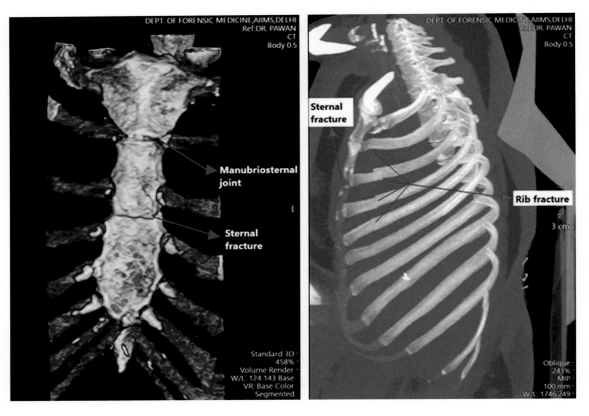

FIGURE 3.40:   Sternal fracture at the level of third rib attachment with adjoining rib fracture in a case of blunt trauma chest due to fall from height.

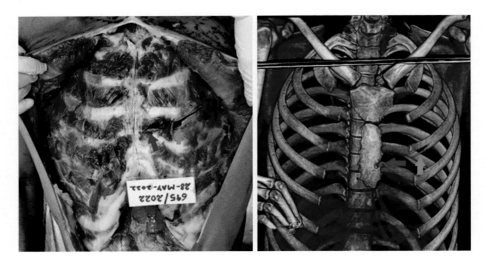

FIGURE 3.41:   Sternum fracture in a case of stab to the chest, the gross and comparative volume rendering 3D reconstruction image of the skeleton shows the fracture of the left side of the sternum in the lower half along with a fracture of the adjoining left third rib.

women, and patients on certain long-term medications like steroid therapy. It can also occur in cases of bone lesions due to tumours or metastasis of the sternum bone. Stress fractures, on the other hand, are seen in cases where people have no acute trauma and occur due to strenuous, repetitive upper body exercise, like in athletes and bodybuilders. Fractures of the sternum also occur due to iatrogenic causes during the peri-mortem or post-mortem period due to the chest compression procedures of cardiopulmonary resuscitation. Fractures of the sternum also show the possibility of underlying internal injuries of vital organs like the heart and lungs.

- Thoracic vertebra fractures

The thoracic vertebra is an important part of the thoracic skeleton. The fracture of these vertebrae occurs due to blunt trauma force commonly and rarely due to penetrating objects like bullets. The vertebra is a strong compact bone, and its fracture requires a significant external force unless the bone has some pathological insufficiency due to osteoporosis, tumour, or metastasis. Fractures of the thoracic vertebra can be classified as follows:

  i.   Compression fracture.
  ii. Burst fracture.
  iii. Flexion-distraction fracture.
  iv. Fracture-dislocation.

Compression fracture

This is usually a type of insufficiency thoracic vertebra fracture, which is usually encountered in cases with a weakened bone condition like osteoporosis or tumours of the bone. The thoracic vertebra can hold and withstand significant external strain and pressure. In cases of weakened bones, any sudden heavy force beyond the threshold of the weakened bone causes a fracture in which the vertebra collapses. If this collapse is limited to the anterior part of the vertebra, it forms a wedge shape and hence is termed a 'wedge fracture'.

Burst fracture

This type of thoracic fracture occurs due to heavy external force due to RTAs. Here the vertebra gets crushed due to the extreme force transmitted in these cases. In a burst fracture, the disruption of the bone occurs at multiple places, contrary to a compression fracture, where disruption occurs at one point. Due to the disruption at multiple places, the tiny bone fragments can also cause injury to the spinal cord, which needs to be examined.

Flexion-distraction fracture

This type of fracture occurs when a person is suddenly pushed forward, like in a decelerating car when the individual is wearing a seatbelt for restriction of ejection. In these cases, the spine bends forward during sudden forward movement, which causes severe stress on the spine and, beyond the threshold limit, causes fracture of either a single vertebra or vertebrae. According to the three-column concept of vertebral fractures, the flexion-distraction type of fracture occurs in the middle and posterior columns.

Fracture-dislocation

This is a category of vertebral fractures where the mechanism involved can be any of the above-mentioned types, but there should be significant movement/dislocation of the vertebral column segment due to the fracture being considered a fracture-dislocation (Figure 3.42). This type of fracture usually involves all three columns of the vertebra and this category of fracture is highly unstable clinically.

Another method of classification of the thoracic, lumbar, or thoracolumbar vertebrae is termed the Denis classification. This method divides the vertebra into three columns (Figure 3.43) to assess the fracture, which is:

  i.   Anterior/front column.
  ii. Middle column.
  iii. Posterior/back column.

This method of classification of the thoracic vertebra fractures helps for the easy visualization and understanding of the severity of fractures and also

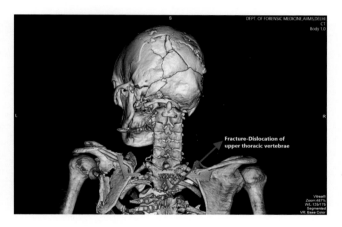

FIGURE 3.42: Volume rendering 3D image in a case of a railway accident showing fracture dislocation of the upper thoracic vertebrae along with fractures of other bones.

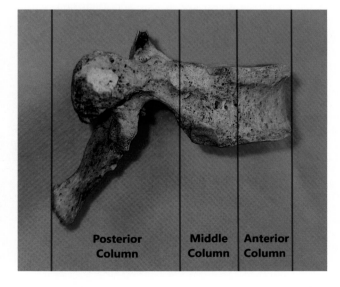

FIGURE 3.43: Denis classification of thoracic vertebra fracture by division of vertebra into three columns: Anterior, middle, and posterior.

the reason for some of these fractures being unstable and damaging the spinal cord more than others.

 - **Anterior/front column**

   This includes the intervertebral disc and the vertebral body's anterior half; it also includes the anterior longitudinal ligament.

 - **Middle column**

   This column is an important segment involved in the stability of the spine and includes the posterior half of the vertebral body, the intervertebral disc, and the posterior longitudinal ligament. Injury in this column is usually associated with damage to the spinal cord due to its close proximity.

 - **Posterior/back column**

   This column includes the parts of the vertebra behind the vertebral body, which includes the pedicles, lamina, facet joints, transverse process, and spinous process.

• Trauma to the lungs

   Lung trauma can be direct or indirect depending upon the type of force applied. In mild cases of trauma, only ribs are fractured, but sometimes it produces minor mechanical injury to the pleura along with contusion or laceration of the lungs produced by the fractured ends of the ribs.

Pulmonary contusion and laceration

A pulmonary contusion is a condition where there is an injury to the interstitium or alveoli of the lung. In simple terms, it is a bruise of the lung parenchyma, usually due to non-penetrating blunt trauma to the chest. This blunt trauma results in damage to the capillaries of the lung, and because of its blood and oedema, fluid accumulates in the lung parenchyma. There is no break or cut in the overlying lung tissue differentiating it from lung laceration. Pulmonary contusion is seen both among adults and children in cases of blunt chest trauma, but children are more prone to develop lung contusions due to the higher flexibility of the chest wall in them. In cases of blunt trauma to the chest, the prevalence of lung contusion ranges from

around 17 to 70%. The lung contusion severity can range from mild to severe, and sometimes these can potentially be lethal. The fatality rate of pulmonary contusion is considered to be between 14 and 40%. In cases where pulmonary contusion is seen, it usually has accompanying injuries. In cases where individuals survive after sustaining pulmonary contusion, they have an increased risk of developing a few complications like pneumonia and acute respiratory distress syndrome (ARDS), and in the long run, they also have a higher risk of developing respiratory disability.

Pathology of pulmonary contusion

The contusion of the lung parenchyma occurs due to disruption of the capillaries present in the alveolar walls and septa of the lung, and this, in turn, causes blood to leak into the alveolar spaces and the interstitium. This disruption of capillaries in the lung can occur due to direct, blunt trauma or even due to the shock waves associated with an explosion. Lung contusions are more common in the posterior part of the lung and also in the lower lobe. The PMCT view of lung contusions looks like focal, non-segmental (typically crescentic) areas of parenchymal opacification (Figures 3.44–3.47), usually peripheral in the location, which are sometimes associated with a surrounding rib fracture, which helps in considering its possibility by PMCT. A CT scan, in comparison to an X-ray, is more sensitive and can identify a pulmonary contusion almost immediately after its occurrence; however, it becomes more appreciable if the individual has survived for 24–48 hours after the injury. If the pulmonary contusion is visible on PMCT but is not appreciable on a chest x-ray then usually it could be a fresh injury or a less severe pulmonary contusion. If the overlying lung tissue remains intact, it is a contusion, and when there is a break in the integrity of the overlying lung tissue, it is called a laceration. A laceration may lead to leakage of air and/or blood into the pleural cavity, causing pneumothorax or haemopneumothorax, respectively.

Mechanism of pulmonary contusion and laceration

The exact mechanism of pulmonary contusion, though poorly understood, is generally considered that the lung tissue gets crushed when there is inward bending of the chest wall

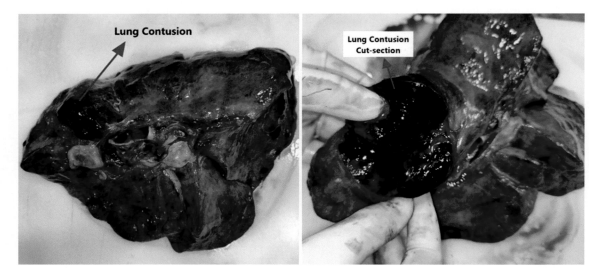

FIGURE 3.44: Lung contusion over the posterior aspect of the right lung in the upper lobe, cut-section showing the accumulation of blood in the lung parenchyma.

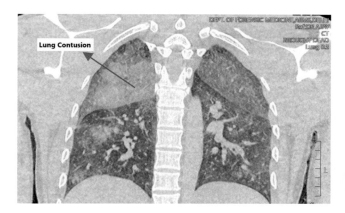

FIGURE 3.45: PMCT image of the chest, lung window in the same case as Figure 3.40 showing the contusion in the upper lobe right lung posterior part next to the vertebrae as a focal opacification of the parenchyma.

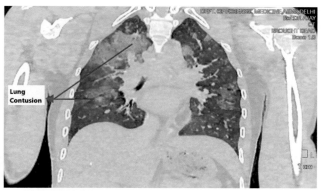

FIGURE 3.47: PMCT image of the chest and lung window in the same case as Figure 3.40 and Figure 3.42 showing the contusion in the lower lobe and upper lobe right lung posterior part next to the vertebrae as a focal opacification of the parenchyma.

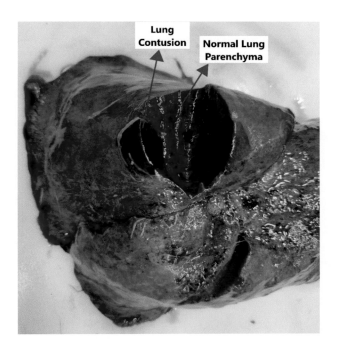

FIGURE 3.46: Cut-section of lung showing the difference between normal lung parenchyma and lung contusion in the lower lobe just below the fissure. The contused part shows the accumulation of blood in the parenchyma.

due to direct, blunt force. This general principle, however, fails to explain pulmonary contusion in cases of explosion victims. The other mechanisms which have been proposed to explain pulmonary contusion include:

    i. The inertial effect.
   ii. The spalling effect.
  iii. The implosion effect.

The inertial effect

In the inertial effect mechanism, it is proposed that as the lung tissue and the hilar tissues have different densities, they will have relatively different rates of acceleration and

deceleration. This difference will cause the lighter alveolar tissue of the lung to get sheared by the heavier hilar structures. This effect is similar to diffuse axonal injury occurring in cases of head injury.

The spalling effect

In the spalling effect mechanism, it is proposed that there exists a gas–liquid type interface with air in the alveoli. When a shock wave hits the lung, the lung tissue bursts or gets sheared at these air–alveoli interfaces. The spalling effect happens at such interfaces where there is a large difference in densities causing the particles of denser tissues, i.e., the alveolar wall, to be spalled (thrown) into the less dense particles that are the air in the alveoli. This bursting effect/spalling effect causes disruption of the capillaries resulting in blood accumulating in the parenchyma and alveoli.

The implosion effect

In the implosion effect mechanism, it is proposed that when a pressure wave hits a lung, the bubbles of air in the parenchyma, especially the alveoli, first implode and, in a rebound phenomenon, expand beyond their original volume, in turn causing tiny explosions which damage the lung tissues. These tiny explosions also cause the disruption of the capillaries, causing bleeding into the parenchyma and pulmonary contusion or laceration.

Pulmonary contusions occurring at the site of the impact is coup injury due to direct positive force and any of the above-mentioned mechanism, and a contrecoup contusion may also occur opposite to the primary impact site. This is due to the shock waves travelling through the chest, hitting the curved end of the chest wall and reflecting back onto the lung tissue in a concentrated manner, thus disrupting the capillaries and causing a pulmonary contusion.

Pulmonary Laceration

Pulmonary laceration occurs due to the macroscopic disruption of the architecture of the lung parenchyma (Figure 3.48). This occurs due to the tear/cut/split of the parenchyma. This cut or break results in blood accumulating at the site, causing a haematoma without any interspersed lung tissue, which is different from the pulmonary contusion, where blood accumulates in the alveoli within the lung tissue.

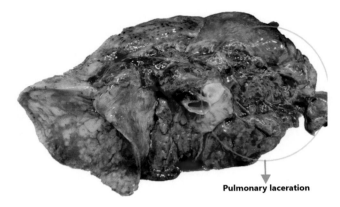

FIGURE 3.48: A gross examination of the lung in a case of a road traffic accident with blunt trauma chest showing the pulmonary laceration over the upper inner aspect of the left lung.

Pulmonary lacerations are mostly associated with surrounding contusions as the mechanism of occurrence is similar. Pulmonary lacerations are also common among children due to the highly flexible rib cage, which yields to external forces. Sometimes after there is a tear in the lung parenchyma causing a laceration, there can be blood filling the disrupted part, which is known as a haematocele; in certain other cases, the disrupted part may be filled with air which is called a pneumatocele (Figures 3.49 and 3.50) or in certain other cases both air and blood may fill the space. In PMCT, due to the accumulation and organization of blood without the intervening lung tissue, lacerations are better appreciated than contusions. If the person survives for 24–48 hours after injury, it is better appreciated.

Pulmonary laceration classification

Wagner et al. in 1988 classified pulmonary lacerations into four categories based on the CT findings of the injury and also the mechanism of injury:

- **Type I – Compression rupture:** This is the most common type of pulmonary laceration recorded, and it usually occurs as a central lung lesion of 2–8 cm in size (Figure 3.51).
- **Type II – Compression shear:** This type of pulmonary laceration is seen in the para-vertebral region of the lung in the lower part. The injury occurs from sudden compression of the lower chest by lateral compression, which causes the lung to suffer from a shear injury against the spine leading to the injury.
- **Type III – Direct puncture/rib penetration:** This type of pulmonary laceration occurs when a fractured rib penetrates the lung disrupting its integrity.
- **Type IV – Adhesion tears:** This type of injury occurs when there is a pre-existing pleuro-pulmonary adhesion, and on sudden chest trauma, pulmonary laceration happens at these sites when the parenchymal attachment part is stretched beyond its elastic limit (Figure 3.52).

Virtual autopsy findings

Pulmonary lacerations are most of the time similar in appearance to pulmonary contusions, but there is additional disruption of the lung parenchyma, which can be observed. This injury is also associated with surrounding rib fractures or pneumothorax, or haemothorax (Figures 3.50–3.52). PMCT shows the areas of pulmonary laceration as a round or oval cavity instead of linear deformity due to the presence of normal pulmonary elastic recoil; this causes the lung tissues surrounding the pulmonary laceration to pull back from the tissue defect caused by disruption.

Lung penetrating injury

A lung penetrating injury occurs due to an abrupt, direct, focal application of mechanical force by an external object which could be a projectile, knife, etc. The damage in this category of injury occurs to all the structures coming in the path of the motion of the projectile or knife; this includes the skin, subcutaneous tissue, muscles, and the underlying lung (Figures 3.53–3.55). The injury's extent depends on the nature of the

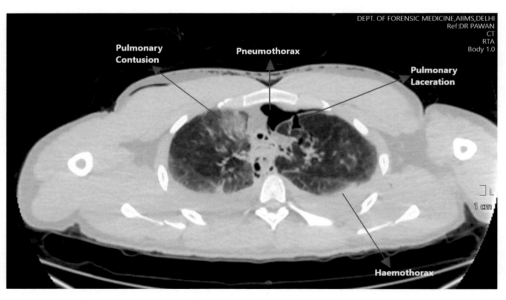

FIGURE 3.49: PMCT image of the axial chest section, lung window in a case of an RTA with blunt trauma chest showing the pulmonary laceration over the anterior aspect of the left lung and pulmonary contusion over the anterior aspect of the right lung. There are associated pneumothorax and haemothorax.

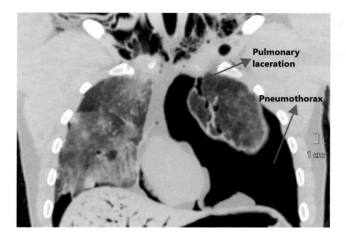

FIGURE 3.50: PMCT image of the axial chest section, lung window in a case of an RTA with blunt trauma chest showing the pulmonary laceration over the upper inner aspect of the left lung in the same case as Figure 3.49, there is associated pneumothorax.

penetrating object, the amount of energy which is transferred to the body tissues by the object, the area of transfer of force, deformability of the body tissue, density of the encountered body structures, etc. The penetrating lung injury may be categorized into low-, medium-, and high-velocity wounds. Low-velocity wounds include injuries due to knives, medium-velocity injuries include those due to bullets or handguns, and high-velocity injuries are due to rifles and military weapons. Bullet injuries cause damage to the tissues along its path, similar to

knife injuries; in addition, bullet injuries cause damage to the adjacent structures due to the mechanism of cavitation and the production of shock waves as the bullet traverses its path.

Pneumothorax

Pneumothorax is an abnormal condition where air collects in the pleural space located between the lung and the chest wall. This collection of air in the pleural space usually causes partial or complete collapse of the lung. This leakage of air into the pleural cavity can occur due to spontaneous leaks or trauma or sometimes due to iatrogenic procedures in the hospital. During the autopsy, pneumothorax is usually encountered in cases of trauma to the chest, which include RTA cases, falls-from-a-height cases, assault cases, penetrating chest injury cases, like stab or gunshot cases, and bomb blast cases.

During the autopsy, there are a few techniques, like creating a small water pool and puncturing the chest wall or using a syringe with water to observe for air bubbles. The drawback of these tests is it is difficult to observe air bubbles or pneumothorax in cases of small air pockets and loculated air pockets. Radiological examination in autopsies like X-ray or PMCT makes identification of pneumothorax very simple and also helps in measuring the volume of pneumothorax and co-relates with overlying and underlying injuries like rib fracture, lung laceration, etc.

Pneumothorax, based on aetiology, is classified into:

i. **Primary spontaneous pneumothorax**: Here, pneumothorax occurs without any apparent cause like trauma or disease of the lungs. It is usually seen in young, thin, and tall men in their 20s.

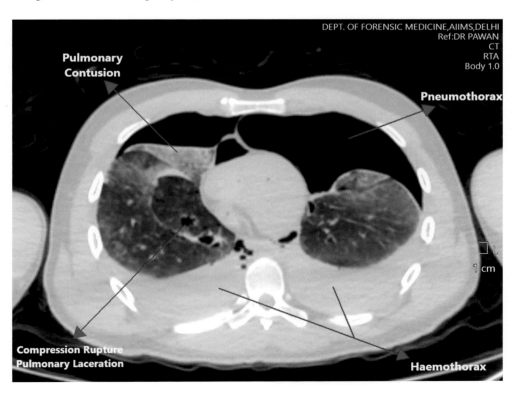

FIGURE 3.51: PMCT image of the axial chest section, lung window in a case of a road traffic accident with blunt trauma chest showing the compression rupture type pulmonary laceration in the central lung region of the right lung. There is pulmonary contusion over the anterior aspect of the right lung along with bilateral pneumothorax and haemothorax.

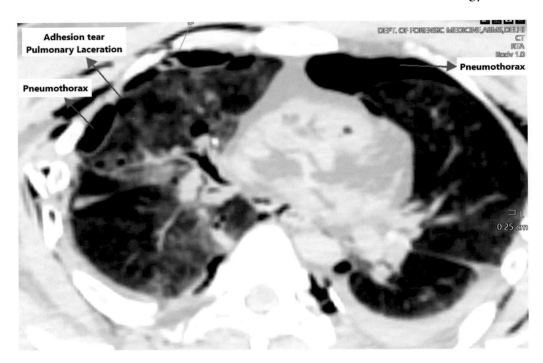

FIGURE 3.52: PMCT image of the axial chest section, lung window in a case of a road traffic accident with blunt trauma chest showing the adhesion tear type pulmonary laceration in the right lung with associated bilateral pneumothorax.

ii. **Secondary spontaneous pneumothorax:** Here, pneumothorax occurs in cases of existing lung diseases, e.g., COPD, asthma, tuberculosis, etc.

    Catamenial pneumothorax: It is a rare type of secondary spontaneous pneumothorax occurring due to intrathoracic endometriosis seen in cases of pre-menopausal women or post-menopausal women on estrogen.

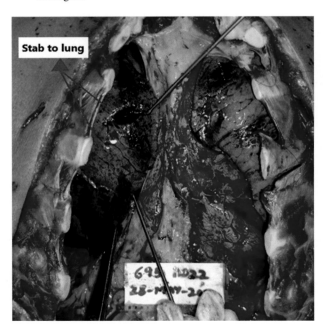

FIGURE 3.53: A gross examination of the lung in a case of a stab to the chest showing two stab injuries over the anterior aspect of the right lung.

iii. **Traumatic pneumothorax:** It is a commonly encountered variety in forensic and general medical practice. It occurs due to injury to the lung parenchyma, causing leakage of air into the pleural cavity. The injury can occur due to blunt trauma or penetrating injuries.

    Iatrogenic pneumothorax: It is a type of traumatic pneumothorax, but here the trauma occurs due to medical interventions like cardiopulmonary resuscitation, transthoracic needle aspiration, mechanical ventilation, etc.

Pathophysiology of pneumothorax

Pneumothorax is abnormal air collection in the pleural cavity as the pleural cavity is usually in negative pressure compared to the atmospheric pressure. Any break in the overlying chest wall and parietal pleura can cause air to enter from the atmosphere, and any break in the lung parenchyma and visceral pleura causes the air to enter from the lungs.

Virtual autopsy interpretation of pneumothorax

X-ray

    Pneumothorax being air in the pleural cavity is appreciated as a dark area in the chest cavity peripheral to the visceral pleura shadow, which appears as a very sharp, thin white line. The dark area peripheral to it lacks lung markings. The collapse of the lung is also appreciated along with the pneumothorax. The pneumothorax is better appreciated in erect X-rays, but the same is not possible in cases of post-mortem radiography.

PMCT

    PMCT examination of the chest in the lung window can help in the easy identification of pneumothorax. The examination of the axial, coronal, and sagittal sections helps in the localization of the pneumothorax, even in cases of loculated pneumothorax. PMCT has the

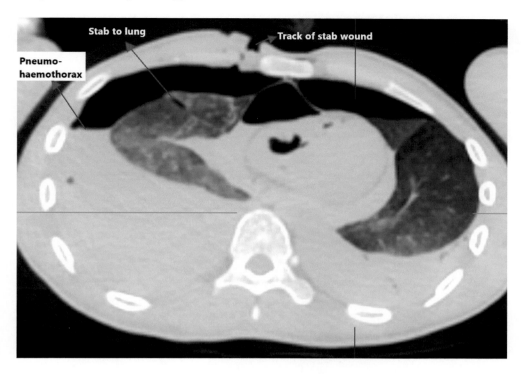

FIGURE 3.54: Axial section of chest PMCT in lung window at the level of an upper stab wound in the same case of Figure 3.53 showing stab injury to right lung along with bilateral pneumohaemothorax.

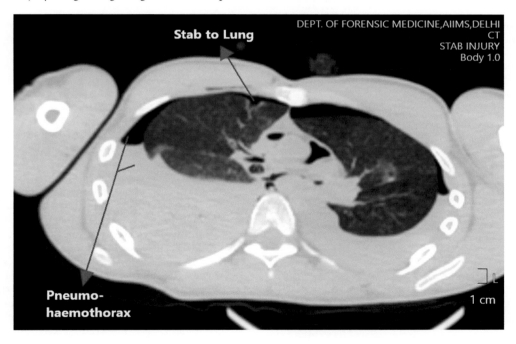

FIGURE 3.55: Axial section of chest PMCT in lung window at the level of a lower stab wound in the same case of Figure 3.53 showing a stab injury to the right lung along with bilateral pneumohaemothorax.

advantage of measuring the volume of pneumothorax as well (Figure 3.56).

Tension Pneumothorax

Tension pneumothorax is a type of fatal pneumothorax where there is a progressive rise in intrapleural pressure, which causes the lung to collapse and also shift the mediastinal structures to the opposite side (Figure 3.57) and also drop in venous return. In tension pneumothorax, the air continues to get into the pleural space with each inspiration, and it fails to exit, similar to a valve mechanism.

Haemothorax

Haemothorax is a condition where blood accumulates in the pleural cavity. Each of the pleural cavities can accommodate

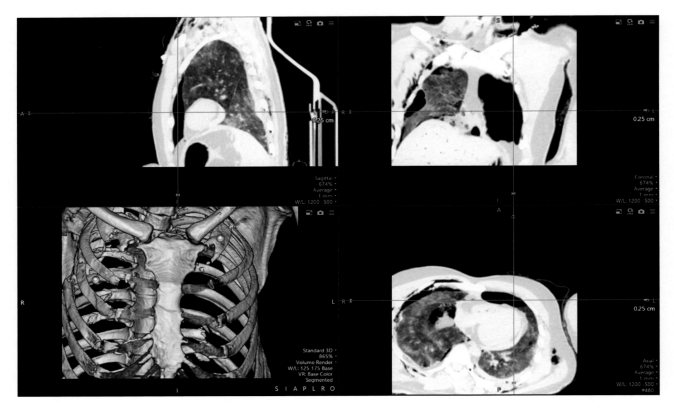

FIGURE 3.56: Volume rendering 3D reconstructed image showing multiple fractures of the ribs and pneumothorax can be appreciated with all three views, i.e., sagittal, coronal, and axial, with full crosshair showing the exact location of pneumothorax.

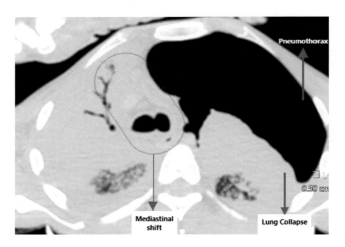

FIGURE 3.57: Axial section of chest PMCT in lung window showing left side tension pneumothorax, the collapse of lung and mediastinal shift to right side appreciated by a shift of tracheal bifurcation.

almost 1500 ml of blood. PMCT examination in the lung window and soft tissue window will help to locate the haemothorax and also in measuring the volume. The haemothorax can be classified based on the aetiology into:

i. **Traumatic haemothorax:** This occurs due to blunt force impact or penetrating trauma to the chest. Blunt trauma to the chest usually causes rib fracture and injury to the intercostal vessels or the lung parenchyma, rarely can

also cause the disruption or transection of large vessels like the aorta leading to massive blood accumulation (Figures 3.58–3.60). In cases of penetrating trauma, the injury directly to blood vessels or the lung parenchyma can cause bleeding into the pleural cavity. In rare cases, people on anti-coagulants or those with bleeding disorders may also develop haemothorax following trivial trauma.

ii. **Iatrogenic haemothorax:** This is a type of traumatic haemothorax where the trauma is induced due to hospital treatment or interventions like venous or arterial catheterization, a biopsy of lung or any mediastinal structures, chest tube placements, etc.

iii. **Non-traumatic haemothorax:** This is a type of haemothorax where blood leaks into the pleural cavity spontaneously due to some pathology in the thoracic structures. The pathology could be a tumour of the thoracic structures, bleeding disorders, or even a spontaneous haemothorax without any identifiable pathology. In certain conditions like Ehler–Danlos syndrome, haemophilia, neurofibromatosis type 1, Rendu–Osler–Weber syndrome, etc., there can be a structural defect of the vessels which can lead to spontaneous disruption or tearing of the blood vessels causing haemothorax. Catamenial haemothorax is yet another variety of non-traumatic haemothorax where due to thoracic endometriosis, there could be blood in the pleural cavity synchronous with the menstrual cycle.

Pneumohaemothorax

Pneumohaemothorax is a combination of pneumothorax and haemothorax, where the pleural cavity contains both air

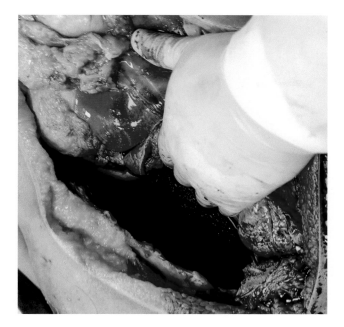

FIGURE 3.58: A gross examination of the chest cavity during autopsy showing massive haemothorax.

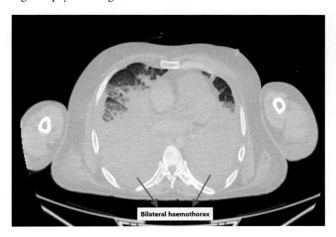

FIGURE 3.59: Axial section of chest PMCT in lung window showing bilateral haemothorax in the same case as shown in Figure 3.58.

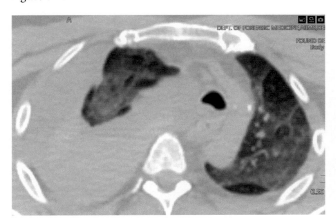

FIGURE 3.60: Axial section of chest PMCT in lung window in a fall from a height case showing right-sided haemothorax and a collapsed right lung.

and blood (Figures 3.61–3.63). Pneumohaemothorax usually occurs due to trauma to the chest which could be blunt trauma or penetrating objects. It occurs due to pathologies of thoracic organs like tumours or bleeding disorders, or endometriosis is very rare in occurrence. Pneumohaemothorax occurring spontaneously is also reported in the literature but is of very rare occurrence.

Pleural effusion

Pleural effusion is a collection of fluid in the pleural space, and it is a very common post-mortem finding. The amount of pleural fluid collected depends on the difference between the hydrostatic pressure and oncotic pressure of the systemic circulation, pulmonary circulation and the pleural space. The fluid collected in the space is also due to dynamic fluid homeostasis involving both the parietal and visceral pleura (Figures 3.64–3.67). The parietal pleura usually plays a major role in the production and absorption of a fluid; however, in cases of left-sided heart failure, the major role is played by the visceral pleura in production. In normal conditions, the rate of production and absorption of the pleural fluid is in equilibrium which is normally 0.2 mL/kg/hr; any disturbance in this equilibrium

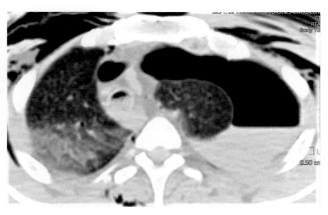

FIGURE 3.61: Axial section of chest PMCT in lung window showing pneumohaemothorax on the left side in a case of blunt trauma chest.

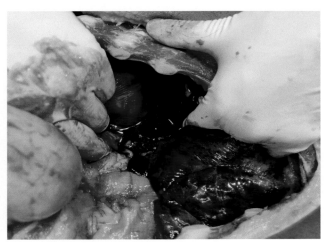

FIGURE 3.62: Gross autopsy examination of the chest in a case of blunt trauma to the chest shows the presence of haemothorax with the collapse of the right lung.

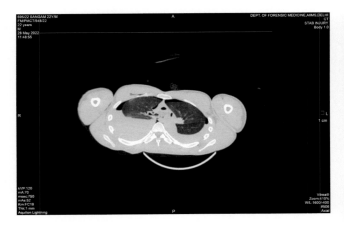

FIGURE 3.63: Axial section of chest PMCT in the lung window in the same case as Figure 3.56 showing pneumohaemothorax on the left side in a case of blunt trauma chest.

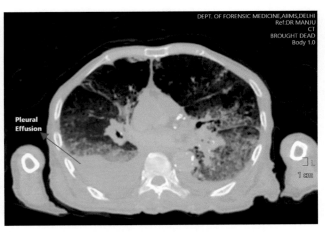

FIGURE 3.65: Axial section of chest PMCT in lung window in the same case as Figure 3.64 showing bilateral pleural effusion with more on the right side.

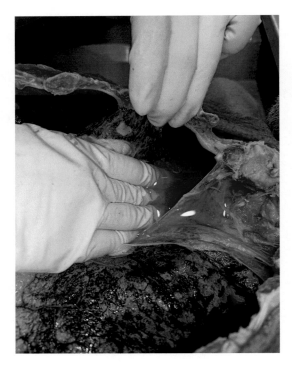

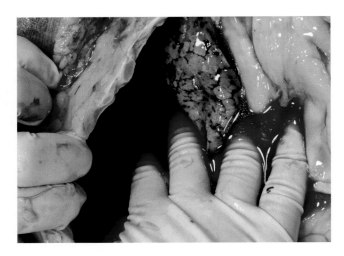

FIGURE 3.66: Gross autopsy examination of the chest in a case of sepsis with bleeding manifestations showing blood-tinged pleural effusion on both sides.

FIGURE 3.64: Gross autopsy examination of the chest in a case showing straw-coloured pleural effusion on the right side.

causes pleural fluid to be accumulated. Pleural effusion is of two types:

- **Transudative pleural effusion:** This is caused by fluid leaking into the pleural cavity due to low oncotic pressure (blood protein count, e.g., in hypoalbuminemia) or due to increased pressure in the blood vessels (e.g., heart failure).
- **Exudative pleural effusion:** This is caused by pathologies like lung infection, injury, tumour, blocked blood vessels, or lymph vessels.

Radiological investigation of the pleural effusion in the post-mortem can be done by X-ray, ultrasound, and PMCT. In the post-mortem, a supine X-ray anteroposterior view is

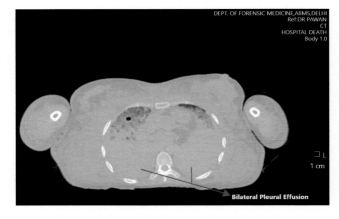

FIGURE 3.67: Axial section of chest PMCT in lung window in the same case as Figure 3.66 showing bilateral pleural effusion.

commonly obtained. In living persons, a posteroanterior is the preferred X-ray view as it can detect a pleural effusion of as low as a volume of 200 mL; if the effusion is even less, then a lateral view is preferred as it can detect effusions of even 50 mL. This view is quite difficult to obtain in post-mortem and also minimal effusion can occur as a post-mortem feature. Ultrasound is a very sensitive technique for pleural effusion detection, but post-mortem ultrasound is rarely used. PMCT is a common technique followed for post-mortem evaluation of the pleural effusion. Transudates have a lower HU compared to the exudates, though this may be useful in considering the autopsy surgeon also should consider the fact that there is a lot of overlap between the HU of transudates and exudates. HU of transudates studies show cutoff value for CHF taken as ≤8.5 HU showed a sensitivity and specificity of 84.6% and 81.2%, respectively; the cutoff value for exudative effusion taken as ≥8.5 HU the sensitivity and specificity was 85% and 86.7% respectively. The entire effusions usually lie in the HU range of 4–15. Pleural effusion can sometimes also be confused with haemothorax on PMCT; this can be differentiated by checking for the settling phenomenon of blood-causing layers, which is better appreciated in the soft tissue window (Figures 3.66 and 3.67).

- **Trauma to the heart**: Trauma to the heart can be due to blunt forces or penetrating injuries. Blunt force can be due to direct transmission of the force to the heart or by compression between the sternum and spine and also due to deceleration injuries. A cardiac contusion is common in blunt trauma but is difficult to appreciate in cases of PMCT in comparison with cardiac laceration, which can be easily recognized due to a breach in the continuity. There may also be pericardial effusion which is fluid collection in the pericardial sac, or cardiac tamponade due to the collection of blood following the laceration. The most common sites for traumatic rupture of the heart are the left ventricles and papillary muscles, while the right auricle has the least probability.

Penetrating injuries such as stab wounds (Figures 3.68 and 3.69) and a gunshot to the heart (Figure 3.70) are easily appreciated on PMCT due to the characteristic break in the continuity in relation to the penetrating object. The track of the wound can also be defined with the help of PMCT.

- **Pericardial effusion and cardiac tamponade**

Pericardial effusion is the accumulation of fluid in the pericardial sac. When a great volume of fluid accumulates in the pericardial sac to a point where it compromises the normal expansion of the heart, usually occurring due to the cardiac rupture is called cardiac tamponade (Figure 3.71). In cardiac tamponade, the raised intrapericardial pressure results in decreased cardiac filling, restricted expansion and decreased cardiac output, causing it to be a fatal condition.

Non-traumatic thorax pathologies

Sudden death is a challenging field in determining the cause of death, and in the thorax cavity, the lungs and heart play a major role as they are vital organs. But PMCT examination is a bit different from the clinical scenario as changes occur in the body after death which resembles some pathologies. These changes are hence to be kept in mind before reaching a

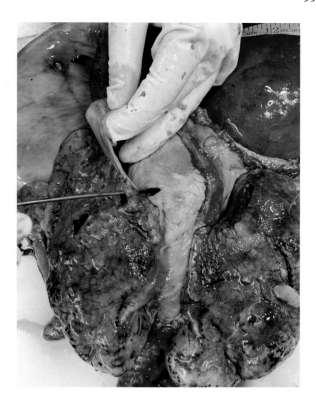

FIGURE 3.68: Gross autopsy examination of the chest in a case of multiple stabs to the chest with a knife.

conclusion. Important normal post-mortem findings of PMCT are hence discussed below.

Normal PMCT findings

1. **Post-mortem hypostasis:** Hypostasis is a commonly seen post-mortem change that affects the whole body, and it is appreciated in the skin as well as internal organs like the lung parenchyma. It appears as ground-glass opacities generally in the dependent part of the organ and is seen as distinct level demarcation, which is seen even near the fissures. Dependent parts of the lung are determined by the position of the body as found, i.e., supine, right and left laterally, or face down. So if the body found was supine, then the post-mortem hypostasis is seen as hyperdense areas of opacification at the posterior aspect of the lung (Figure 3.72).

2. **Decomposition-related pneumothorax:** It can also occur as a normal PMCT finding in decomposed cases and should not be confused with pathological pneumothorax. This could be differentiated by the presence of other signs of decomposition seen in the PMCT, like the presence of decomposition gas in other cavities, blood vessels, muscles, subcutaneous tissues, etc., and also by the external examination to check for the degree of decomposition (Figure 3.73). Mild pneumothorax may also be seen in cases with a history of cardiopulmonary resuscitation attempts with or without rib fractures which need to be considered.

3. **Layered separation of blood clots in great vessels:** Sedimentation or layering separation of the blood from its cellular components as a result of gravity creates a fluid level of different densities (Figure 3.74). This pattern

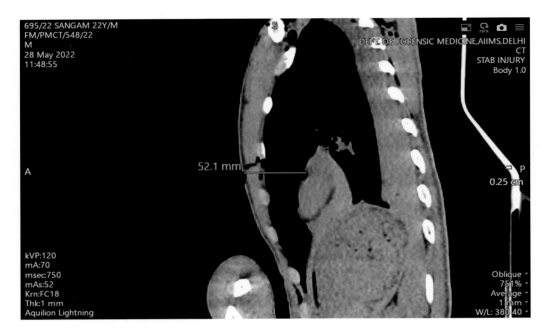

FIGURE 3.69: Axial section of chest PMCT in soft tissue window in the same case as Figure 3.68 showing the stab injury to the heart as a break in the continuity.

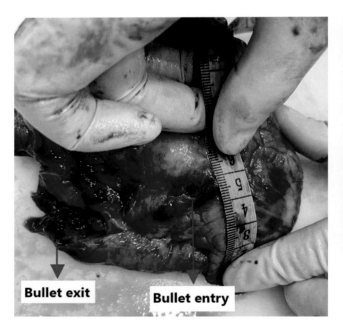

FIGURE 3.70: Gross autopsy examination of the heart in the case of a gunshot to the chest; the heart shows the entry and exit wound of the bullet.

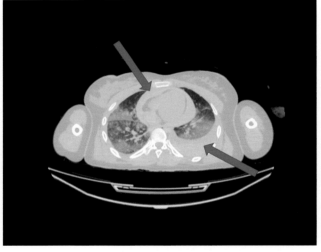

FIGURE 3.71: Axial section of PMCT showing hemoperi-cardium and left hemothorax in a case of stab to the chest.

of sedimentation is commonly seen in the aorta and pulmonary vessels.

4. **Hyperdense aortic wall:** Hyperdensity in the aortic wall is seen as a normal post-mortem finding, as a result of lack of artefact due to movement of the wall as seen in live patients' CT (Figure 3.75).

Abnormal patterns in PMCT

Non-traumatic lung pathologies on PMCT can be identified by assessing different abnormal patterns in the lung parenchyma, bronchoalveolar tract, pulmonary vessels, and pleura.

Abnormal patterns refer to the different attenuations observed as:

- **Consolidation:** On CT, consolidation is described as the presence of homogeneous lung opacity due to the replacement of air within the alveoli with underlying obscuration of pulmonary vessels and the bronchial wall (Figure 3.76). Air bronchograms are often present. It is one of the most common findings observed on PMCT, and its differential diagnosis depends upon the duration of the symptoms.
  - Consolidation associated with acute symptoms usually represents pneumonia, severe pulmonary oedema or haemorrhage, aspiration, or diffuse alveolar damage associated with acute respiratory distress syndrome.

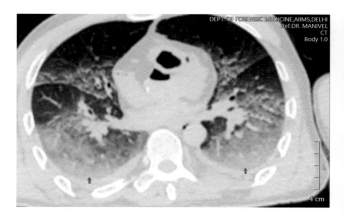

FIGURE 3.72: Axial image of chest PMCT in lung window showing post-mortem hypostasis (red arrows) in the dependent areas of the lung parenchyma, i.e., fissures and posterior aspect of the lungs.

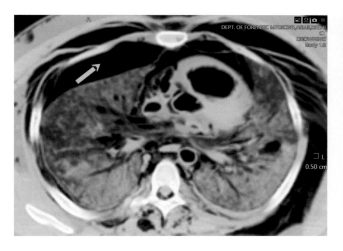

FIGURE 3.73: Axial section of chest PMCT in lung window showing pneumothorax (yellow arrow) as a result of decomposition gases.

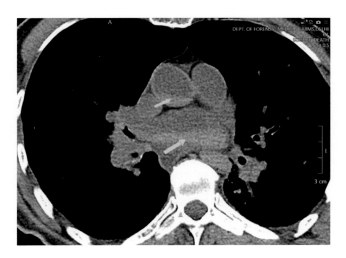

FIGURE 3.74: Axial section of chest PMCT in soft tissue window showing post-mortem layered separation of a blood clot in the aorta and pulmonary artery.

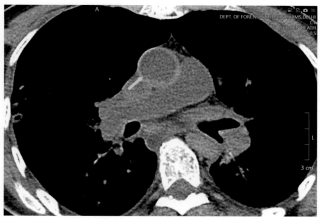

FIGURE 3.75: Axial section of chest PMCT in soft tissue window showing post-mortem hyperdensity in the aortic wall (yellow arrow).

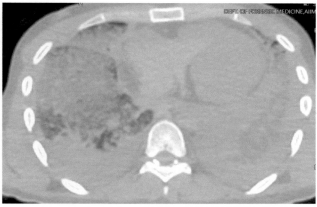

FIGURE 3.76: Axial section of chest PMCT in lung window showing bilateral opacification with obscuring vessels, i.e., consolidation with minor lung parenchyma visibility on the right side.

- Consolidation and chronic symptoms (i.e., longer than 4 to 6 weeks), common causes include organizing pneumonia, invasive mucinous adenocarcinoma, and chronic eosinophilic pneumonia.
- **Ground-glass opacity (GGO):** It is defined as increased haziness without obscuring underlying pulmonary vessels (Figure 3.77). GGO is non-specific and can be seen in a variety of diseases. Similar to consolidation, the differential diagnosis of GGO is primarily based on the duration of symptoms.

  - **GGO with acute symptoms:** Seen in pneumonia, pulmonary haemorrhage, pulmonary oedema, aspiration, or acute hypersensitivity pneumonitis
  - **GGO with chronic symptoms (i.e., longer than 4 to 6 weeks):** Seen in bronchoalveolar carcinoma, organizing pneumonia, pulmonary alveolar proteinosis (PEP), sub-acute hypersensitivity pneumonitis, non-specific interstitial pneumonia (NSIP), desquamative interstitial pneumonia (DIP), organizing pneumonia, invasive mucinous

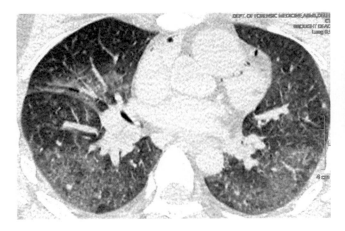

FIGURE 3.77: Axial section of chest PMCT in lung window showing diffuse GGO in bilateral lungs.

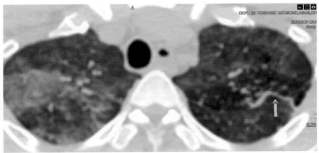

FIGURE 3.78: Axial section of chest PMCT in lung window showing thickened interlobular septa (yellow arrow) along with surrounding ground-glass opacity.

adenocarcinoma, lipoid pneumonia, and pulmonary alveolar proteinosis.

- **GGO with fibrosis (honeycombing, reticulation, and traction bronchiectasis):** It represents fibrosis rather than active disease and is seen in usual interstitial pneumonia (UIP) and Interstitial pulmonary fibrosis (IPF).

Ground-glass opacities	Consolidation
1. Increase haziness in the lung without obscuring vessels	Increased haziness in the lung, obscuring vessels

- **Thickened interlobular septa:** Interlobular septal thickening can be seen in patients with a variety of interstitial lung diseases. Septal thickening can appear smooth, nodular, or irregular in different diseases. It is an important component for the diagnosis of pulmonary oedema (interstitial oedema) (Figures 3.78–3.80).
- **Nodules:** A lung nodule is commonly called a 'spot on the lung' or a 'shadow'. It appears as a round white spot on CT and is denser than normal lung tissue (Figures 3.81 and 3.82). It can be single or multiply clustered and can be present in one or both lungs. These are usually caused by scar tissue, a healed infection, or some irritant in the air. When infection or illness causes inflammation of lung tissue, it can cause the formation of a small clump of cells (granuloma). The granuloma can eventually calcify or harden in the lung, causing a lung nodule. Sometimes, a nodule can be an early sign of lung cancer, but most lung nodules are benign (not cancerous). A nodule has a higher likelihood of being cancer if a person is a smoker, older than 65 years and has a family history of cancer or has received radiation therapy to the chest. Nodules usually spread through the haematogenous route, so they will predominate in the lower lobe as the blood flow is more towards the base.
- Distribution of lung nodules

Lung nodules are present in three different patterns:

1. **Peri-lymphatic nodules:** Nodules are present in an area which has an abundant lymphatic channel and are seen in cases of sarcoidosis, silicosis, and lymphangitic carcinoma. The main lymphatic channel areas are:

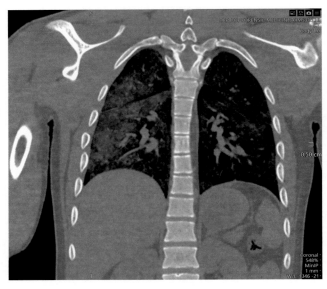

FIGURE 3.79: Coronal section of chest PMCT in lung window showing thickened interlobular septa along with surrounding ground-glass opacity.

- Pleural surfaces.
- Adjacent to bronchi and large.
- Within interlobular septa.
- Centrilobular region.
2. **Random nodules:** As the name suggests, these nodules are randomly distributed with respect to lung structures and are in a diffuse and uniform fashion. It also involves pleural surfaces. Most commonly seen in miliary tuberculosis.
3. **Centrilobular nodules:** These nodules tend to be visible in relation to small vessels, with the most peripheral nodules located a few millimeteres away from the pleural surface (an important point for differentiating from random nodules). It usually reflects diseases that occur in relation to centrilobular bronchioles and are most commonly associated with the endobronchial spread of infection, as seen in TB or bronchiolitis.

In view of differentiating the types of nodules, to start, the involvement of the pleural surface is looked for. If the nodules involve a pleural surface; centrilobular nodules can be excluded easily. Then further, if it had a specific distribution in relation

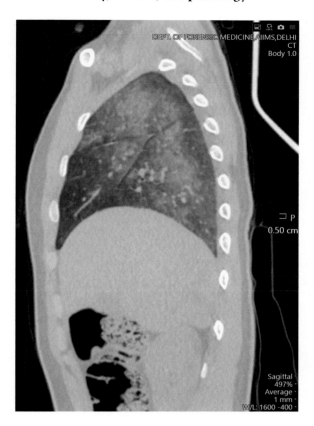

FIGURE 3.80: Sagittal section of chest PMCT in lung window showing thickened interlobular septa along with surrounding ground-glass opacity.

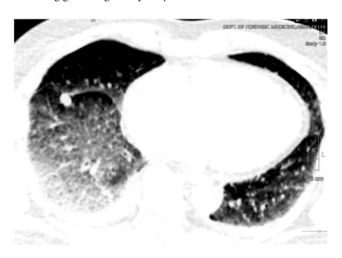

FIGURE 3.81: Axial section of chest PMCT in lung window showing nodule (red arrow) in the right lung.

to a particular lung structure, then it is peri-lymphatic nodules and if it has a diffuse and uniform distribution it indicates it is a random nodule pattern.

• **Lung Cyst**

A pulmonary cyst is a low-attenuating air-filled lucency of several millimetres to 1 cm in diameter (Figure 3.83), bordered by thick, clearly definable walls, and typically appears in rows and clusters in the peripheral and subpleural lung, with

adjacent cysts sharing a wall. Usually, cysts are seen in a combination of various other patterns. Honeycombing is a specific pattern in which a cluster of cysts is visible in the subpleural lung, and its presence signifies pulmonary fibrosis. If the lucent areas lack visible walls, then it is known as emphysema.

Several rare lung diseases where lung cysts are the primary manifestation. These include:

1. Langerhans cell histiocytosis.
2. Lymphangiomyomatosis.
3. Lymphocytic interstitial pneumonia.

The nomenclature of air-filled lucency depends upon the size:

- **Cyst:** Gas-filled structure with a thin perceptible wall (<2–4 mm) diameter <1 cm.
- **Cavity:** Gas-filled structure with wall >4 mm.
- **Bulla:** Focal region of emphysema measuring <1–2 cm without imperceptible wall.
- **Bleb:** Focal region of emphysema measuring >1–2 cm with imperceptible walls.
6. **Crazy paving:** It is a combination of GGO and superimposed septal thickening. It indicates a concomitant alveolar filling process. The term 'crazy paving' is used because the pattern resembles paths made from broken pieces of stone or concrete (Figure 3.84). It is a non-specific finding seen in pulmonary oedema, pulmonary haemorrhage, bronchoalveolar carcinoma, and organizing pneumonia.
7. **Honeycombing:** Honeycombing is a specific pattern where rows and a cluster of cysts are visible in the subpleural lung, and its presence signifies pulmonary fibrosis.

Interpretation of the finding

In order to reach a specific diagnosis finding on PMCT, different abnormal patterns, i.e., consolidation, GGO, nodules, cyst, reticulation, etc., are to be evaluated along with their location and distribution. Sometimes there are overlapping findings; in that scenario, the case history should be considered in order to reach a conclusion.

1. **Appearance of a pattern:** On PMCT, different abnormal patterns like consolidation, GGO, cyst, nodule, honeycombing, traction bronchiectasis, crazy paving, reticulations, and thickened septa appear as a result of evidence of pathologies. Appreciating these hyper- and hypodense areas assist in the diagnosis of the disease.
2. **Location of the pattern:** The four major locations to be observed while viewing CT are the lung parenchyma, bronchoalveolar tract, pulmonary vessels, and pleura. Sequentially observing the location for any abnormal patterns or specific signs helps us in reaching a specific diagnosis. Some specific signs in a specific location are as follows:
   • **Lung parenchyma**
      – **Air crescent sign:** The air crescent sign has been described as a complete or partial circumferential rim of radiolucent airspace within a parenchymal consolidation or nodular opacity. Seen in immunocompromised persons, bronchogenic carcinoma, and invasive aspergilloma.

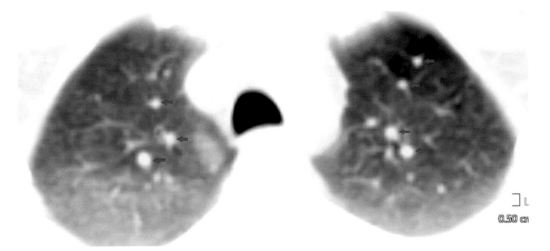

FIGURE 3.82: Axial section of chest PMCT in lung window showing multiple nodules (red arrow) in both lungs.

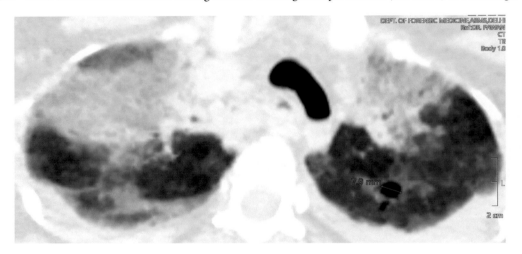

FIGURE 3.83: Axial section of chest PMCT in lung window showing a lung cyst of size 7.9 mm, i.e., cavity.

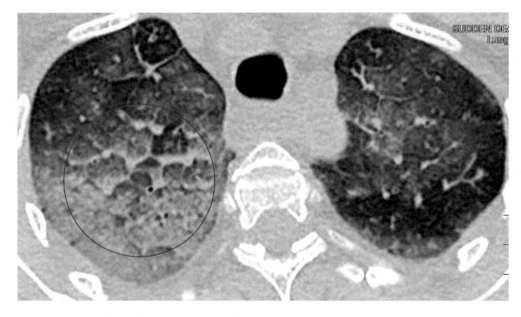

FIGURE 3.84: Axial section of PMCT in lung window showing crazy paving, i.e., GGO and superimposed septal thickening.

- **Halo sign:** In this, a solid pulmonary nodule is surrounded by a circumferential GGO. These have classically been described in pulmonary aspergillosis and pulmonary mucormycosis in immunocompromised hosts. The central nodule represents a focus of pulmonary infarction, and the surrounding GGO corresponds to the areas of pulmonary haemorrhage. Other non-infectious causes include granulomatosis with polyangiitis, amyloidosis, sarcoidosis, and metastatic cancers.
- **Atoll sign (Reverse Halo sign):** It is characterized by a central GGO surrounded by a crescentic or circumferential rim of dense consolidation. It has been classically described in cryptogenic organizing pneumonia but is not specific to the disease. It can also be seen in a wide range of pulmonary diseases, including invasive fungal infections, Pneumocystis jirovecii pneumonia (PJP), sarcoidosis, and adenocarcinoma of the lung.
- **Head Cheese sign:** The head cheese sign is characterized by radiographic areas of low, normal, and high attenuation (Figure 3.85). It was considered pathognomonic for sub-acute hypersensitivity pneumonitis and can also be appreciated in other conditions like sarcoidosis, respiratory bronchiolitis, and atypical infections (e.g., mycoplasma pneumoniae). It represents areas of consolidation (high attenuation, i.e., white), interspersed with areas of low attenuation (i.e., black), suggestive of mosaic perfusion and normal lung parenchyma (normal attenuation, i.e., grey)
- **Cheerios sign:** The Cheerios sign, also called the open bronchus sign, is characterized by a pulmonary nodule with a lucency at its centre. It occurs due to the proliferation of neoplastic or non-neoplastic cells around a patent airway, seen in conditions such as lung adenocarcinoma and pulmonary Langerhans cell histiocytosis, respectively.
- **Comet Tail sign:** The comet tail sign has been classically described in rounded atelectasis of the lung. It consists of a curvilinear opacity that originates from a pleural-based opacity towards the ipsilateral hilum. The opacities resemble a comet tail and comprise vessels and adjoining airways that get pulled into a mass-like opacity as the lung collapses. The main differential diagnosis includes bronchogenic carcinoma.
- **Corona Radiata sign:** The corona radiata, also called the sunburst sign, is used in reference to a solitary pulmonary nodule or mass with spiculated and irregular margins and distortion of surrounding blood vessels. It is highly suggestive of lung malignancy.
- **Galaxy sign:** This refers to tiny satellite nodules at the periphery of a pulmonary nodule, giving the appearance of a galaxy seen in sarcoidosis
- **Bronchoalveolar tract**
  - **Air bronchogram sign:** The air bronchogram sign refers to patent airways seen through an opacified lung (Figure 3.86). The airways appear

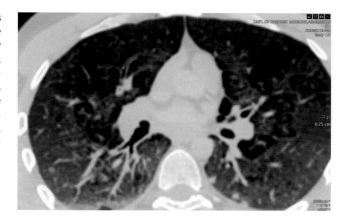

FIGURE 3.85: Axial section of chest PMCT in lung window showing head cheese sign which is the presence of low, normal, and high attenuation areas in the lung.

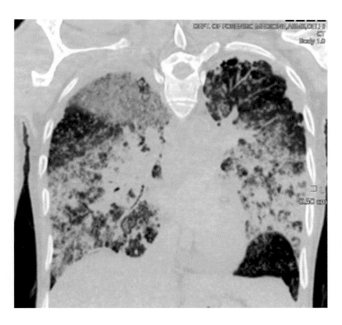

FIGURE 3.86: Coronal section of chest PMCT in lung window showing air bronchogram sign which is a patent airway made prominent by opacification of surrounding alveoli.

as air-filled, hyper-lucent tubular structures made prominent by the opacification of the surrounding alveoli. It is most commonly seen in consolidative processes of the lung, such as pneumonia but can also be seen in pulmonary oedema, severe interstitial lung disease, and neoplasms, such as adenocarcinoma.
- **Positive bronchus sign:** There is representative of an airway leading directly to a peripheral lung nodule or mass. It is a powerful clue in predicting the success of a transbronchial lung biopsy when a positive bronchus sig is identified at the level of the fourth-order bronchi in this series.
- **Signet ring sign:** The signet ring is a common sign in bronchiectasis (Figure 3.87). The dilated airway is prominently larger than its accompanying pulmonary artery on axial images,

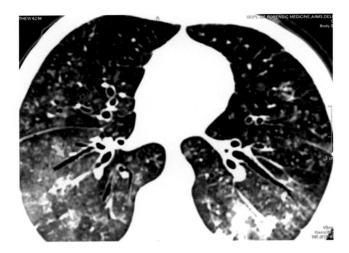

FIGURE 3.87: Axial section of chest PMCT showing signet ring (red arrow) and tram track sign (yellow arrow).

resembling a signet ring. Normally, the airway and the blood vessel must be of equal calibre. A broncho-arterial ratio >1 is suggestive of bronchiectasis.

- **Tram track sign:** The tram track sign refers to the parallel, non-tapering airways seen extending to the lung periphery in bronchiectasis (Figure 3.87). The bronchial walls are always thickened, denoting airway inflammation.

- **Tree-in-bud sign:** The tree-in-bud sign refers to the presence of mucus or pus-filled dilated centrilobular bronchioles. They are arranged in a linear branching pattern, as in buds on a tree. It is indicative of the endobronchial spread of inflammation or bronchiolar infection in the vast majority of cases. It is now recognized in a variety of lung disorders like TB, bacterial bronchopneumonia, focal bronchiolitis, infections such as non-tuberculous mycobacteria, and aspiration pneumonia.

• **Pulmonary vessels**
- **Feeding vessel sign:** The feeding vessel sign consists of a distinct pulmonary vessel leading into a lung nodule (Figure 3.88) or mass (Figure 3.89). The sign has also been described in pulmonary infarctions, metastasis, and pulmonary arteriovenous malformations.

- **Polo mint sign:** The Polo mint sign is used to describe a partial filling defect in a blood vessel surrounded by a rim of contrast material in a CT angiogram on images acquired perpendicular to the long axis of a vessel. This sign was described with reference to pulmonary embolism, but it can be seen in venous thrombosis at other sites, such as portal vein thrombosis.

• **Pleural**
- **Split pleura sign:** The split pleura sign is evident on a contrast-enhanced CT scan of the chest. It is seen in empyema and in some malignant effusions. It is considered a reliable CT sign to differentiate an empyema from a lung abscess. The split pleura sign is formed due to contrast enhancement of the parietal and visceral pleura,

separated by the exudative effusion, as a result of fibrin deposition along the opposing pleural surfaces and the ingrowth of blood vessels.

4. **Distribution of the pattern**

Abnormal patterns can be confined in the acute phase as later, with the advancement of the diseases, they may occupy the whole of the lung. The distribution of the pattern can be diffuse or patchy, upper lobe or middle lobe predominance, peripheral or central predominance, etc.

The lungs have a major physiological variation which results in location-specific diseases. The upper lobe of the lungs has a few basic variations which make it prone to various infections such as:

• It only receives 5% of the total volume of blood in comparison to the lower lobe.

• Ventilation is 30% of that provided to the lower lobe.

• Decreased lymphatic clearance because of which in chronic conditions, enhanced lymphatic clearance in the lower zone leaves retained particles in the upper zone.

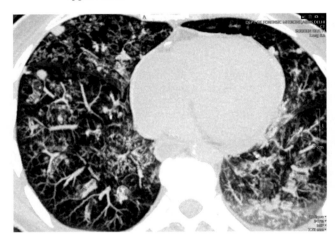

FIGURE 3.88: Axial section of chest PMCT 8 mm thickness with maximum intensity projection showing feeding vessel sign (red arrow) with a distinct pulmonary vessel leading to a nodule.

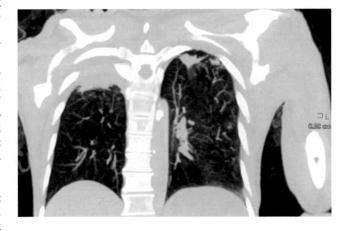

FIGURE 3.89: Coronal section of chest PMCT 8 mm thickness with maximum intensity projection showing feeding vessel sign (red arrow) with a distinct pulmonary vessel leading to a mass.

- It is an alkaline (high pH) and oxygen-rich environment in comparison to other areas of the lung.

Major upper lung zone diseases include sarcoidosis, silicosis, TB, PCP, cystic fibrosis, etc. Different patterns in the upper zone are as follows:

- **GGO:** GGO in the upper zone is quite common, and the duration of the disease plays a vital role in diagnosis. Cause of upper zone GGO:
  1. **Acute:** neurological pulmonary oedema, laryngeal spasm, or high altitude pulmonary oedema.
  2. **Sub-acute:** *Pneumocystis carnii* infection (B/L symmetric).
  3. **Chronic:** Allergic alveolitis.
- **Fibrosis:** It is also an important and most frequently found pattern in PMCT. The location of the fibrosis gives clues regarding the diagnosis like:
  1. **Fibrosis in upper and middle lobe:** Sarcoidosis, Langerhans cell histiocytosis, silicosis, and other pneumoconioses.
  2. **Fibrosis in peripheral areas:** Non-specific interstitial pneumonia, interstitial lung diseases (ILD).
  3. **Fibrosis in broncho-vascular area:** Sarcoidosis, chronic aspiration.

Specific lung diseases with pathognomonic findings

In day-to-day experiences, the most common findings in the lungs are pulmonary oedema, aspiration pneumonia active, or old pulmonary tuberculosis. Less common cases include all other pathologies like ILD, malignancy, haemorrhage, infection, etc.

1. Pulmonary oedema

Pulmonary oedema is a broad descriptive term. It is an abnormal accumulation of fluid in the extravascular compartments of the lung, i.e., interstitium and alveoli (Figure 3.90). It is seen in a number of diseases. Major causes can be broadly classified as cardiogenic and noncardiogenic (fluid overload).

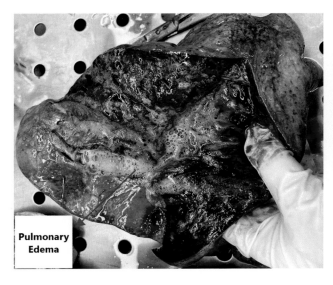

FIGURE 3.90: A gross examination of a cut-section of the lung showing froth oozing out due to pulmonary oedema.

Pulmonary oedema can occur either as a result of increased hydrostatic pressure or increased permeability with or without diffuse alveolar damage. In cardiogenic pulmonary oedema, as soon as the pressure in the left ventricle increases or in fluid overload conditions, it is redistributed towards pulmonary veins, which leads to dilatation of the pulmonary vasculature and is termed vascular congestion, i.e., congested lung, which further increases in pressure and will lead to leakage of fluid in the interstitium and termed as interstitial oedema. The further increase in pressure or increased permeability will also lead to leakage of fluid in the alveolar space and is termed alveolar oedema. Interstitial and alveolar oedema can be considered pulmonary oedema. Radiologically on CT scan (Figure 3.91):

1. Vascular congestion is demonstrated as:
   - Dilated pulmonary vasculature.
2. Interstitial pulmonary oedema is demonstrated as:
   - Ground-glass opacification.
   - Broncho-vascular bundle thickening (due to the increased vascular diameter).
   - Interlobular septal thickening.
3. Alveolar oedema is demonstrated as:
   - Airspace consolidation + above findings of interstitial oedema.

Pleural effusions are a frequent accompanying finding in cardiogenic/hydrostatic pulmonary oedema, which is usually bilateral. It helps to differentiate pulmonary oedema from pulmonary haemorrhage and pulmonary alveolar proteinosis, both of which do not have pleural effusion.

2. Tuberculosis

Tuberculosis (TB) is a contagious infection caused by *Mycobacterium tuberculosis* that usually infects the lungs, which is termed pulmonary tuberculosis. It can also infect or spread to any other part of the body like the brain, vertebra, spine, testis, abdomen, etc. There are two forms of the disease:

- **Latent TB:** In this form, germs are present in the body, but the immune system keeps them under check and prevents it from spreading. Usually, the person does not manifest any symptoms, nor is it contagious.

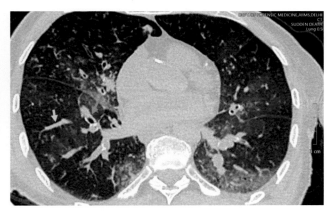

FIGURE 3.91: Axial section of chest PMCT in lung window showing interstitial pulmonary oedema, i.e., dilated vessels (yellow arrow), broncho-vascular bundle thickening (blue arrow), and GGO (red arrow).

- **Active TB**: In this form, the germs present inside the body, and the immune system fails to keep them under check; hence, the microbe multiplies and the condition is contagious. Active TB can be primary (affecting lungs) or disseminated (affecting other parts of the body).

Pulmonary manifestations of tuberculosis are variable and depend on if the tubercular infection is the primary or the post-primary. The primary infection by tuberculosis commonly involves the lungs, and they are a major source of the spread of the disease.

- Primary infection

Primary infection is usually asymptomatic in the majority of cases, but sometimes the patient becomes symptomatic due to haematological dissemination, which may result in miliary TB. In children, infections can be anywhere in the lung; in adults, there is a predilection for the upper or lower zone. The initial focus of infection can be anywhere in the lung and can have non-specific appearances, which can range from being too small to be detected to being a patchy area of consolidation or even lobar consolidation. Cavitation is uncommon in primary TB. In children, there is ipsilateral hilar and contiguous mediastinal (paratracheal) lymphadenopathy, usually right-sided. Pleural effusions are more frequent in adults. In most cases, the infection gets localized and forms a caseating granuloma (Figures 3.92 and 3.93) (tuberculoma) which eventually calcifies and is known as a Ghon lesion.

- Post-primary pulmonary tuberculosis

It is also referred to as reactivation TB or secondary TB, which occurs years later, most commonly because of the decreased immune status of the host. Post-primary TB in the lungs usually develops in either the upper lobe's posterior segments or the lower lobe's superior segments. The typical appearance of post-primary TB is that of patchy consolidation or poorly defined linear, nodular opacities, and cavitations (Figures 3.93 and 3.94). Post-primary infections usually cavitate as compared to primary infections. Endobronchial spread in nearby airways is common, which causes well-defined nodules of size 2–4 mm or branching lesions (tree-in-bud sign) identifiable on CT.

Hilar lymph node enlargement is seen in only one-third of cases. Post-primary TB can also result in lobar consolidation, tuberculoma formation, or miliary TB, which are less common. Tuberculomas in cases of post-primary TB appear as a well-defined rounded mass typically located in the upper lobes. They are usually single and can range up to a size of 4 cm. In most cases, small satellite lesions can be seen along with superimposed cavitation.

- Miliary pulmonary tuberculosis

Miliary tuberculosis is less commonly encountered, and it carries a poor prognosis. It is due to uncontrolled TB infection disseminating through the hematogenous route. It can occur in both primary and post-primary TB. Miliary deposits are nodules of 1–3 mm in diameter, which are uniform in size and uniformly distributed.

- Pleural Involvement in TB

Tuberculous involvement of the pleura presents as pleural effusion, empyema, or pleural thickening. In the acute stages, the most common form of extrapulmonary TB is TB pleural effusion. Diffuse pleural thickening and adhesions, often with calcification, occur in chronic cases.

- **Diagnosis of TB**

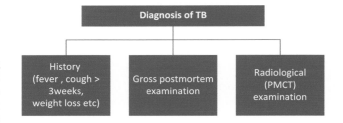

Gross history or PMCT (radiological examination) history is sufficient for the diagnosis of TB. On PMCT, if primary TB is there affecting only the lungs, features of pneumonia appear, but if it is disseminated through the endobronchial pathway or

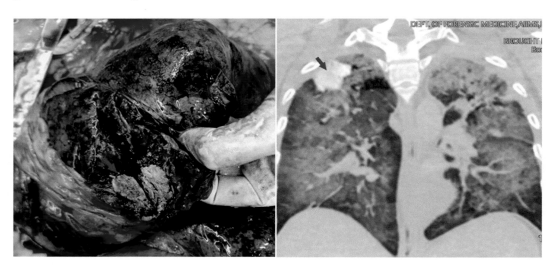

FIGURE 3.92: A gross examination of TB infected lung showing caseous granuloma in the apex of the right lung along with congestion and oedema. The hyperdense area is at the same location on the coronal image of the chest PMCT in the lung window.

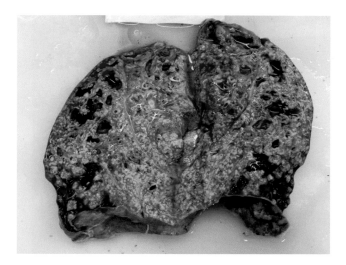

FIGURE 3.93: A gross examination of the lung showing multiple caseous granulomas throughout the right lung along with multiple cavitary lesions with haemorrhages.

the miliary (through the blood) pathway, the findings are more specific:

- Tree-in-bud pattern.
- Fibrosis with traction bronchiectasis.
- Fibro cavitary changes.
- Destruction of lung parenchyma
- Centrilobular nodules.

In severe complicated form, various other findings can be easily ascertained:

- The fungal colonization of cavities, e.g., aspergilloma.
- Bronchiectasis (dilatation of bronchi).
- Empyema – tuberculous empyema, i.e., pus.
- Bronchopleural fistula.

3. Pneumonia

It is a general term with widespread use, defined as infection within the lung parenchyma. It is usually due to purulent material filling the alveoli. It is a form of acute respiratory infection that affects the lungs; usually, alveoli are filled with air in a healthy person, but when an individual has pneumonia, the alveoli are filled with fluid and pus, which makes breathing painful and limits oxygen intake. It commonly affects older age groups, and it sometimes leads to severe or life-threatening illness and or even death. India contributes to more than 50% of the world's pneumonia deaths.

On the basis of the spread of infection, it is classified as:

1. **Lobar pneumonia:** It is a type of pneumonia which consists of inflammatory exudate and consolidation, which involves a lobe of the lung. (Figures 3.95–3.97)
2. **Bronchopneumonia:** It is a type of pneumonia where there is the involvement of usually more than one secondary lobule of the lung (Figures 3.98 and 3.99). The distribution can occur in both lungs asymmetrically, but there is a common tendency to involve the lower lobes.

On the basis of the infective agent, it is classified as:

1. **Bacterial:** Streptococcus pneumonia is the most common cause of bacterial pneumonia in children, followed by *Haemophilus influenza* type B (HiB), which is the second most common cause of bacterial pneumonia.
2. **Viral:** Respiratory syncytial virus is the most common viral cause of pneumonia.
3. **Fungal:** Pneumocystis, cryptococcus, and aspergillus are the common causes of fungal pneumonia.

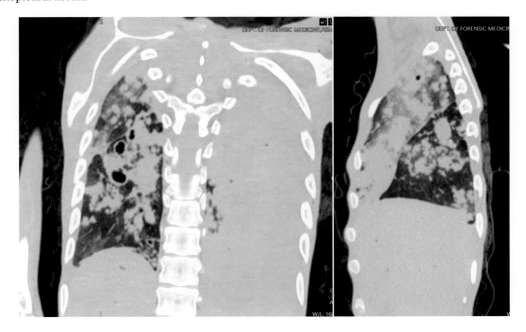

FIGURE 3.94: Coronal and sagittal section of chest PMCT in lung window showing tuberculous pneumonia lung in the same case with multiple granulomas and cavitary lesions in a background of pneumonic consolidation in the middle and upper lobe.

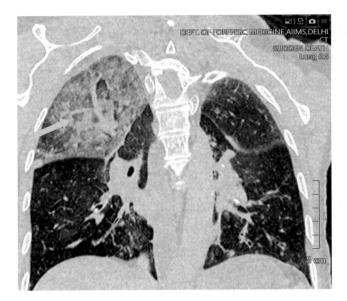

FIGURE 3.95: Coronal section of chest PMCT in lung window showing right upper-lobe consolidation, i.e., lobar pneumonia.

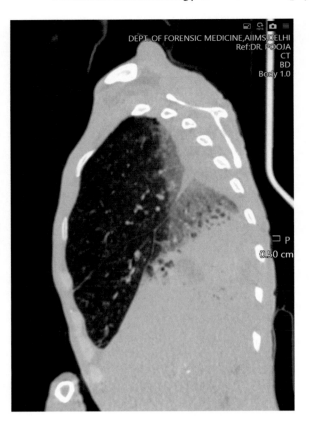

FIGURE 3.97: Sagittal section of chest PMCT in lung window showing right lower lobe consolidation, i.e., lobar pneumonia.

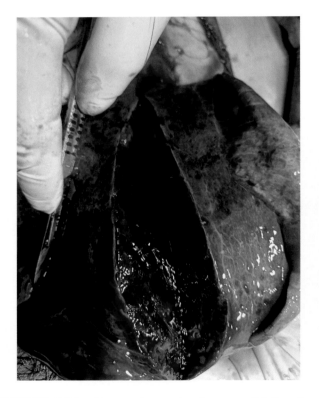

FIGURE 3.96: Gross autopsy showing consolidation features in a case of pneumonia.

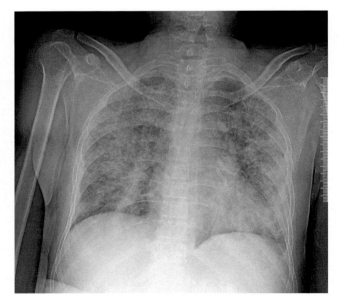

FIGURE 3.98: Chest X-ray AP showing multiple nodular patterns and diffuse ground-glass opacity in both lungs involving more than one secondary lobule, i.e., bronchopneumonia.

Sometimes findings of pneumonia are not associated with known diseases or exposures associated with a histologic pattern; that category is known as idiopathic interstitial pneumonia, and it includes:
– Usual interstitial pneumonia (UIP).
– NSIP (non-specific interstitial pneumonia).

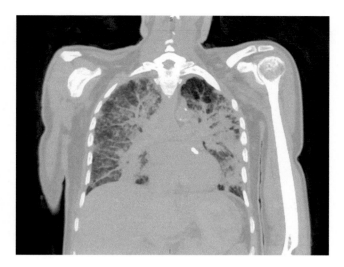

FIGURE 3.99: Coronal section of chest PMCT in lung window showing multiple nodules and diffuse GGO involving more than one secondary lobule, i.e., bronchopneumonia.

– Organizing pneumonia (OP).
– Desquamative interstitial pneumonia (DIP).

A. **Atypical pneumonia**

Mycoplasma pneumoniae is the most common cause of atypical pneumonia. In atypical pneumonia, the inflammation is often confined to the pulmonary interstitium and the interlobular septa; this causes the characteristic radiological features of atypical pneumonia. As there is often no exudate in the alveolar air spaces, consolidation is a less common sign in atypical pneumonia than in bacterial pneumonia of more typical causative organisms.

Important PMCT findings of pneumonia:

• Focal GGO in a lobular distribution is often diffuse and bilateral.
• Evidence of pleural effusion.
• Bronchial wall thickening is another common CT finding.
• Diffuse ground-glass nodules in a centrilobular pattern.

B. **Usual interstitial pneumonia (UIP):** UIP pattern on HRCT is characterized by:
1. Subpleural and basal predominance.
2. Reticulation (with traction bronchiectasis).
3. Honeycombing.
4. Absence of inconsistent features, including the following: a) Upper, mid-lung, or peribronchial predominance, b) Extensive GGO (>reticulation in extent), c) Profuse micronodules (bilateral, upper lobe), d) Discrete cysts not representing honeycombing, e) Mosaic perfusion or air trapping (bilateral, ≥ three lobes), and f) Segmental or lobar consolidation.

If these four criteria are met, a UIP pattern should be diagnosed based on an HRCT.

C. **NSIP (non-specific interstitial pneumonia):** It has a variable appearance but often has the following characteristics:

1. Predominance in the peripheral, posterior, and basal lung regions, with a concentric distribution.
2. Sparing of the immediate subpleural lung.
3. GGO.
4. Reticulation.
5. Traction bronchiectasis (usually but not always in fibrotic NSIP).
6. Rare honeycombing, which, if present, is of a limited extent.

NSIP	UIP
1. Reticulations	
2. Traction bronchiectasis	
3. GGO	3. Honeycombing
4. Patchy distribution	4. Basal predominance
5. Subpleural sparing	5. Subpleural involvement

D. Organizing pneumonia

HRCT features are nonspecific and include the following:
1. Patchy or nodular consolidation/GGO.
2. A peripheral and peribronchial distribution.
3. The atoll sign or reversed halo sign, in which a ring of consolidation surrounds GGO, a sign that is uncommonly seen in other diseases.

E. Hypersensitivity pneumonitis (HP) is a common lung disease resulting from exposure to one of a number of organic dust.

In the sub-acute stage, HRCT typically shows the following:
1. Patchy GGO.
2. Poorly defined centrilobular GGO nodules.
3. Upper- or mid-lung predominance, with involvement of the entire cross-section of the lung (i.e., there is no subpleural predominance).
4. Mosaic perfusion caused by bronchiolar obstruction.
5. Air trapping.
6. A combination of patchy GGO and patchy mosaic perfusion (termed the headcheese sign because of its resemblance to a sausage of the same name), the headcheese sign is typical of HP.

In the chronic or fibrotic stage, HP typically shows the above signs, along with honeycombing and traction bronchiectasis.

4. Bronchiectasis

Bronchiectasis is a condition characterized by irreversible damage to part of the airway, seen as bronchial dilatation. It is commonly associated with chronic infection and sputum production. In a normal lung, a bronchus and its adjacent pulmonary artery, as they travel together, are about the same size. In patients with bronchiectasis, the dilated bronchus appears larger than its adjacent artery, and together they appear as a signet ring in which the internal diameter of a bronchus exceeds the diameter of the adjacent artery. The bronchioles normally taper off while travelling to the periphery, but in the case of bronchiectasis, as they are dilated, so in spite of the tapering, the parallel walls of the bronchi are seen, which is termed as tram track sign.

Important features are:

1. Bronchial dilatation.
2. Bronchial wall thickening.
3. Atelectasis with some air trapping.
4. Mucus retention.
5. Lack of normal tapering with visibility of airways in peripheral lungs.

Causes:

1. Childhood infection.
2. Chronic airway infection.
3. Immunodeficiency.
4. Cystic fibrosis, which shows bilateral bronchiectasis involving the upper lobes.

Some lung infections also have a pattern of bronchiectasis specific to a region of the lung. Asymmetrical upper-lobe bronchiectasis is seen in TB. Middle lobes and lingual bronchiectasis are seen in Mycobacterium avium complex (MAC) infection. Lower lobe bronchiectasis is typically associated with Immune deficiency, childhood infections, and ciliary dysmotility.

Important airway signs on CT in case of bronchiectasis:

1. **Signet ring sign:** Usually, the airway and blood vessels are of equal calibre, but if the broncho-arterial ratio is >1, it is suggestive of bronchiectasis (Figures 3.100 and 3.101).
2. **Tram track sign:** Dilated, non-tapered bronchi extend to the lung periphery (Figures 3.100 and 3.101).

5. **Lung cancer**

   Adenocarcinoma is the most common cell type of lung cancer presenting as a lung nodule, but any cell type can present in this manner. Although a definite diagnosis of lung cancer cannot be made on CT, findings that strongly suggest malignancy in a patient with a solitary nodule include the following:

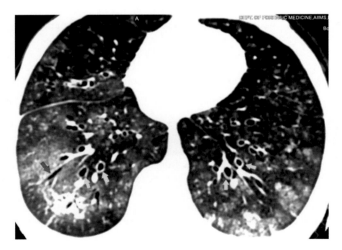

FIGURE 3.100: Axial section of chest PMCT showing bronchial dilatation with thickened walls (yellow arrows) and lack of normal tapering, causing visibility of airways in the periphery of the lungs (red arrow).

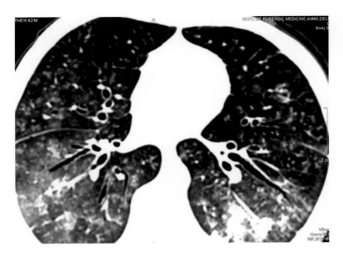

FIGURE 3.101: Axial section of the chest PMCT showing signs of bronchiectasis, i.e., tram track sign (yellow arrow) and signet ring sign (red arrow).

1. An irregular or spiculated nodule margin, usually caused by fibrosis or invasion of the surrounding lung (90% of nodules with a spiculated edge are malignant).
2. Air bronchograms present.
3. A nodule exceeding 5 mm with solid attenuation (two-thirds are malignant).
4. Cavitation with a nodular cavity wall or a wall exceeding 15 mm in greatest thickness.

Lung cancers may present as an atypical radiological pattern. Squamous cell cancer may present as a cavitating lesion. Adenocarcinoma may present as a dense consolidation. Bronchoalveolar carcinoma (adenocarcinoma *in situ*) presents as ground-glass opacity and mixed density, solid, and ground-glass nodules

Metastasis in the lung

Metastasis in the lungs occurs due to the spread of the tumour cells from different organs where the primary tumour is located, and this spread commonly occurs through the haematogenous or lymphatic route. Some of the common cancers which metastasize to the lungs include:

- Breast cancer
- Bladder cancer
- Renal cancer (Figures 3.102 and 3.103)
- Prostate cancer
- Colon cancer

6. **Emphysema**

   It is a condition where there is air sacs (alveoli) wall damage. With this damage, the alveoli cannot support the bronchial tubes. The tubes collapse and cause an obstruction/blockage, which traps air inside the lung. It is commonly associated with smoking, which damages the alveoli and the rest of the lung parenchyma (Figure 3.104). Chronic obstructive pulmonary disease (COPD) comprises both emphysema and chronic bronchitis. Emphysema can be easily differentiated from honeycombing or cystic lung disease because, in most cases, the lucent (black) areas lack visible walls (also called a cyst with no wall). Emphysema is classified as:

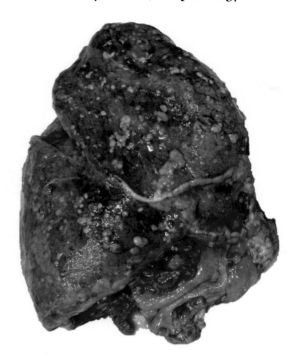

FIGURE 3.102: Lung metastasis in a case of renal cell carcinoma.

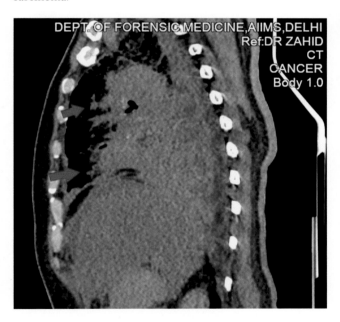

FIGURE 3.103: Chest PMCT chest in soft tissue window showing Lung metastasis in a case of renal cell carcinoma.

- **Centrilobular emphysema:** It is the most common type and is usually associated with smoking. It usually affects the upper lobe severely. The presence of spotty upper-lobe lucencies without visible walls is diagnostic.
- **Paraseptal emphysema:** It involves the subpleural lung adjacent to the chest wall and mediastinum, more in the upper lobe. Emphysematous spaces several centimetres in diameter are typical, and their walls are seen easily. It can occur as an isolated abnormality in young patients or may be associated with centrilobular emphysema (Figure 3.105).

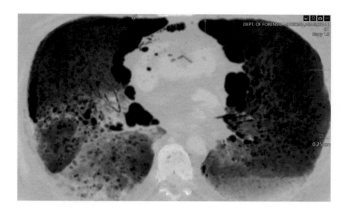

FIGURE 3.104: Axial section of chest PMCT showing para septal emphysema, subpleural lucency typical of para septal emphysema is appreciated. It is similar to a honeycomb but present in a single layer. The image is with minimum intensity projection, i.e., MinIP with increased slice thickness.

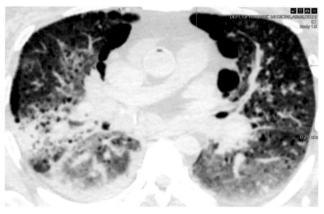

FIGURE 3.105: Axial section of chest PMCT showing para-septal emphysema of the same case as in Figure 3.104 without MinIP and in 1 mm thickness.

- **Pan lobular emphysema:** Less common and is often related to α1-antitrypsin deficiency. It is diffuse or most severe at the lung bases and is manifest as an overall decrease in lung attenuation and in the size of pulmonary vessels.
- **Bullous emphysema:** It is said to be present when bullae predominate. It is most often associated with paraseptal emphysema. Large bullae can be seen, particularly in young men. Bullae sometimes contain fluid as well as air, which may indicate infection.

7. **Pulmonary fibrosis**

It is a condition where the lung tissue is scarred and fibrosis over a period of time. There are three important patterns which individually or in combination will define pulmonary fibrosis, and these are:

- **Reticulations:** Appearing as a network of linear opacities, is commonly present in patients with lung fibrosis and is typically associated with architectural distortion and displacement of vessels or fissures (Figure 3.106).

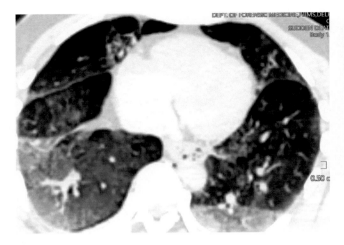

FIGURE 3.106: Axial section of the chest PMCT in lung window showing diffuse reticulations pattern.

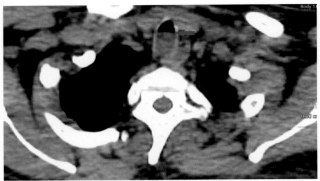

FIGURE 3.107: Axial section of chest PMCT showing air–fluid levels in trachea suggestive of retrograde aspiration of blood in a case of stab to the lung parenchyma.

- **Traction bronchiectasis:** Traction bronchiectasis (dilatation of bronchi because of surrounding lung fibrosis) is a common finding in patients with fibrotic lung disease and reticulation. It is commonly present in patients with honeycombing. In traction bronchiectasis, large or small airways are dilated and have a very irregular appearance
- **Honeycombing:** Honeycombing represents lung fibrosis associated with cystic areas of lung destruction. It results in a characteristic coarse reticular pattern or cystic appearance on HRCT that is typical. Cystic spaces are usually several millimetres to 1 cm in diameter, are marginated by thick, clearly definable walls, and typically appear in rows and clusters in the peripheral and subpleural lung, with adjacent cysts sharing walls. Unless a row or cluster of cysts is visible in the immediate subpleural lung, honeycombing cannot be diagnosed with certainty. The presence of honeycombing on HRCT means that fibrosis is present and is essential for a diagnosis of UIP.

8. **Blood in the respiratory tract**

The presence of blood deep in the respiratory tract is traditionally considered a vital phenomenon. Blood can reach the intrapulmonary airways in two ways:

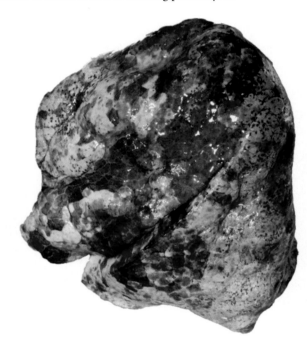

FIGURE 3.108: Gross examination of blood aspiration lung.

- **Anterograde manner:** As in traumatic injuries involving fractures of the skull base causing bleeding into the nasopharynx and oropharynx
- **Retrograde manner:** As seen in an injury located beneath the bronchial tree in the pulmonary parenchyma.

Moreover, depending on the volume of blood aspirated, it may be interpreted as the primary or, more frequently, contributing cause of death. Expiratory and inspiratory movements involve not only the central regions of the lungs but also the periphery. Thus, in cases of pulmonary contusion, laceration, or destruction of the lung tissue structure, blood escapes from the damaged parenchyma into the alveoli and bronchioles. Fluid in the large airways was considered blood when its density was measured to be between 40 and 60 HU (Figures 3.107–3.109).

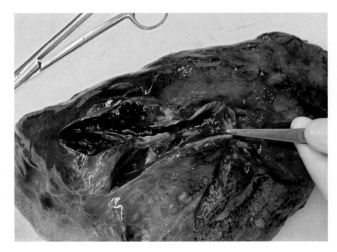

FIGURE 3.109: Dissection showing aspiration of blood in lungs, in a case with middle cranial fossa fracture.

Heart

Non-traumatic cardiac deaths are most commonly observed among the general population, so their detection seems to be of utmost importance. PMCT can be used to find morphological abnormalities like calcification, pericardial effusion, hypertrophy of the walls, valvular pathologies, etc. Various pathologies detected on PMCT are as follows:

a. **Calcification:** Calcium is radiopaque and is therefore hyperdense on CT. The presence of calcium in arteries left coronary artery, left anterior descending artery, left circumflex artery, and right coronary artery can easily be detected in PMCT (Figures 3.110–3.114). Valvular (Figures 3.115 and 3.116) and great vessel calcification are also frequently observed. The arterial wall calcification may serve as an objective marker of atherosclerotic disease. The detection of calcium is also noted in valves,

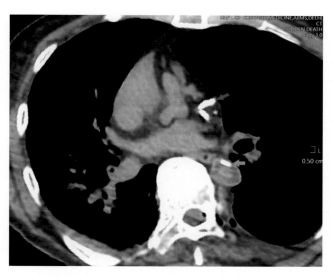

FIGURE 3.112: Axial section of chest PMCT showing calcification at the bifurcation of left anterior descending artery (red arrow) and left circumflex artery (blue arrow). Calcification in descending aorta is also seen (green arrow).

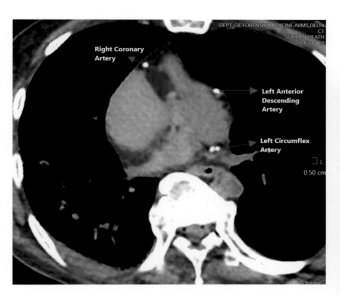

FIGURE 3.110: Axial section of chest PMCT showing calcification in all three coronary arteries.

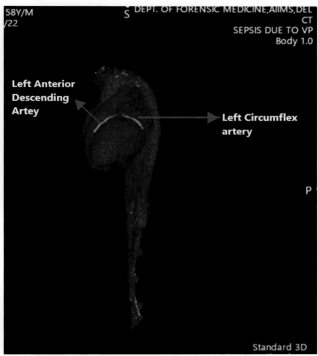

FIGURE 3.113: Volume rendering standard 3D CT reconstruction of the heart showing a calcified left anterior descending artery and left circumflex artery in a case with triple previous PCI stents which were calcified.

myocardium, pericardium, and other arteries, including the aorta.

b. **Cardiomegaly:** Cardiomegaly on PMCT is detected with the help of the cardiothoracic ratio. The cardiothoracic ratio is the ratio between the cardiac diameter and the transverse diameter of the chest wall, which is used as a radiological tool to assess cardiomegaly, which helps

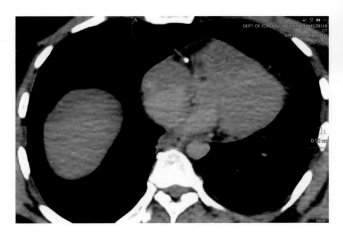

FIGURE 3.111: Axial section of chest CT showing isolated calcification in right coronary artery (red arrow).

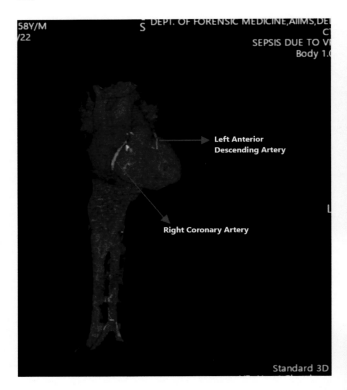

FIGURE 3.114: Volume rendering standard 3D CT reconstruction of the heart showing calcified left anterior descending artery and right coronary artery in a case with triple previous PCI stents which were calcified.

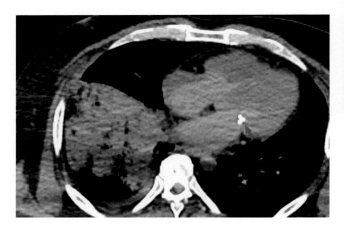

FIGURE 3.115: Axial section of chest PMCT showing calcification of a mitral valve.

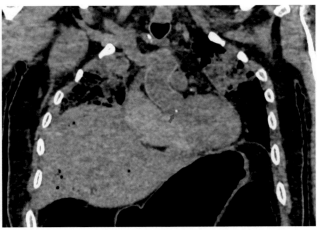

FIGURE 3.116: Axial section of chest PMCT showing calcification of an aortic valve.

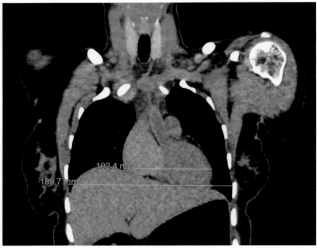

FIGURE 3.117: Coronal view of chest PMCT showing a method of calculating the cardiothoracic ratio, i.e., cardiac diameter with the transverse diameter of the chest wall.

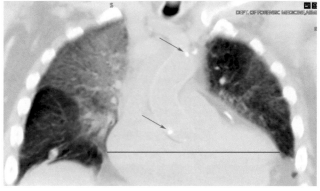

FIGURE 3.118: Coronal section of chest PMCT in lung window showing cardiomegaly with aortic calcifications.

in the estimation of heart size and the pathology related to it (Figures 3.117 and 3.118). The clinically used criteria are modified from 0.50 to 0.57 to calibrate the post-mortem setting and therefore find the abnormality. A ratio of 0.57 is set as the cut-off to define cardiomegaly, but this is not conclusive but only suggestive of the cardiomegaly. The thickness of the right ventricle and left ventricle is normally defined as 5 mm and 15 mm, respectively. Variation of the value for the normal cut-off is an abnormality to detect the pathology of the ventricular wall. The presence of calcium suggests previous infarction, which is visualized in PMCT.

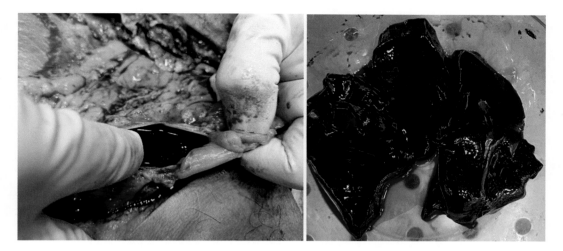

FIGURE 3.119: Gross autopsy examination of the pericardial sac showing cardiac tamponade with fluid and blood clots in a case of ruptured heart post-myocardial infarction.

c. **Cardiac rupture:** Cardiac rupture in non-traumatic cases occurs due to softening or thinning of the layers because of previous infarctions, which leads to pericardial effusion/cardiac tamponade. Rupture is commonly seen over the left ventricle (Figures 3.119–3.123).

d. **Coronary occlusion:** Coronary occlusion occurs due to multiple pathologies like thrombus (Figure 3.124), emboli, atherosclerotic occlusion, spasm, myocardial bridging, etc., which is difficult to identify with PMCT. Adjunctive procedures like PMCT angiography can help in better identification of occlusion. It helps in demonstrating the lumen and, therefore, the thrombus or any other occlusion.

Aorta

The thoracic section of the aorta is divided into three parts, namely: Ascending aorta, aortic arch, and descending aorta. It

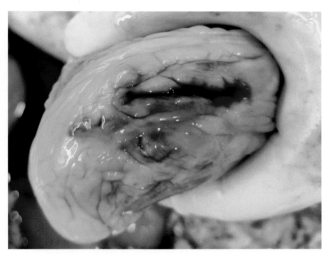

FIGURE 3.121: A gross examination of the heart showing cardiac rupture leading to cardiac tamponade in a case of myocardial infarction.

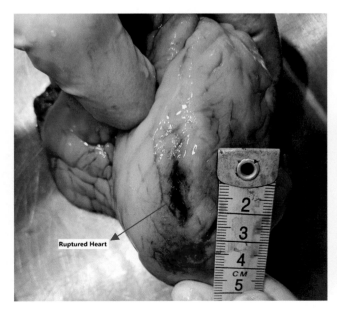

Ruptured Heart

FIGURE 3.120: Gross autopsy examination of the heart showing the ruptured site in a case of myocardial infarction.

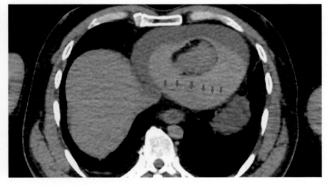

FIGURE 3.122: Axial section of chest PMCT in soft tissue window showing sedimentation effects in a case of haemopericardium in the same case as Figure 3.121.

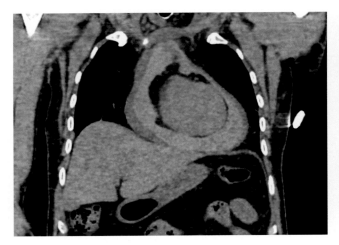

FIGURE 3.123: Coronal section of chest PMCT in soft tissue window showing sedimentation effects in a case of haemopericardium in the same case as Figure 3.121.

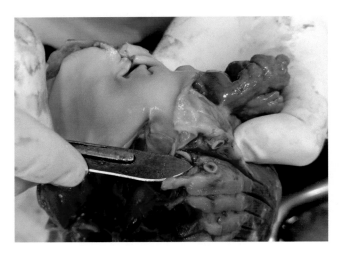

FIGURE 3.124: Thrombus occluding the left anterior descending artery, which is difficult to appreciate in PMCT.

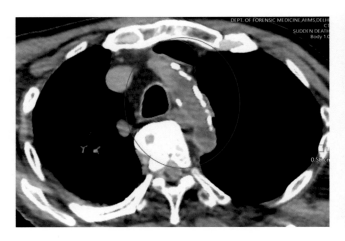

FIGURE 3.125: Axial section of chest PMCT showing aortic arch calcification.

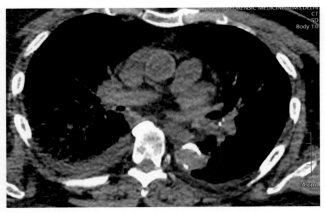

FIGURE 3.126: Axial section of chest PMCT showing descending aortic calcification.

begins at the aortic valve and ends as it exits the thorax to enter the abdomen through the median arcuate ligament between the diaphragmatic curare anterior to the twelfth thoracic vertebral body. The most commonly detected pathologies are aortic calcification (Figures 3.125 and 3.126) and aortic rupture.

Lymph nodes

CT is a preferred radiologic modality for visualizing lymph nodes; the normal mediastinal nodes are seen as soft tissue structures with a fatty hilum. Normal lymph nodes in the thorax typically measure less than 10 mm by a short axis. Healthy lymph nodes can be larger as a result of acute infection or chronic lung diseases such as emphysema or pulmonary fibrosis; however, enlarged lymph nodes are most worrisome for a pathologic process such as lymphoma, malignant metastases, or sarcoidosis. Lymphadenopathy is a common and non-specific sign. Many enlarged mediastinal nodes will be pathological, but not all. Common causes include:

- Metastatic malignancies to the mediastinum from other sites.
- Autoimmune.
- Infective aetiology like pneumonia and pulmonary TB.
- Occupational lung disease, silicosis.
- Interstitial lung disease.
- Congestive cardiac failure.

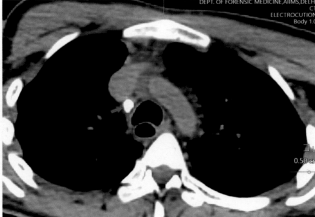

FIGURE 3.127: Axial section of chest PMCT showing paratracheal lymph node calcification.

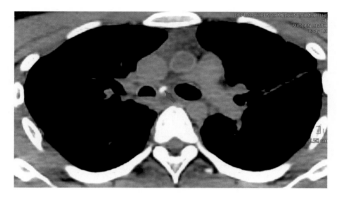

FIGURE 3.128: Axial section of chest PMCT showing subcarinal lymph node calcification.

Apart from increased size, calcification of lymph nodes are also an important finding detected on CT (Figures 3.127 and 3.128). Lymph node calcifications are easily seen on PMCT, and the usual pathology causing lymph node calcifications is prior granulomatous infections like TB. There are other less common causes of lymph node calcification like sarcoidosis, silicosis, and calcifications secondary to radiation therapy or chemotherapy.

Bibliography

Abramowitz Y, Simanovsky N, Goldstein MS, Hiller N. Pleural effusion: Characterization with CT attenuation values and CT appearance. *AJR Am J Roentgenol.* 2009;192:618–623.

Allen GS, Coates NE. Pulmonary contusion: A collective review. *Am Surg.* 1996 November 1;62(11):895–900.

Allen GS, Cox Jr CS. Pulmonary contusion in children: Diagnosis and management. *South Med J.* 1998 December 1;91(12):1099–1106.

Bastos R, Baisden CE, Harker L, Calhoon JH. Penetrating thoracic trauma. *Semin Thorac Cardiovasc Surg.* 2008;20:19–25.

Bintcliffe O, Maskell N. Spontaneous pneumothorax. *BMJ.* 2014 May 8:348.

Clark GC, Schecter WP, Trunkey DD. Variables affecting outcome in blunt chest trauma: Flail chest vs. pulmonary contusion. *J Trauma.* 1988;28:298–304.

Cohn SM. Pulmonary contusion: Review of the clinical entity. *J Trauma Acute Care Surg.* 1997 May 1;42(5):973–979.

Dogrul BN, Kiliccalan I, Asci ES, Peker SC. Blunt trauma related chest wall and pulmonary injuries: An overview. *Chin J Traumatol.* 2020 June 1;23(03):125–138.

Kaewlai R, Avery LL, Asrani AV et al. Multidetector CT of blunt thoracic trauma. *Radiographics.* 2008;28(6):1555–1570.

Kissling S, Hausmann, R. Morphology of direct and indirect rib fractures. *Int J Legal Med.* 2021;135:213–222.

Klein Y, Cohn SM, Proctor KG. Lung contusion: Pathophysiology and management. *Curr Opin Anesthesiol.* 2002 February 1;15(1):65–68.

Lardi C, Egger C, Larribau R, Niquille M, Mangin P, Fracasso T. Traumatic injuries after mechanical cardiopulmonary resuscitation (LUCAS™2): A forensic autopsy study. *Int J Legal Med* 2015;129(5):1035–1042.

Lewis B, Herr K, Hamlin S et al. Imaging manifestations of chest trauma. *Radiographics.* 2021;41(5):1321–1334.

Light RW, Macgregor MI, Luchsinger PC, BALL JR WC. Pleural effusions: The diagnostic separation of transudates and exudates. *Ann Intern Med.* 1972 October 1;77(4):507–513.

Moloney JT, Fowler SJ, Chang W. Anesthetic management of thoracic trauma. *Curr Opin Anesthesiol.* 2008 February 1;21(1):41–46.

Nandalur KR, Hardie AH, Bollampally SR, Parmar JP, Hagspiel KD. Accuracy of computed tomography attenuation values in the characterization of pleural fluid: An ROC study. *Acad Radiol* 2005;12:987–991.

O'Connor AR, Morgan WE. Radiological review of pneumothorax. *BMJ.* 2005 June 23;330(7506):1493–1497.

O'Connor JV, Adamski J. The diagnosis and treatment of noncardiac thoracic trauma. *JRAMC.* 2010;156:5–14.

Pearson EG, Fitzgerald CA, Santore MT. Pediatric thoracic trauma: Current trends. *Semin Pediatr Surg.* 2017;26:36–42.

Požgain Z, Kristek D, Lovrić I, et al. Pulmonary contusions after blunt chest trauma: Clinical significance and evaluation of patient management. *Eur J Trauma Emerg Surg.* 2018;44:773–777.

Sasser SM, Sattin RW, Hunt RC, Krohmer J. Blast lung injury. *Prehosp Emerg Care.* 2006 Jan 1;10(2):165–72.

Shorr RM, Crittenden M, Indeck M, Hartunian SL, Rodriguez A. Blunt thoracic trauma: Analysis of 515 patients. *Ann Surg.* 1987;206:200–205.

Simon B, Ebert J, Bokhari F, Capella J, Emhoff T, Hayward III T, Rodriguez A, Smith L. Management of pulmonary contusion and flail chest: An Eastern Association for the Surgery of Trauma practice management guideline. *J. Trauma Acute Care Surg.* 2012 November 1;73(5):S351–361.

Strange GR, Ahrens WR, Schafermeyer R, Wiebe R, Prendergast H, Dobiesz V. *Pediatric emergency medicine.* McGraw Hill Medical; 2009, pp. 92–100.

Thomas DO, Bernardo LM, Herman B, editors. *Core curriculum for pediatric emergency nursing.* Jones & Bartlett Learning, 2003, p. 446.

Ullman EA, Donley LP, Brady WJ. Pulmonary trauma: Emergency department evaluation and management. *Emerg Med Clin.* 2003 May 1;21(2):291–313.

Wagner R, Crawford W, Schimpf P. Classification of parenchymal Injuries of the lung. *Radiology.* 1988;167(1):77–82.

Weinberger SE, Cockrill BA, Mandel J. Principles of pulmonary medicine e-book. *Elsevier Health Sci.* 2017 December 26:215–216.

4 ABDOMEN – ANATOMY, TRAUMA, AND PATHOLOGY

The abdomen is a critical part of the human body that houses many of the vital organs of the body, including the stomach, small intestine, large intestine, liver, pancreas, spleen, adrenal, and kidneys. The abdomen is protected by the abdominal muscles and the spine. Post-mortem computed tomography (PMCT) of the abdomen is a diagnostic imaging technique used to visualise the abdominal organs and tissues of a deceased individual and also to identify and diagnose various conditions. A few of these include abdominal injuries, internal bleeding, and disease processes, which help in evaluating the cause of death, especially in cases of sudden or unexpected death. For understanding the detailed anatomy and pathologies, the abdomen is classified under the following four headings:

1. Peritoneum
2. Muscles and bones
3. Accessory organs: Liver with gall bladder, spleen, kidneys, adrenals, and pancreas
4. Gastrointestinal tract

Peritoneum

The peritoneum is a membranous inner lining of the abdominal cavity and covers the abdominal wall and the viscera. It acts as a support and provides pathways for blood and lymph vessels. The peritoneum consists of two layers, i.e., visceral and parietal peritoneum, which are in continuation with each other. The potential space between the two layers is known as the peritoneal cavity and normally contains a small amount of lubricating fluid. Abdominal organs based on relation to peritoneal covering are divided into two categories, namely intraperitoneal organs and retro-peritoneal organs.

Intraperitoneal organs

Intraperitoneal organs are organs enveloped or covered by the visceral peritoneum. The peritoneum covers these organs both anteriorly and posteriorly, e.g. stomach, liver and spleen (Figure 4.1).

Retro-peritoneal organs

Retro-peritoneal organs are not in association with the visceral peritoneum; they are only covered by the parietal peritoneum, and only on their anterior surface. Retro-peritoneal organs include the kidneys (Figures 4.2 and 4.3), adrenals, pancreas, and parts of the colon and rectum, which can be easily visualised on PMCT.

Retro-peritoneal organs are further classified as primary and secondary retro-peritoneal organs:

- Primary retro-peritoneal organs: These organs develop and remain outside of the parietal peritoneum, e.g., the oesophagus, rectum, adrenals, and kidneys.
- Secondary retro-peritoneal organs: These organs are initially intraperitoneal and suspended by the mesentery. During embryogenesis, they become retroperitoneal as their mesentery fuses with the posterior abdominal wall,

e.g., the duodenum, except for the proximal segment, the ascending and descending colon, and the pancreas (head, neck, and body).

The peritoneum is a highly folded complex structure, and each of its folds and spaces is described by several terminologies. There are three categories of peritoneal formations with specific terms: mesentery, omentum, and peritoneal ligaments (Figure 4.4).

1. Mesentery: It is a double layer of peritoneum formed by the invagination of an organ into the peritoneum; it holds the organ with the body wall and also forms a channel for the blood vessels, nerves, and lymphatic ducts between the organ and the body wall. It is named according to the viscera it connects, for example, the transverse and sigmoid mesocolons, the mesoappendix, etc.
2. Omentum: The omentum is the visceral peritoneum in layers extending from the stomach and proximal part of the duodenum to the other abdominal organs. They are classified into the greater omentum and lesser omentum.
   - Greater omentum: It is the larger of the two omentums. It extends from the proximal part of the duodenum and greater curvature of the stomach (Figure 4.1) to the transverse colon and transverse mesocolon and hangs down freely from the transverse mesocolon anterior of the intestines (Figure 4.4). It is referred to as the policeman of the abdomen as it migrates to cover the inflamed or infected organs to separate them from the other non-infected abdominal organs.
   - Lesser omentum: It is considerably smaller than the greater omentum; it extends from the stomach's lesser curvature and the initial segment of the duodenum to the liver (Figure 4.1). It is divided into hepatogastric and hepatoduodenal ligaments and they form the anterior border of the epiploic foramen.
3. Peritoneal ligaments: These are the peritoneal layers organised in a way that they connect an organ with another organ or with the body wall. The peritoneal ligaments which interconnect two organs are named based on both the organs, e.g., gastrocolic ligament – connecting the stomach and colon, hepatogastric ligament – connecting the liver and stomach, and splenorenal ligament – connecting the spleen and the kidney, etc.

Peritoneal cavity

The peritoneal cavity is a potential space in the abdomen lying between the parietal peritoneum and visceral peritoneum. It is a space which is derived from the coelomic cavity of the embryo, similar to other spaces like pleural cavities surrounding the lungs and the pericardial cavity surrounding the heart. The peritoneal cavity is separated into two compartments by the transverse colon and its mesocolon, separating them into an upper supra-colic compartment and a lower infra-colic compartment. The supra-colic compartment hosts

DOI: 10.1201/9781003383703-4

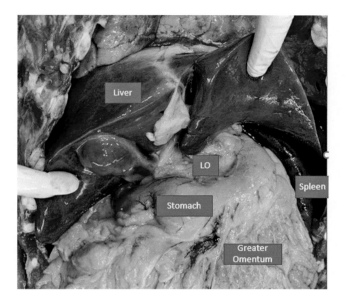

FIGURE 4.1: Image showing intraperitoneal organs, i.e., liver, spleen and stomach, along with peritoneal folds dropping from the stomach and proximal part of the duodenum, i.e., greater omentum (from the greater curvature of the stomach) and lesser omentum (LO) from the lesser curvature of the stomach

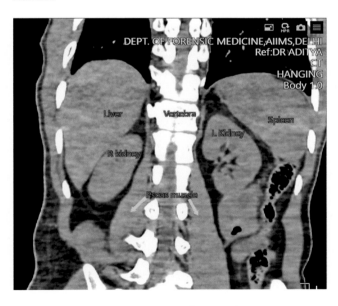

FIGURE 4.2: Coronal section of PMCT (posterior to anterior view) showing retroperitoneal organ, i.e., kidney, along with intraperitoneal organs, i.e., liver and spleen and also the psoas muscles (yellow arrows).

vital organs like the liver, spleen, stomach, and lesser omentum. The infra-colic compartment of the peritoneum hosts the small intestine, ascending colon, descending colon, and paracolic gutters. The distal portion of the peritoneal cavity differs between both sexes due to different pelvic organs. In males, the peritoneal cavity is completely closed, while in females, the peritoneal cavity is not completely closed as the uterine tubes open into the peritoneal cavity. This provides a potential pathway between the female genital tract and the abdominal cavity which can transmit infections of the vagina, uterus, or

uterine tubes into the peritoneal cavity and cause infection and inflammation of the peritoneum called peritonitis.

Pathology of the peritoneum
The important pathologies of the peritoneum include the following:

1. Peritonitis: Peritonitis is a condition in which the peritoneum, the membrane lining the abdominal cavity and covering the organs, becomes inflamed. This inflammation can be caused by a bacterial infection, a fungal infection, chemical irritants, or other factors. Peritonitis can be a serious and life-threatening condition if left untreated. The symptoms of peritonitis can include abdominal pain, tenderness, and swelling, as well as fever, nausea, and vomiting. In severe cases, the patient may develop sepsis (Figure 4.5), a condition in which the body's immune response to the infection can cause organ failure and even death. On a PMCT scan, peritonitis may be identified by several characteristic findings, such as:
   - The peritoneum itself may appear thickened or inflamed, and there may be an accumulation of fluid within the peritoneal cavity, known as ascites. This fluid may appear as low-density areas on the scan.
   - Presence of abscesses or collections of pus within the abdominal cavity. These abscesses may appear as rounded, fluid-filled areas with thick, irregular walls.

   Peritonitis may be caused by a perforation or rupture of the gastrointestinal tract, such as a perforated ulcer or a ruptured diverticulum or a rupture of the stomach in case of corrosive poisoning (Figure 4.6). These conditions may be identified by the presence of free air or gas within the abdomen, causing pneumoperitoneum. Free air appears as black areas on the PMCT scan and is a concerning finding, as it suggests that perforation has occurred and the infection may be spreading rapidly.

2. Tubercular peritonitis: Tubercular peritonitis is an infectious condition commonly seen in patients with risk factors such as an immunocompromised state, chronic kidney disease, or cirrhosis/liver disease. The spread is usually haematogenous from pulmonary foci but rarely also from intestinal tuberculosis from the ingested source of infection. Peritoneal tuberculosis is a form of abdominal tuberculosis in which the deceased presents with a history of abdominal pain and distention due to ascites; apart from that, there are constitutional symptoms like weight loss and fever. Laboratory investigations are primarily helpful in diagnosing, including the analysis of the peritoneal fluid. On PMCT, loculated ascites or peritoneal fluid may be appreciated with no evidence of perforation, and tubercles may also be noted.

3. Peritoneal metastasis/peritoneal carcinomatosis: This is the intraperitoneal dissemination of any form of cancer that does not originate from the peritoneum itself. It is seen mostly in abdominopelvic malignancies. Computed tomography (CT) is an important radiological tool for the detailed assessment of peritoneal metastasis and has high sensitivity in the detection process. The peritoneal metastasis can be seen as multiple large masses/nodules (Figure 4.7) and sometimes maybe grossly invisible. The PMCT appearance of these metastases can include

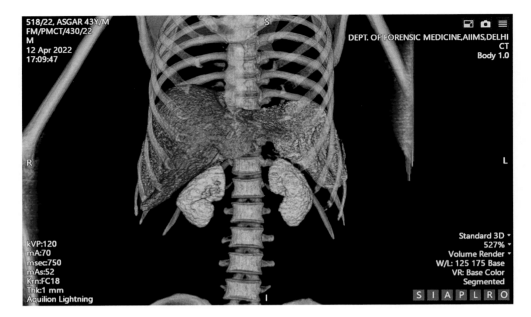

FIGURE 4.3: Volume rendered 3D PMCT image showing intraperitoneal organs, i.e., liver (orange) and spleen (purple) and retroperitoneal organ, i.e., kidney (sea green).

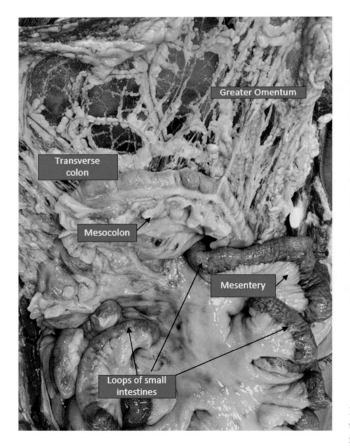

FIGURE 4.4: Autopsy examination of the abdomen showing the mesentery and the omentum, which are parts of the peritoneum.

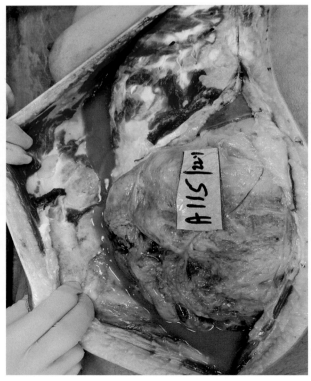

FIGURE 4.5: Autopsy examination of a case of peritonitis with sepsis, abdominal examination on opening showing inflamed peritoneum straw-coloured foul-smelling fluid in the peritoneal cavity.

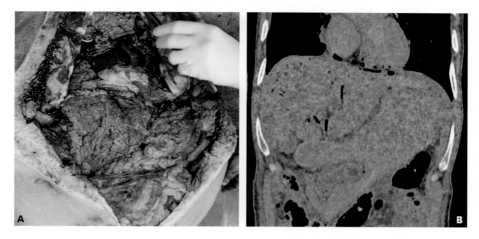

FIGURE 4.6: A case of perforation of the stomach after acid ingestion: (A) Gross image of a case showing a ruptured stomach in a case with content spilt inside the peritoneal cavity causing peritonitis. (B) The coronal section of PMCT in the case shows mixed attenuation of hypo and hyperdensity inside and surrounding areas of the stomach.

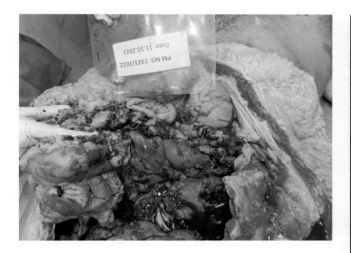

FIGURE 4.7: Peritoneal metastasis seen in a case of renal cell carcinoma seen as multiple nodules distributed throughout the peritoneal cavity.

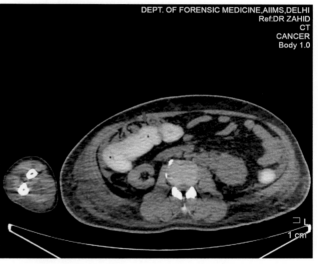

FIGURE 4.8: Axial section of PMCT in soft tissue window of the same case as Fig. 7 showing peritoneal metastasis as irregular thickenings of the peritoneum. In this case, the deceased had been given a contrast prior to death which is seen in the colon.

thickening and enhancement of peritoneal reflections, which is usually seen as a nodular appearance (Figure 4.8), thickening of the omentum, fluid collection in the abdominal cavity causing ascites, and calcification of the metastasis.

4. Ascites: This is a condition characterised by abnormal fluid accumulation in the abdominal cavity (Figure 4.9). This fluid build-up occurs when the body is unable to properly regulate the production and absorption of fluid within the peritoneal cavity. Ascites are commonly associated with liver disease, heart failure, kidney disease, and certain types of cancer. On PMCT scans, ascites appear as a collection of fluid within the peritoneal cavity, between the abdominal organs and the abdominal wall (Figure 4.9). It can also be associated with features, such as thickening or nodularity of the peritoneal lining or the presence of masses or tumours. The Hounsfield unit (HU), i.e., the density of the fluid, helps to differentiate simple fluid from a haemorrhagic fluid.

5. Adhesions: Peritoneal adhesions are bands of scar tissue that can form between the peritoneum and organs within the abdominal cavity. These adhesions can be caused by surgery, infection, inflammation, etc. On a PMCT scan, peritoneal adhesions may be identified by several characteristic findings, such as:
   - The adhesions themselves may appear as thin/thick irregular linear bands of tissue on the scan, connecting two or more organs or the peritoneum to the abdominal wall.
   - Complications related to the adhesions, such as bowel obstruction, may appear as a dilated, fluid-filled loop of bowel upstream from the obstruction and a collapsed or empty loop of bowel downstream on PMCT.

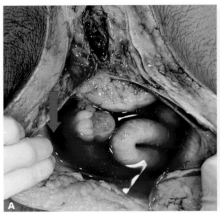
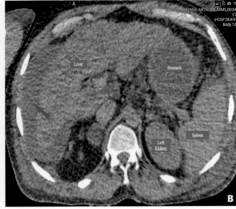

FIGURE 4.9: A case of chronic liver disease with macronodular cirrhosis showing ascites; A: Autopsy examination of the abdomen showing straw-coloured ascitic fluid in the peritoneal cavity; B: Axial section of same case showing peritoneal fluid (marked with red arrow) along with liver showing irregular surface and parenchyma showing mixed attenuation.

6. Hernias: This is a condition where internal organs or tissues protrude through a weak area in the covering muscle or connective tissue. The common types of hernias are inguinal, femoral, umbilical, and incisional. Direct inguinal hernia (Figure 4.10) is a common type of abdominal hernia. A direct inguinal hernia occurs due to protrusion of abdominal viscera or tissues through a weak area in the inguinal canal's posterior wall, medial to the inferior epigastric vessels and more specifically through the Hesselbach's triangle. On a PMCT, a round or oval shape bulge or protrusion of tissue through the muscle or connective tissue is seen (Figure 4.10). Direct hernia can be differentiated from indirect hernia by lateral crescent sign in which the fat and the other inguinal canal contents are flattened by the herniated fat and omentum into a thin lateral 'moon-like' crescent while the common femoral artery and vein are seen coursing laterally and posteriorly to the hernia. Complications,

such as bowel obstruction or strangulation, can also be detected on a PMCT.

7. Peritoneal cysts: A peritoneal cyst is a fluid-filled sac that develops in the lining of the abdominal cavity. These cysts are relatively rare and can be asymptomatic. On a PMCT, a peritoneal cyst appears as a well-defined fluid-filled structure within the peritoneal cavity. The cyst may be in any part of the abdomen and can range in size from a few mm to several cm in diameter.

8. Spontaneous haemoperitoneum: Usually, haemoperitoneum is seen in traumatic cases, but still without a trauma, it can also be seen in conditions like ectopic pregnancy (Figures 4.11 and 4.12), non-traumatic rupture of the liver, spleen, or abdominal vasculature with underlying pathology, which is fatal.

9. Non-traumatic spontaneous retro-peritoneal haemorrhage: Spontaneous retro-peritoneal haemorrhage is a rare entity but has a high degree of morbidity and

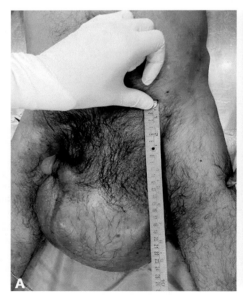
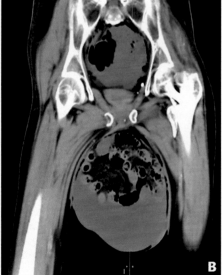

FIGURE 4.10: A case of inguinal hernia: (A) Autopsy examination of the case showing inguinal hernia (B) Coronal section of PMCT showing oval shape bulge or protrusion of tissue containing the loops of intestine and fluid.

The blood in the cavity accumulates between the abdominal wall's inner lining and the internal abdominal organs (Figure 4.13). Haemoperitoneum is generally classified as an emergency, and in most cases, urgent laparotomy is done to secure the bleeding point. Excessive loss of blood will be fatal and leads to haemorrhagic shock. Causes of hemoperitoneum include:

- Penetrating trauma or blunt trauma to the abdomen causes injury to the solid organs such as the liver (Figure 4.14), spleen, and kidney or to vascular structures like the mesentery (Figure 4.15).
- Vascular ruptures due to weakening of the wall of the vessels like an abdominal aortic aneurysm or common iliac aneurysm, even after trivial trauma.
- Perforation of the colon or stomach due to blunt trauma abdomen.
- Haemorrhage due to rupture of a vascular intra-abdominal neoplasm like hepatoblastoma by a trivial trauma.

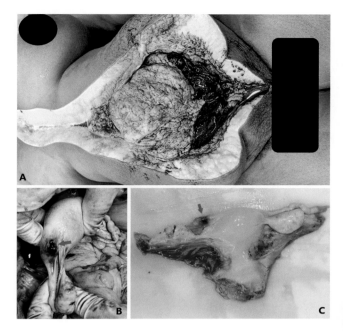

FIGURE 4.11: A case of ectopic rupture causing death due to haemorrhagic shock. A: Abdominal examination of the case during autopsy showing haemoperitoneum due to spontaneous rupture of the ectopic pregnancy. B: The examination of the internal reproductive organs in situ shows the ectopic rupture site on the right fallopian tube. C: Virchow's technique of examination of the uterus, fallopian tubes, and ovary shows the rupture site in the right fallopian tube.

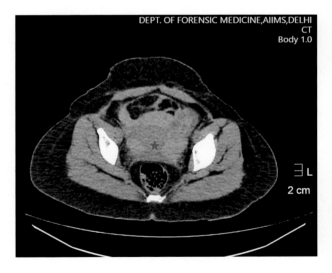

FIGURE 4.12: PMCT examination in the case of spontaneous haemoperitoneum due to ectopic pregnancy rupture showing blood collection in the abdomen and pelvis; the rupture site cannot be identified due to blood masking the rupture site.

mortality. It is commonly seen in an elderly patient on anticoagulation therapy and those with underlying coagulopathy and sometimes as a result of rupture of parenchymal lesions or underlying vascular malformations.

Traumatic pathology
- **Haemoperitoneum:** Haemoperitoneum is the presence of blood in the peritoneal cavity of the abdomen.

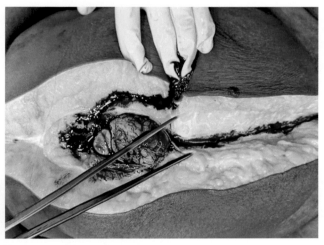

FIGURE 4.13: Anterior abdominal wall incision showing blood in peritoneal cavity in a case of traumatic hemoperitoneum.

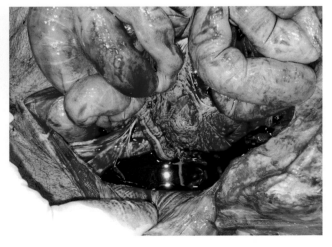

FIGURE 4.14: Haemoperitoneum case in which abdominal examination during the autopsy showed blood over the right side of the abdomen in case of gunshot injury to the liver.

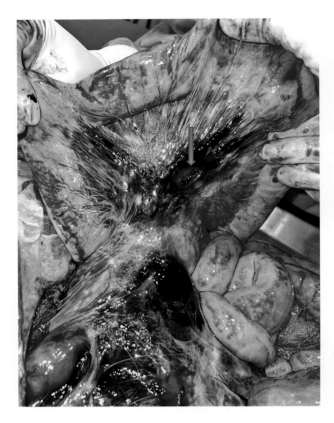

FIGURE 4.15: Hemoperitoneum case in which abdominal examination during the autopsy showed blood along with blood clots in the mesentery due to gunshot injury to the mesentery.

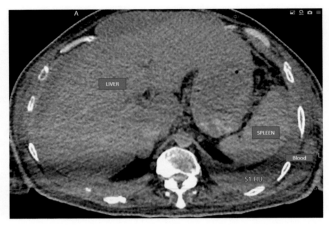

FIGURE 4.16: Axial section of PMCT in soft tissue window showing haemoperitoneum in case of a road traffic accident with multiple ribs and vertebra fracture (at a different level). Collection of blood is seen with a varied HU from 20 to 60 on the left side of the abdomen along with fluid-fluid level.

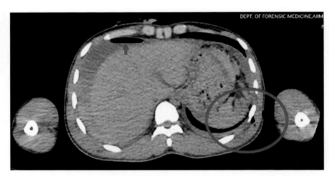

FIGURE 4.17: Axial section of PMCT in soft tissue window of a case of stab to the left side lower chest entering the abdomen (red circle) causing pneumoperitoneum, the air is seen over the anterior abdomen due to supine posture of the dead body at the time of PMCT capturing.

- Traumatic rupture of the uterus, especially in cases of criminal abortions.

  On a PMCT, the HU will suggest its composition, i.e., ascites fluid or haemorrhage fluid. A recent haemorrhage (acute bleed) measures about 30–45 HU. Clotted blood measures about 45–70 HU, and old blood products or blood in patients measures roughly <30 HU. A collection of blood products can be homogeneous or heterogeneous (mix of hypo- and hyperdensities) fluid–fluid levels are often present (Figure 4.16).

- Pneumoperitoneum: Pneumoperitoneum is defined as an abnormal collection of air or other gas within the peritoneal cavity. A few of the common causes include the following:
  - Penetrating trauma (Figure 4.17).
  - Perforated duodenal ulcer, peptic ulcer or inflammatory bowel disease (e.g., megacolon).
  - After laparotomy or laparoscopy.
  - Bowel injury after endoscopy.
  - Peritoneal dialysis (PD).
  - Colonic or peritoneal infection.

  On a PMCT examination, the HU of air is around −1000. It should be differentiated from decomposition. The history of the case is to be assessed properly for analysing the PMCT findings.

Muscles and bones of the abdomen

The abdominal wall encloses the abdominal cavity and protects the abdominal viscera. It also keeps the abdominal viscera in its anatomical position against gravity and assists in forceful expiration by pushing the abdominal viscera upwards. It also plays a vital role in actions like coughing, vomiting, and defecation that require increased intra-abdominal pressure.

The muscles of the abdominal wall can be divided into two main groups:

- Posterior abdominal wall muscles include – the psoas muscle, erector spinae, and quadratus lumborum muscle (Figure 4.18).
- Anterior abdominal wall muscles include – the rectus abdominis (R), external oblique (EO), internal oblique (IO), and transverse abdominis (TA) (Figure 4.18).

The abdominal cavity is supported by the lumbar spine, which is the third region of the vertebral column, located below the thoracic and above the sacral vertebral segment. It consists of five distinct vertebrae (Figure 4.19), which are the largest vertebrae of the entire vertebral column. It has an important role as a weight-bearing structure. It extends up to the pelvic cavity, with is bounded by pelvic bones

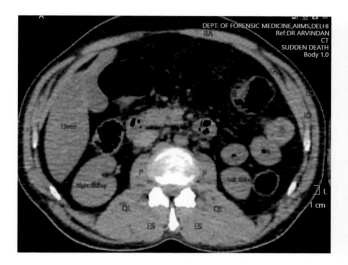

FIGURE 4.18: Axial image of the lower abdomen showing anterior abdominal muscles, i.e. Rectus abdominis (R), External oblique (EO), Internal oblique (IO), Transverse abdominis (TA) and posterior abdominal muscles, i.e., Psoas muscle (P), Erector spinae (ES) and Quadratus lumborum (QL) muscle.

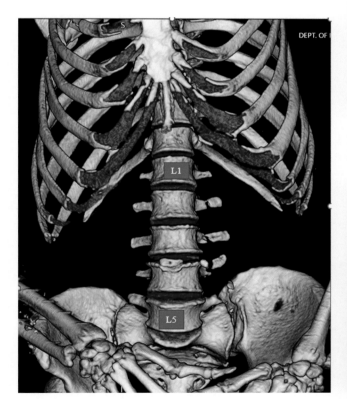

FIGURE 4.19: Volume rendering 3D image showing the L1 – L5 vertebra; in this case, there is also a fracture of the transverse process of L2- L4 on the left side.

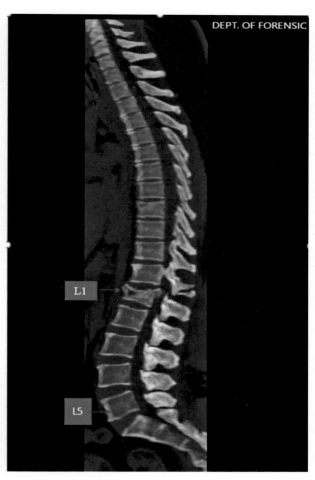

FIGURE 4.20: Sagittal section of PMCT showing fracture of L1 vertebra body and spinous process of T12 vertebra

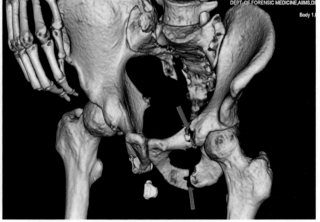

FIGURE 4.21: Volume rendering 3D image showing fracture of the left superior and inferior pubic ramus (red arrows).

Traumatic pathology

1. Fracture: During trauma like an RTA, fall from a height, gunshot wound, etc., a fracture of the vertebral column (Figures 4.19 and 4.20) or the pelvis (Figure 4.21) is a common finding, especially if the person landed on their foot or buttock. These are difficult to identify by dissection and also to expose the full extent of fracture lines. These fractures remain concealed in cases where conventional dissection techniques are being used casually. Detailed dissection and demonstration of these

bony injuries expose the pathologist to injuries by sharp concealed edges of fractured segments. These fractures are readily identifiable with PMCT, with the 3D reconstruction giving a complete view, along with the position of the displaced fragments helping in demonstrating a mechanism of causation of these injuries.

Accessory organs

Accessory organs of the abdomen include solid organs and hollow organs. Solid organs include the liver with the gall bladder, kidneys, adrenals, spleen, and pancreas. The hollow organs include parts of the gastrointestinal tract like the oesophagus, stomach, small intestine, and large intestine. A PMCT is useful for assessing the shape, size, and homogeneity and identifying abnormal densities of solid organs. It is also useful in assessing the wall thickness and lumen patency of hollow organs. Here we will be discussing the anatomy and pathology along with the traumatic pathology of all the accessory organs in brief.

Liver

The liver is the largest abdominal organ, it is also wedge-shaped (Figure 4.22). It is located just below the diaphragm and topographically occupies the right upper quadrant of the abdominal cavity extending into the epigastric quadrant as well. It is mostly covered by the right lower ribs over the posterior and lateral aspects and the costal cartilage in the anterior aspect. The liver in adults generally measures 10–12.5 cm craniocaudally and around 20–23 cm transversely, but the size is variable from one individual to another and is dependent on multiple factors like build, genetic background, gender, presence of any pathology, etc. It is almost entirely covered by the visceral peritoneum except for the posterosuperior aspect, which is spared, and this area is called the bare area (area nuda).

Surfaces: The liver has two surfaces, namely the diaphragmatic surface and the visceral surface, which are sharply demarcated from each other anteriorly by the inferior margin.

- Diaphragmatic surface: It is the large, smooth surface which has a peritoneal covering area that faces superiorly, laterally, and anteriorly but also includes the bare area over the posterosuperior region.
- Visceral surface: It faces inferiorly and posteriorly and is covered by the peritoneum; it is marked by the structures of the porta hepatis. It is in direct contact with important abdominal structures like the oesophagus, stomach, and lesser omentum on its left. The pancreas and duodenum occupy the midline position. On the right end, there are structures like the right kidney, hepatic flexure of the colon and right adrenal.

Ligaments: Major ligaments associated with the liver are:

- Falciform ligament: It is a ligament which attaches anteriorly and separates the right and left liver lobes (Figure 4.23).
- Ligamentum teres (round ligament): It is the ligament formed from the remnant of the umbilical vein. Its attachment extends from the inferior border of the liver near the lower end of the falciform ligament, and its attachment continues posteriorly up to the porta hepatis, where it attaches to the left portal vein (Figure 4.23).
- Ligamentum venosum: It is the remnant of ductus venosum and continues from the ligamentum teres into the superior part of the porta hepatis.

Segmental anatomy: The liver is covered by a shiny, fibrous layer known as Glisson's capsule. The liver consists of a larger right lobe and a smaller left lobe anatomically divided by the falciform ligament. There are two other accessory lobes of the liver which arise from the right lobe located over the visceral surface, which are:

1. Caudate lobe: It is located on the upper aspect of the visceral surface and lies between the inferior vena cava, ligamentum venosum, and bare area of the liver and the porta hepatis (Figure 4.24).
2. Quadrate lobe: It is located on the lower aspect of the visceral surface and lies between the gall bladder, round ligament, and porta hepatis (Figure 4.24).

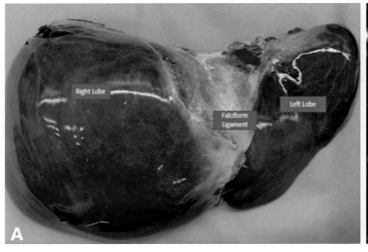
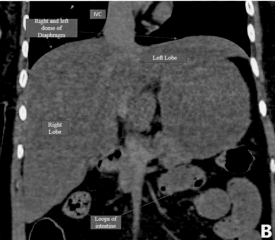

FIGURE 4.22:   A: The gross image of the liver showing the right and left lobe of the liver along with the falciform ligament. B: Coronal section of PMCT in soft tissue window showing right and left lobe of the liver.

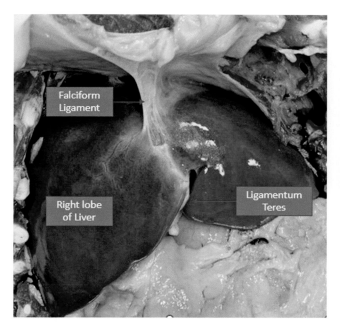

FIGURE 4.23: Abdominal examination during autopsy showing the diaphragmatic surface of the liver with a shiny covering capsule called Glisson's capsule along with the attachment of the falciform ligament anteriorly and ligamentum teres inferiorly.

Porta hepatis: The porta hepatis, also known as the transverse hepatic fissure, is a deep fissure in the inferior surface of the liver, separating the caudate and quadrate lobe. It transmits to the hepatic artery, common bile duct and portal vein.

As per the Couinaud classification (Figure 4.25), the liver is divided into eight segments which have an individual segmental hepatic artery, portal veins, and bile ducts. The middle hepatic vein, which also represents Cantlie's line, separates the right and left liver lobes according to the Couinaud classification. The right liver lobe is divided into anterior and posterior

segments by the right hepatic vein, while on the other hand, the left lobe of the liver is divided into medial and lateral segments by the left hepatic vein. The vascular anatomy is more relevant in PMCT imaging as it helps in the identification of the lesion location in a more scientific and precise form. It provides standardised identification and localisation of hepatic segments. Eight segments method of division of the liver is on the basis of considering two transverse planes and three longitudinal planes. The first longitudinal plane, which traverses through the gallbladder fossa, inferior vena cava and the middle hepatic vein, separates the right and left lobes of the liver. The second longitudinal plane traversing through the right hepatic vein separates the right lobe of the liver into anterior and posterior segments. The third longitudinal plane, which traverses through the left hepatic vein, separates the left liver lobe into medial and lateral segments. The first transverse plane, which traverses through the left portal vein, separates the left lobe into superior and inferior segments. The second oblique transverse plane, which traverses through the right portal vein, separates the right liver lobe into superior and inferior segments. The caudate lobe is considered segment I, and it extends from the inferior vena cava to the fissure of the ligamentum venosum.

Pathology of the liver

Liver disease is a broad term describing a number of anatomical and pathological irregularities that can affect the functional capacity of the liver, which in turn affects the other organs of the body. Confirmation of the hepatic pathology can be done by a combination of investigation, gross examination, and histopathological and radiological evaluation. In the initial stages of liver disease, the inflammation of the hepatic cells is seen and is termed hepatitis, and when there is fat deposition in the hepatic cells, it is called steatosis, or a combination of both is referred to as steatohepatitis. This damage to the hepatocytes can continue and culminate in the non-reversal phase of fibrosis and eventually causing cirrhosis of the liver if the cause of liver injury is not removed at the appropriate time. Liver pathologies are described as follows:

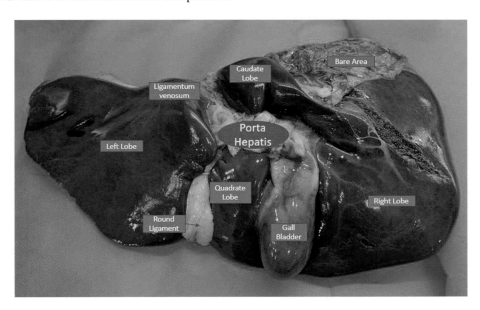

FIGURE 4.24: Visceral Surface: Examination of the posterior aspect (visceral surface) of the liver with lobes and ligaments along with porta hepatis which consists of the common bile duct, hepatic artery and portal vein.

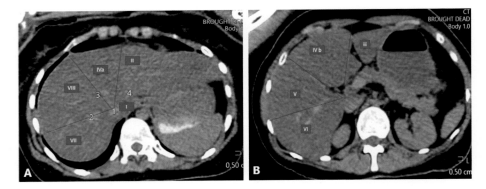

FIGURE 4.25: Couinaud Liver Segments. A: Axial section of the PMCT abdomen at the superior portion of the liver showing inferior vena cava (1) and the three longitudinal planes (marked as red lines) across the right hepatic vein (2), middle hepatic vein as (3) left hepatic vein((4). B: Axial section at the inferior portion of the liver. CT scans illustrate the Couinaud classification of the numbering of liver segments. The longitudinal plane (marked as red arrows) of the right hepatic vein divides VIII from VII in the superior portion of the liver and V from VI in the inferior portion of the liver. The longitudinal plane of the middle hepatic vein through the gallbladder fossa separates IVa from VIII in the superior liver and IVb from V in the inferior liver. The longitudinal plane of the left hepatic vein separates IVa from II in the superior liver and IVb from III in the inferior liver.

1. **Hepatomegaly:** Hepatomegaly is a condition characterised by the enlargement of the liver. Hepatomegaly is considered a sign of an underlying pathology, more than a disease, like liver disease or congestive heart failure or cancer. It is a non-specific medical sign and often presents with an abdominal mass. The mechanism of hepatomegaly consists of vascular swelling and inflammation as a result of the infectious cause or due to the deposition of fat or other matter inside the hepatic cells. It can be seen in certain conditions, such as:
   - Infections like hepatitis, malaria, liver abscess hydatid cyst, etc.
   - Heart failure.
   - Tumours like hepatocellular carcinoma or leukaemia.
   - Anaemias.
   - Congenital heart diseases, sickle cell anaemia or polycystic liver disease, and other metabolic disturbances.

   On a PMCT the following linear measurements of the liver (Figure 4.26) are important in diagnosing hepatomegaly:
   1) Maximum diameter mediolateral (CT max ML): This distance is taken in the coronal plane and is the maximum distance between the medial and the lateral ends of the liver.
   2) Maximum diameter craniocaudal (CT max CC): This distance is also taken in the coronal plane and is the maximum distance between the cranial and caudal ends of liver
   3) Maximum diameter dorsoventral (CT max DV): This distance is also taken in the axial plane and is the maximum distance between the anterior and posterior ends of liver

2. **Liver failure**: The most severe clinical consequence of liver disease is liver failure. It is divided into two categories depending on the onset of the disease:
   1) Acute liver failure:
      Acute liver failure (ALF), also known as fulminant hepatic failure, refers to sudden severe

liver dysfunction from injury without underlying chronic liver disease. It is defined as acute liver illness associated with encephalopathy and coagulopathy that occur within 2 weeks of initial liver injury in the absence of pre-existing liver disease. It is most commonly caused by drugs or toxins, e.g., accidental or deliberate ingestion of acetaminophen, suicidal ingestion of aluminium phosphide (Figure 4.27), or zinc phosphide, which is available as rat killer poison, etc. Apart from these metabolic disorders, viral infections like hepatitis B and hepatitis E also predominate as a cause of acute liver failure. The deceased will present with a history of nausea, vomiting, and jaundice followed by life-threatening encephalopathy and coagulation defects. Macroscopically acute liver failure depicts as smaller and shrunken liver with massive hepatic necrosis. On a PMCT the liver shows a heterogenous enhancement pattern (Figure 4.28).

2) Chronic liver disease (CLD):
   Chronic liver disease is a pathological condition of the liver where the organ is dysfunctional, and this condition persists for a period of more than six months. The main pathological event is permanent structural changes within the liver due to long-standing hepatocyte damage. Leading causes are chronic hepatitis B, chronic hepatitis C, non-alcoholic fatty liver disease and alcoholic liver disease. Macroscopically, cirrhosis occurs diffusely throughout the liver parenchyma (Figures 4.29 and 4.30).

3) **Alcoholic liver disease**
   Excessive consumption of alcohol (ethanol) is one of the leading causes of liver disease. Alcoholic liver disease gives rise to three distinctive appearances depending upon the exposure time of alcohol to the liver; they are: steatosis (fatty liver), alcoholic hepatitis and progressive fibrosis, and marked derangement leading eventually to cirrhosis (Figure 4.31.1).
   Alcohol undergoes an oxidative metabolic pathway in the hepatocytes, leading to a reduced ratio of the nicotinamide adenine dinucleotide (NAD) to nicotinamide

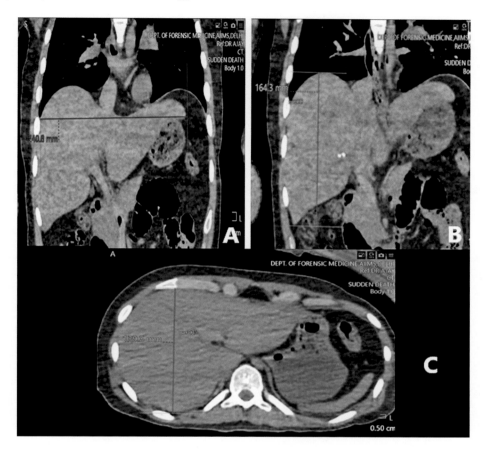

FIGURE 4.26: (A) Coronal section of PMCT showing Maximum diameter mediolateral (ML). (B) Coronal section of PMCT showing Maximum diameter craniocaudal (CC). (C) Axial section of PMCT showing Maximum diameter dorsoventral (DV).

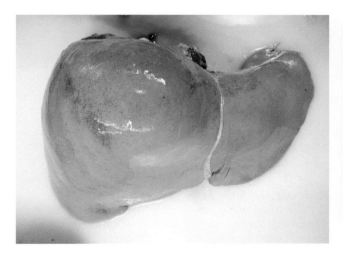

FIGURE 4.27: Steatosis and hepatic necrosis in a case of acute liver failure due to rat poison (aluminium phosphide).

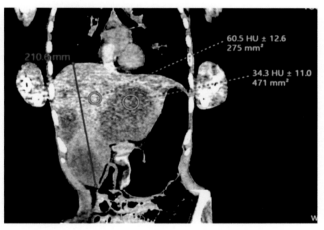

FIGURE 4.28: PMCT Coronal section of the abdomen in soft tissue window showing the altered densities of the liver due to fatty changes in the liver parenchyma. Measurement of the liver span using PMCT.

adenine dinucleotide + hydrogen (NADH). This promotes lipogenesis by inhibiting the oxidation of triglycerides and fatty acids. Another known mechanism of alcohol-induced liver injury is the translocation of endotoxins in the form of lipopolysaccharides from the intestines into the hepatocytes. In the hepatic cells, the lipopolysaccharides bind to the protein CD14 and toll-like receptor

4 to release a barrage of reactive oxygen species, which activates the release of cytokines such as tumour necrosis factor-alpha, interleukin-8, monocyte chemotactic protein 1, and platelet-derived growth factor. This leads to the accumulation of neutrophils, macrophages, and systemic clinical features of alcohol injury.

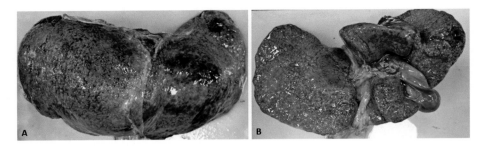

FIGURE 4.29: Autopsy image of the liver parenchyma of a 68-year-old female showing macro-nodules due to chronic liver failure. Note the haemorrhagic liver parenchyma involving the left lobe. (A&B)

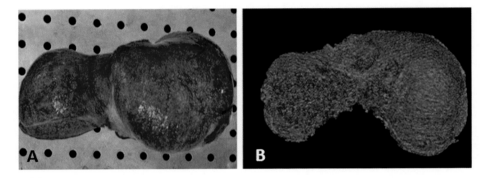

FIGURE 4.30: A: The gross image of liver parenchyma with multiple nodules and rounded borders due to cirrhosis. B: 3D Volume Rendered Technique of the liver in PMCT showing the liver parenchyma with nodules and rounded borders.

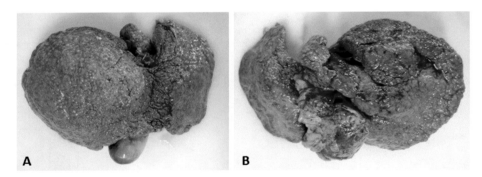

FIGURE 4.31.1: Autopsy image of a case 79-year-old male with macronodular cirrhosis with chronic liver failure, liver parenchyma showing macro-nodules and nodular irregular borders. Anterior (A) and posterior (B) views show the diffuse distribution of the pathology.

Histopathological examination: Alcoholic liver disease is characterised by steatosis, hepatocellular ballooning representing steatohepatitis, cholestasis, fibrosis, cirrhosis in severely ill patients, neutrophilic and lymphocytic infiltration, and Mallory–Denk bodies.

PMCT examination: A PMCT is not very sensitive to detect cirrhosis in its early stages, but the fatty changes can be identified by the parenchymal heterogeneity. In the advanced cirrhosis stage, the nodules may be appreciated as isodense or hyperdense in comparison to the rest of the liver parenchyma, along with a nodular margin owing to the cirrhotic pattern. A few signs of portal hypertension may also be seen, like an enlarged portal vein, splenomegaly, enlarged superior mesenteric vein and splenic vein.

Grading Alcoholic Liver Disease

The grading of the disease is essential to understand the progress of the disease. In the end stage of chronic liver disease, the pathognomic change seen in autopsy is cirrhosis with clinical history and signs of decompensation. The liver parenchyma is very hard to feel, with evidence of macro- or micro-nodules or both. The earlier stages have minor degrees of fibrosis or cirrhosis along with the fatty deposition of the parenchyma, which makes the liver greasy on touching. When the liver cells are injured or insulted by external agents like pathogens or toxins, it causes the liver to respond by a reparative response which includes the inflammatory stage causing hepatitis. The liver cells heal or recover in different modes; one such visible mode is the deposition of fat in cells, causing fatty(steatosis) changes. In certain cases, both inflammatory response and fatty deposition can be seen together, which is termed steatohepatitis. This

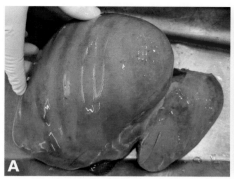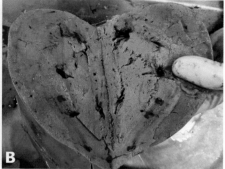

FIGURE 4.31.2: A case of severe fatty changes in the liver, A: liver is enlarged and has a smooth, shiny appearance. B: Cut-section in the case shows yellowish discolouration of parenchyma due to steatosis of liver parenchyma.

is the stage of liver disease where the organ still has its regenerative power, and if the external agent causing the injury is removed, it can revert back to normal functioning. If the external agent continues to cause injury or insult to the hepatocytes, then it may progress to a stage of fibrosis and cirrhosis.

1. Steatosis

The gross appearance of the liver in fatty liver is pale yellow-brown due to the increased lipid content within hepatocytes. The capsule is smooth, and on the cut surface, the parenchyma has a uniform texture. There may be associated hepatomegaly where the liver is twice to thrice the span and weight of normal liver size (Figure 4.31.2). Increased lipid biosynthesis from the generation of more NADH and deranged lipoprotein synthesis and its secretion along with an increased peripheral fat catabolism is the pathophysiology of hepatic steatosis. The most common cause is excessive alcohol consumption. The toxic injury from drugs like methotrexate or corticosteroids may also produce steatosis.

Histopathological examination: The cytoplasm of the hepatocytes is filled with large, clear lipid droplets with associated macrovesicular steatosis (Figure 4.31.3). This process is potentially reversible in weeks to months with cessation of exposure to causative factors like alcohol, drugs, etc. Portal fibrosis is an essential feature of chronic injury to the liver parenchyma. Some degree of steatosis accompanies all cases of chronic alcohol abuse, but only about 10–15% of these patients go on to develop cirrhosis.

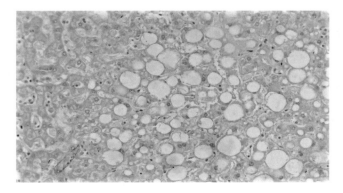

FIGURE 4.31.3: Histopathological examination of a fatty liver with H&E staining in 20X showing cytoplasm of the hepatocytes are filled with large, clear lipid droplets, with associated macro-vesicular steatosis.

On PMCT: A non-pathological liver has the same attenuation as the spleen. In steatosis (fatty liver), the liver attenuation will be lesser than that of the spleen by usually at least 10 HU or will have an absolute liver attenuation of less than 40 HU (Figure 4.31.4).

2. Fibrosis

Liver fibrosis refers to the accumulation of fibrous scar tissue in the liver. This occurs due to necrosis of hepatocytes as a result of the release of cytokines, growth factors, and various unknown chemicals by the immune cells, which causes the hepatic stellate cells to activate and produce collagen, glycoproteins, and proteoglycans along with other substances. These end products are deposited in the liver parenchyma, which causes them to be non-functional connective tissue. In a healthy liver, the fibrogenesis and fibrinolysis of the matrix tissue are equally carried out in balance, but fibrosis here occurs due to an imbalance in the process (Figure 4.31.5).

3. Cirrhosis

Cirrhosis occurs when diffuse chronic hepatic injury leads to the formation of fibrous septa that extend between portal tracts, disrupting the normal hepatic architecture with the formation of regenerative nodules of parenchyma. The normal vascular inflow and outflow patterns are disturbed, leading to the condition called portal hypertension. Fibrous septa surround regenerative hepatocyte nodules. Cirrhosis requires at least a decade to develop from chronic liver injury. A cirrhotic liver has rounded borders due to shrinkage of the liver parenchyma due to fibrosis. This is classified as micronodular and macronodular cirrhosis based on the size of the nodules.

    I. Micronodular cirrhosis: In micronodular cirrhosis, the average size of the nodules is 3 mm or less. The yellow-brown appearance of these nodules is due to hepatic steatosis. Chronic alcohol abuse is the most common cause of micronodular cirrhosis and steatosis. A fine reticulin network of type IV collagen is normally present in the liver, but with cirrhosis, there is an extensive deposition of type I and III collagen generated from activated perisinusoidal stellate cells. Cirrhosis may remain clinically silent for many years until complications of portal hypertension, such as oesophageal varices or ascites, develop (Figure 4.32).

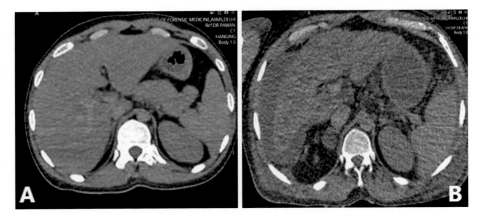

FIGURE 4.31.4: A: Axial section of PMCT in a normal case showing similar attenuation of liver and spleen. B: On the axial section of PMCT in a case with fatty liver, there is hypo attenuation of liver parenchyma as compared to spleen depicting fatty changes in the liver.

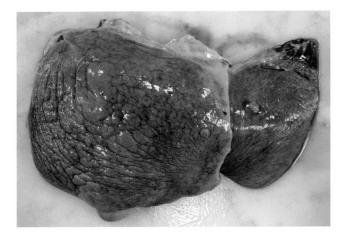

FIGURE 4.31.5: Autopsy examination of a 60-year-old female showed a liver with fibrotic changes, and the liver parenchyma admixed with macronudules.

II. Macronodular cirrhosis: Macronodular cirrhosis is characterised by nodules larger than 3 mm in size (Figure 4.33). There is an extensive deposition of tan-appearing collagen surrounding these regenerative nodules. The most common cause of macronodular cirrhosis is viral hepatitis. Most causes of cirrhosis can produce both patterns and mixed micronodular and macronodular cirrhosis (Figure 4.34).

4. **Metabolic liver disease**

I. Non-alcoholic fatty liver: In non-alcoholic fatty liver, the hepatocytes are filled with triglycerides even when there is an absence of a history of alcohol consumption. This steatosis can cause hepatocyte inflammation, which can give a combined picture referred to as non-alcoholic steatohepatitis (Figure 4.35). The most common metabolic disorder associated with non-alcoholic fatty liver disease is metabolic syndromes like obesity, type 2 diabetes mellitus or other syndromes with impairment of insulin responsiveness, dyslipidemia and hypertension.

Non-alcoholic fatty liver disease may show all the changes associated with alcoholic liver disease: Steatosis, steatohepatitis, and steatofibrosis, but they are less prominent.

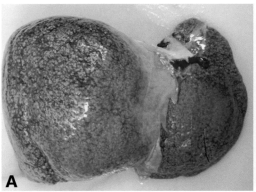
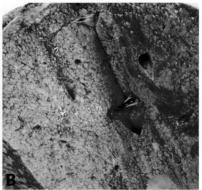

FIGURE 4.32: A: Micronodular cirrhosis admixed with fatty changes in the liver parenchyma of a 50-year-old male. B: Cut-section of the liver showing a similar pattern in the liver parenchyma.

II. Haemochromatosis: It is caused due to absorption of excessive amounts of iron from the diet, which later gets deposited in various organs. The iron stored in the hepatocytes of the liver results in damage to the cells, which is seen progressing from simple hepatitis to irreversible liver cirrhosis in the end.

III. Wilson's disease: It happens due to the accumulation of copper in the body organs, mainly the liver and the brain causing hepatitis, fibrosis, and cirrhosis. It is a genetic condition due to the mutation in the Wilson disease protein gene (ATP7B).

5. **Infection**

Viruses are a common cause of hepatitis; among them, the Hepatitis A–E virus is commonly seen. In these infective cases, the usual histopathological examination shows features like the expansion of the portal triad by mononuclear inflammatory cell infiltrates and the breach of the hepatocyte margins along with piecemeal necrosis of the hepatocytes (Figure 4.36).

6. **Malignancy**

Hepatocellular carcinoma is the most common primary malignant tumour of the liver. The most important underlying factors in hepatocarcinogenesis are viral infection (HBV, HCV) and toxic injuries like alcohol. Alcohol is probably by itself an important risk factor for HCC, but it also synergises with a viral infection and even with cigarette smoking. This malignancy is also reported to occur secondary to infective conditions like viral hepatitis (B or C) or chronic conditions like cirrhosis.

The gross appearance of hepatocellular carcinomas (Figures 4.37 and 4.38 A) typically appear as well-defined masses within the parenchyma of the liver, and they may vary from being unifocal, multifocal, or diffusely infiltrative. The macroscopic growth of hepatocellular carcinoma is usually categorised into three subtypes:

I. Nodular: It appears as multiple masses of variable attenuation.

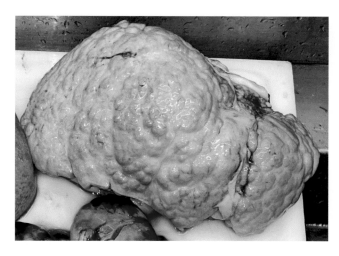

FIGURE 4.33: A gross examination of the liver showing a macronodular surface of the liver.

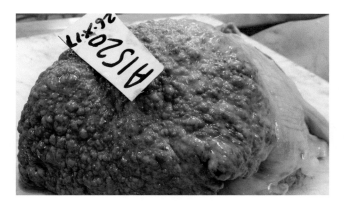

FIGURE 4.34: A gross examination of the liver showing a macronodular surface of the liver admixed with micro-nodules.

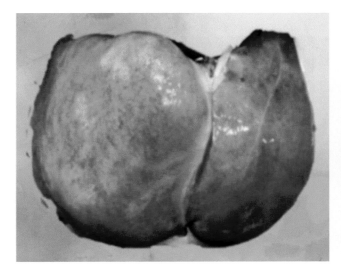

FIGURE 4.35: The autopsy examination of the liver showed liver parenchyma being yellowish and greasy in a deceased who had no habit of consumption of alcohol.

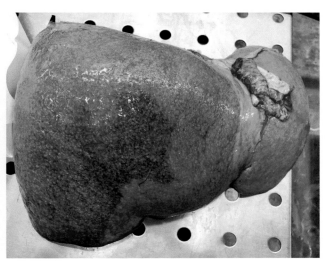

FIGURE 4.36: Autopsy examination of the liver in a case of Hepatitis B infection showing a yellowish discolouration of the parenchyma with areas of hepatic necrosis.

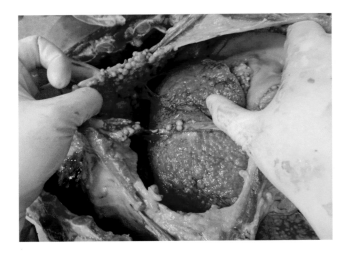

FIGURE 4.37: A case of hepatocellular carcinoma with evident macronodular cirrhosis over the liver parenchyma and secondary metastasis to the inferior surface of the diaphragm and the abdominal wall.

II. Massive: It appears as a large mass.

III. Infiltrative: In the infiltrative subtype, there are multiple tiny nodules throughout the liver parenchyma or a complete liver segment. In certain cases, it may be difficult to differentiate them from the associated cirrhosis of the liver.

On a PMCT, several patterns can be seen, depending on the subtype of hepatocellular carcinoma. A focal fatty change in the normal liver with decreased attenuation, i.e., hypodense, is seen as compared to the unaffected liver (Figure 4.38 B and C).

7. **Hepatic abscess**

A liver abscess is defined as a pus-filled mass in the liver (Figures 4.39 A and B, and 4.40) that can develop from injury to the liver or an intra-abdominal infection disseminated from the portal circulation. These abscesses are mostly pyogenic, and few are due to parasites and fungi. Most amoebic infections are caused by *Entamoeba histolytica*. The pyogenic abscesses are

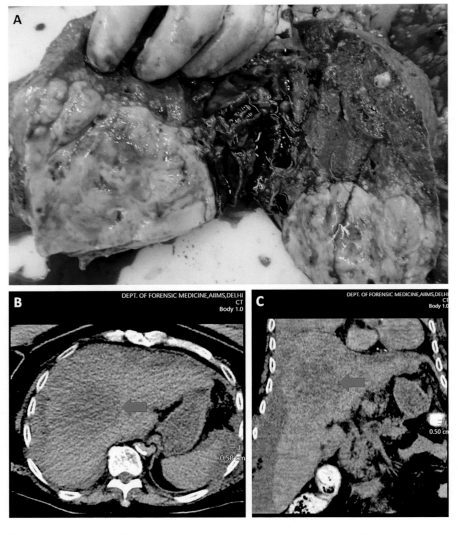

FIGURE 4.38: A: The cut section of the liver shows the presence of the well-demarcated hard tumour growth in a known case of hepatocellular carcinoma. (B-Axial, C-Coronal) The tumour growth seen on the gross image looks hypodense (blue arrows) in the PMCT abdomen.

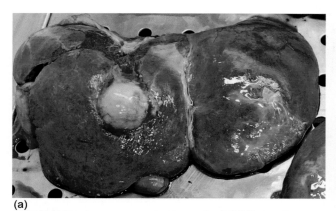

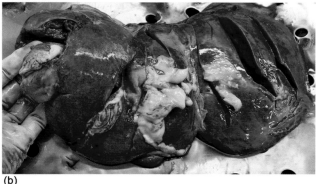

FIGURE 4.39 A: Autopsy gross image of the liver with a liver abscess in a case of abdomen tuberculosis. B: Liver abscess in the right lobe, which on cut section contained thick white paste-like pus.

usually polymicrobial, caused by microorganisms like *Klebsiella, Streptococcus, Staphylococcus,* or anaerobes. The usual pathophysiology for pyogenic liver abscesses is bowel content leakage and peritonitis. Bacteria travel to the liver via the portal vein and reside there. Infection can also originate in the biliary system, while the haematogenous spread is also a potential route.

On PMCT, the appearance of liver abscesses on CT is variable. Important signs seen in hepatic abscess are:

I. Double target sign: It is a characteristic imaging feature seen on contrast-enhanced PMCT with a low central attenuation as it is fluid-filled and it is surrounded by a high attenuated inner ring and low attenuated outer ring.

II. Cluster sign: It is a feature which is specific to pyogenic hepatic abscesses. It is characterised by aggregation of multiple low attenuation liver lesions in an area forming a solitary larger abscess cavity.

8. **Hepatic cyst**

These cysts are usually incidental findings in the autopsy, and in most cases, the deceased would have been asymptomatic. They are usually known for slow growth, but a rapid increase in size should always raise the suspicion of an internal haemorrhage in the cyst.

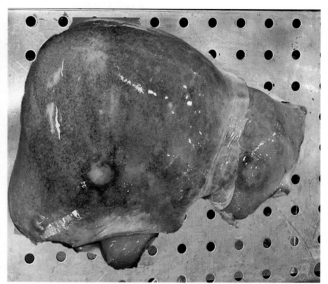

FIGURE 4.40: Liver abscess in a deceased presented with abdomen pain who had died due to perforation of the small intestine. The abscess is present in both the right and left lobes.

True hepatic cysts contain serous fluid (Figure 4.41), which are lined by a thin wall. They can be detected in any part of the liver; however, they have a greater predilection to be found in the right lobe of the liver. The hepatic cyst may be associated with autosomal dominant polycystic kidney disease. On a PMCT, a hepatic cyst is usually well-circumscribed and demonstrates homogeneous hypoattenuation (water attenuation) around 0–10 HU. The wall is usually imperceptible, and the cyst does not enhance after intravenous administration of contrast material.

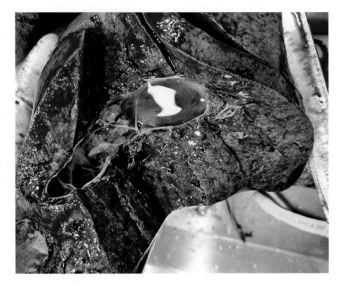

FIGURE 4.41: An incidental finding of a simple benign cyst in a case of hanging. On the cut section, serous fluid was present inside the cyst.

9. Chronic venous congestion

Chronic venous congestion of the liver has a nutmeg appearance with the altered red and brown colour of the liver parenchyma. The dark red areas depict the congestion due to the accumulation of red blood cells within the centrilobular regions. The nutmeg pattern results from congestion around the central veins, usually from right-sided heart failure. If the passive congestion is pronounced and heart failure leads to ischaemia, there can be centrilobular necrosis because the oxygenation in zone three of the hepatic lobule is diminished (Figures 4.42 and 4.43).

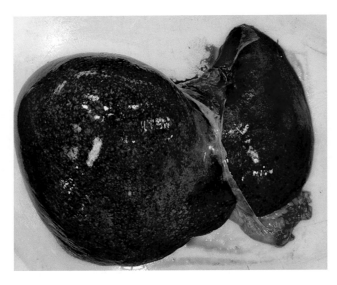

FIGURE 4.42: Autopsy image of chronic venous congestion of liver parenchyma, the liver showing a nutmeg appearance with red and brown areas.

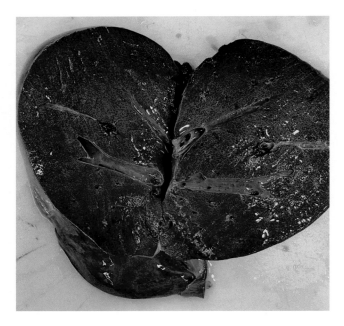

FIGURE 4.43: Autopsy image of chronic venous congestion of liver parenchyma, on the cut section of the liver showing the nutmeg appearance with red and brown areas.

10. Hepatic calcification

Hepatic calcifications may be found in cases with inflammatory hepatic lesions or even in cases with a benign or malignant liver neoplasm. The calcified hepatic lesions are also commonly found in cases with granulomatous diseases (e.g., tuberculosis). The calcification usually involves the entire lesion, and on a PMCT, it appears as a hyperdense mass in the liver parenchyma (Figure 4.44).

11. Intraparenchymal hepatic haemorrhages

A spontaneous hepatic haemorrhage (SHH) is a rare condition that results from a breach in the hepatic parenchyma that occurs without an external cause. It is an acute surgical emergency as it results in intra-abdominal bleeding that, if untreated, will progress to haemorrhagic shock and death. Few cases of spontaneous intraparenchymal hepatic haemorrhage as a sequela of COVID-19 are reported in the literature. The most common causes of non-traumatic hepatic haemorrhage are hepatocellular carcinoma (HCC) and hepatocellular adenoma (Figure 4.45).

Kidneys

The kidneys are a pair of bean-shaped retro-peritoneal organs that lie obliquely at the level of the T12 to L3 on either side of the vertebral column (Figure 4.46). The liver pushes the right kidney making it usually lie slightly lower than the left kidney. The normal adult kidney measures about 10–14 cm in length in males and about 9–13 cm in females; width varies from about 3–5 cm, and antero-posterior thickness is usually about 3 cm; and it normally weighs about 150–260 g. On a PMCT, the length of a normal kidney is roughly estimated to be around not less than the length of three vertebral bodies and not more than the length of four vertebral bodies (Figure 4.46). The kidney has two poles, namely the superior and inferior poles, two surfaces namely the anterior and posterior surfaces, and two borders namely the lateral and medial borders (Figure 4.47). It is wrapped by a thick fibrous capsule called the Bowman's capsule, which is in turn surrounded by a layer of fat which protects the kidney called the perirenal fat.

The kidneys, on a cut cross-section, can be divided into two regions called renal parenchyma and renal sinus:

1. Renal parenchyma: It is the outer region which is subdivided into an outer cortex layer and an inner medulla layer. The outer cortex layer is directly in contact with the Bowman's capsule, and any pathology or scarring results in the tight adherence between them, causing stripping the capsule difficult during an autopsy examination. The medulla is the inner layer consisting of 10–14 renal pyramids, which are separated by an invagination of the cortex layer called renal columns (Figure 4.48).
2. Renal sinus: It is the inner region which contains the renal pelvis, calyces, renal vessels, nerves, and lymphatics. The renal hilum is the point where the vessels and ureter enter and leave the renal sinus; it is located on the anteromedial aspect of the kidney. The kidneys receive their arterial supply directly from the aorta through renal arteries; the venous drainage is by renal veins, which drain directly into the inferior vena cava (Figure 4.48).

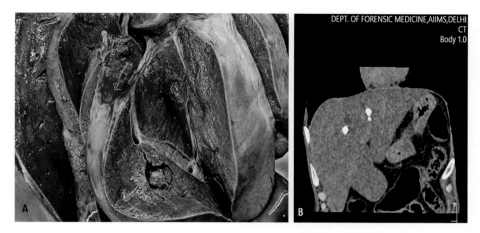

FIGURE 4.44: A: Autopsy gross examination of the liver showing intraparenchymal calcification (red arrow) in the liver's right lobe in a case of hanging. B: In PMCT, two intraparenchymal calcifications (red star) are visualised as hyperdense lesions in the liver parenchyma.

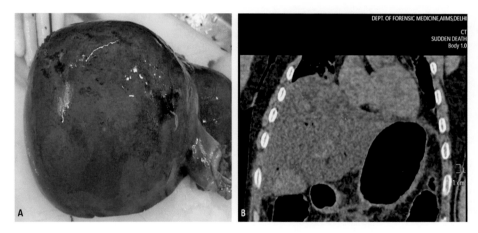

FIGURE 4.45: A: Autopsy examination of the liver showing multiple intraparenchymal haemorrhages (red stars) over the right lobe of the liver in a case of Disseminated intravascular coagulation. B: In PMCT, the intraparenchymal haemorrhages (red stars) are visualised as multiple hyperdense areas in the liver parenchyma.

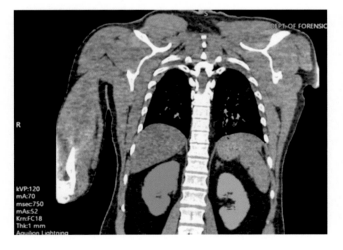

FIGURE 4.46: Coronal section of PMCT in soft tissue window showing right kidney (blue) and left kidney (yellow) on either side of the vertebral column. A rough estimate of the length of a normal kidney is estimated to be around not less than the length of three vertebral bodies and not more than the length of four vertebral bodies

Pathology of the kidney

Various renal pathologies, along with renal size in reference to vertebral body lengths, can be assessed on a PMCT. Gas, calculi, renal parenchymal calcifications, haemorrhage, and masses can be easily revealed with unenhanced CT. However, a contrast material-enhanced study is essential for the complete evaluation of renal inflammatory diseases, vascular obstruction, or stenosis. The most commonly encountered pathologies are:

1. Chronic kidney disease (CKD): It is also referred to as chronic renal failure, and it is characterised by progressive loss of glomerular function, possibly due to a longstanding renal parenchymal disease. A variety of diseases or conditions can cause damage to the kidney, which include diabetes mellitus, hypertension, glomerulonephritis, polycystic kidney disease, etc. PMCT is a useful tool in assessing aetiology.

2. Urolithiasis: The presence of calculi anywhere along the course of the urinary tract is known as urolithiasis. The composition of urinary tract stones varies widely depending upon metabolic alterations; the most common are calcium oxalate/calcium phosphate calculi. On

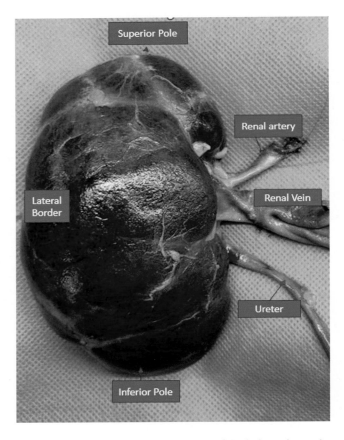

FIGURE 4.47: Autopsy examination of the kidney shows the shiny Renal capsule covering the kidney; it has superior and inferior poles and medial and lateral borders. The anterior surface is seen in the image.

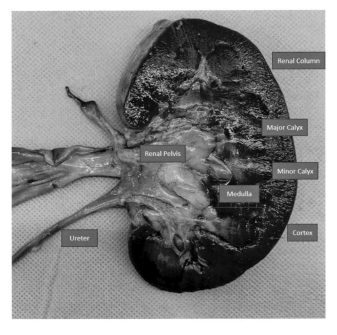

FIGURE 4.48: Autopsy examination of kidney on cut section showing the cortex, medulla and the renal pelvis along with vessels and ureter near the hilum.

a CT, almost all stones are opaque and visible. Low fluid intake, urinary tract malformation, and infection are a few of the important risk factors (Figure 4.49).

3. Inflammatory renal disease: Inflammatory diseases of the kidney are a broad group of renal pathologies. The aetiology of inflammation may be diverse, e.g., infections or autoimmune diseases. It includes acute pyelonephritis (APN), renal and perinephric abscesses, emphysematous pyelonephritis (EPN), emphysematous pyelitis (EP), chronic pyelonephritis (CPN), and glomerulonephritis (GN). Confirmatory pathology can be assessed by histopathological examination of the tissue (Figure 4.50).

4. Simple cyst: Cysts in the kidney are also called simple kidney cysts, which are a collection of fluid in pouches either on the surface or in the parenchyma of the kidney (Figure 4.51). It usually occurs due to injury or microscopic blockages in the tubules. Renal cysts are graded based on the complexity of their structure; a simple cyst is mostly benign in nature, while complicated or complex cysts which some enhancing components that raise the suspicion of malignancy. Most of the parenchymal cysts are benign; however, rarely, renal cell carcinoma can also present as a cystic lesion. On a PMCT, it is identified as a hypo/hyperattenuated area which is well-marginated (Figure 4.51). Hypo- (Figure 4.51) and hyper- (Figure 4.52) attenuation are described on the basis of contents inside the cyst. Confirmation of the nature of the lesion can be done by histopathological examination.

5. **Polycystic kidney disease:** Polycystic kidney disease is broadly divided into two forms:

   1. Autosomal dominant polycystic kidney disease (ADPKD): It is more common than autosomal recessive polycystic kidney disease (ARPKD). ADPKD is a hereditary disorder characterised by multiple expanding cysts of both the kidney and which ultimately destroy the renal parenchyma. It is autosomal dominant and universally bilateral. It occurs as a result of a mutation in PKD1 (85%) and is associated with more severe disease, end-stage renal disease or death occurring at an average age of 53 years. Macroscopically the kidneys are enlarged bilaterally and demonstrate many cysts of variable size (from a few mm to a few centimetres) in both the cortex and medulla (Figure 4.53). They are filled with fluid of variable colour (from clear or straw-coloured to altered blood or chocolate-coloured to purulent when infected). People with ADPKD have a history of pain in the flanks, high blood pressure and kidney failure at some point in their lives. Apart from renal complications, i.e., rupture of a cyst or infection, non-renal complications such as liver cysts (extremely common), pancreatic cysts, heart valve abnormalities, colonic diverticula, and aneurysms are also seen. Cerebrovascular bleeding following aneurysm rupture is also seen in cases with uncontrolled hypertension and a family history of aneurysm rupture.

   2. Autosomal recessive polycystic kidney disease (ARPKD): It is a rare developmental anomaly with serious manifestations, which are usually present at birth; young infants might succumb rapidly to renal failure in this condition. Macroscopically, kidneys are enlarged and have a smooth external

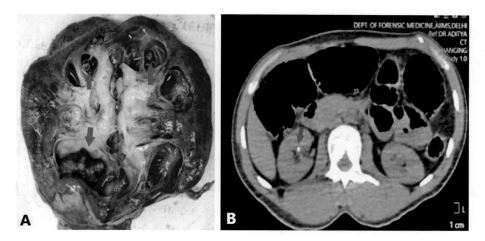

FIGURE 4.49: A: Autopsy examination of a cut section of a kidney showing multiple calculi in the renal pelvis (red arrows). B: PMCT axial section in soft tissue window showing the calculi near renal pelvis (red arrow) of the right kidney.

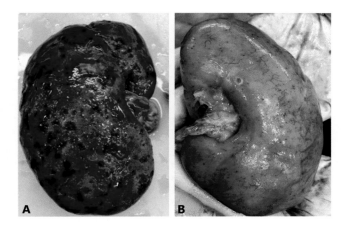

FIGURE 4.50: A: Gross examination showing pus-laden kidney suggestive of pyelonephritis. B: Gross examination showing swollen kidney with multiple punctate haemorrhagic points.

appearance. On the cut section, numerous small cysts in the cortex and medulla give the kidney a sponge-like appearance. Lung complications may be present at birth due to abnormal pressure present on the lungs by the enlarged kidneys during intrauterine life. A patient who survives infancy may present later with a hepatic picture (portal hypertension and splenomegaly).

On a PMCT, polycystic kidney disease will appear as multiple hypoattenuated rounded structures with near water attenuation and thin, regular walls (Figure 4.54). Any complications to the cyst, like haemorrhage or infection, raise the attenuation of the cyst contents.

6. Flea-bitten kidney: The pattern of small, pinpoint petechial haemorrhages may appear on the cortical surface from rupture of arterioles or glomerular capillaries. This gives the kidney a peculiar, flea-bitten appearance. It is typically seen in cases with malignant HTN caused by thromboses (Figure 4.55).
7. Fatty kidney: Deposition of fatty tissue occurs in several areas of the kidney, including the retro-peritoneal

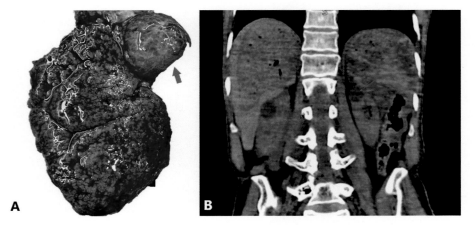

FIGURE 4.51: A: Autopsy examination of the kidney showing a single cyst at the superior pole of the left kidney. B: Coronal section of PMCT in soft tissue window showing hypoattenuated, well-demarcated and well-marginated cyst in bilateral kidneys (red arrow).

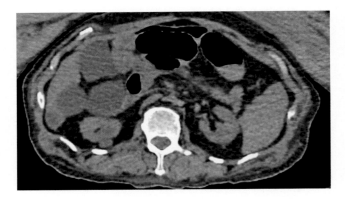

FIGURE 4.52: Axial section of PMCT in soft tissue window showing localised hyperattenuated area, i.e., single cyst on right kidney

space, the perinephric space outside the renal capsule, the hilum, and the sinus area is termed 'fatty kidney'. It is associated with both hypertension and CKD. The accumulation of renal sinus fat is important as there is direct physical compression of the renal vein and artery passing through the renal sinus, which may interfere with renal function (Figure 4.56)

8. Renal cell carcinoma: Renal cell carcinoma (RCC) is an important tumour which was previously called hypernephroma or Grawitz tumour. They are primary malignant adenocarcinomas originating commonly from the renal tubular epithelial cells. They are malignant renal tumours. It usually occurs in the elderly in the age range of 50–70 years, and they commonly present with a history of haematuria, flank pain, or palpable mass. Smoking and hypertension are important risk factors.

Macroscopically, renal cell carcinomas are variable in appearance, ranging from solid and relatively homogeneous to markedly heterogeneous with areas of necrosis, cystic change, and haemorrhage.

On a PMCT, renal cell carcinoma appears with a soft tissue attenuation between 20–70 HU. Larger or more complicated

lesions are present with areas of necrosis and calcification. It appears as a renal mass (Figure 4.57) with irregularly thick and enhancing septae.

9. End-stage renal disease: End-stage renal disease corresponds to the last stage of chronic kidney disease (stage 5) when the kidneys' function is no longer sufficient to sustain life. In end-stage kidney disease, the kidneys are small or shrunken bilaterally, with scarring of the parenchyma (Figure 4.58). This condition is associated with chronic renal failure, and the patient's blood urea nitrogen (BUN) and serum creatinine are raised, which can be confirmed from the hospital records, if available. The microscopic appearance of the end-stage kidney disease is similar regardless of the aetiology, which is why a biopsy in a patient with chronic renal failure yields little useful information. PMCT can identify shrunken kidneys with scarring of the parenchymal tissue.

Anatomical variants of kidneys

1. Lobulated kidney

The lobulated kidney is characterised by the persistence of fetal lobulations of the kidney, which is an uncommon condition which gives the surface of the kidney a peculiar lobulated appearance. Embryologically, the kidneys originate as distinct lobules that disappear as a result of fusion by the end of the fetal period. It appears as a variant occasionally seen in adult kidneys (Figure 4.59).

2. Horseshoe-shaped kidney

The horseshoe kidney is a variant that is rarely encountered. It is more common in males as compared to females. During fetal development of kidneys, they migrate from a lower position upwards to reach their normal position. If these kidneys get fused or attached commonly in the lower pole, it results in the formation of the U-shaped or horseshoe-shaped kidney. This also interferes with the normal fetal migration of the

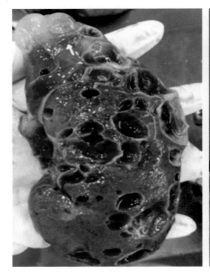
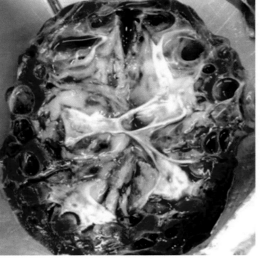

FIGURE 4.53: Autosomal dominant adult polycystic kidney disease(ADPKD) viewed from cut surface showing multiple cysts in cortex and medulla. The kidney is enlarged with numerous dilated cysts.

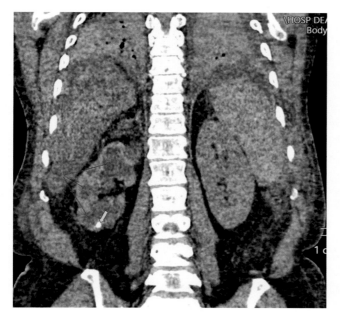

FIGURE 4.54: Coronal section of PMCT in soft tissue window showing multiple hypoattenuated areas in the right kidney (red arrows) along with the irregular surface. A hyperattenuated area in the right kidney at the lower pole shows urolithiasis (yellow arrow).

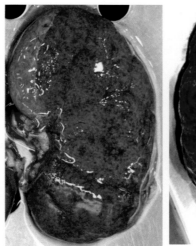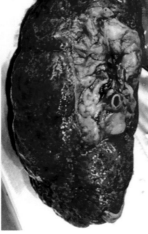

FIGURE 4.55: Autopsy examination of kidneys in these two cases shows multiple small, pinpoint petechial haemorrhages giving it a granular appearance.

kidney resulting in locating these kidneys at ectopic locations (Figure 4.60).

Spleen

The spleen is an oval-shaped organ present in the abdomen located in the left upper quadrant, just below the diaphragm and protected laterally by the ninth to eleventh left ribs. The spleen is ensheathed by the peritoneum on all surfaces except at the hilum; a few ligaments form the attachment. They are:

1. The gastrosplenic ligament, which attaches the spleen to the greater curvature of the stomach.

2. Splenorenal ligament, which attaches the spleen to the left kidney.

The size and weight of the spleen vary from individual to individual, but on average, in an adult, they measure approximately 2.5 cm in thickness, 7.5 cm in width, and 12.5 cm in length. The spleen has two poles/extremities (anterior and posterior), three borders (superior, inferior, and intermediate) and two surfaces (diaphragmatic and visceral) (Figure 4.61).

The spleen is a highly vascular abdominal organ. It receives its arterial supply from the splenic artery, and its venous drainage is into the splenic vein. The spleen, apart from its vital role in removing old red blood cells from circulation (red pulp), also plays an important role in both cell-mediated and humoral immune responses (white pulp).

On a PMCT, the normal spleen measures approximately 40–60 HU; on an unenhanced CT, it is about 10 HU less than that of the average normal liver attenuation. Spleen size is evaluated using CT scans in the axial and coronal sections. (Figures 4.62 and 4.63), linear measurements of the spleen are important in diagnosing splenomegaly.

1. Maximum length: It is the longitudinal dimension between the two poles of the spleen in the axial section (Figure 4.62).
2. Maximum thickness: It is the widest dimension perpendicular to the long axis of the spleen (Figure 4.62).
3. Vertical height: It is the longest vertical dimension between the cranial and caudal borders of the spleen in the coronal section (Figure 4.63).

Anatomical variants of the spleen: There are various anatomical variations of the spleen that are essential to recognise so as not to mistake them for pathologies, such as a splenic laceration or enlarged lymph node. The anatomic variants are as follows:

1) Splenules or splenunculus: It is an anatomical variant with an accessory spleen along with the main spleen. It is also referred to as supernumerary spleen or splenule, or splenunculus. It is a non-pathological and asymptomatic condition where the splenic tissue is found in place apart from the normal region. They are round masses of splenic tissue measuring up to several centimetres in size that are separate from but usually close to the main spleen, most commonly seen at the splenic hilum (Figure 4.64).
2) Splenic cleft: Splenic clefts are invaginations of the splenic capsule, which create septations in the splenic parenchyma or may mimic traumatic laceration.
3) Wandering spleen: Without gastrosplenic and splenorenal ligament supports, the spleen can move around the abdomen, a condition known as wandering spleen. A wandering spleen is at increased risk for torsion.
4) Polysplenia: It refers to the association of two or more multiple spleens with multiple congenital abnormalities in the abdomen and chest. It is different from the accessory spleen by the part that there are multiple splenules without a parent spleen.
5) Asplenia: It is a condition where the spleen is absent. It can be due to the anatomical absence of the spleen or functional asplenia secondary to a variety of disease states. A few of the important secondary causes

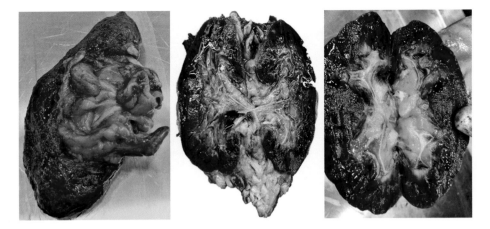

FIGURE 4.56:   Autopsy examination of the kidneys in these cases shows fat accumulation at the renal pelvis area.

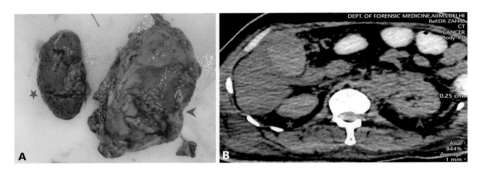

FIGURE 4.57:   A case of Renal cell Carcinoma of the left kidney. A: Autopsy examination showing the enlarged left kidney with renal cell carcinoma. B: Axial section of PMCT showing left side renal mass with an irregular surface.

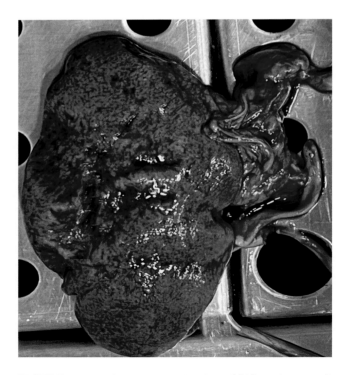

FIGURE 4.58:   Autopsy examination of kidney in an end-stage renal disease case showing shrunken kidney with scarring of the parenchymal tissue.

resulting in asplenia are trauma, infarction, or surgery. Asplenic individuals are highly susceptible to infections, especially from capsulated pathogens like *Streptococcus pneumoniae*.

Pathology of the spleen

1. **Splenomegaly:** It is a condition where the spleen increases in size (Figure 4.65). The most common cause of splenomegaly include:
   1. Infections such as HIV, tuberculosis, endocarditis, malaria, toxoplasmosis, etc.
   2. Liver diseases like chronic hepatitis or cirrhosis.
   3. Leukaemia or lymphomas.
   4. Autoimmune diseases.
   5. Blood disorders.
2. **Splenic calcifications**: The causes of splenic calcification include pathologies like histoplasmosis, tuberculosis, candidiasis, *Pneumocystis jiroveci*, sickle cell disease, systemic lupus erythematosus (SLE), etc. It can also be seen following trauma, ischaemia/infarction. Splenic calcification may precede auto splenectomy and hyposplenism. The pattern of calcification can be diffuse, as seen in SLE or segmental calcification. Peripheral calcifications can occur after splenic infarct. Curvilinear calcifications along the capsule are visible with old resolved haematomas.
3. **Spleen atrophy:** It is an acquired anatomical diminution of the size of the spleen. If both the red and white pulp

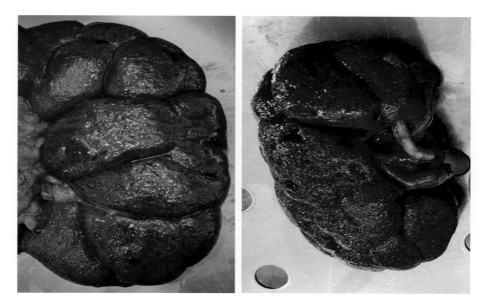

FIGURE 4.59: Autopsy examination of a kidney showing incidental finding of lobulated kidney in both cases due to persistence of fetal lobulations.

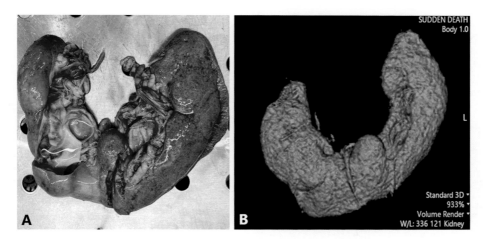

FIGURE 4.60: A case of horseshoe-shaped kidney: A. Autopsy examination showing the fused lower poles. B: Volume rendering 3D CT image of PMCT showing the horseshoe-shaped kidney.

of the spleen are involved, then it is diagnosed as spleen atrophy (Figure 4.66).

4. **Splenic infarct:** It characteristically presents on PMCT as a peripheral wedge-shaped hypodense lesion. The causes of splenic infarcts include cardioembolic events, vasculitis, haematologic phenomena, splenic vein thrombosis, pancreatitis, and iatrogenic causes. Chronic infarct results in notching of the normally smooth splenic contour and peripheral calcifications.

5. **True cysts:** They are congenital epithelial-lined fluid-filled structures. On a PMCT, they appear as rounded, non-enhancing, hypodense lesions with internal attenuation like that of water.

Pancreas

The pancreas is a retro-peritoneal organ, 12–15 cm in length, located in the epigastric region. It has both endocrine and exocrine functions. Pancreases consist of four main parts (Figure 4.67):

1. Head: It is the thickest part with an extension known as the uncinate process and is in close approximation with the duodenum. The common bile duct traverses through the head of the pancreas and joins with the pancreatic duct at the ampulla of Vater to empty bile into the second or descending part of the duodenum.

2. Neck: It is the thinnest part that lies anterior to the superior mesenteric artery and vein

3. Body: It is the main part that lies to the left of the superior mesenteric artery and vein. Its anterior surface is covered with peritoneum forming the posterior surface of the lesser sac

4. Tail: It is located between the layers of the splenorenal ligament near the splenic hilum.

On a CT a normal pancreas is of the same width as the abdominal aorta, i.e., around 2.5 cm; if the pancreas is greater than this, it suggests its enlargement. Along with contrast enhancement the pancreas has the same density as the liver

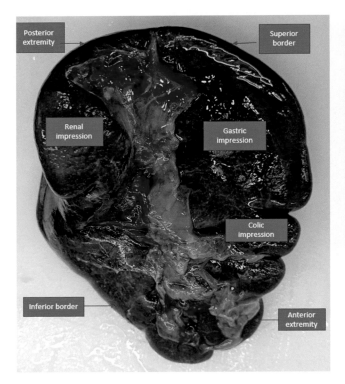

FIGURE 4.61: Autopsy examination of the spleen, the visceral surface of the spleen showing renal, colic, and gastric impressions due to their close proximity with the spleen. The borders and extremities can also be appreciated in the image.

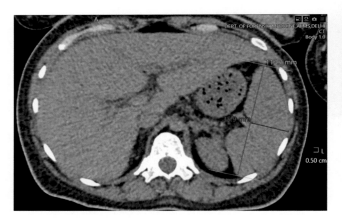

FIGURE 4.62: Axial section of PMCT spleen showing maximum length (dimension between the two poles) and maximum thickness (dimension perpendicular to the long axis) at the level of hilum.

and spleen. It is recognisable by the splenic vein running along its inferior posterior groove.

Pathology of the pancreas

1. **Acute pancreatitis:** Acute pancreatitis is a condition where there is acute inflammation of the pancreas. This is a medical emergency and is a potentially life-threatening condition. In this, there is an activation of pancreatic enzymes within the pancreas, which causes pancreatic tissue inflammation along with the disruption of small

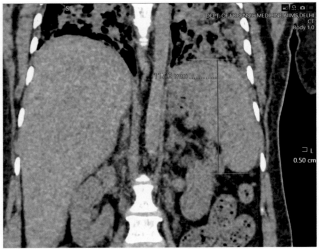

FIGURE 4.63: Coronal section of PMCT spleen showing longest vertical dimension.

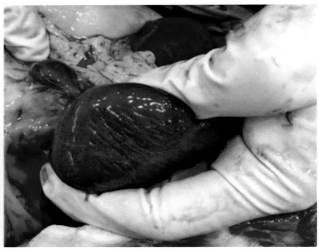

FIGURE 4.64: Autopsy examination of the spleen incidentally showing an accessory spleen found outside the normal spleen at the region of splenic hilum.

pancreatic ducts and leakage of pancreatic secretions. As the pancreas lacks a capsule, the pancreatic juices spread to surrounding tissue, and it can easily digest the fascial layers, which in turn spreads the inflammatory process to multiple other anatomic compartments. There are two subtypes of acute pancreatitis:

1. Interstitial edematous pancreatitis: It is often referred to as acute pancreatitis or as uncomplicated pancreatitis.
2. Necrotising pancreatitis: It is a condition where necrosis occurs within the pancreatic tissue and/or peri-pancreatic tissues.

The most common causes of acute pancreatitis are alcohol abuse, gallstones in adults, and trauma in children.

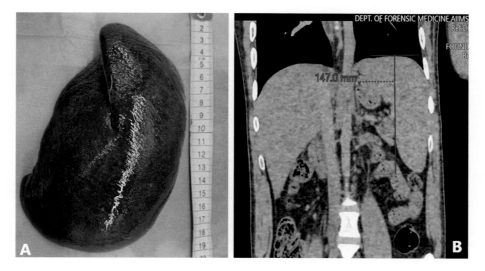

FIGURE 4.65: A: A gross examination of the spleen showing splenomegaly. B: PMCT examination of the spleen in the coronal section showing splenomegaly

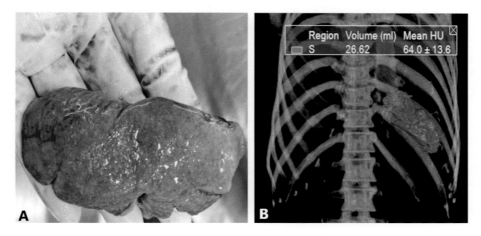

FIGURE 4.66: A: Gross examination showing atrophic spleen. B: On PMCT volume, the reconstructed image of the atrophic spleen.

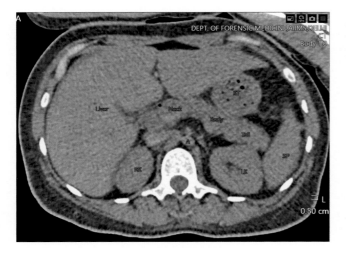

FIGURE 4.67: Axial section of PMCT showing the anatomical location of various parts of the pancreas (tail, body and neck) in this section in reference to the vertebral body, aorta (A). stomach (ST), spleen (SP), right kidney (RK) and left kidney (LK).

In medicolegal cases of sudden death, the deceased may have a history of acute onset of severe central epigastric pain, which was exacerbated by sleeping in the supine position or having a pain which was radiating to the back.

On a PMCT following findings can be seen:

1. The pancreas is focal or diffusely enlarged because of oedema.
2. With IV contrast, the density of the pancreas is less than the liver and spleen.
3. The necrotic part of the pancreas shows decreased or no enhancement with IV contrast when compared with normal enhancing tissue (necrotising pancreatitis).
4. Increased attenuation of fluid (hyperdensity) is seen in the area of haemorrhage (blood) with the enlarged pancreas (acute haemorrhagic pancreatitis) (Figure 4.68).

2. **Chronic pancreatitis:** It represents the end result of a continuous, prolonged, inflammatory, and fibrosing process that affects the pancreas. This results in irreversible morphologic changes and permanent endocrine

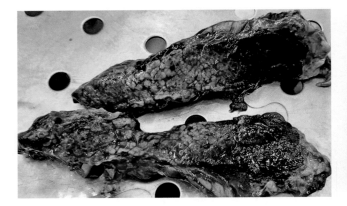

FIGURE 4.68: Autopsy examination of the pancreas in a case of acute hemorrhagic pancreatitis showing the areas of haemorrhage along with the enlarged pancreas.

and exocrine pancreatic dysfunction. A common cause for this among adults is excessive alcohol consumption. Medical history and radiological findings can play an important role in identifying this condition.

The clinical history of the deceased shows multiple exacerbations (episodes of acute pancreatitis) where the person may have had epigastric pain with medical attention. These may have recurred over several years.

1. As a result of biliary obstruction, jaundice will be seen.
2. Due to a chronic decrease in exocrine function, malabsorption will be present, and the deceased will have a thin build.
3. Due to a chronic decrease in endocrine function, the deceased may have a history of diabetes mellitus.

Radiological features on a PMCT suggest:

1. Dilatation of the main pancreatic duct.
2. Calcification of the pancreatic tissue (Figure 4.69).
3. The size, shape, and contour of the pancreas changes may be seen as atrophy of the pancreas.

Traumatic pathology to accessory organs

Laceration and rupture of abdominal organs are commonly seen in blunt force injuries to the abdomen, which include lacerations of the liver, pancreas, spleen, and kidneys accompanied by surrounding tissue contusions. The liver (Figures 4.70 and 4.71) and kidneys (Figure 4.72) are the most commonly affected organs. Stabs to the abdomen are also frequently encountered, where it commonly affects the liver (Figure 4.73) or intestine with its mesentery due to its large surface area. This morphologic tissue disruption, and if it is deep-seated, the associated intraparenchymal blood collections are identifiable with PMCT imaging. Subscapular haematomas give a hyperdense contained lesion with blood density (~40 HU). Ruptures of hollow viscus like that of the stomach, intestine, and urinary bladder, if it is of reasonable size, are demonstrable by CT imaging. Associated haemorrhages (haemoperitoneum) and air leaks (pneumoperitoneum) into the peritoneal cavity are easy to be demonstrated, along with soft tissue lacerations, which are seen as tissue disruption. Traumatic herniations of intestinal loops into potential spaces can also be visualised easily. Muscle and

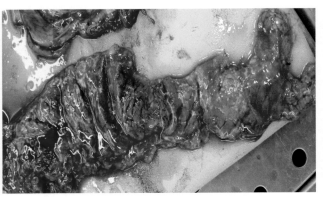

FIGURE 4.69: A gross examination of pancreas showing oedematous pancreas with diffuse pin point calcification on the cut section in a case of chronic pancreatitis.

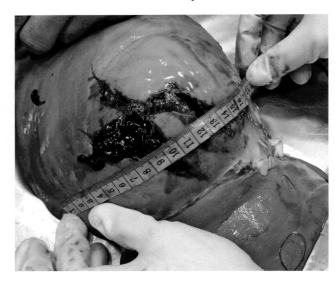

FIGURE 4.70: Gross image showing traumatic cruciate-shaped laceration of the liver with hemoperitoneum in case of a roadside accident with a laceration measuring size 11x 10cm.

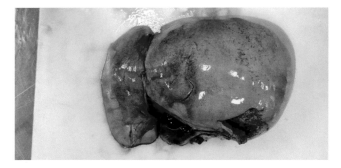

FIGURE 4.71: The gross image of the liver with lacerations on the right lobe along with parenchymal haemorrhage in case of fall from a height, the liver appears pale due to blood loss.

soft tissue contusions, if large enough, may be recognisable as hyperdense regions. The pancreas is an abdominal organ which is rarely injured in blunt trauma to the abdomen, but in cases where they are injured, it has a high morbidity and mortality rate (Figure 4.74).

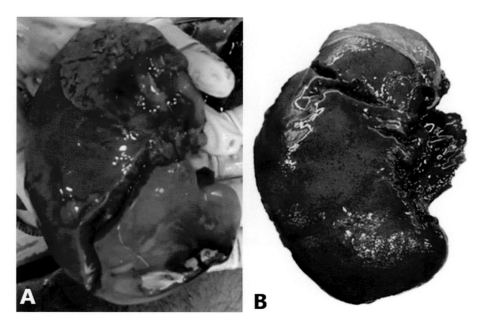

FIGURE 4.72: Kidney lacerations due to blunt trauma abdomen, A: Gross image showing kidney laceration with a contusion at the lower pole in case of road traffic accident. B: Gross image showing kidney laceration near the upper pole and hilar region in a case of road traffic accident.

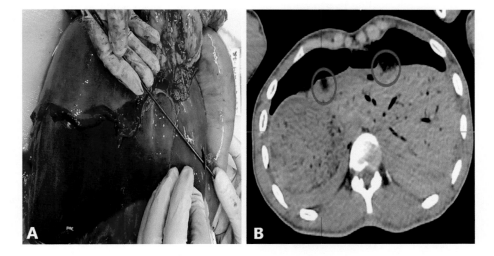

FIGURE 4.73: Liver stab injury, A: The gross image of stab injury to the liver in a case of stab injury to the abdomen. B: Axial section of PMCT in the same case showing breach in the continuity of liver at two places (marked with a red circle) accompanied with pneumoperitoneum.

Gastrointestinal system

After solid accessory organs now comes the hollow viscera in the abdomen that includes the stomach and intestine. Gastrointestinal conditions are rare causes of sudden and/or unexpected death as compared to cardiovascular diseases, motor vehicle trauma, or suicide, and may involve an array of fatal mechanisms. The gastrointestinal system starts from the neck region at the level of C6 as the oesophagus and extends through the thorax and abdomen, and ends at the pelvic cavity anal canal. It includes:

1. Oesophagus.
2. Stomach.

3. Small intestine.
4. Large intestine (caecum, appendix, colon, rectum, and anal canal).

1. Oesophagus

The oesophagus is a fibromuscular tube with an approximate length of 25 cm (Figure 4.75) that begins in the neck at the level of C6. It starts at the level sixth cervical vertebra corresponding to the inferior border of the cricoid cartilage positioned between the trachea and the vertebral bodies of T1 to T4 and enters the abdomen via the oesophagal hiatus (an opening in the right crus of the diaphragm) at T10. The abdominal portion

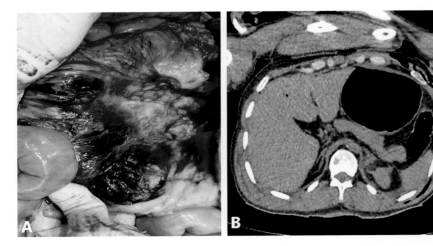

FIGURE 4.74   Pancreatic hematoma in a case of blunt trauma to the abdomen, A: Gross examination of pancreas showing pancreatic hematoma with the indistinct region of parenchymal oedema. B: Axial section of PMCT of the same case.

of the oesophagus is short and about 1.25 cm long, which ends by joining the cardiac end of the stomach at the level of T11.

The oesophagus is lined with adventitia, the muscle layer, submucosa and mucosa, which are similar to many of the organs in the alimentary tract except in the distal and intraperitoneal portion of the oesophagus that has an outer covering of serosa, instead of adventitia. Food is transported through the oesophagus by peristalsis movement. There are two sphincters present in the oesophagus at its extremities, referred to appropriately as the upper and lower oesophagal sphincters.

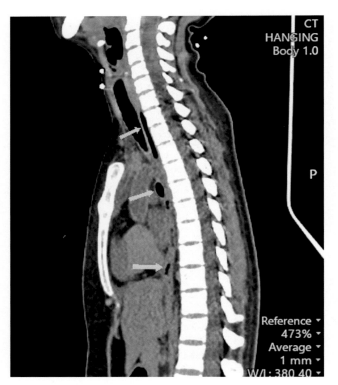

FIGURE 4.75:   Sagittal section of PMCT showing oesophagus (marked with yellow arrow).

1. **Upper Esophageal Sphincter:** The upper sphincter is an anatomical produced by the cricopharyngeal muscle located at the junction between the pharynx and oesophagus.
2. **Lower Esophageal Sphincter:** It is a rather physiological (or functional) sphincter located at the gastro–oesophagal junction that allows food to enter the stomach. And to prevent the reflux of acidic gastric contents into the oesophagus.

There are four physiological constructions in the lumen of the oesophagus where foreign bodies/food are most likely to get impacted. They are:

1. Arch of aorta.
2. Bronchus.
3. Cricoid cartilage.
4. Diaphragmatic hiatus.

The thoracic and abdominal part of the oesophagus receives its arterial supply mainly from the branches of the thoracic aorta and left gastric artery (a branch of the coeliac trunk) artery respectively, and the venous drainage is via a portosystemic anastomosis. Oesophagal varices are visible on contrast-enhanced cross-sectional imaging as torturous, enlarged tubular structures. They, depending on size and pressure, may protrude into the oesophagal lumen accompanied by thickened oesophagal wall, but autopsy examination of these varices is difficult as the pressure in the vessels drops after death.

2. **Stomach**

The stomach is an important part of the gastrointestinal tract, which is intraperitoneally located between the oesophagus and the duodenum. The stomach, when empty its volume is about 45 mL in adults and is divided into four main anatomical divisions, i.e., the cardia, fundus, body, and pylorus (Figure 4.76).

1. **Cardia**: It is the first division of the stomach around the upper opening of the stomach where the oesophagus opens (gastroesophageal junction).

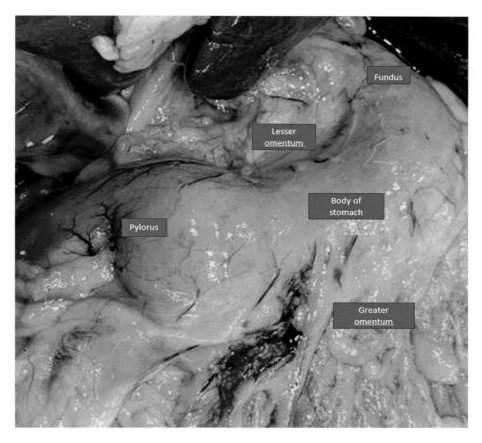

FIGURE 4.76: A gross examination of the stomach showing different parts of the stomach with peritoneal fold, i.e., greater omentum and lesser omentum.

2. **Fundus**: It is the second part of the stomach, which is usually rounded, and it is often filled with gas.
3. **Body**: This is the third part of the stomach, a large central portion that is inferior to the fundus.
4. **Pylorus**: It is the fourth and last part of the stomach, where it continues as the duodenum.

The medial border of the stomach is curved and forms the shorter and is also known as the lesser curvature of the stomach. The lateral border is long and convex and is known as the greater curvature. The greater and lesser omentum are two peritoneal folds that are attached to these curvatures, respectively. The stomach has two sphincters located at its ends. They control the passage of material entering and exiting the stomach.

1. **Inferior oesophageal sphincter:** It is a physiological sphincter. It allows food to enter the stomach, and any dysfunction of this sphincter can result in reflux of gastric into the oesophagus, causing a condition like gastro-esophageal reflux disease.
2. **Pyloric sphincter:** It is an anatomical sphincter. It lies between the pylorus and the first part of the duodenum and controls the exit of chyme (food and gastric acid mixture) from the stomach.

PMCT scans can reveal structural abnormalities, abnormal growths, gastric perforation and the presence of any foreign body inside the stomach.

Pathology of the stomach

1. **Gastric perforation**: Gastric perforation is the rupture of the gastric wall. The most common site for perforation in the case of peptic ulcers is the gastric antrum and duodenal bulb. Other important causes for gastric perforation are as follows:
   1. Corrosive acid poisoning (Figure 4.77).
   2. Spontaneous gastric perforation.
   3. Malignancy-related gastric perforation.
   4. Endoscopy-related gastric perforation.

The findings interpreted at CT could be graded as normal appearing organs, wall lesions in the form of thickening, soft tissue infiltrations, extraluminal air in the mediastinum, and peritoneal cavity (pneumoperitoneum) as a sign of perforation.

2. **Foreign body in the stomach:** Any radiopaque material inside the stomach creates a doubtful situation to analyse. It can be undissolved medicines or illegally packed drugs. Body packing symbolises the concealment of illegal substances in a person's body with the motive of smuggling. People practising body packing are referred to as body packers, (drug) mules, or swallowers. Drugs may be packed with non-digestive materials like condoms, foil, latex, or cellophane. Body packers either swallow drug-filled packets or introduce drug-filled packets into their bodies while the body stuffers place the drugs rectally or vaginally with the purpose of concealing them. The main smuggled drugs are cocaine,

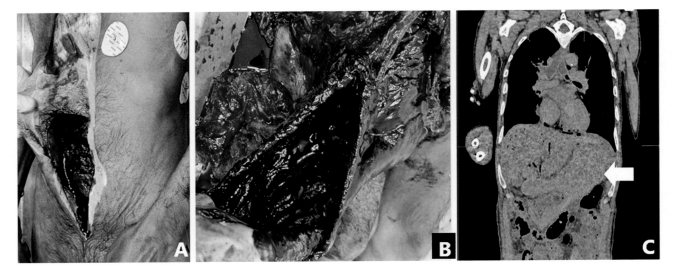

FIGURE 4.77: Corrosive acid poisoning case A: Blood collection inside the peritoneal cavity. B: Haemorrhagic stomach wall with clots. C: Coronal section of PMCT showing hyperdense stomach with poorly differentiated borders

heroin, and cannabis products. Sometimes body packers sustain a serious risk of acute narcotic toxicity from drug exposure as a result of the rupture of the packets. It can also lead to intestinal obstruction owing to pellet impaction and bowel perforation with consequent abdominal sepsis. Macroscopically (Figure 4.78), drug packets appear as round to oval shape structures tightly wrapped with latex or plastic material.

Radiological evaluation by plain abdominal radiography is a commonly adopted approach for screening and diagnosing body packing of illicit drugs. On abdominal radiograph signs of this are:

• Tic-tac sign: the presence of multiple homogeneous radiopaque oval/round-shaped foreign bodies with sharp borders and clear air–substance interface on the plain abdominal radiography.

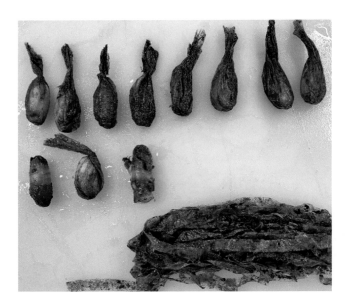

FIGURE 4.78: Foreign body in stomach, examination of packed illicit drugs evacuated from a body packer

• Double condom sign: the radiolucent rim of air trapped between the multiple layers of packing surrounding each drug packet in a well-defined shape.

PMCT has been advocated for evaluating suspected body packers for its superior sensitivity and specificity. Drug packets on a PMCT will appear as multiple radiopaque foreign bodies with various signs (Figure 4.79). It can accurately determine size, number, and location and assess for complications.

3. **Gastric carcinoma:** Gastrointestinal stromal tumours (GISTs) tend to appear as well-defined masses that arise from the gastric wall and may be exophytic when large. GISTs are usually not associated with significant adenopathy.

4. **Peptic ulcers:** Peptic ulcers correspond to defects in the digestive tract mucosa, which extend through the muscularis mucosa. The most common risk factors include smoking, obesity, and non-steroidal anti-inflammatory drug use, including low-dose aspirin. There are no specific PMCT scan findings associated with peptic ulcer disease. However, a PMCT scan detects a few of the common complications of peptic ulcer disease, such as perforated peptic ulcer, by detecting pneumoperitoneum, seen as free air in the abdomen.

3. Small intestine

The small intestine is an organ that is around 6.5 metres long and located within the gastrointestinal tract and plays an important role in the digestion and absorption of food. It starts near the pylorus of the stomach and ends at the ileocaecal junction. The small intestine has three sections namely the duodenum, jejunum, and ileum.

4. Large intestine

The large intestine comprises five major parts::

1. **Caecum:** It is the most proximal part between the end of the ileum and the ascending colon. The caecum is continuous as the ascending colon. Unlike the ascending colon, the cecum is intraperitoneal.

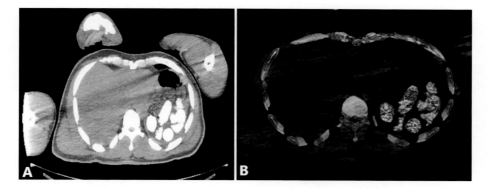

FIGURE 4.79:   Foreign body in the stomach in a case of body packing. A: Axial PMCT scan showing multiple hyperdense/ radioopaque foreign bodies in the stomach. B: Multiplanar reconstructed image showing drug-laden packets.

2. Appendix: The appendix is a vestigial part of the gastrointestinal tract, which is a narrow blind-ended tube attached to the caecum. The most common position is retrocaecal.

3. Colon: The colon or the large intestine extends from the cecum to the anal canal. Colon principally functions by reabsorbing water and electrolytes, and the remnants make the faeces. The colon is divided into four sections which are – the ascending colon, the transverse colon, the descending colon and the sigmoid colon. These sections form an arch, which encircles the small intestine.

4. Rectum: The rectum is the most distal segment of the large intestine and has an important role as a temporary store of faeces. It is continuous proximally with the sigmoid colon and terminates into the anal canal.

5. Anal canal: It is the last segment of the gastrointestinal tract and has an important role in the process of defecation and maintaining faecal continence. The anal canal has internal and external anal sphincters, which help in proper faecal continence.

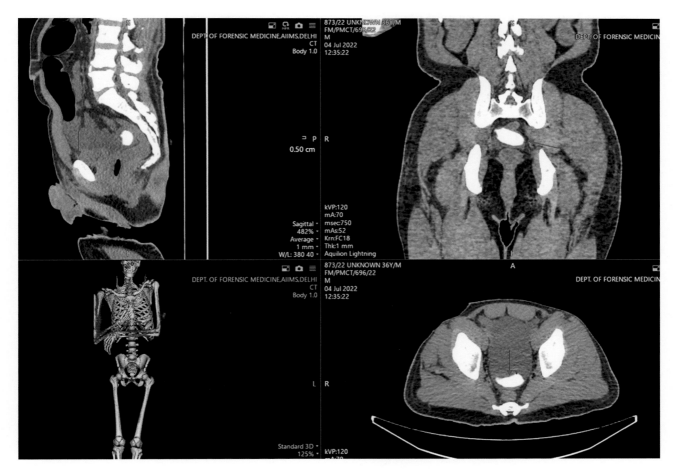

FIGURE 4.80:   Drug packet in Rectum: Four windows, i.e., sagittal, coronal, axial section with volume reconstructed image showing the location of the drug packet (marked with red arrow) in the rectum.

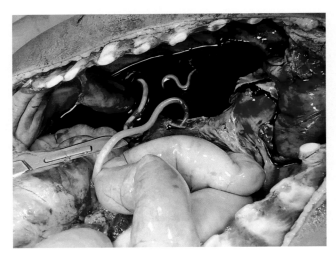

FIGURE 4.81: Autopsy examination of the intestines of a child showing intestinal worms as an incidental finding.

Pathology of small and large intestine

1. **Foreign body**: Body packers by swallowing and body stuffer by placing drug packets in the anal area with the intention of concealment of drugs can be easily detected on a PMCT (Figure 4.80).
2. **Appendicitis:** Inflammation of the appendix is known as appendicitis and is a common cause of acute severe abdominal pain; if it is not removed, it can cause rupture, leading to peritonitis.
3. **Haemorrhoids:** They are the vascular cushions found within the anal canal of a healthy individual, which help with the maintenance of faecal incontinence. If they are swollen or distended, they refer to as pathological.

4. **Anal canal tear:** In cases of sexual assault history or a suspicious one, the anal canal is to be examined for any local injury, i.e., contusion, swelling, or tearing.
5. **Intestinal worms:** Intestinal worms are common in children and are responsible for many nutritional disorders. They can also cause complications like intestinal obstruction when they are present in large numbers. During the autopsy, it can be an incidental finding, especially in children (Figure 4.81).

Bibliography

Mirilas P, Skandalakis JE. Surgical anatomy of the retroperitoneal spaces, Part III: Retroperitoneal blood vessels and lymphatics. *Am Surg.* 2010 February;76(2):139–144.

Mirilas P, Skandalakis JE. Surgical anatomy of the retroperitoneal spaces, Part IV: retroperitoneal nerves. *Am Surg.* 2010 March;76(3):253–262.

Pannu HK, Oliphant M. The subperitoneal space and peritoneal cavity: Basic concepts. *Abdominal imaging.* 2015 October;40:2710–2722.

Rajiah P, Sinha R, Cuevas C, Dubinsky TJ, Bush WH, Kolokythas O. Imaging of uncommon retroperitoneal masses. *Radiographics.* 2011 July–August;31(4):949–976.

Selçuk İ, Ersak B, Tatar İ, Güngör T, Huri E. Basic clinical retroperitoneal anatomy for pelvic surgeons. *Turk J Obstet Gynecol.* 2018 December;15(4):259–269.

Stallard DJ, Tu RK, Gould MJ, Pozniak MA, Pettersen JC. Minor vascular anatomy of the abdomen and pelvis: A CT atlas. *Radiographics.* 1994 May;14(3):493–513.

Tirkes T, Sandrasegaran K, Patel AA, Hollar MA, Tejada JG, Tann M, Akisik FM, Lappas JC. Peritoneal and retroperitoneal anatomy and its relevance for cross-sectional imaging. *Radiographics.* 2012 March–April;32(2):437–451.

Vesselle HJ, Miraldi FD. FDG PET of the retroperitoneum: Normal anatomy, variants, pathologic conditions, and strategies to avoid diagnostic pitfalls. *Radiographics.* 1998 July–August;18(4):805–823; discussion 823–824.

5 NECK – ANATOMY AND ASPHYXIAL DEATHS

Pathophysiology of asphyxial death

'Asphyxia' is a condition that results in a lack of oxygen in the blood, which may be due to a mechanical disturbance in oxygen uptake, transport, or cellular utilization, i.e., cellular oxidation. In the forensic literature, asphyxia is considered a mode of death, the other two being coma and syncope. In almost all centres performing forensic autopsies in India, deaths due to asphyxia account for most cases. A similar scenario is seen in countries with a similar sociodemographic profile. Although there is no clear classification system or detailed treatises on asphyxia deaths in forensic medical practice, deaths due to asphyxia are the cases that routinely present the most ambiguity at each step of the forensic death investigation. Relatives, neighbours, or friends of the deceased, society at large, and even the officials of the investigative agencies involved often frown at the conclusions of the autopsy surgeon. Such incidents occur even when one has performed a complex autopsy by carefully and systematically documenting and interpreting the post-mortem findings. He may have preserved viscera to rule out poisoning and supported his opinion by reliable forensic analysis of the fibres recovered to clearly attribute them to the material allegedly used, which has been examined for tensile strength by qualified forensic scientists. All of this must be confirmed with due consideration of all available circumstantial evidence, including the testimony of all persons involved and a detailed examination of the crime scene. While there are numerous demonstrable signs in cases of fatal asphyxia, most are not exclusively attributable to a single cause of death. Therefore, a holistic and cautious approach is needed in suspicious asphyxia deaths to arrive at an evidence-based and scientifically sound opinion of the cause and manner of death. There are numerous causes of the asphyxial mode of death, but suicide by hanging is the most common worldwide. Both rural and urban populations commit suicide through the method of hanging most commonly. This is probably due to the widespread belief that hanging is quick and painless, as well as the easy availability of ligature materials and suspension points. Hanging is a form of mechanical asphyxia in which the body is suspended around the neck by a ligature, the constricting force being the weight of the entire or a portion of the body. The possible features that are observed during an autopsy are determined by a variety of factors, including the degree to which the neck was compressed, the kind of ligature material used, the type of noose, where the knot is placed, the individual's weight acting as a constricting force, the individual's position, and the height of the drop. The autopsy features must be analyzed holistically rather than individually because of the dynamic and interdependent nature of this process.

Cross-sectional anatomy of the neck

The neck is a region of the body which is a relatively small area but has considerable complexity with its anatomy and functions. With the help of advancements in imaging techniques, neck structures and their anatomy can be well differentiated. Identification of the following structures is vital in autopsy examination: Skin, hyoid bone, thyroid cartilage, cervical vertebrae, respiratory passage, muscles of the neck, arteries, and veins of the neck.

The skin of the neck

Lines observed in external examination and cross-sectional anatomy are termed relaxed skin tension lines. The next layer consists of the adipose tissue and platysma, which is the superficial cervical fascia. Muscles and other structures of the neck, to a varying extent, are surrounded by the deep cervical fascia. The carotid sheath is a condensed part of the deep fascia that encloses the structures like carotid arteries, the vagus nerve, and the internal jugular vein. Blood supply to the neck skin includes the facial, occipital, posterior auricular, and subclavian arteries, and venous drainage of skin is into the jugular and facial veins.

Skeletal support of the neck

The skeletal support of the neck includes the cervical vertebrae and hyoid bone along with the laryngeal cartilages comprising of the thyroid, cricoid, epiglottis, arytenoid, corniculate, and cuneiform.

Cervical Vertebrae (Figures 5.1–5.3)

There are seven cervical vertebrae which support the neck. Among them, the third to sixth vertebrae have some characteristic features, which include:

- Spinous processes, which are short and bifid.
- Articular facets, which are flat and oval.
- The transverse process, which contains the foramen transversarium.

The rest of the cervical vertebrae are distinct, with each one having peculiar features like:

- The first vertebra lacks a spinous process and is more of a ring with anterior and posterior arch and is called the atlas.
- The second vertebra (axis) acts as a pivot on which the atlas and the skull move, and it also has an odontoid process that forms a joint with the atlas.
- The seventh vertebra is called the vertebra prominence and has a very long and prominent spinous process, making it easily palpable under the skin.

Radiological examination, either with an X-ray or CT scan, is very useful for the determination of fracture–dislocations of cervical vertebrae, which could be fatal.

Hyoid bone (Figure 5.4)

The hyoid bone is a U-shaped bone located anteriorly in the neck which is seen at the midline below the mandible. It consists of five parts: a central body, two greater cornua, and two lesser cornua.

Forensic relevance

1. Anatomical variants may be related to age, sex, and ethnicity. They may be important when using hyoid bone for establishing a biological profile.

DOI: 10.1201/9781003383703-5

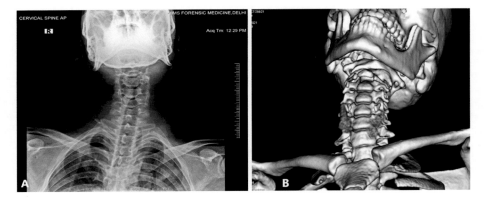

FIGURE 5.1 A: Post-mortem X-ray antero-posterior view of the neck showing neck skeletal structures. B: Volume-rendering 3D PMCT image showing the skeletal structures of the neck in the anterior view.

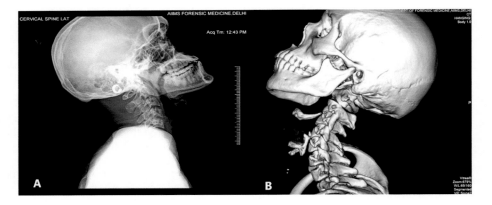

FIGURE 5.2 A: Post-mortem X-ray lateral view of the neck showing neck skeletal structures including the spinous process of the vertebrae. B: Volume-rendering 3D PMCT image lateral view of the neck showing the intact skeletal structures.

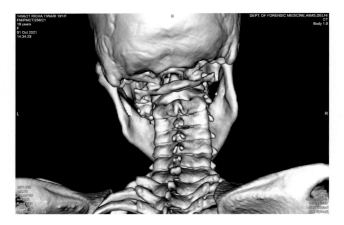

FIGURE 5.3: Volume-rendering 3D PMCT image posterior view of vertebrae showing the spinous processes.

2. Anatomical variants resembling fractures should be kept in mind when examining the hyoid–larynx complex.
3. Untimely fusion of joints may occur in younger age groups, in which, if fractures occur, chances of being missed are high.
4. Similarly, fusion in older age groups may not have occurred, and thus, a mistaken diagnosis of a fracture in the case of joint mobility should not be made.

5. Each anomaly may affect the way they are mobilized during neck injuries, which may not always give expected consequences in the autopsy findings.

Muscles of the neck
Platysma (Figure 5.5)
The superficial muscle of the neck, which also covers the upper parts of the pectoralis major and deltoid muscle, is known as the platysma. The fibres of the platysma go upwards and medially on either side of the neck. The anterior fibres of the contralateral muscle interlace across the midline. The rest of the fibres are attached to the lower lip or lower border of the mandible or across the mandible.

Sternocleidomastoid (Figure 5.6)
Sternocleidomastoid goes downwards and obliquely across either side of the neck and gives an elevation when it contracts. The central belly is thick, and the end parts are narrow. Two heads are there in the inferior aspect of the muscle, namely the clavicular and sternal head. In which the sternal head is rounded and tendinous, whereas the clavicular head is muscular and broad.

Supra-hyoid muscles
It is a pharyngeal muscle which consists of digastric (Figure 5.7), stylohyoid, geniohyoid, and mylohyoid muscles (Figures 5.8 and 5.9). These muscles play a vital role in swallowing. Together helps in the elevation of the hyoid bone and widening the oesophagal opening apart from its individual actions.

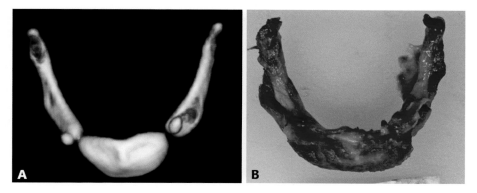

FIGURE 5.4 A: Volume-rendering 3D image of the hyoid bone with greater cornua not fused with the body. B: Autopsy examination of the hyoid bone after removal of all the muscular attachments.

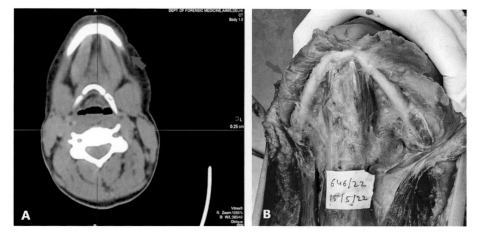

FIGURE 5.5 A: Axial section of neck PMCT in soft tissue window showing the platysma muscle. B: Layer-wise neck dissection showing the platysma muscle.

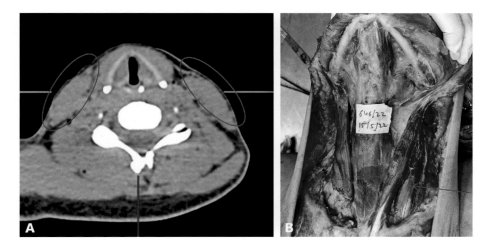

FIGURE 5.6 A: Axial section of neck PMCT in soft tissue window showing the sternocleidomastoid muscle (red circle). B: Layer-wise neck dissection showing the sternocleidomastoid muscle (red arrow).

Infra-hyoid muscles

It consists of sternohyoid (Figure 5.10), sternothyroid, thyrohyoid, and omohyoid muscles, altogether named strap muscles and are present over the anterior aspect of the neck. These muscles are long and flat. It helps in lowering the hyoid bone apart from their generic action. For better visualization,

layer-wise dissection of both supra and infrahyoid muscles is done in a bloodless field.

Carotid sheath contents (Figure 5.11)

The carotid sheath is situated over the anterolateral aspect of the neck on both sides, which is lateral to the trachea and it is a

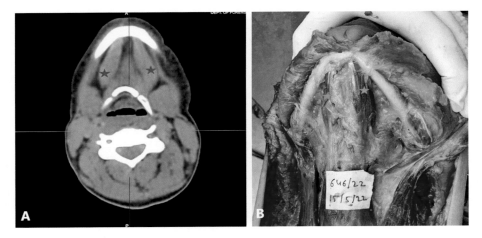

FIGURE 5.7   A: Axial section of the neck showing the digastric muscle (red star). B: Layer-wise neck dissection showing the digastric muscle (blue star).

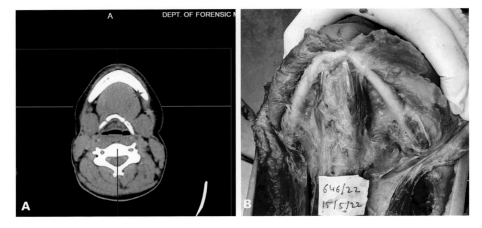

FIGURE 5.8   A: Axial section of the neck in soft tissue window showing the mylohyoid muscle (red star) and the submandibular gland (blue star). B: Layer-wise neck dissection showing the mylohyoid muscle (red star) and submandibular gland (blue star).

part of the deep cervical fascia. Contents of the carotid sheath are as follows:

1. Carotid artery – the common carotid artery, which bifurcates at the level of the fourth vertebra.
2. Internal jugular vein.
3. Vagus nerve.
4. Part of recurrent laryngeal nerve.
5. Deep cervical lymph nodes.

Full-body PMCT evaluation

If a facility for PMCT examination is available, a CT scan of the whole body should be done in all possible cases. It also ensures the radiological documentation, and it helps us to avoid the loss or leaving unnoticed any foreign materials/personal belongings of the dead body. In asphyxial deaths, PMCT examinations are useful in identifying any fracture of the hyoid bone, thyroid, or other laryngeal cartilage and vertebral column, any foreign body within the airway, any gag in place, and any injury over the face and neck. PMCT

helps the autopsy surgeons in finding out the direction of force applied over the neck by assessing the direction of the distal portions of the fractured structures.

If a PMCT facility is not available, then a post-mortem X-ray (PM X-ray) examination to identify the fracture pattern can be used. For better visualization of bony and cartilaginous structures of the neck, we can incorporate micro CT after the removal of the tissues from the body; it gives a better image because of the absence of vertebral structures. PM X-ray is also helpful for identifying any foreign bodies in the airways in cases of choking and aspiration. It also helps to examine the skeletal framework of the neck in asphyxia death cases which includes vertebrae, ribs, and small bones like hyoid. The presence of foreign objects in the airway can also be appreciated well.

Visual autopsy in asphyxial deaths

A visual autopsy is essential in asphyxial deaths as the major finding in asphyxial deaths could be mere abrasion or contusion over the neck, lips or even just a congested face. These findings are poorly appreciable with radiological tools and

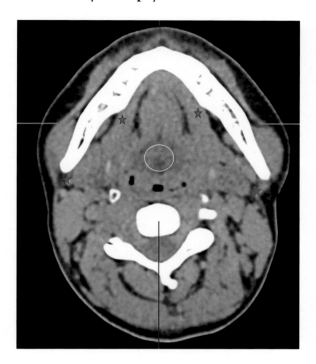

FIGURE 5.9: Axial section of the neck showing the mylohyoid muscle (blue star), sternocleidomastoid muscle (red star), and oropharynx (yellow circle).

visual autopsy, with the external examination, photographic documentation, clothes examination, and ligature examination playing a vital role. Virtual autopsy helps in ruling out other possible causes of death and concluding asphyxial deaths.

External examination

In all cases of death by asphyxia, a systematic examination should be performed from head to toe.

Scalp

The hair on the head should be examined for stains or breakage. The scalp should be palpated for hidden lesions. If necessary, doubtful areas should be shaved to make the scalp lesions more visible.

Face

The face should be carefully examined. The entire face should be examined for pallor, congestion, petechiae, oedema, and cyanosis. All of these findings may be present in varying degrees in choking deaths. Congestion and petechiae are present throughout the face and extend to the ears. Examination of the neck is the most important measure in choking death congestion, petechiae, or severe subconjunctival haemorrhage. The cornea should be examined for transparency, and haemorrhages inside the eyeball should be assessed with an ophthalmoscope. Tache noir (Figure 5.12), the colour change of the exposed conjunctiva, should not be misinterpreted as a haemorrhage or other lesion.

Nose
Examination Technique

Externally, the bridge of the nose, nostrils, and adjacent cheeks must be thoroughly examined in all cases of asphyxia. Injuries to the soft tissues are common in cases of asphyxia. The bridge of the nose may have fractures in rare cases. Abrasions, contusions, and lacerations may be visualized in many cases of asphyxia. The external visual examination should follow palpation to avoid misdiagnosis of nasal bone fractures. The inside of the nostrils must be examined in detail, preferably with a nasal speculum, to obtain a better view. Nasal bleeding, mucosal lesions, etc., can be detected by this examination. The nose is palpated to detect abnormal movements suggestive of a fracture. A nasal speculum is inserted into the nostrils and then released to visualize the inside of the nose.

Findings

Alae and the bridge of the nose should be examined for any injuries. Routinely, the bridge of the nose should be examined by palpation. The nostrils should be examined thoroughly with a nasal speculum. If asphyxia is suspected, mucosal lesions should be examined. Bloodstains, frothy fluids, vomited stomach contents, any foreign bodies, etc., must be identified and documented. Adjacent cheeks must be examined for external injuries.

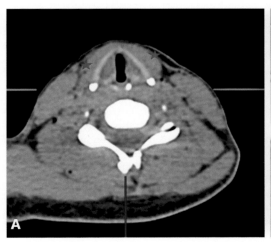
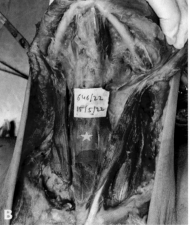

FIGURE 5.10 A: Axial section of the neck PMCT in soft tissue window showing the sternohyoid muscle (red star). B: Layerwise neck dissection showing the sternohyoid muscle (yellow star).

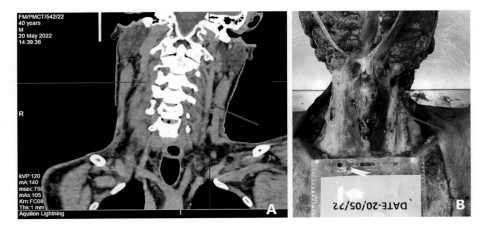

FIGURE 5.11:   A: Carotid sheath in a coronal section of neck PMCT in soft tissue window (red arrow). B: Autopsy examination showing carotid sheath during neck dissection.

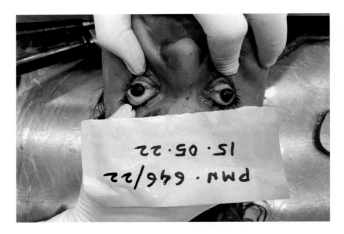

FIGURE 5.12:   Tache noir seen in a hanging case.

Mouth

External examination of the lips must be performed in detail in all cases of asphyxia. The inside of the lips can be examined by turning them upside down with a pair of tweezers that are not toothed. The inside of the cheeks, gums, teeth, tongue, hard and soft palate, tonsils, and tonsil bed may be examined if the temporomandibular joints are forcibly disrupted. Injuries to these structures are common, especially in cases of asphyxiation and other violent deaths. The inside of the lips and mouth can be further examined by specular examination of the facial flap, which is described in detail at the end of this chapter. In this method, the facial flap can be created as a continuation of the upper skin flap of the V-shaped neck incision. The flap can be elevated to the tip of the nose without disfiguring the face. This method of facial dissection allows clearer visualization of soft tissue lesions on the face, including those on the inside of the lips. Temporomandibular cutting of the fibres of the masseter muscle. This helped disarticulate the mandible, allowing better access to the oral cavity and protected upper airways, i.e., the nasopharynx and oropharynx. This method of dissection is useful in the treatment of choking cases, especially choking attacks and retching. Injuries to the soft tissues around the pharynx, mouth, and tongue can be clearly demonstrated using this method.

Examination Technique

Both lips are held with non-toothed forceps and inverted to view the gums, frenulum, and teeth to determine if the tongue is protruding and trapped between the teeth. The oral cavity should be examined as much as possible. Because of rigor mortis, opening the mouth will be difficult. Rigor mortis can be overcome by cutting the masseter muscle so that rigor mortis is released and visibility is improved.

Findings

In all cases of asphyxia, the external and internal aspects of the upper and lower lip should be examined. Mucosal congestion, cyanosis, and injuries in the form of abrasions, contusions, and lacerations should be noted and documented. These injuries are common in homicides and may be the only positive findings suggestive of the manner of death. The frenulum of the upper and lower lip should also be examined and documented in all cases of death by asphyxiation. If injuries are present on the inner surfaces of the lips, they should be correlated with the sharp, pointed edges of the teeth. Hygiene of the oral cavity, discolouration of the gums and teeth, signs of infection, and the presence of liquid discharge or pus should also be noted. Protrusion of the tongue should be checked for hanging teeth but need not be noted in all cases. Drying of the exposed portions of the lips and tongue results in a dark reddish or blackish discolouration of the exposed areas. This may confuse inexperienced autopsy surgeons and be misinterpreted as ante-mortem lip or tongue lesions.

Chin

The chin should be examined for external injuries, i.e., abrasions, bruises, nail marks, or other injuries. Placement of the knot near the chin is observed in cases of hanging; the knot marks are generally seen as isolated pressure abrasions. The autopsy surgeon must correlate the overall pattern of ligature signs and examine the ligature material before settling on the nature of the causation of these lesions.

Dribbling of saliva

In general, signs of excessive salivation show up in cases left suspended from the ligature. Saliva drips from the mouth, usually from the corner of the mouth, which is in the lower region because of a possible tilt of the head. This is thought to be due to direct pressure and stimulation of the submandibular salivary glands due to the compressive force of the ligature. The autopsy surgeon should assess the direction of the ligature marking and ensure that the salivary track follows the laws of gravity and anatomy. The pattern of drying should be consistent with post-mortem duration. The autopsy surgeon should be aware of the possibility of staging by artificially introducing dried stains that resemble saliva drip marks. In this case, swabs can be taken from the suspect site and sent for analysis (e.g., amylase test). DNA matching is also possible with saliva stains. In many cases, these rivulets extend to the front of the torso and can be seen on the ground just below the body. The direction and placement of these marks can be analyzed holistically before a conclusion is drawn. Intense pulmonary oedema, mucosal congestion, etc., may result in post-mortem fluid collections in the throat, mouth, and nostrils. These fluids may seep out through the mouth during transport or other manipulations of the cadaver. These wet or dry fluid trickles are rarely misinterpreted as salivary trickles. In such cases, the trickling is almost horizontal. The author believes that the direction of salivary traces should be analyzed in all cases of alleged or suspected deaths after hanging before a conclusion is drawn. If in doubt, the stains should be collected and sent for further forensic evaluation.

Ears

An otoscope can be used for a detailed examination of the external auditory canal, tympanic membrane, and middle ear in the case of a ruptured eardrum. The otoscope can also be used to take photographs of these findings. The anterior and posterior aspects of the earlobes should be examined for any lesions. The external auditory canal should be examined for any injuries or bleeding. The tympanic membrane may also be examined, as many cases of mechanical asphyxia may have tympanic membrane haemorrhage, but this is considered a non-specific finding by many authors.

Neck

The neck is the most important region of the body to examine in all cases of choking. The neck should be stretched as much as possible by placing a wooden board, block, or neck support under the shoulder. The neck should be examined for abnormal range of motion due to a fracture of the spine. Any injury to the neck following traumatic neck compression should be described in detail as to type, size, shape, location, and direction. Vivid descriptions of restraint marks, fingernail marks, fingertip bruises, cuts inflicted with sharp weapons, defensive wounds, and injuries indicative of a last stand for life or an attempt to escape, etc., should be made. These should be recorded with appropriate photographs. Magnifying hand lenses, flashlights, and infrared or ultraviolet photography may be useful for further evaluation of ligature marks.

Ligature mark (Figures 5.13–5.16)

Areas of erythema above and below the ligature marks should be identified and documented. One of the most important features of a ligature mark is its direction. Although there are some exceptions, hanging marks inevitably have a slant due to the downward gravity of the body. Neck injuries from manual strangulation, ligature strangulation, palmar strangulation, and other forms of mechanical compression of the neck vary. These injuries range from intact skin to obvious abrasions, contusions, and/or lacerations. The course of the ligature should be examined in detail in terms of its course, continuity on either the anterior, lateral, or posterior aspect of the neck,

multiple ligature marks due to multiple loops, pattern, dimensions, wide or thin appearance, texture, accompanying injuries such as blisters, abrasions, etc. The width of the ligature mark at various locations on the neck should be noted in relation to anatomical landmarks. The total length of the ligature mark should be noted in the report. The total circumference of the neck must be reported in all cases of asphyxia for later comparison and correlation with the presumed ligature material. If an obvious pattern of ligature marks is evident, this must be mentioned in the autopsy report and recorded photographically.

Upper limb

The inside of the arms and forearms must be examined in all cases of asphyxia. Bruising of the pads of the fingers indicates the involvement of another person who clasped the upper limbs of the deceased while alive. These injuries should be interpreted with caution because they may occur during the agonal phase of the rescue.

Hesitation cuts

Fresh, transverse parallel cuts on the anterior and internal aspect of the forearm of the non-dominant upper limb represent the classic picture of hesitation cuts. These injuries must also be properly documented and interpreted. Multiple linear, transverse, hypopigmented scars also suggest suicidal ideation or intentional self-injury in the past. Gradually tapering and tapering scarring are often seen on the medial aspects of these superficial or even deeper lacerations. In the author's experience, razor blades are the most common weapon used to cause these injuries, and counter-injuries are observed on the insides of the first two or three fingers of the dominant hand, resulting from holding the razor blade. These injuries are generally very shallow, obliquely incised wounds on the thumb and index finger of the right hand. The pattern of these injuries must be analyzed, taking into account the possibility of staging hesitation cuts by an intelligent offender. The investigating officer should be informed of these injuries, and the weapon can be examined by experts. Many cases of suicide by hanging have multiple hypopigmented transverse scars on the front of the non-dominant forearm. Many of these indicate previous failed attempts at intentional self-harm.

Examination of hands and fingers

In all cases of death by asphyxiation, any injuries to the hands should be noted, and the autopsy physician should evaluate the possible mechanisms behind them. Any possible defensive wound should be investigated and must be detailed in the autopsy report for possible later evaluation by an expert witness. In all cases of alleged or suspected asphyxiation deaths, the hands should be searched for possible evidence of another cause of death, such as burns from electrocution, etc., taking into account the possibility of post-mortem exposure and staging. Rigor mortis prevents full opening of the hands, thus complicating the examination. For a proper and complete examination, the flexor tendons at the front of the wrist must be severed to allow proper extension of the palm and fingers.

Fingernail beds and cyanosis

In living individuals, cyanosis represents an increased concentration of reduced or deoxyhaemoglobin in the blood. It is noticeable by a bluish discolouration of the mucous membrane of the lips and peripheral areas, such as the tips of the fingers and toes. This bluish discolouration is noticeable when the concentration of reduced haemoglobin rises above 5 g/100 ml of

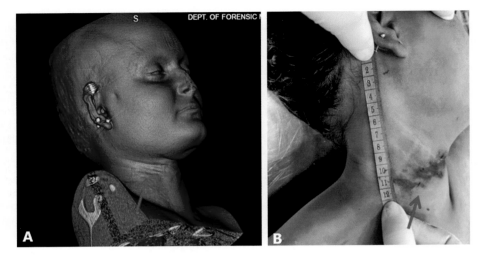

FIGURE 5.13:   A comparative image of ligature mark over the lateral aspect of the neck (red arrow) in a hanging case with A: 3D reconstruction image and B: external examination.

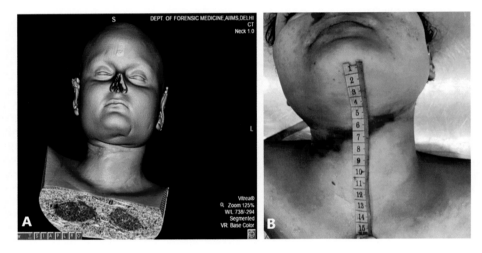

FIGURE 5.14:   A comparative image of ligature mark over the anterior aspect of the neck in a hanging case with A: 3D reconstruction image and B: external examination.

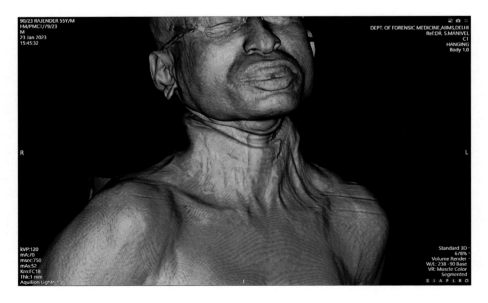

FIGURE 5.15:   3D reconstruction image shows ligature mark compressing the neck

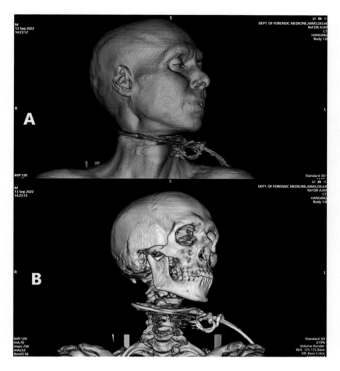

FIGURE 5.16 A and B: Shows ligature material in situ in a hanging case in volume-rendering 3D images of PMCT; it also shows the relation of ligature material to skin and underlying hyoid and vertebral bones.

liquid blood. The total amount of haemoglobin is not relevant to the occurrence of cyanosis. Oxygen utilization occurs at the tissue level even after somatic death. Thus, 'cyanosis' on mucous membranes and fingertips does not necessarily correspond to the exact oxygen content of haemoglobin at the time of death. However, it has been observed that asphyxiation deaths show marked cyanosis in most cases. Because the nails are transparent, discolouration of the fingernails can be seen at autopsy. Examination of the fingernails is an essential component of asphyxia. Freshly broken nail tips indicate some type of hand grip immediately prior to death, and the broken pieces must be preserved for the detection of extraneous traces, including extraneous DNA.

Hanging

Hanging is an asphyxial death which is usually suicidal in nature. The height of the hanging point should always be analyzed and compared to the alleged method used to achieve the desired height of the hanging. The availability of the restraint material to the deceased must be verified. In most cases, the restraints used for hanging have cracks depending on the strength and direction of the tensile force. Suppose a discrepancy is found regarding the type of restraint material used; a detailed investigation should be conducted before we reach a conclusion in cases of suicide by hanging. A simple hand lens is of great use in investigating the direction of pull by analyzing the needle pattern of the ligature material. Any stains found on the ligature material should be examined in detail and preserved for further biological and chemical analysis. The pattern of post-mortem staining should be photographed at the scene in all possible cases. This will provide information on the

duration of the suspension and the presence of a primary pattern of post-mortem staining. The posture of the lower limbs during partial hanging after the onset of rigor mortis provides information about the degree of hanging and the type of hanging. From these observations, a rough estimate of the time since death or the duration of suspension can be derived. If any of these findings differ, the autopsy examiner should thoroughly investigate the possibility of extraneous fault. Such doubts arise, especially in cases of partial hanging when the legs touch the ground, and they raise doubts in the minds of relatives and friends. The scene should be searched for signs of scuffle or violence. Any foreign material, biological stains, including bloodstains, etc., must be identified and should be sent for further examination. For bodies found in remote locations, the possibility of post-mortem exposure should be ruled out, especially if the person is intoxicated.

Causes of death in hanging

Based on the author's experience with hanging cases, observation of autopsy results in relation to the position of the ligature, knot, and point of hanging, and research of the existing literature, the author would like to draw the conclusion that one of the primary causes of death in a hanging case is obstruction of the posterior pharynx as a result of pressure on the soft structures of the neck and floor of the mouth, which eventually results in respiratory asphyxia. The most important part of the respiratory system is the oropharynx, which connects the nasopharynx and oral cavity to the larynx and laryngopharynx (Figure 5.17). The base of the tongue, the tonsillar region, and the lateral and posterior oropharyngeal walls make up the oropharynx.

Over 30 muscles, numerous motor and sensory nerves, and coordination through the brainstem, cortex, and subcortical structures are required for each of them to play an important part in inhalation, exhalation, swallowing, and speech. The oropharyngeal function is paralyzed, and the brain receives no oxygen due to mechanical blockage or ligature pressure obstructing the pharynx. Necrosis and death of the respiratory centres' neurons in the pons and medulla result in apnea, loss of spontaneous breathing, and death of the brainstem. The natural and outward tongue muscles and different muscles answerable for opening/shutting the jaws and pharynx, particularly those innervated by the hypoglossal nerve, which keeps the tongue from gnawing or falling back and impeding the aviation route, additionally become deadened at times. Airway obstruction, asphyxia, and unconsciousness due to the impairment and collapse of the pharynx are almost immediately caused by the constriction and forward pull of the posterior pharyngeal wall and the backwards displacement of the tongue's dorsum caused by the mechanical constriction of the oropharynx caused by the pressure of the ligature. The author would like to provide evidence for this by contrasting the PMCT findings of the neck in a hanging case with the ligature material still present in situ enclosing the neck, which shows that the critical passage of the oropharynx is obstructed by the pressure exerted by the ligature, even when the vertical traction of the ligature is removed at hanging during the recovery of the dead body at the scene (Figures 5.18 and 5.19), with the PMCT findings of the neck in a control case without compressive force across the neck where the oropharynx is open (Figure 5.20). The obstruction of this critical passage by this mechanical force results in the loss of speech and the ability to scream or make sounds, and this is the reason for the cases in which a person commits suicide by

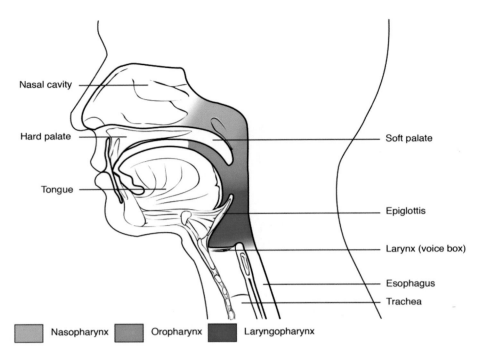

FIGURE 5.17: The various sub-divisions of the pharynx, and it is seen that the oropharynx connects the oral cavity, nasopharynx, and laryngopharynx.

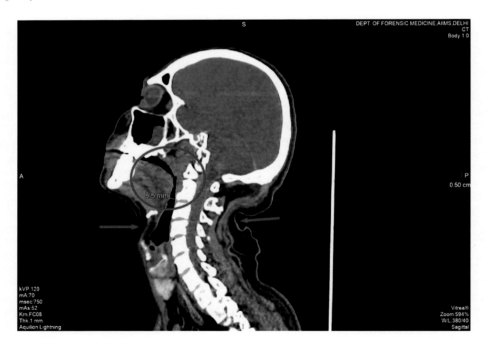

FIGURE 5.18: PMCT examination of the neck in a case of hanging with ligature present in situ, compressing the neck (red arrows) and causing constriction and occlusion of the oropharynx (red circle), even when the vertical traction of the hanging ligature is removed during recovery of the dead body at the scene.

hanging and remains unnoticed/unheard by the wife/husband/ sleeping in the same room.

Manual strangulation

Manual strangulation, also known as throttling, is compression to the neck by a perpetrator's hands. It is a common method of homicide because the perpetrator only needs to use his or her bare hands to commit the crime. When compared to deaths caused by ligature strangulation, throttling has a higher death rate. Homicide throttling typically takes place between two people whose physical characteristics are reasonably different. The majority of victims are women, while the perpetrators are typically men. The typical victim of a female

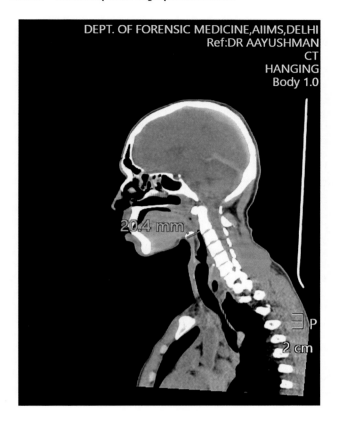

FIGURE 5.19: PMCT examination of the neck in a case of hanging with ligature present in situ, compressing the neck and causing constriction and occlusion of the oropharynx.

perpetrator is a child. It is difficult to diagnose throttling deaths due to the high variability of the injuries, especially when findings are unusual. In a case of homicide, one of the many approaches taken may be manual strangulation. In cases of a suspected violent homicide, a thorough examination for other causes of death should be conducted despite the presence of injuries consistent with manual strangulation.

Mechanism of injury

All of the death mechanism combinations that have been described for hanging are also possible in manual strangulation. The larynx and windpipe are compressed obstructing the lumen completely. In most cases, jugular veins are compressed. Compression of the carotid artery is also common, but the fluctuating grip may permit some arterial blood flow in between. Adult victims typically cannot have their vertebral arteries completely occluding if there is only one offender. As a result, above the level of neck constriction, the majority of cases of manual strangulation exhibit signs of congestion. There are a lot of cases of manual strangulation where there are no visible external injuries or facial congestion. The most plausible explanation for these cases is the possibility of carotid sinus stimulation followed by reflex cardiac arrest as a result of stimulation of the brain stem's tenth cranial nerve centre.

Findings from the autopsy external examination

Typical Fingernail Abrasion: The 'typical' external injuries on the neck are abrasions in the shape of crescents and oval or circular dermal contusions (Figure 5.21).

In general, there are two types of neck abrasions caused by manual strangulation. One is abrasions caused by the static pressure applied by the fingernail tips as they penetrate the neck's soft tissues. Typically, abrasions in the shape of a crescent represent the perpetrator's injury from the act. A correlation between the perpetrator's handedness and the location of these curvilinear abrasions has been attempted but without success. The concavity of the fingernail abrasion typically points toward the pulp of that finger, but it can also be linear, crescent-shaped, or even 'S'-shaped. In most cases of manual strangulation, fingernail cuts are more likely to be on the sides of the neck, above the thyroid cartilage. They are less common but can be seen on the front and back of the neck.

The dragging effect of nail tips over the victim's or assailant's neck skin is the cause of the second category of abrasions. The victim's fingernail tips typically cause abrasions that are linear and vertical, and if multiple fingertips are involved, they are parallel. These dragging abrasions, also known as struggle marks, can also indicate a variety of orientations. Many authors believe it is unrealistic to be able to distinguish between the nail tip abrasions caused by the victim's struggle and those

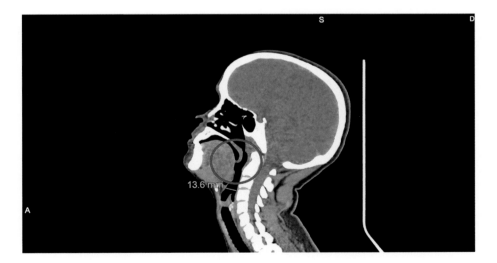

FIGURE 5.20: PMCT examination of a control case in which no pressure was applied to the neck. The oropharynx remains open, with neither the base of the tongue pushed back, nor the posterior pharyngeal wall pushed forward (red circle).

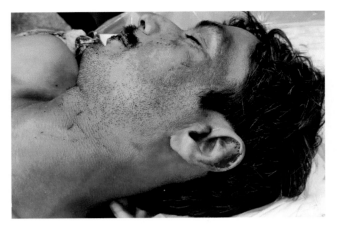

FIGURE 5.21: Typical fingernail abrasion is seen during external examination over the anterolateral aspect of the neck in a case of manual strangulation.

caused by the perpetrator's nails by simply analyzing the objective findings from the autopsy. During an examination with the naked eye, moist skin may not reveal all of these abrasions. Therefore, the neck examination should be performed only after the body surface has become dry in those instances. The assailant's distinctive nail tips may leave impressions that can be reproduced. If the identity of the assailant is in question, it may be helpful to analyze the shapes of fingernail tips and scientifically compare them to the abrasions during the investigation and trial. Within a few days of the incident, the perpetrator was examined for similar nail tip abrasions, typically on the upper limbs. For further comparative analysis of physical or biological trace evidence, fingernail clippings or nail scrapings must be preserved in any case of suspected manual strangulation. It has been demonstrated that these comparative forensic analyses are helpful in determining the identity of the perpetrators and the exact location of the crime. Detail should be taken of the shape of the nail tips and any breakage that may be present.

Haemorrhages on an internal examination: Even minor external neck injuries can reveal significant underlying tissue bleeding. Subcutaneous fat, platysma, and neck muscles (Figure 5.22) frequently experience bleeding. In many instances, contusions can also be seen in the structures of the carotid sheet, lymph nodes, salivary glands in the under-chin area, and the outer aspect of the larynx. In some cases, the thyroid gland parenchyma (Figure 5.23) and subcapsular regions contain

areas of bleeding. Additionally, there are numerous superficial haemorrhages at the base of the tongue.

Thyro-hyoid complex fractures: Direct pressure on the larynx is the most common method of manual strangulation. Compared to hanging and ligature strangulation, manual strangulation results in a greater number of thyrohyoid complex fractures because it involves a larger area at the front of the neck. The fractures are caused by direct pressure or pressure that is transmitted through the thyrohyoid membrane, the same mechanisms as in hanging or ligature strangulation. Although these fractures do not directly result in death, they do indicate that force was applied to the voice box. The most prevalent fracture is a unilateral isolated fracture of the superior horn of the thyroid. The second most normal break in manual strangulation is that of more noteworthy cornua of the hyoid bone.

There is a lot of variation in the scientific literature regarding the absolute frequency of these fractures. In most cases, these fractured segments exhibit an inward displacement. However, in many instances, both inward and external fractures occur together. Fractures are more common on the side where the thumb's pulp is thrust. It is not appropriate to speculate about the assailant's handedness or cause of death based solely on the fracture pattern, given the variability of these fractures. Premortem fractures typically reveal haemorrhagic infiltration of the soft tissues surrounding the fracture. The essentialness of these breaks ought to be affirmed terribly and minutely if all else fails. Post-mortem fractures may exhibit some artefact haemorrhage around the fracture site, which the autopsy surgeon should be aware of. A fracture site must be dissected for minute details, like where the tear is in the periosteum and if there is subperiosteal bleeding. In manual strangulation, laminar fractures of the thyroid cartilage and cricoid cartilage are uncommon. However, if they do occur, they indicate severe anteroposterior compression of the neck structures between the external force and the anterior aspect of the bodies of cervical vertebrae. Hyoid bone and laryngeal cartilage ossification start late, so these structures are flexible early in life, and fractures are less common in younger people. Due to the calcification of the bone, hyoid bone fractures are more prevalent in victims of throttling and hanging who are over 40 years old.

There are three types of hyoid bone fractures:

1. **Fracture of inward compression (Figure 5.24):** This kind is frequently used in throttling situations; The hyoid bone's inward compression is the primary force that causes the fracture. The greater horns of the hyoid

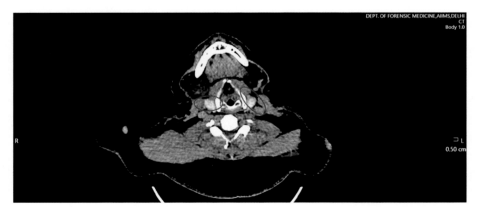

FIGURE 5.22: PMCT of the neck showing haemorrhage of neck muscles (hyperdense area inside red circle).

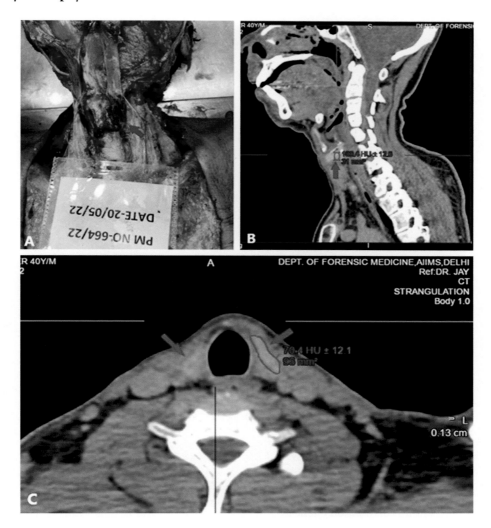

FIGURE 5.23 A: Bloodless neck dissection shows haemorrhage in the thyroid gland in case of strangulation. B and C: PMCT of the neck shows a haemorrhage of the thyroid gland in both images (hyperdense area inside the pink circle with HU of more than 60).

are compressed inward, resulting in a fracture and tear of the periosteum on the outer surface of the bone. The fractured ends are then displaced inward. Holding the hyoid's body in one hand and its distal portion between the fingers of the other hand can demonstrate this. The distal portion can be bent inwards, but not outwards, due to the intact periosteum on the medial surface.

2. **Fracture of compression in the front and back:** The greater cornu is impacted over the cervical vertebra, compressing the hyoid bone backwards, resulting in a fracture with the fractured ends moving outward. The inner side of the periosteum is torn here, causing the fragment to move outward. It can be seen in hanging, ligature strangulation, and other situations.

3. **Fracture of an avulsion:** It results from traction on the thyrohyoid ligament brought on by neck hyperextension or violent movement brought on by lateral or downward compression. The hyoid bone is dragged up here. It is not possible to mistake the joints that connect the body and the greater/lesser cornu for fractures. Additionally, the presence of haemorrhage in the affected area should

support the ante-mortem nature of the hyoid bone fracture and should be confirmed by the presence of haemorrhage at the affected area.

PMCT examination furnishes us with many subtleties in asphyxia cases. This method is exceptionally useful in figuring out wounds over little designs in the neck, which are encircled by many little delicate tissues and, along these lines, hard to be valued in a customary post-mortem examination. By 3D reconstruction, PMCT reveals ligature marks, fractures of the greater horns of the hyoid bone, and fractures of the superior horn of the thyroid cartilage. MSCT is an important tool for finding injuries like fractures caused by trauma to the larynx. Ossification of tristichous cartilage and fractures of thyroid horns as displaced fragments or discontinuities are revealed by 3D reconstruction. Because it provides us with an idea for selecting the appropriate dissection technique, many forensic surgeons recommend performing PMCT prior to the conventional autopsy, paying particular attention to strangulation cases. The laminae of the thyroid cartilage and fractured greater horns of the hyoid bone are visible on the reformatted MSCT.

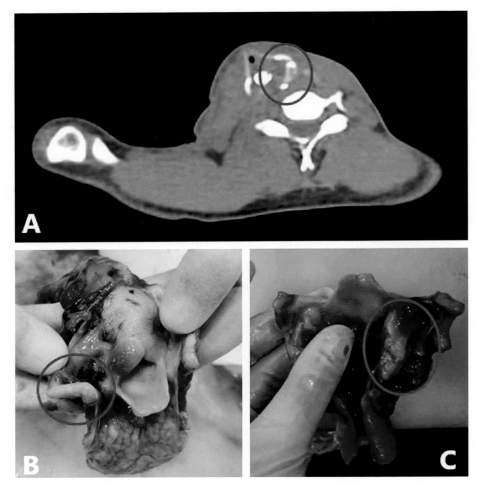

FIGURE 5.24   A: Shows inward compression fracture of the hyoid bone in a case of manual strangulation in the axial section neck PMCT (red circle). B and C: Shows fracture of hyoid bone with surrounding tissue infiltration and haemorrhage in a case of manual strangulation (red circle).

In cases of strangulation, magnetic resonance imaging (MRI) is an important tool for detecting soft tissue haemorrhage. Muscle haemorrhage in the posterior crico-arytenoid muscles and the retropharyngeal regions can be seen on MRI. Both cases of ligature strangulation and manual strangulation result in lymph node haemorrhage. In short tau inversion recovery (STIR) – weighted MRI, haemorrhages appear as hyperintense areas. The muscle that seems tumid and hyper-extraordinary is reminiscent of discharge and enlarging. Lymph node haemorrhage, soft tissue, and muscular haemorrhage resembling drowning can be detected with the help of an MRI.

Ligature strangulation

The fatal compression of the neck by a ligature, where the constricting force is applied externally and is not the body's weight, is referred to as ligature strangulation. The majority of these cases fall under the category of homicide. However, there have been very few reports of accidental and suicidal deaths. The source, magnitude, and direction of the constricting force are the primary distinctions between ligature strangulation and hanging. Typically, in hanging, the body's gravitational drag constricts vital neck structures, resulting in death through various mechanisms previously discussed. The constricting force in ligature strangulation is typically lower and insufficient to compress all neck arteries, particularly the well-protected vertebral arteries. Unless reflux is the cause of death, strangulation with ligatures always results in some degree of visible congestion above the ligature mark.

Mechanism of death in ligature strangulation

All possible combinations of mechanisms of death that can occur in hanging are also possible. The ligature used typically transmits the constriction force from the attackers' upper limbs. The majority of times, venous flow obstruction and subsequent upstream congestion are caused by neck veins' easy compressibility. The majority of times, carotid artery compression and complete occlusion do not occur. With the normal forces of ligature strangulation, tracheal, or laryngeal compression may cause airway obstruction. The ligature strangulation's compressive force typically does not obstruct the vertebral arteries; As a result, the 'pale face' image of hanging appears in cases of reflex cardiac inhibition. In ligature strangulation, each of these mechanisms contributes to death to varying degrees, either individually or collectively.

External examination after the death

The ligature mark: The transmitted force during neck compression results in the appearance of a depressed mark, or pressure abrasion, as well as a clearly defined groove on the neck (Figures 5.25–5.27). The traditional description of a ligature strangulation mark is a transverse, complete ligature mark, but the majority of cases do not exhibit this typical finding. A pale, compressed area with some erythematous margins is seen in many cases. Reddish dermal contusions are visible in some cases. Pressure abrasions may occur if the friction is greater, as in the case of rough materials like ropes. At first, these pressure abrasions are pale and yellowish, but as they dry, they turn brownish. These abrasions have a texture similar to parchment when dried after death. Most of the time, the underlying subcutaneous tissues do not exhibit a 'dried, whitish, or glistening appearance' because the pressure is not maintained continuously like in hanging. On the other hand, ligature strangulation marks usually cause bleeding. The manner of death and the type of ligature material used determine the mark's presence and appearance. Due to friction, hard materials make it simple to cause cuts and abrasions on the skin. In many cases, materials like soft clothing do not leave any visible marks.

In many instances, ligature impressions can be identified by thorough examination with the aid of a hand lens, oblique illumination, infrared photography, and UV lamps. Engrave examples of the ligature can be valued with unaided eyes or with the assistance of these extra apparatuses and whenever laid out, can be utilized as proof in the courtroom. The material for the ligature and the mark ought to be the same depth and width. A deep grooved ligature mark, also known as the cheese-cutter method, is produced when very thin ligature materials like chains, strings, or narrow electric wire or cord are used. The skin and other underlying structures are frequently cut by these thin materials. If the pressure is released immediately following death, the mark may not always be visible because broad materials leave shallow impressions. Erythematous lines are frequently visible on the ligature mark's upper and lower margins. The mechanical displacement of blood as a result of the compressive force transmitted through the noose is the explanation for these reddish areas

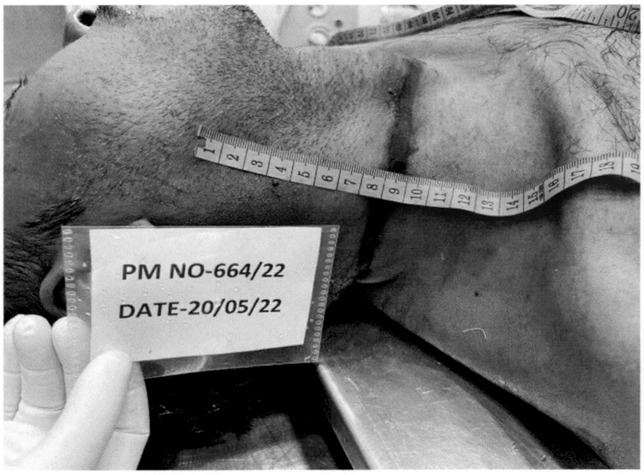

FIGURE 5.25: Shows a depressed mark, or pressure abrasion, as well as a clearly defined groove on the neck which is transverse and complete around the neck in a case of ligature strangulation.

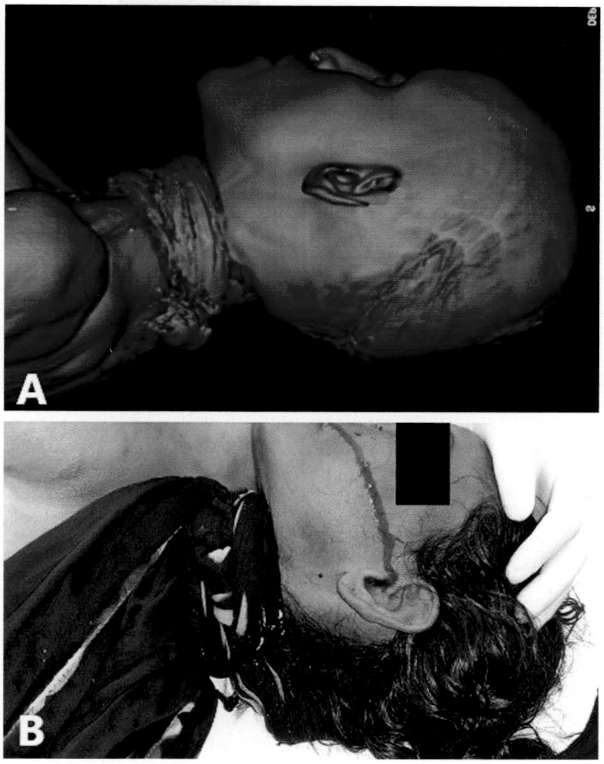

FIGURE 5.26: A and B: Shows knot position of ligature in 3D reconstruction image and external examination in a ligature strangulation case.

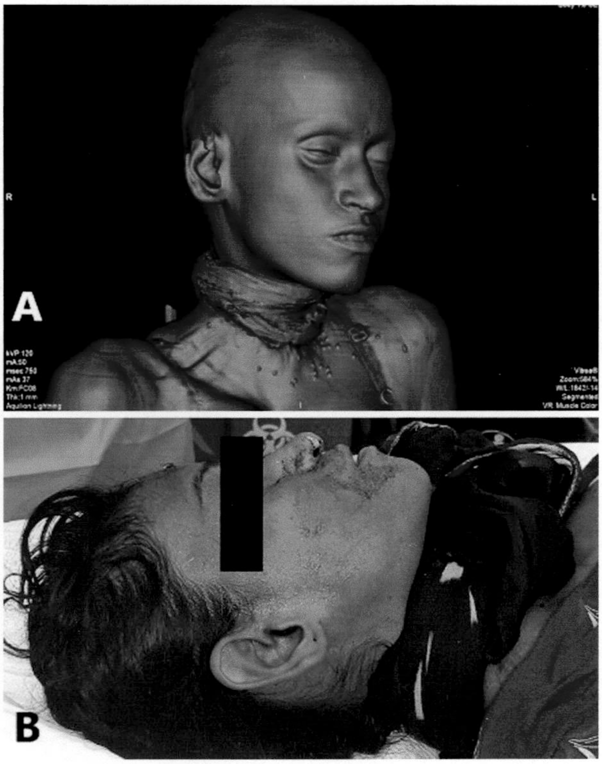

FIGURE 5.27: A and B: Shows the position of ligature in 3D reconstruction image and external examination in a ligature strangulation case.

that can occur in ligature compression of the neck even after death. Thus, it is not viewed as an indication of imperativeness. In opposition to hanging, the ligature mark is crossed over in the majority of the instances of ligature strangulation in the event that there is no extraordinary divergence between the levels of the person in question and the aggressor. The absence of vertical draw because of gravity, as if there should arise an occurrence of hanging, makes sense of this cross-over situation of ligature mark. The mark is oblique, like hanging, when the victim is a child or when the attacker is at a relatively higher level, like when the victim is lying down. A component of 'homicidal hanging' is present in many of these cases due to the fact that the victim's weight acts as the constricting force. Multiple slippage abrasions are the result of ligature material sliding upwards frequently as a result of the victim's physical struggle and pull. In contrast to hanging, there is no vertical dragging force, so the mark is usually at the level of the larynx or lowers down on the neck. Tissues beneath the ligature mark remain as a relatively bloodless field if the ligature is in place and the pressure is maintained. In many decomposed cases, therefore, ligature marks with in situ material demonstrate a high degree of preservation.

Linear scratches: The victim tries to grab the ligature and release the constriction, usually violently. Fingernail tips above the ligature mark typically result in multiple vertical, linear abrasions on the neck from these attempts. There may be dermal abrasions or contusions underneath these abrasions. The ligature typically slides upward, causing skin abrasions, and then settles higher, causing slippage abrasions. Although fingernail marks and finger poke contusions are less common than in manual strangulation, they can still occur in some instances. The possibility of ligature strangulation in conjunction with throttling should be taken into consideration in the event that fingertip contusions and nail marks are present.

The entire face shows extensive congestion, cyanosis (Figure 5.28), oedema, and multiple petechiae throughout the face and the portion of the neck above the compression level. These findings persist if the ligature compression is not relieved until post-mortem examination. Delivering the narrowing outcomes in the vanishing of the clog, oedema and cyanosis by and large, while the petechiae will generally continue. Fluid evaporation as a result of tissue hypoxia and subsequent membrane dysfunction leads to tissue oedema. Even after death,

the constriction continues to cause some oedema. In ligature strangulation, severe oedema of the peri-orbital region causes the eyes to bulge out.

Blood in the mouth and nostrils: Nasal, mouth, and ear bleeding can result from smaller blood vessels breaking apart as a result of intense congestion and increased pressure.

Other injuries: A normal adult's homicidal ligature strangulation exhibits multiple injuries from physical struggle and defence. In ligature strangulation, attempts to silence or smother the victim are not uncommon, and the lips exhibit the corresponding contusions and lacerations. When multiple attackers are involved, various restraint attempts result in abrasions and contusions commonly affecting the limbs.

Non-specific findings include the following: The genital organs are stuffed full. Urine, faeces, and sperm may be secreted uncontrollably. Some cases of ligature strangulation do not display any of the aforementioned signs of asphyxia, such as congestion, cyanosis, oedema, or petechiae. Cadaveric spasms of the hands may be observed because the victim's death may be in defence.

These cases may be explained by the vagal reflex mechanism's inhibition of the heart. If it is present, the ligature mark is typically situated at the C3 vertebral level over the anatomical position of the carotid bifurcation. Due to a constant, localized constricting force, suicide cases typically exhibit fewer muscle and dermal contusions. Usually, self-destruction cases show extreme facial blockage and oedema, which propose a slower beginning of death by complete venous hindrance and fractional blood vessel patency. In some cases, asphyxia may occur because the airway is completely blocked. Because the tongue's muscular belly and surfaces are in close contact with the hard palate and other bony structures like teeth, ligature strangulation can result in contusions and abrasions.

From a medico-legal perspective, internal neck injuries must be identified and interpreted during the internal examination. The best correlation results are obtained by layer-wise dissection of the neck in a field without blood. Dissection may reveal a dried, parchment-like ligature mark. Other than this, the most significant internal findings are as follows:

- **Perforation:** Without the dried, parchment-like appearance on dissection, the ligature mark may appear as a reddish dermal contusion. Multiple streaks of bleeding in the subcutaneous tissues immediately below the ligature mark are commonly regarded as a sign of vitality. In many instances, the platysma has layers of bleeding. There are also bleeding pockets between the torn fibres in the neck muscles. The absence of a lot of loose tissue and relatively thicker fascia on the posterior aspect of the neck explains why there are typically few dermal and muscular injuries there.
- **Laryngeal and thyroid-hyoid complex fracture:** Fractures typically manifest themselves on the superior horn of the thyroid in laryngeal cartilage. In many instances of ligature strangulation, the greater cornua of the hyoid bone are fractured, despite the fact that the hyoid bone is in a more secure and elevated position. In the majority of these instances, fractures are caused by forces transmitted through the thyrohyoid ligament. When the anteroposterior compression occurs directly over the larynx, the thyroid lamina rarely fractures. In this group, cricoid fractures are the least common. The larynx directly presses against the cervical vertebrae's

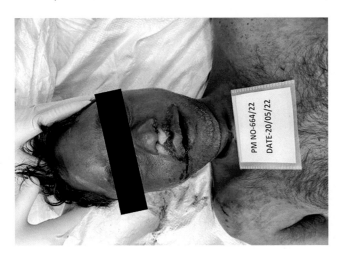

FIGURE 5.28: Shows congestion of the face and lips in a ligature strangulation case.

anterior aspect during neck compression. Manual strangulation must be considered in the event of a fracture of the thyroid laminae or cricoid. The autopsy surgeon may sometimes mistake the subluxation of the joint between the body and the greater horn of the hyoid bone for a fracture due to inexperience. Due to the changes in decomposition, subluxation of the joint frequently occurs in post-mortem examinations. Extraordinarily, the injury on the neck might be one-sided. In cases of ligature strangulation, multiple peri cartilaginous and submucosal haemorrhages are possible.

- **Petechiae:** It is possible to have sub-pleural petechiae on the surfaces of the lungs as well as subpericardial petechiae on the surfaces of the heart, but neither of these conditions is specific to ligature strangulation.
- **The tracheobronchial tree's froth:** The fluid leak from the alveolar capillaries and epithelial cells that causes pulmonary oedema as a result of parenchymal hypoxia and increased respiratory struggle can explain why the tracheobronchial tree frequently contains blood-stained froth.

Ligature strangulation does not reveal any particular findings in any of the other internal organs.

The majority of instances of ligature strangulation involve female victims and a sexually explicit motive. In many cases, injuries such as bite marks, fingernail abrasions, and genital and perineal injuries suggest sexual assault. Injuries caused by unsuccessful attempts, such as smothering, throttling, stabbing, etc., could be seen.

In cases of strangulation or hanging, a CT scan or X-ray can be used to look for larynx fractures and dislocations. It has the unique advantage of being able to record even the tiniest fractures, distinguish between ante-mortem fractures and dissection artefacts, and provide a permanent record for use in court in the future. Delicate tissues around the crack site will likewise show swelling much of the time, which could be deciphered during virtual examination practice and, furthermore, would be an indication of risk mortem break.

Some post-mortem findings may occasionally resemble ligature strangulation. A ligature mark can be created by superimposing patches of post-mortem staining over folds of skin on the anterior side of the neck. Sharp edges of these purplish sores raise questions about the use of ligature material. This artefact is frequently found in refrigerated bodies, particularly those of children or obese people with short necks. The soft tissues of the neck are compressed against clothing that is too tight around the neck as a result of decomposition swelling. In most of these instances, a pressure band is visible right after the tight cloth is removed. Inexperienced eyes frequently mistakenly interpret this artefact as a ligature mark. In disintegration, inside neck structures, particularly those with quick area to veins, show ruddy staining because of shades of haemolysis. These pigmentations that copy haemorrhages of muscles and other delicate tissues of the neck need a mindful assessment before understanding. Due to the post-mortem phenomenon of gravitational pooling of blood and fluids, the face exhibits features of congestion and oedema if the head is in the dependent position after death for a longer period of time, particularly when it is in a prone position. Multiple petechiae over the face are also present in these cases if they are severe, but this is a post-mortem phenomenon. Congestion, oedema, and strangulation-related petechiae should not be confused with these post-mortem artefacts.

If such haemorrhagic lividity develops in the necks of bodies that have ventral lividity as a result of lying down during and after death, substantial medical and legal issues may arise. This phenomenon may resemble strangulation-related internal injuries as well as soft tissue injuries (also known as 'pseudo-bruising'). When diagnosing strangulation and distinguishing between hanging and ligature strangulation in bodies with anterior neck lividity, caution must be exercised.

Ligature strangulation's medico-legal impact

Homicidal: It is an overall assumption in the general set of laws that strangulation is murderous in nature except if and until the opposite is demonstrated based on post-humous discoveries and fortuitous confirmations of legitimate examination. Due to the possibility that the assailants. Fingers may have come into contact with the victim's neck while applying the ligature; the majority of victims exhibit injuries during post-mortem examination, such as scratch abrasion. These crescent-shaped abrasions or nail marks are signs of murderous strangulation. In some cases, the victim also tries to defend against the assailant's tightening of the ligature around the neck. Nail marks on the victim's neck are a crucial medical and legal finding in determining whether or not a case of homicidal strangulation has been committed.

Drowning

When a corpse is recovered from a water collection or washed ashore, and the fatal event was not witnessed, it is typically difficult for any practising forensic surgeon to determine the cause and manner of death. This exercise is even harder because of the changes caused by putrefaction. Although it is one of the areas in which extensive research has been conducted, there are no established diagnostic criteria for drowning deaths that can be put into use. In the context of forensics, the term 'drowning' refers to asphyxiated death caused by the obstruction of respiratory orifices or air passages by water or any other fluid. Since inundation of the nose and mouth for an adequate period can cause demise, complete submersion of the individual isn't required for suffocating. Relatives' disbelief following a death in shallow water frequently leads to disputes and litigation, prompting a second investigation. 'Suffocation and death resulting from filling the lungs with water or other fluid so that gas exchange becomes impossible' is another definition of drowning. According to this point of view, deaths resulting from 'laryngeal spasm' and 'vagal mediated reflex cardiac inhibition-immersion syndrome' are not included in the definition of 'drowning'. As a result, numerous researchers have questioned the existence of 'dry lung' drowning deaths over the past few decades. Traditionally, the term 'near drowning' refers to both immediate deaths following an episode of submersion and non-fatal incidents. Additionally, these postponed deaths have forensic significance. Even though the majority of these cases provide a clear picture of what happened, many forensic surgeons still consider drowning to be an exclusionary diagnosis.

Incidence: During the summer months, it occurs more frequently in males than in females. The age group with the most involvement is young children and adults.

Pathophysiology of drowning

When someone falls into water, the force of the fall initially propels them to a predetermined depth. Alongside this energy, the explicit gravity of the body of that singular assumes a part in the span and profundity of submersion. The victim sinks until the medium's upwards thrust on the body and the momentum of the fall reaches equilibrium. Due to the person's natural buoyancy and the body movements of struggling, the individual then begins to return to the surface. The victim, who does not know how to swim, is struggling to stay afloat despite his desperate efforts. Typically they consume some water through aspiration and drinking. The breath-holding spell is followed by sinking, in which the victim vigorously tries to resurface with their mouth shut. When the victim is incapacitated by drugs, alcohol, or injury, or when there is a deliberate attempt to inhale water, as in some suicides, the period of breath-holding is often negligible. The victim's mental preparedness and the temperature of the drowning media are two additional factors that influence the duration of the breath-holding spell. The breath-holding stops when hypoxemia and hypercapnia reach a certain level, and the medium rushes into the respiratory tract. An unexpected flood of liquid into the aviation route quickly brings about laryngospasm and the conclusion of glottis as a defensive measure to limit unfamiliar material from arriving at the lower aviation routes. Hypoxia and hypercapnia are exacerbated throughout the entire breath-holding and laryngospasm episode, causing respiratory and metabolic acidosis. The fluid medium is inhaled into the alveoli by continuing respiratory movements, leaving the alveoli without enough air for effective gas exchange. Following a period of tonic–clonic seizures brought on by cerebral hypoxia, the victim eventually passes away.

Surfactant dysfunction, atelectasis, and decreased lung compliance are additional effects of aspirated hypotonic media. As a result of these changes in ventilation and perfusion, cerebral hypoxia and decreased oxygenation of haemoglobin occur. By drawing plasma fluid into the alveolar cavity in hypertonic media, pulmonary surfactants become dysfunctional, eventually leading to atelectasis and end-organ hypoxia. Transmembrane osmosis of the drowning medium was the cause of electrolyte imbalances in blood in earlier animal studies. This 'electrolyte imbalance – cardiac arrhythmia' theory is not supported by recent blood samples taken from immediate survivors of non-fatal submersion incidents. Electrolyte imbalance is not considered the primary cause of drowning deaths in many recent studies. The mechanism discussed in terminal stages is similar to that of the drowning of swimmers due to fatigue, and it generally takes longer. There is a possibility of an underlying natural disease, injury, or drug if a swimmer sinks and drowns.

- Case 1: A 13-year-old boy drowned in the Yamuna River, following which the body was recovered and was brought to AIIMS Hospital, New Delhi, by the police. A post-mortem examination was done in the Department of Forensic Medicine AIIMS, New Delhi. Examination showed a swollen face with fine lathery foam along with blood-tinged fluid oozing from the nostrils (Figure 5.29). Marbling and swelling were present over the chest, abdomen and, limbs (Figure 5.30). Examination of the brain showed dilated congested vessels in the brain along with decomposition changes (Figure 5.31). Examination of the sinus shows fluid in the frontal sinus (Figure 5.32)

and maxillary sinus (Figure 5.33). PMCT examination of the lungs shows a mosaic pattern (Figure 5.34) and PMCT also helps in ruling out other possible causes of death like trauma or assault.

- Case 2: 14-year-old boy with an alleged history of going for a swim with his friends in a river suddenly went missing in the water, and after a search operation, his body was found on the second day. He was taken to AIIMS Hospital, where he was declared dead on arrival. Postmortem examination was done in the Department of Forensic Medicine AIIMS, New Delhi. Examination showed a swollen face with fine lathery foam along with blood-tinged fluid oozing from the nostrils (Figure 5.35). Marbling and swelling were present over the chest, abdomen, and limbs (Figure 5.36). Examination of the hand of the deceased shows soddening, wrinkling, and bleaching along with mud particles (Figure 5.37). Examination of the brain showed dilated congested vessels in the brain along with decomposition changes (Figure 5.38). PMCT examination of the lungs shows a mosaic pattern (Figure 5.39), and PMCT also helps in ruling out other possible causes of death like trauma or assault. Examination of the trachea revealed mud particles (Figure 5.40), and stomach examination revealed mud particles (Figure 5.41).

Gagging

This is a form of asphyxia that occurs when a foreign object is forced into the mouth or throat. Most of the time, it is used to stop the victim from screaming for help, and the death that results is usually not intentional. As a result, the victim may also have their hands and legs tied in order to prevent them from removing the gag and escaping. However, the gagging may occasionally be homicidal, particularly in the cases of infants, people who are incapacitated by alcohol or drugs, the elderly, and the infirm, among other groups. Papers, ties, scarves, rolled-up clothing, and other items are common gagging materials. False dentures, on the other hand, are known to have been used as a gag. Some authors prefer to include gagging as a form of smothering or, in some cases, choking because they do not see it as a separate type of asphyxia. The gag not only prevents air from entering the body through the back of the throat but also blocks the mouth. Once in place, saliva, mucus, and oedema fluid quickly moisten the gag, and inspiratory gasps may further pull it in, eventually causing a complete obstruction. The pathophysiology of the gag is influenced by its size and position; The gag can either directly occlude the nasopharyngeal space, or it can cause the base of the tongue to move upwards, causing the occlusion. In order for gagging to result in death, the upper airways –the oral and nasal cavities that meet at the pharynx –must be completely blocked. As a result, the gag should extend all the way up to the pharynx's posterior wall to cause fatal obstruction; this is alluded to as finish choking. In complete gagging, on the other hand, the gag is pushed into the mouth but does not reach the posterior pharyngeal wall. Because the airway behind the gag is still open, death typically does not occur right away. However, the gag absorbs saliva and other secretions and swells over time, especially given that the majority of commonly used gags are made of fluid-absorbent materials. This causes a complete obstruction, which ultimately results in death. A person may tolerate the gag's volume obstruction of up to 100 millilitres,

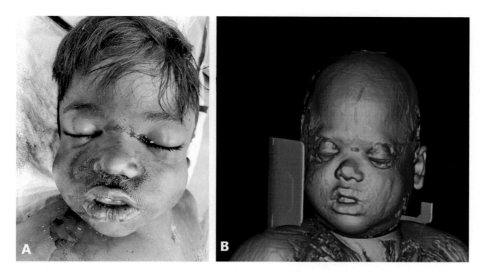

FIGURE 5.29: A: Shows swollen face with fine, blood-tinged, lathery foam around nostrils due to drowning during the external examination. B: shows swollen face in volume-rendering technique image using PMCT.

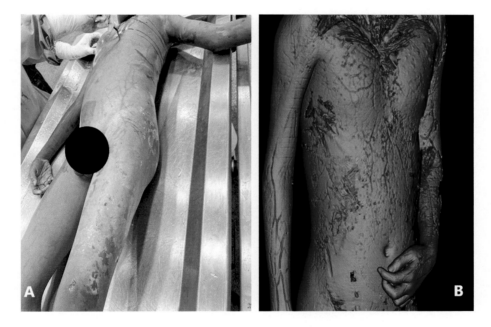

FIGURE 5.30: A: Shows marbling in external examination. B: Shows marbling in volume-rendering technique image using PMCT in drowning case.

but if it obstructs 150 to 200 millilitres or more, the internal airways will close, and asphyxia will occur due to respiratory obstruction. Pharyngeal obstruction is commonly the cause of gagging-related deaths. In addition, if the gag prevents nasal respiration more proximally, the fatal situation may develop earlier.

The results of the autopsy will vary depending on how hard it was for the victim to breathe, which could range from negligible to absent at times. If the material that caused the gagging has since been removed, blunt mucosal injuries, such as, individually or in a variety of combinations, bruising, abrasions, or cuts may be visible on the lips, soft palate, and/or over the pharynx. If adhesive tapes were used to hold it in place, injuries like peri-oral abrasions and gag marks on the angles of the

mouth and over the cheeks might also be visible. Smear samples taken from the oral cavity can be used to examine the gag for evidence of the textile material used for gagging. There may even be traces of the gag in the mouth and between the teeth. The presence of buccal epithelial cells can be checked to see if a particular material was used in the smothering or gagging process. If the material has come into contact with the mouth, it may be possible to observe the approximately 200–2000 buccal epithelial cells that are present in normal saliva per cubic millimetre. However, there are instances in which the gagging material is only attached to the face or occludes the oral cavity partially but is still sufficient to cause death. In such instances, the gag initially admits air and becomes impermeable as saliva is absorbed, expanding the material. The pressure effect and

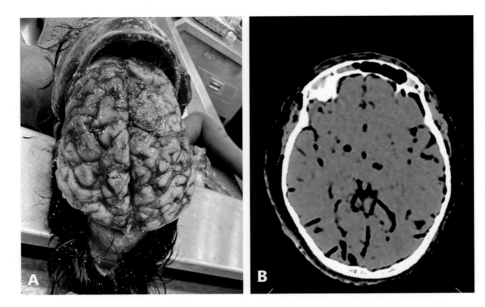

FIGURE 5.31: A: Shows dilatation of cerebral vessels and decomposition in the internal examination. B: Shows air inside brain vessels sign of decomposition in the axial section of the brain PMCT in a drowning case.

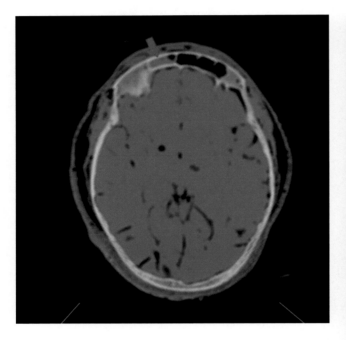

FIGURE 5.32: Shows air–fluid demarcation in the right frontal sinus in a case of drowning.

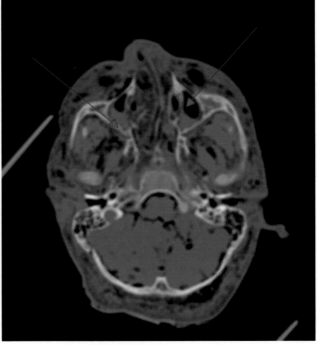

FIGURE 5.33: Shows air–fluid demarcation in both maxillary sinuses in a case of drowning (red arrows).

the onset of mucosal oedema further narrow the nasal cavity. Some authors have even described cases in which only adhesive tape was applied to the mouth, obstructing the nasal orifices, but oedema in the nasal mucosa developed, occluding the airways and resulting in asphyxia

Death by gagging

Gagging has also been documented in sexual asphyxia and suicides, typically in conjunction with other means of ensuring death. When someone dies from gagging, forensics usually look at the gagging material to see who owns it, especially if it

can not be traced back to the victim. They also look at the gag for volatile poisons, foreign DNA, and other things. If adhesive tape was used to fix the gag, even fingerprints could sometimes be recovered from the material. As a result, the material that is gagging should be removed carefully to avoid destroying any potential evidence. The method of death in most of these cases is asphyxia; however, at times, the demise might happen because of a reflex vagal hindrance.

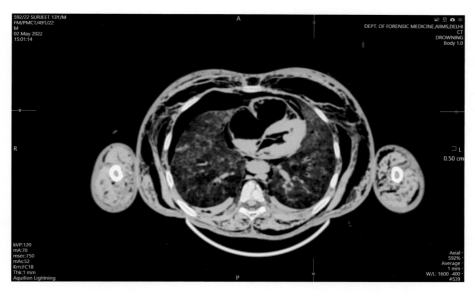

FIGURE 5.34: PMCT chest in lung window showing a mosaic pattern of lungs seen in PMCT in cases of drowning. There is pneumothorax due to the decomposition of gas.

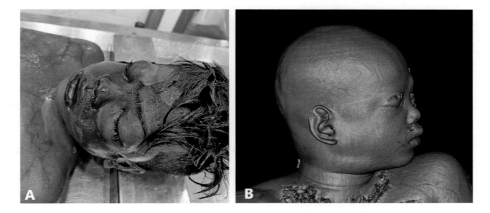

FIGURE 5.35: A: Shows a swollen face with skin peeling in a drowning case. B: Shows swollen face in PMCT volume-rendering technique image.

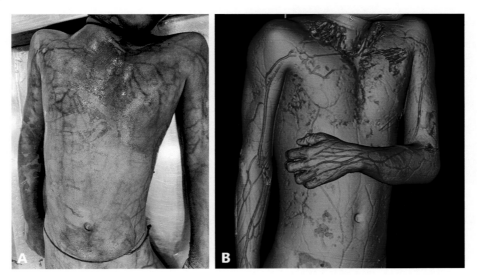

FIGURE 5.36: A: Shows marbling in external examination. B: Shows marbling in volume-rendering technique image using PMCT in a drowning case.

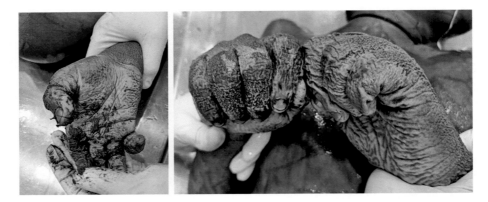

FIGURE 5.37: Shows soddening, wrinkling and bleaching suggestive of washerwoman's hands along with mud particles in the hand of the deceased.

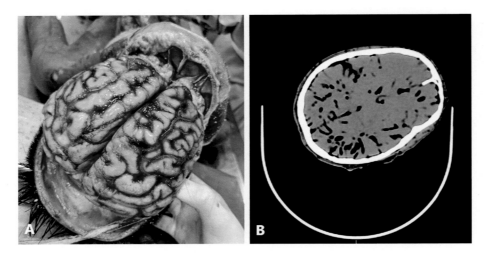

FIGURE 5.38: A: Shows dilatation of cerebral vessels and decomposition in internal examination B: Shows air inside brain vessels sign of decomposition in the axial section of the brain PMCT in drowning case.

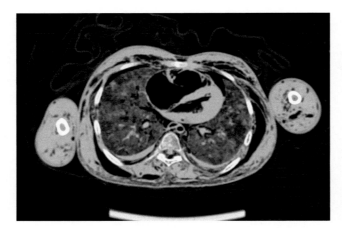

FIGURE 5.39: Mosaic pattern of the lung seen in case of drowning with air inside chambers of heart due to decomposition.

Post-mortem examination findings in gagging

During the autopsy, the typical signs of asphyxia, namely, cyanosis, petechial haemorrhages, congestion, especially over the face, and occasionally facial swelling, may be present. Most of the time, the petechial haemorrhages are small, dispersed, and present all over the face, including the sclera and conjunctiva. These are uncommon in young people, but they are more prevalent in elderly victims. However, these findings are not specific and can be observed in any kind of asphyxia as well as in other types of deaths that are not caused by asphyxia. On the assessment of the oral depression, the gag will, as a rule, be available inside, and in the wake of checking for the fulfilment of impediment, the choking material should be painstakingly taken out, inspected and depicted exhaustively and afterwards be sent for examination to the measurable science research facility. In addition, the oral cavity may display petechiae and mucosal congestion, typically over the soft palate. Injuries such as abrasions, contusions, and sometimes even mucosal lacerations and nasal bone fractures should be checked out in the oral and nasal cavities and orifices. These injuries may have occurred when the gag was forced into the mouth or was tightly applied to the face.

- The actual gag might be tracked down to the oral pit or in the oropharynx.
- Injuries to the lips, tongue, oral mucosa, hard and soft palates, or both.

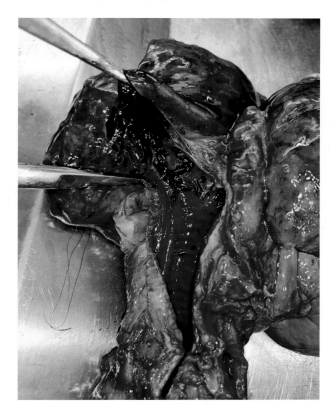

FIGURE 5.40: Shows mud particles inside the trachea and bronchi, evidence of ante-mortem drowning.

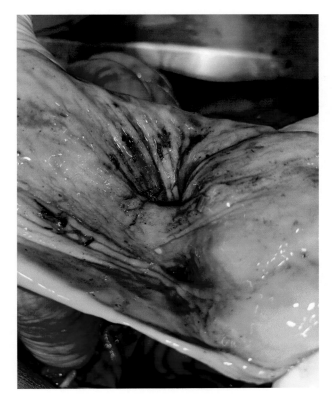

FIGURE 5.41: Shows mud particles inside the stomach wall, evidence of ante-mortem drowning.

- Injuries to the nose and peri-oral area.
- General and non-specific signs of asphyxia include facial congestion and bleeding over the base of the tongue and the auxiliary muscles of respiration.

An incision can be made from the corners of the mouth and transversely extending until the cheeks on both sides so as to expose the oral cavity and nasopharynx in order to determine the extent of gagging and thus help in confirming whether or not it is the cause of death if the gag is present in situ and is left as such during the autopsy after describing and photographically documenting the facial injuries.

Medico-legal significance

To prevent victims from shouting, rolled papers or rags are frequently thrown down their throats.

- Stuffing the gag in one's own mouth to stifle cries of pain and prevent any potential rescue attempts may be suicidal.
- This is evident in combined suicides, where it is one of the various methods employed.
- It is rarely associated with autoerotic asphyxia deaths.

Choking

The term 'choking' refers to the obstruction of the internal respiratory passages by a solid or semi-solid material, typically in the area between the pharynx and the bifurcation of the trachea. Pieces of food, such as meat lumps or corn kernels, false teeth, coins, buttons, marbles, haemorrhages, aspirated vomitus, etc., are common causes of this obstruction. Young children and the elderly typically fall victim to choking, with the extremes of age reporting the highest rates. In situations where a person dies while eating, choking should be considered one of the possible causes of death. A special mention must be made of food debris or bolus choking. It is possible for food to enter the larynx either by passing through the mouth during swallowing or by being regurgitated from the stomach. The airways may also contain food that has not been digested. Although it can occur at any age, this typically affects elderly or mentally ill individuals. When the food bolus is too big, it may get stuck in the posterior hypopharynx and block the oesophagus and glottis at the same time. In such situations, the person may only be able to exhale air and cannot inhale due to the obstruction. The bolus will typically become lodged in either the trachea or the bronchi if it is smaller and passes through the glottis. Choking is more likely if a person has any neurological problems like epilepsy, brain tumours, dementia, cerebrovascular accidents, multiple sclerosis, mental retardation, organic brain syndromes, cerebral palsy, or any condition that has anatomical and/or physiological problems swallowing like dysphagia, pharyngeal tumours, laryngeal cancers, or oesophagal dysmotility. The simultaneous presence of upper aerodigestive structural abnormalities like Treacher–Collins syndrome, which presents with cleft palate and mandibular hypoplasia, also further increases this risk. Infants and young children, especially those with only the incisors emerging and the molar teeth, which are the main masticators, are at an increased risk of asphyxial choking incidents. The contents of the stomach and any food particles found in the respiratory tract must be thoroughly examined in order to determine whether food entered the respiratory tract during swallowing or by regurgitation of stomach contents. Checking to see if the particles are partially digested food mixed with gastric acid is the first step in this process. This can be accomplished by analyzing the contents' pH, as gastric contents have an acidic pH, and respiratory secretions have a slightly basic pH. According to Knight's study from 1975, gastric contents were found in the airways in 25% of deaths from various causes. Gardner came to the conclusion that the presence of gastric contents in the bronchi or even the alveoli cannot be accepted as evidence of ante-mortem aspiration unless immediate post-mortem handling precautions are taken to prevent gastric contents from spilling into the lungs. He also demonstrated that even after somatic death has occurred, microscopic differentiation between post-mortem and ante-mortem aspirations is extremely challenging due to ongoing cellular reactions in the lungs (until molecular death).

The respiratory tract may contain food debris for the following reasons:

1. Food enters the larynx during gulping.
2. Regurgitation ante-mortem that occurred shortly before or a significant amount of time prior to death, resulting in aspiration pneumonia (Mendelson's syndrome).
3. Agonal reflux during the course of death or the peri-mortem period.
4. During the post-mortem period, the contents of the stomach were passively sucked into the airways.

Classification based on the place of the obstruction
- **Laryngeal obstruction (bolus death):** By striking the larynx, the bolus material that has become lodged in the throat initiates the reflex.
- **Tracheal and bronchial obstruction:** Aspiration of a substance from within the body or from a foreign body can result in asphyxiation due to obstruction of the trachea and/or bronchi.

Reasons for choking
1. By accident, foreign bodies:
   - Small toys, gags, meat, dummies, and other objects are placed by children and mentally ill people in their gullets.
   - Adults occasionally do the same thing by accident.
2. Food items: Several mechanisms can bring food into the larynx:
   - While passing through the mouth during the swallowing process: Because whole, undigested food can be found in the airways and there is usually a history of people dying while eating, this situation could be misinterpreted.
   - Inhaled through the stomach: This is most common in elderly, mentally ill, and drowsy individuals.
   - Cafe cardiomyopathy: Haugen came up with the term in 1963.
   - A 'cafe coronary' is a sudden, unplanned, accidental death caused by food bolus obstructing the upper airway and resulting in choking. In 1963, Dr. Roger Haugen, who worked for the Office of the Broward County Medical Examiner and investigated nine such cases over the course of several years, coined the term. The attending physicians had reported the cases as natural deaths, most likely caused by coronary artery disease. In his paper titled 'The Café Coronary Sudden Deaths in Restaurants', Dr. Haugen wrote about these. Haugen's initial observation was that the majority of victims were healthy, well-nourished individuals who died suddenly and

unexpectedly, typically at a party, without showing any of the 'classical' signs of asphyxia. Autopsies later revealed that boluses of food were lodged in the pharynx or larynx, despite the fact that such deaths had previously been misdiagnosed as occurring due to coronary heart disease. A contributory role has also been established due to the fact that alcohol has an inhibitory effect on the sympathetic nervous system and an activating effect on the parasympathetic nervous system.

Additionally, a sizeable portion of the subjects has been known to have consumed alcohol during the bolus event. He regarded these instances as accidental deaths caused by food obstruction of the airway. He also regarded alcoholism, poor dental health, and poor table manners as some of the factors that contributed to the victims' erratic deaths, most of whom were middle-aged or elderly. Despite the fact that alcohol suppresses the gag reflex, the original study found that it was a significant factor in the majority of cafe coronary deaths. However, more recent research has shown that many other drugs, including psychotropic, particularly sedatives and hypnotics, anticholinergics, and dopaminergic, also have a similar effect on increasing the risk of choking.

3. Exogenous:
   - Dental implants and bleeding: blood clots and frank haemorrhages following dental or ear, nose, and throat surgical procedures like a tonsillectomy, as well as false teeth (especially partial plates).
   - Short-term obstructions: lesions of the glottis or other parts of the larynx, like the swelling caused by acute hypersensitivity to a drug or other substances.
   - Lesions that obstruct the airway: oedema or inflammatory response to infectious conditions, such as diphtheria and haemophilic influenza epiglottis in children, are the most dangerous lesions of the glottis larynx or upper respiratory tract.
   - Stings from insects/short-term obstructive lesions: Oedema over the glottis or larynx may develop as a result of a sudden hypersensitivity reaction to insect stings.
   - Intentional inhalation: Intentional inhalation of hot gases and irritant vapours can also result in obstruction due to oedema of the upper respiratory tract.
4. Suicide:
   - There have been a few documented instances of suicide by choking deaths. The individual had pushed a closed pill bottle into his pharynx in one of these cases.
   - A case of self-inflicted gagging by a schizophrenic subject was documented by Forster and Schulz (1964), which evidently resulted in death by bolus mechanism choke.
5. Homicidal:
   - Older or disabled patients with dysphagia have been, on occasion, wrongly or hurriedly taken care of the ingested bolus of food, which has caused their demise. These might be regarded as careless actions that led to a person's death.
   - There have been reports of adult homicide by choking; according to Kurihara et al., one such death occurred in a mental hospital with tissue paper

inserted into the patient's mouth. In that case, further investigation revealed that his roommate, another male inpatient, choked him to death with a large amount of tissue paper after making him semi-conscious by applying pressure to his neck.

6. Sudden infant death syndrome (SIDS): Before considering an accident, it is necessary to rule out the possibility of negligence. In this scenario, parents may fall into the trap of thinking that their child's death was caused by their own carelessness, such as not noticing vomiting.

7. Dysphagia infant death syndrome (DIDS): 'The consistent intracranial venous hypertension resulting from feed aspiration, violent coughing, or a high intrathoracic pressure which is necessary for attempted cardiopulmonary resuscitation following apnea,' Talbert defined the term 'dysphagia infant death syndrome.'

Choking can be ruled out as a diagnosis during a sudden collapse if there is coughing, as coughing requires an open airway, which is not possible in the case of choking.

Presentation of choking

1. Difficulty or inability to speak.
2. Difficulty breathing.
3. Vomiting.
4. The person may begin to clutch the throat.
5. Cyanosis.
6. The person may become unconscious and die. However, choking can be ruled out as a diagnosis during a sudden collapse

Component of death in choking

The typically expected component of death in stifling cases is mechanical asphyxia as there is a check of the respiratory section, and there are clear elements of hypoxia with enormous unfamiliar bodies getting affected in the pharynx and shutting the larynx making demise due to hypoxic hypoxia or anoxic anoxia. Witnesses to choking deaths have frequently stated that the victim did not struggle a great deal while dying, and in some instances, the examination of the crime scene has implied that the victim died while sitting without any obvious signs of struggle. The obstructed food material may have stimulated tenso-receptors in the wall of the respiratory passage, resulting in increased vagal outflow to the medulla and these overlapping impulses to the cardiovascular and respiratory centres, causing bradycardia, dysrhythmia, and/or bronchospasm. This may explain the mode of death, which may be reflex neurogenic cardiovascular failure leading to cardiac arrest. Impacted foreign material at the bifurcation of the trachea, which causes irritation and parasympathetic cardiac inhibition, is another hypothesized mechanism. Laryngeal spasm has been observed to cause complete obstruction even when the food material only partially obstructs the laryngeal lumen due to its irritant nature.

Management of choking

1. A person should encourage a conscious victim of choking to cough.
2. If the victim is unable to cough, one should blow on the sternum or back to induce coughing and, by extension, the expulsion of the impacted foreign object.
3. Giving abdominal thrusts (the Heimlich manoeuvre) should be done if the victim is still not feeling better.

4. If the victim is obese or pregnant, chest thrusts should be administered because abdominal thrusts are ineffective.
5. Cardiopulmonary resuscitation (CPR) should be started if a person chokes unconscious.
6. If this fails, the foreign object should be removed from the hypopharynx using forceps or the middle and index fingers.

Finding seen in autopsy: Usually found lying with clothes stained with gastric contents or vomitus.

1. External results:
   1. Vomit stains the mouth and nostrils.
   2. Petechiae are extremely uncommon or absent entirely from the conjunctivae.
2. Findings from within:
   1. The laryngeal inlet will be obstructed by the thickening of the epiglottis and aryepiglottic folds as a result of inflammatory tissue and jelly-like oedema.
   2. All of the asphyxial signs, including congestion, cyanosis, and possibly even petechiae, may be present when the victim struggles to breathe for a significant amount of time in hypoxia caused by an obstruction of the airway.
   3. Death occurs abruptly in the majority of cases prior to any of the possible hypoxic manifestations. Neurogenic cardiac arrest, which may be accelerated by excess catecholamine release as a result of an adrenaline response, may be the cause of these fatalities.
   4. In some cafe coronary cases, cardiac arrest is clearly the cause of death. This is probably because stimulation of the laryngeal or pharyngeal mucosa over activates the parasympathetic nervous system, also known as the 'vasovagal reflex' or 'reflex cardiac inhibition'.

Radiological Finding

1. In an experiment that was carried out by Gardner, barium was placed in the stomachs of hospital patients who had recently passed away. X-rays were taken after the patients were first moved to the mortuary and then again when they were moved into the autopsy room. In the majority of the cases, barium was found in the tracheo-bronchial tree, demonstrating that the phenomenon of post-mortem over-spilling is very common.
2. The upper airway obstruction caused by food was the subject of a post-mortem CT study by Lino et al. They could confine the place of food definitively in every one of the 14 cases.

Medico-legal significance

1. Incidental stifling is the most widely recognized. Choking by suicide or homicide is extremely uncommon. Children under the age of five are most likely to choke accidentally. Due to aspiration of the gastric contents, elderly people, people under the influence of alcohol or drugs, and people with status epilepticus can also become choked. However, even after death, these might reach the bronchi. Microscopy will reveal alveoli filled with debris, red cells, macrophages, and a few polymorphs if the aspiration is ante-mortem and unexplained diffuse haemorrhagic areas in the dependent parts of the

lung, possibly with interstitial emphysema and signs of asphyxia will also typically be evident (Gardner, 1958).

2. Reflex cardiac inhibition may occasionally result in sudden death from food inhalation into the airway. These situations are referred to as "cafe coronaries" because they can be mistaken for coronary artery death.

Case 1: A middle-aged man was found in an unconscious state in a public place. He was taken to AIIMS Hospital, New Dehli, where he was declared as brought dead and subsequently referred to the Department of Forensic Medicine for autopsy. On PMCT the author found a solid particle blocking the airway (Figures 5.42 and 5.43), and on minimal invasive autopsy, neck dissection revealed the 'food particle', which was an intact *momo* (a kind of dumpling) in the trachea (Figure 5.44). The cause of death was given as asphyxia due to choking.

Case 2: A teenage girl with Down's syndrome was brought to the causality in an unconscious state, with an alleged history of collapse after having food at her residence. She was declared as brought dead and referred to the Department of Forensic Medicine, AIIMS, New Delhi, for post-mortem examination. On examination, PMCT showed some solid objects blocking the airway (Figures 5.45 and 5.46). Subsequently, a minimally invasive autopsy was done, and upon neck dissection food, a solid soya chunk was found in her tracheal opening (Figure 5.47). The cause of her death was given as asphyxia due to choking on food particles.

Aspiration

Aspiration can be caused by food entering the lungs while eating, or it can be caused by stomach contents moving back up the food tube (oesophagus) and spilling over into the person's airway. Most people cough violently when they aspirate, but some people do not. Their cough reflex has been weakened. When a person aspirates but does not cough, this is called a silent aspiration. Choking refers to an obstruction or blockage of the airway of a person, which interferes with breathing. This is an emergency if the person is unable to clear their airway on their own by coughing. The aspiration of food fragments

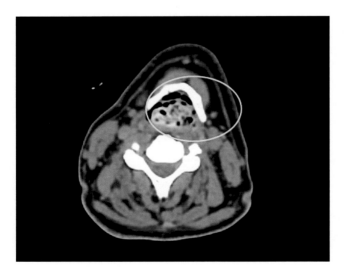

FIGURE 5.42: Shows some solid object obstructing the airway in the axial section of neck PMCT in soft tissue window (yellow circle).

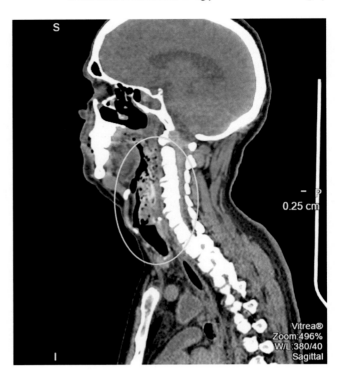

FIGURE 5.43: Shows some solid object obstructing the airway in the sagittal section of neck PMCT in soft tissue window (yellow circle).

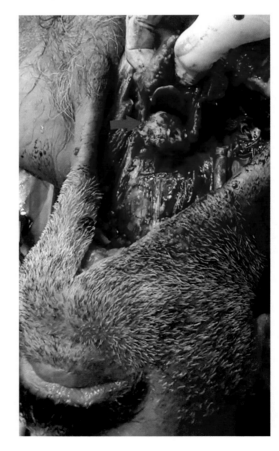

FIGURE 5.44: Autopsy examination shows an intact momo in the tracheal opening in a case of choking.

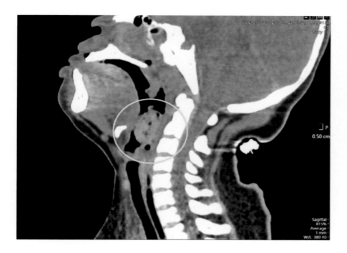

FIGURE 5.45: Shows a solid object obstructing the airway in the sagittal section of neck PMCT in soft tissue window (yellow circle).

into the distal airways/alveolar ducts is another cause of sudden death. Notably, aspiration is either unsuspected before autopsy or misdiagnosed clinically as acute myocardial infarction or cardiac arrest. Aspiration, at times, may not cause sudden death but may lead to pulmonary pathologies such as partial airway obstruction, pneumonia, chemical pneumonitis, or acute respiratory distress syndrome, which causes morbidity or mortality. The final outcome after aspiration of stomach contents depends on multiple factors like volume of content aspirated, chemical composition of the aspirant, particle size, presence of infectious agents in the aspirated material, health condition of the individual, conscious state of the person to evoke a protective cough reflex, presence of any intoxicating agents, under the influence of drug or anaesthesia, etc. These foreign particles can be clearly seen on PMCT as a foreign body obstructing the airway, the same can be confirmed on traditional autopsy, but there is a high chance of foreign particles getting dislodged or moved or leaked out due to the process of handling and dissection.

Risk factors for aspiration

1. **Age:** all age groups are susceptible, but young children and elderly people are at higher risk.
2. **Gender:** It equally affects both genders.
3. **Cognitive impairment:** Due to intoxication, developmental delay, or any other cognitive impairment disorders.
4. **Central neurologic impairment:** Due to stroke, seizure, raised intracranial pressure, intracranial haemorrhages, tumours, etc.
5. **Focal neurologic impairment:** Due to injury of nerves involved in deglutition, pharyngeal muscle injury, neuromuscular disorders, oesophagal dysmotility, muscular dystrophies, etc.
6. **Pulmonary diseases:** Those requiring mechanical ventilation, diseases causing poor cough reflex, or poor expiratory effort.
7. **Mechanical causes:** Trauma to the neck, base of the skull or due to the presence of an NG tube, tracheostomy, iatrogenic procedures like endoscopy, bronchoscopy, etc.
8. **Miscellaneous causes:** Poisoning by CNS depressants, overuse of proton pump inhibitors, high volume vomiting, poisoning by hydrocarbons, and position changes can cause aspiration even in healthy people.

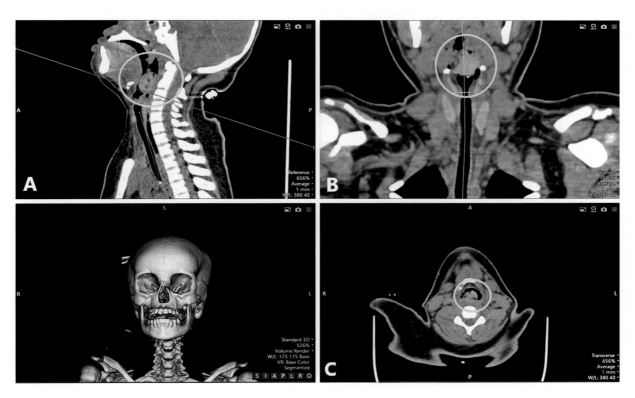

FIGURE 5.46: Shows airway obstruction by some solid object in A: Sagittal section, B: Coronal section, and C: Axial section of PMCT.

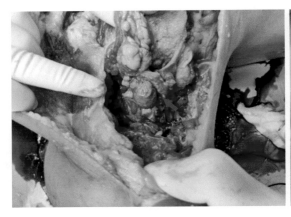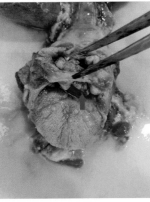

FIGURE 5.47:   Shows an intact soybean chunk in the tracheal opening, causing choking.

Pathophysiology of aspiration

A litmus test can be performed to differentiate whether the aspirate is from the stomach or from swallowing; gastric contents are acidic in nature. Aspiration of gastric contents, which are acidic in nature, into the respiratory tract can lead to chemical pneumonitis. Commonly due to the position of the right bronchus, which is less acutely angled at the carina, aspirate enters it and affects the right lower lobe. When the volume of aspirate is large, it can involve one or both sides. The position of the individual at the time of aspiration also can determine the lobe that gets affected. In cases where the aspirate is large enough to block the airway completely, it can cause immediate death. Such cases need immediate clearance of the airway;

even then, the acidic nature of the aspirate results in immediate damage to the mucosa of the respiratory tract. The pH of the aspirate is also an important determinant of the outcome, and any pH below 2.5 is highly fatal.

Case 1: A middle-aged man brought to causality with a history of brick fell over his face and collapsed suddenly. He was declared brought dead and referred to the Department of Forensic Medicine, AIIMS, New Delhi, for post-mortem examination. The author observed fractures of the mandible and pneumonitis in the lungs in post-mortem computed tomography (Figures 5.48–5.50). Subsequently, a traditional autopsy was done, and the aspiration of blood was found due to trauma over the face, which led to death.

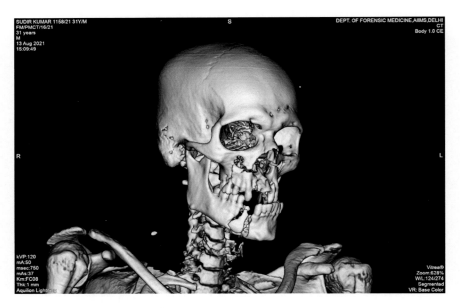

FIGURE 5.48:   Fracture of the mandible seen in the case.

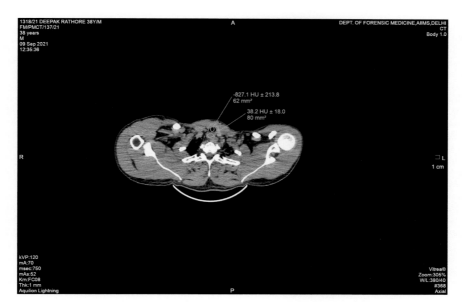

FIGURE 5.49: Shows occluded trachea due to aspiration.

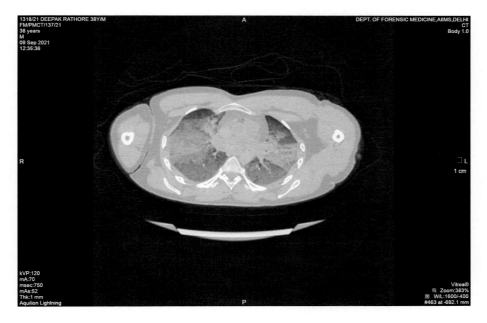

FIGURE 5.50: Shows ground glass opacities in both lungs due to aspiration pneumonitis.

Bibliography

Advenier AS, De La Grandmaison GL, Cavard S, Pyatigorskaya N, Malicier D, Charlier P. Laryngeal anomalies: Pitfalls in adult forensic autopsies. *Med Sci Law.* 2014 January;54(1):1–7.

Ahmad M, Hossain MZ. Hanging as a method of suicide: Retrospective analysis of postmortem cases. *J. Armed Forces Med. Coll. Bangladesh.* 2010 December;6(2): 37–39.

Ali E, Maksud M, Zubyra SJ, Hossain MS, Debnath PR, Alam A, Chakrabarty PK. Suicide by hanging: A study of 334 cases. *Bangladesh Med J.* 2014 May;43(2):90–93.

Ambade VN, Tumram N, Meshram S, Borkar J. Ligature material in hanging deaths: The neglected area in forensic examination. *Egypt J Forensic Sci.* 2015;5(3):109–113.

Badkur DS, Yadav J, Arora A, Bajpayee R, Dubey BP. Nomenclature for knot position in hanging: A study of 200 cases. *J Indian Acad Forensic Med.* 2012 January–March;34(1):34–36. ISSN 0971-0973 36.

Bamousa MS, AL-Madani OM, Alsoway KS, Madadin MS, Mashhour MM, Aldossary M, Kharoshah M. Importance of tissue biopsy in suicidal hanging deaths. *Egyptian Journal of Forensic Sciences.* 2015;5:140–143.

Behera C, Chauhan M, Sikary AK. Body coloration artifacts encountered at medicolegal autopsy in India. *Am J Forensic Med Pathol.* 2019 June;40(2):129–135.

Ben Dhiab M, Jdidi M, Nouma Y, Ben Mansour N, Belhadj M, Souguir MK. Accidental hanging: A report of four cases and review of the literature. *J Clin Pathol Forensic Med*. 2014 February;5(1):1–5.

Bhosle SH, Batra AK, Kuchewar SV. Violent asphyxial death due to hanging: A prospective study. *J Forensic Med, Sci and Law*. 2014 January–June;23(1):1–8.

Bohnert M, Faller-Marquardt M, Lutz S, Amberg R, Weisser H-J, Pollak S. Transfer of biological traces in cases of hanging and ligature strangulation. *Forensic Sci Int*. 2001;116:107–115.

Bohnert M, Pollak S. Complex suicides—A review of the literature. *Archiv fur Kriminologie*. 2004;213(5–6):138–153.

Bolliger SA, Thali MJ. Imaging and virtual autopsy: Looking back and forward. *Phil Trans R Soc B*. 2015 August 5;370(1674):20140253. http://dx.doi.org/10.1098/rstb.2014.0253

Bowen D. Hanging – a review. *Forensic Sci Int*. 1982;20:247–249.

Carlson BM. *Human embryology and developmental biology*, 3rd ed. New York: Elsevier, 2004, pp. 317–349.

Chatzaraki V, Heimer J, Thali M, Dally A, Schweitzer W. Role of PMCT as a triage tool between external inspection and full autopsy – Case series and review. *J Forensic Radiol Imaging*. 2018 December;15:26–38. http://dx.doi.org/10.1016/j.jofri.2018.10.002

Christe A, Flach P, Ross S, Spendlove D, Bolliger S, Vock P, et al. Clinical radiology and postmortem imaging (Virtopsy) are not the same: Specific and unspecific postmortem signs. *Legal Med*. 2010 September;12(5):215–222. http://dx.doi.org/10.1016/j.legalmed.2010.05.005

Cirielli V, Cima L, Bortolotti F, Narayanasamy M, Scarpelli M, Danzi O, et al. Virtual autopsy as a screening test before traditional autopsy: The verona experience on 25 Cases. *J Pathol Inform*. 2018;9(1):28. http://dx.doi.org/10.4103/jpi.jpi_23_18

Clement R, Guay J-P, Redpath M, Sauvageau A. Petechiae in hanging: A retrospective study of contributing variables. *Am J Forensic Med Pathol*. 2011;32:378–382.

Clément R, Redpath M, Sauvageau A. Mechanism of death in hanging: A historical review of the evolution of pathophysiological hypotheses: Mechanism of death in hanging. *J Forensic Sci*. 2010 September;55(5):1268–1271.

Dayapala A, Samarasekera A, Jayasena A. An uncommon delayed sequela after pressure on the neck: An autopsy case report. *Am J Forensic Med Pathol*. 2012 March;33(1):80–82.

de Bakker BS, de Bakker HM, Soerdjbalie-Maikoe V, Dikkers FG. The development of the human hyoid-larynx complex revisited. *Laryngoscope*. 2018 Aug;128(8):1829–1834.

de Bakker BS, de Bakker HM, Soerdjbalie-Maikoe V, Dikkers FG. Variants of the hyoid-larynx complex, with implications for forensic science and consequence for the diagnosis of Eagle's syndrome. *Sci Rep*. 2019 November 4;9(1):15950.

Delbreila A, Gambierc A, Lefrancqd T, Tarisa M, SaintMartinc P, Sapaneta M. Pathology diagnosis of an atypical thyroid cartilage lesion. *Legal Med*. 2019;36:47–49.

Dirnhofer R, Jackowski C, Vock P, Potter K, Thali MJ. VIRTOPSY: Minimally Invasive, Imaging-guided Virtual Autopsy. *RadioGraphics*. 2006 September;26(5):1305–1333. http://dx.doi.org/10.1148/rg.265065001

Fisher E, Austin D, Werner HM, Chuang YJ, Bersu E, Vorperian HK. Hyoid bone fusion and bone density across the lifespan: Prediction of age and sex. *Forensic Science, Medicine and Pathology*. 2016 June;12(2):146–157.

Gadkaree SK, Hyppolite CG, Harun A, Sobel RH, Kim Y. An unusual case of bony styloid processes that extend to the hyoid bone. *Case Rep Otolaryngol*. 2015 June 22:780870.

Garetier M, Deloire L, Dédouit F, Dumousset E, Saccardy C, Ben Salem D. Postmortem computed tomography findings in suicide victims. *Diagn Interv Imaging*. 2017 February;98(2):101–112. http://dx.doi.org/10.1016/j.diii.2016.06.023

Gnanadev R, Iwanaga J, Loukas M, Tubbs RS. An unusual finding of the hyoid bone. *Cureus*. 2018 September;10(9):e3365.

Hayakawa M, Yamamoto S, Motani H, Yajima D, Sato Y, Iwase H. Does imaging technology overcome problems of conventional postmortem examination? *Int J Legal Med*. 2005 October 12;120(1):24–26. http://dx.doi.org/10.1007/s00414-005-0038-x

Howard RS, Holmes PA. Koutroumanidis M. Hypoxicischaemic brain injury. *Pract Neurol*. 2011;11:4–18.

Inanir NT, Bülent ER, Çetin S, Filiz ER, Gündoğmuş ÜN. Anatomical variation of hyoid bone: A case report. *Maedica*. 2014 September;9(3):272.

Ishida M, Gonoi W, Hagiwara K, Okuma H, Shintani Y, Abe H, et al. Fluid in the airway of nontraumatic death on postmortem computed tomography. *Am J Forensic Med Pathol*. 2014 June;35(2):113–117. http://dx.doi.org/10.1097/PAF.0000000000000083

Ito K, Ando S, Akiba N, Watanabe Y, Okuyama Y, Moriguchi H, Yoshikawa K, Takahashi T, Shimada M. Morphological study of the human hyoid bone with three-dimensional CT images -Gender difference and age-related changes. *Okajimas Folia Anat Jpn*. 2012;89(3):83–92.

Jian J, Wan L, Shao Y, Zou D, Huang P, Wang Z, et al. Postmortem chest computed tomography for the diagnosis of drowning: A feasibility study. *Forensic Sci Res*. 2019 February 23;6(2):152–158. http://dx.doi.org/10.1080/20961790.2018.1557386

Kanchan T, Atreya A, Raghavendra Babu YP, Bakkannavar SM. Putrefaction, hanging and ligature mark. *Int J AJ Inst Med Sci*. 2014 November;3(2).112–117.

Kanchan T, Menon A, Menezes RG. Methods of choice in completed suicides: Gender differences and review of literature. *J Forensic Sci*. 2009;54(4):938–942.

Kasahara S, Makino Y, Hayakawa M, Yajima D, Ito H, Iwase H. Diagnosable and non-diagnosable causes of death by postmortem computed tomography: A review of 339 forensic cases. *Legal Med*. 2012 September;14(5):239–245. http://dx.doi.org/10.1016/j.legalmed.2012.03.007

Kempter M, Ross S, Spendlove D, Flach PM, Preiss U, Thali MJ, et al. Postmortem imaging of laryngohyoid fractures in strangulation incidents: First results. *Legal Med*. 2009 November;11(6):267–271. http://dx.doi.org/10.1016/j.legalmed.2009.07.005

Khan MK, Hanif SA. Accidental hanging on loaded sugarcane trolley – A case report. *Egypt J Forensic Sci*. 2012;2:139–141.

Klovning JJ, Yursik BK. A nearly circumferential hyoid bone. *Am J Otolaryngol*. 2007;28(3):194–195.

Kodikara S, Alagiyawanna R. Accidental hanging by a T shirt collar in a man with morphine intoxication: An unusual case. *Am J Forensic Med Pathol*. 2011 September;32(3):260–262.

Kodikara S. Attempted suicidal hanging: An uncomplicated recovery. *Am J Forensic Med Pathol*. 2012 December;33(4):317–318.

Koebke J. Some observations on the development of the human hyoid bone. *Anatomy and Embryology*. 1978 January 1;153(3):279–286.

Krywanczyk A, Shapiro S. A retrospective study of blade wound characteristics in suicide and homicide. *Am J Forensic Med Pathol*. 2015 December;36 (4):305–310.

Leth P, Vesterby A. Homicidal hanging masquerading as suicide. *Forensic Sci Int*. 1997 February 7;85(1):68–70.

Lino M, O'Donnell C. Postmortem computed tomography findings of upper airway obstruction by food. *J Forensic Sci*. 2010 Sep;55(5):1251–1258.

Lupascu C. Letter to the editor/legal. *Medicine*. 2003;5:110–111.

Maiese A, Gitto L, dell'Aquila M, Bolino G. When the hidden features become evident: The usefulness of PMCT in a strangulation-related death. *Legal Med*. 2014 November;16(6):364–366. http://dx.doi.org/10.1016/j.legalmed.2014.06.009

Makino Y, Yokota H, Nakatani E, Yajima D, Inokuchi G, Motomura A, et al. Differences between postmortem CT and autopsy in death investigation of cervical spine injuries. *Forensic Sci Int*. 2017 December;281:44–51. http://dx.doi.org/10.1016/j.forsciint.2017.10.029

Marcus P, Alcabes P. Characteristics of suicides by inmates in an urban jail. *Hosp Community Psychiatry*. 1993;44(3):256–261.

Matsumoto S, Iwadate K, Aoyagi M, Ochiai E, Ozawa M, Asakura K. An experimental study on the macroscopic findings of ligature marks using a murine model. *Am J Forensic Med Pathol*. 2013 March;34(1):72–74.

McClane GE, et al. A review of 300 attempted strangulation cases part II: clinical evaluation of the surviving victim. *J Emerg Med*. 2001;21(3):311–5.

Mugadlimath AB, Sane MR, Kallur SM, Patil MN. Survival of a victim of Isadora Duncan syndrome: A case report. *Med Sci Law.* 2013;53(4):219–222.

Nanci A. *Ten Cate's oral histology: Development, structure, and function*, 7th ed. St. Louis, MO: Mosby Elsevier, 2008.

Nouma Y, Ben Ammar W, Bardaa S, Hammami Z, Maatoug S. Accidental hanging among children and adults: A report of two cases and review of the literature. *Egypt J Forensic Sci.* 2016;6:310–314.

Parsons FG. The topography and morphology of the human hyoid bone. *J Anat Physiol.* 1909 July;43(Pt 4):279.

Patel JB, Bambhaniya AB, Chaudhari KR, Upadhyay MC. Study of death due to compression of neck by ligature. *Int J Health Sci Res.* 2015 August;5(8): 76–81.

Pathak AK, Sinha US. A study of findings in asphyxial deaths due to external compression of neck. *Sch J Appl Med Sci.* 2020 February;8(2):481–485.

Pinto DC. The laryngohyoid complex in medicolegaldeath investigations. *Acad Forensic Pathol.* 2016;6(3):486–498.

Porrath S. Roentgenologic considerations of the hyoid apparatus. *Am J Roentgenol.* 1969 January;105(1):63–73.

Radunovic M, Vukcevic B, Radojevic N. Asymmetry of the greater cornua of the hyoid bone and the superior thyroid cornua: A case report. *Surg Radiol Anat.* 2018 Aug;40(8):959–961.

Rao D. An autopsy study of death due to suicidal hanging – 264 cases. *Egypt J Forensic Sci.* 2016;6:248–254.

Rao VJ, Wetli CV. The forensic significance of conjunctival petechiae. *Am J Forensic Med Pathol.* 1988 March;9(1):32–34.

Roberts IS, Benamore RE, Benbow EW, Lee SH, Harris JN, Jackson A, Mallett S, Patankar T, Peebles C, Roobottom C, Traill ZC. Post-mortem imaging as an alternative to autopsy in the diagnosis of adult deaths: A validation study. *Lancet.* 2012 January 14;379(9811):136–142. http://dx.doi.org/10.1016/S0140-6736(11)61483-9. Epub 2011 Nov 21. PMID: 22112684; PMCID: PMC3262166.

Russo MC, Antonietti A, Farina D, Verzeletti A. Complete decapitation in suicidal hanging – A case report and a review of the literature. *Forensic Sci Med Pathol.* 2020;16:325–329.

Saternus KS, Maxeiner H, Kernbach-Wighton G, Koebke J. Traumatology of the superior thyroid horns in suicidal hanging – An injury analysis. *Legal Med.* 2013;15:134–139.

Sauvageau A, Godin A, Desnoyers S, Kremer C. Six-year retrospective study of suicidal hangings: Determination of the pattern of limb lesions induced by body responses to asphyxia by hanging. *J Forensic Sci.* 2009;54(5):1089–1092.

Sauvageau A, LaHarpe R, King D, Dowling G, Andrews S, Kelly S, Ambrosi C, Guay JP, Geberth VJ. Agonal sequences in 14 filmed hangings with comments on the role of the type of suspension, ischemic habituation, and ethanol intoxication on the timing of agonal responses. *Am J Forensic Med Pathol.* 2011 June;32(2):104–107.

Sharma BR, Sharma BR, Harish D, Singh VP, Singh P. Ligature mark on neck: How informative? *J Indian Acad Forensic Med.* 2005;27(1):10–15.

Shiotani S, Kohno M, Ohashi N, Yamazaki K, Nakayama H, Watanabe K, Oyake Y, Itai Y. Non-traumatic postmortem computed tomographic (PMCT) findings of the lung. *Forensic Sci Int.* 2004 January 6;139(1):39–48. http://dx.doi.org/10.1016/j.forsciint.2003.09.016. PMID: 14687772

Simonsen J. Patho-anatomic findings in neck structures in asphyxiation due to hanging. *Forensic Sci Int.* 1988;38:83–91.

Singh V, Priya K, Bhagol A, Kirti S, Thepra M. Clicking hyoid: A rare case report and review. *National J Maxillofacial Sur.* 2015 July;6(2):247.

Sittel C, Brochhagen HG, Eckel HE, Michel O. Hyoid bone malformation confirmed by 3-dimensional computed tomography. *Arch Otolaryngol Head Neck Surg.* 1998 July 1;124(7):799–801.

Standring S. *Gray's anatomy the anatomical basis of clinical practice*, 41st ed. 2016. Philadelphia: Elsevier, pp. 442–474.

Suárez-Peñaranda JM, Alvarez T, Miguéns X, RodríguezCalvo MS, De Abajo BL, Cortesão M, Cordeiro C, Vieira DN, Munoz JI. Characterization of lesions in hanging deaths. *J Forensic Sci.* 2008 May;53(3):720–723.

Talbert DG. Dysphagia as a risk factor for sudden unexplained death in infancy. Med Hypotheses. 2006;67(4):786–791.

Talukder MA, Mansur MA, Kadir MM. Incidence of typical and atypical hanging among 66 hanging cases. *Mymensingh Med J.* 2008 July;17(2):149–151.

Thali MJ, Dirnhofer R, Vock P. *The Virtopsy Approach 3D optical and radiological scanning and reconstruction in forensic medicine*, 1st ed. Boca Raton. 2009. 261–263.

Tumram NK, Ambade VN, Bardale RV, Dixit PG. Injuries over neck in hanging death and its relation with ligature material: Is it vital? *J Forensic Leg Med.* 2014;22:80–83.

Tumram NK, et al. Injuries over neck in hanging deaths and its relation with ligature material: Is it vital? *J Forensic Leg Med.* 2014;22:80–83.

Warren S. Strangulation: A full spectrum of blunt neck trauma. *Ann Otol Rhinol Laryngol.* 1985;94:542–546.

Weustink AC, Hunink MGM, van Dijke CF, Renken NS, Krestin GP, Oosterhuis JW. Minimally invasive autopsy: An alternative to conventional autopsy? *Radiology.* 2009 March;250(3):897–904. http://dx.doi.org/10.1148/radiol.2503080421

6 TRAUMA TO THE LIMBS

Trauma to the limbs by an external unbalanced mechanical force occurring unintentionally or intentionally is termed a limb injury. Damage to the tissues occurs when the physiological tolerance of the tissues is exceeded. Limb injuries range from any minor injury like abrasions, bruises, etc., to major injuries involving the limbs like broken bones, dislocations, or crush injuries, and this could involve the whole limbs or just the arms, legs, fingers, or even just the toes. Limb injuries can be broadly categorized into upper limb injuries and lower limb injuries. Upper limb injuries usually constitute a major source of cases seen in casualty and mortuary, and it commonly occurs due to road traffic accidents, workplace injuries, etc. Lower limb injuries are very common among the athletic group, such as road traffic accidents and falls from height cases. The National Crime Records Bureau (NCRB) of the government of India collects national data on all crimes, and one such important aspect recorded is injury-related information. The study of these data over the years shows the fact that due to factors like rapid urbanization and motorization in India, the cases of injury to limbs have increased.

Anatomy of the limbs

Upper limbs

Bone and joints: The bones of the upper limb consist of the clavicle, scapula, humerus, radius, ulna, and bones of the hand, i.e., the carpals, metacarpals, and phalanges. The joint includes the shoulder, elbow, wrist, and interphalangeal joint. The glenohumeral joint or shoulder joint (Figure 6.1), which is a ball-and-socket type of joint, allows movement of the upper limb in all three orthogonal planes, while the elbow joint (Figure 6.1), which is a hinge joint restricts movement to a single plane. However, the wrist joint (Figure 6.1) is a gliding joint, which allows movement of the hand in both anteroposterior and lateral to medial directions.

Clavicle

The clavicle is the first bone to appear in intrauterine life at the gestational age of five to six weeks, with two primary centres which later fuse with each other at the junction of the middle and lateral third after one and a half months of a full-term birth. The clavicle lies almost horizontally at the root of the neck and is subcutaneous throughout its course; the medial two-thirds are convex anteriorly, and the lateral third is convex posteriorly (Figure 6.2). The medial end of the bone articulates with the manubrium portion of the sternum near the sternal notch and forms the sternoclavicular joint which is a synovial sellar joint and is the only skeletal articulation between the upper limb skeleton and the axial skeleton. The lateral end, also called the acromial end, articulates with the acromial process of the scapula to form the acromioclavicular joint, a synovial plane joint (Figure 6.3). The junction between the medial two-thirds and lateral third of the clavicle is the weakest portion and is the most common site of fracture. A shorter, thinner, less curved, and smoother clavicle is characteristic of the female clavicle. The mid-shaft circumference is one of the most reliable single indicators to determine the sex from the clavicle; however, a combination of weight and length gives a better result.

Scapula

The scapula, also referred to as the shoulder blade, is a large flat triangular bone situated at the posterolateral aspect of the chest wall and also connects the clavicle with the humerus. The scapula has two surfaces, namely costal and dorsal surface; it has three borders, namely medial, lateral and superior border (Figure 6.4); it has three angles, namely inferior, superior, and lateral angles; and it has four processes, namely spine, acromion, coracoid, and glenoid processes. The lateral angle modifies to form a glenoid cavity which articulates with the head of the humerus to form the shoulder joint, which allows the arm to have a wide range of movements and to move along a three-dimensional axis.

Humerus (Figure 6.5)

The humerus is the largest bone of the upper limb. It has two ends and a shaft. The upper or proximal end consists of the head, anatomical neck, and greater and lesser tubercle. The head of the humerus articulates with the glenoid cavity of the scapula and faces medially, backwards, and upwards in its resting anatomical position. The shaft is cylindrical in the upper half and is compressed anteroposteriorly in its lower half, having three borders and three surfaces. The lower or distal end is called 'condylar', which has articular and non-articular parts. The articular part consists of the capitulum laterally and trochlea medially, which articulates with the forearm bones. The non-articular parts are medial and lateral epicondyles which are seen as the eminences of the elbow joint. The lower end of the humerus also consists of the olecranon, coronoid, and radial fossa, which articulates with the corresponding process of the forearm bones. The elbow joint is a complex synovial joint as a result of a combination of the humeroulnar and humeroradial joints. The complexity increases due to its continuity with the superior radioulnar joint.

Radius (Figure 6.6A)

The radius is a forearm bone anatomically situated on the lateral side of the forearm. It has proximal and distal ends and a shaft. The proximal end is expanded to contain the head, neck, and tuberosity, which articulates superiorly with the capitulum of the humerus and medially with the radial notch of the ulna, respectively. The shaft is convex laterally and triangular in cross-section with one sharp edge towards the medial aspect, making an interosseous border except for the proximal and distal medial surface. The anterior and posterior border of the shaft of the radius is situated over the lateral side, which is rounded and indefinite. It has three surfaces, namely the anterior surface between the interosseous and anterior border, the posterior surface between the interosseous and posterior border, and the lateral surface between the anterior and posterior border. The distal end is the most expanded part of the radius and is quadrangular in cross-section. A projection from the lateral surface of the distal end forms a styloid process. The inferior surface articulates with the carpal bones, and the medial surface of the distal end articulates with the head of the ulna.

Ulna (Figure 6.6B)

Anatomically, the ulna is situated on the medial side of the forearm. Like the radius, it has proximal and distal ends and a shaft. The proximal end contains two processes, namely the

DOI: 10.1201/9781003383703-6

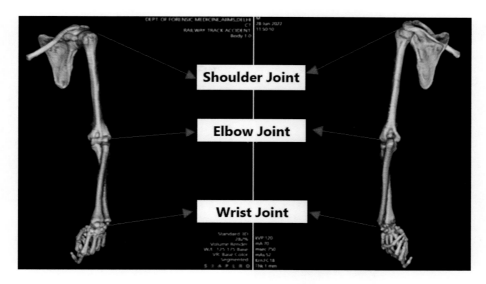

FIGURE 6.1: Volume rendering 3D image of the upper limb showing the shoulder, elbow and wrist joints.

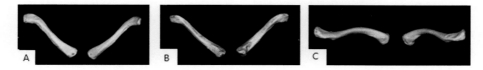

FIGURE 6.2: Volume rendering 3D image of clavicle bone A: anterior view, B: posterior view and C: superior view.

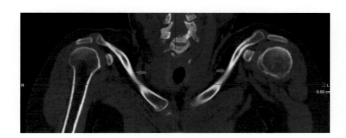

FIGURE 6.3: Coronal section of PMCT in the bone window showing clavicle bone, the medial and lateral end articulating with manubrium and scapula, respectively.

olecranon and coronoid, and two notches, namely the trochlear notch and radial notch. The olecranon process is a large hook-like structure with anterior concavity and articulates with the olecranon fossa of the humerus. The coronoid process is distal to the olecranon process and projects anteriorly; it articulates with the head of the radius (Figures 6.6–6.8). The trochlear notch of the ulna articulates with the trochlea of the humerus, while the radial notch articulates with the peripheral part of the radial head. The shaft of the ulna is triangular in the proximal but cylindrical in the distal part in cross-section. Like the radius, the ulnar shaft also has three borders, namely the interosseous, anterior, and posterior borders; it has three surfaces, namely the anterior, posterior, and medial surfaces.

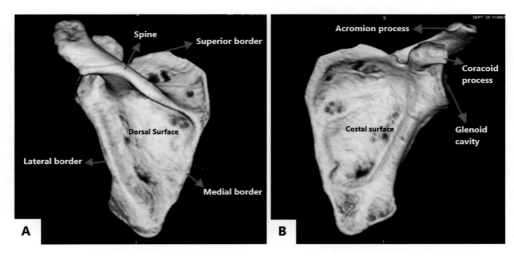

FIGURE 6.4: Volume rendering 3D image of A: dorsal surface and B: the costal surface of scapula bone showing the important anatomic landmarks like borders and processes.

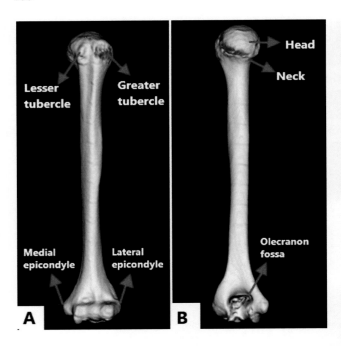

FIGURE 6.5: Volume rendering 3D image of humerus bone A: anterior and B: posterior view showing important anatomical landmarks.

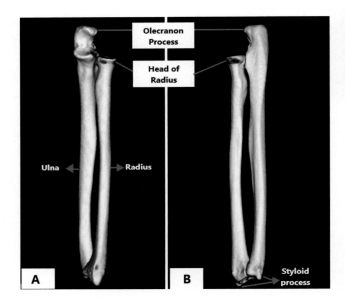

FIGURE 6.6: Volume rendering 3D image of forearm bones radius and ulna A: anterior view and B: posterior view.

The expanded distal end of the ulna consists of a head and a projection in its medial aspect, known as the styloid process. Its inferior smooth surface is separated with an articular disc from the carpel bone, while the lateral articular surface fits with the ulnar notch of the radius.

Bones of hand (Figure 6.9)
The hand bone consists of the carpals, metacarpals, and phalanges in proximal to distal order. The carpal bones contain eight bones arranged in two rows. The proximal row contains

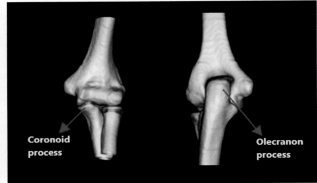

FIGURE 6.7: Volume rendering 3D image of elbow joint anterior and posterior view showing olecranon process and coronoid process.

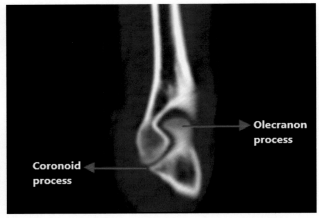

FIGURE 6.8: PMCT sagittal section of the elbow joint in the bone window showing the olecranon process and coronoid process.

the scaphoid, lunate, triquetrum, and pisiform from lateral to medial; while the distal row contains the trapezium, trapezoid, capitate, and hamate arranged from lateral to medial. Except for the pisiform bone, all other proximal row bones articulate with the forearm bones, the radius and the articular disc of the distal radioulnar joint. The distal row bones articulate with the metacarpal bones. There are five metacarpal bones conventionally numbered in radioulnar/lateral to medial order. All the metacarpals have a distal head, shaft, and proximal expanded base. The base articulates with the distal row of carpal bones and with each other except the first metacarpal. The heads articulate with the proximal phalanges and form knuckles. There are 14 phalanges, three in each finger except in the thumb, which contains two phalanges. Each phalanx has a distal head, shaft, and proximal base. The base of each proximal phalanx articulates with the distal head of corresponding metacarpals. The head of the distal phalanges is non-articular and has palmar tuberosity to which the pulps of fingertips are attached.

Integument and soft tissue
The thickness of the skin of the upper limb varies from one segment to another. Anteriorly, it is thinner and hairless,

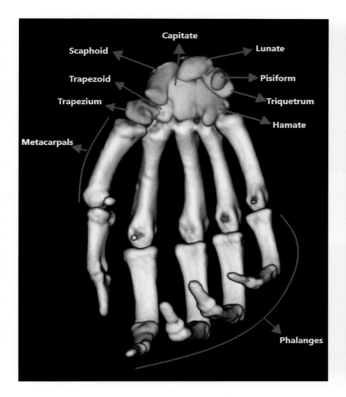

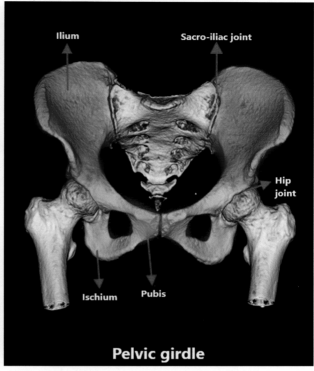

FIGURE 6.9: Volume rendering 3D image of hand bones showing carpals, metacarpals and phalanges.

FIGURE 6.10: Volume rendering 3D image of pelvis girdle/ hip bone and its joints; lower limb bones and joints.

making it easy to injure than the thicker, hairier skin at the posterior aspect, where comparatively higher force is required to produce injury. The palm has the thickest skin layer in the upper limb, and it is most resistant to any external force to produce injury. The musculature of the arm and forearm are organized into groups or compartments, namely flexors and extensors, and they are separated into the compartment by the fascia. The internal injury of the vasculature in a compartment causing extravasation and oedema produce an intense increase in intra-compartmental pressure, which impedes the flow of blood to and from the affected tissue, which is known as compartment syndrome. This is an emergency condition requiring surgery to prevent permanent injury.

Lower limbs
Bones and joints

The bones of the lower limbs comprise the pelvic girdle, which is made up of the innominate bones, which are formed by three fused bones, namely the ilium, pubis, and ischium; the femur and patella (thigh); the tibia and fibula (leg); and the tarsals, metatarsals, and phalanges (foot) (Figure 6.10). The pelvic girdle is the component which connects the lower limbs to the axial skeleton through a stable and strong synovial joint called the sacroiliac joint. A slightly movable secondary cartilaginous joint, namely pubic symphysis, is formed anteriorly by the articulation of the pubis of bilateral innominate bones, which helps the pelvic outlet to widen while childbirth and provides a minimal degree of movement during hip and sacroiliac movement. The hip joint is a type of ball-and-socket variety of synovial joints which allows movement in three orthogonal planes but also helps in maintaining the stability of the joint. The knee joint is the articulation between the femur and tibia and is a

synovial joint which allows mainly flexion and extension movement but also slight medial and lateral rotation. Apart from the tibiofemoral joint, the knee joint also consists of patellofemoral articulation, which is responsible for the gliding movement of the patella over the distal femur. The superior plane synovial joint and inferior fibrous joint of the tibia and fibula allow slight gliding movement near the knee joint and fibular rotation at the ankle joint, respectively. The ankle joint is formed by the articulation of the distal end of the tibia and fibula with the talus and allows movement into dorsiflexion and plantar flexion. The tarsal, metatarsal, and phalanges of the foot consist of multiple joints, and it helps in the complex movement required to fulfil its functional role in standing, as a shock absorber and in gait propulsion. The ankle is a major load-bearing joint, even though the incidence of significant degenerative arthritis is low as compared to the hip and knee joints. The knee joint is more susceptible to open injury and infection because of its superficial location. Both knee and ankle are prone to closed injuries.

Pelvic girdle

The pelvic girdle/hip bone consists of three parts, namely the ilium, ischium, and pubis, which articulate with each other by cartilage in young and are united as a bone in adults, principally in the acetabulum region (Figure 6.11). Posteriorly, each hip bone articulates with the sacrum to form a fixed and stable sacroiliac joint (Figure 6.12), while anteriorly it articulates with its contralateral part and forms pubic symphysis (Figure 6.13). A lateral radiological view of the acetabulum in young gives a tri-radiate pattern due to the cartilaginous part of articulation between the ilium and pubis superiorly, ilium and ischium in the posteroinferior, and pubis and ischium in the antero-inferior in young people which disappears in adults due to its

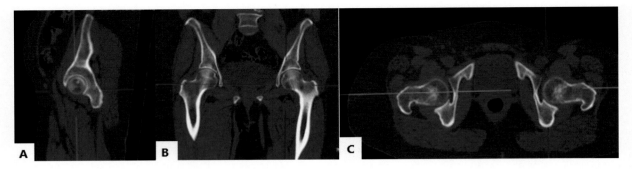

FIGURE 6.11:   PMCT of the pelvic region in the bone window showing acetabulum and hip joint in the A: sagittal section, B: coronal section, and C: axial section.

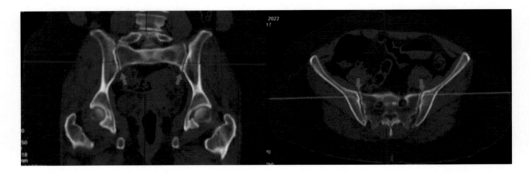

FIGURE 6.12:   PMCT of the pelvic region in the bone window showing sacroiliac joint in A: coronal section, B: axial section.

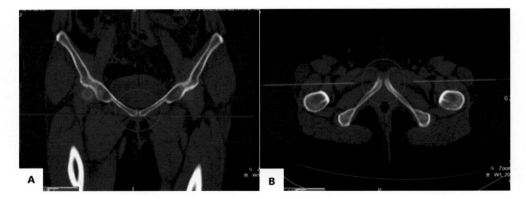

FIGURE 6.13:   PMCT of the pelvic region in the bone window showing pubic symphysis in A: coronal section, B: axial section.

transformation into bony tissue. The acetabulum is an approximately hemispherical cavity that faces anteroinferior and covers the part of the head of the femur circumferentially, forming the hip joint (Figure 6.11).

Femur (Figures 6.14 and 6.15)

The femur is the longest of all bones in the human body, mainly consisting of a proximal rounded head which articulates medially with the acetabulum, a short neck, an almost cylindrical shaft bowing forward and a distal expanded double condyle which articulates with the tibia. The femoral neck connects the head with the shaft and, at the junction, forms an angle called the neck shaft angle, which facilitates movement at the hip joint. This angle is widest at birth and reduces gradually until adolescence, and is smaller in females

compared to males. The neck of the femur is a common site of fracture, especially among the elderly. The shaft is narrowest at its central part, and its middle third has three borders, namely medial, lateral, and broad posterior border, also known as linea aspera; it has three surfaces, namely anterior, posterolateral, and posteromedial surfaces. Distally, the posterior surface of the shaft presents a popliteal surface which is triangular in outline; the popliteal vessels pass just behind this surface. The articular surface of the distal end is a broad area presented as an inverted U-shape for the articulation of the patella and tibia. The trochlear groove situated at the lower end helps stabilize the patella. The patella is the largest sesamoid bone situated over the anterior aspect of the knee joint and helps to strengthen and prevent the joint from external injury.

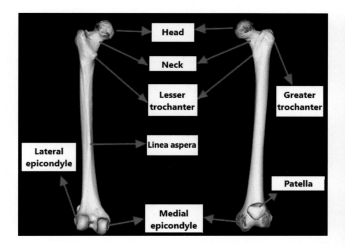

FIGURE 6.14: Volume rendering 3D image of the femur along with patella bone posterior and anterior view showing various parts.

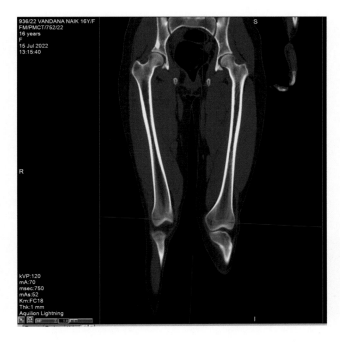

FIGURE 6.15: Coronal section of PMCT of thigh region in the bone window showing bilateral femur bones forming hip joint above and knee joint below.

The knee joint is a complex synovial joint formed by tibiofemoral and femoropatellar articulation. The superior surface of the tibia has a lateral and medial articular surface for the corresponding condylar surface of the distal end of the femur. The medial articular surface is oval and longer in comparison to the circular lateral articular surface, which gives more instability in the lateral aspect. The joint is separated by the medial and lateral meniscus, a fibrocartilaginous lamina at their corresponding parts, which helps the tibial articular surface to be wider and deep. The periphery of the meniscus is vascular, while the inner part is avascular, where the tear is common and seldom heals spontaneously. With reference to tibial attachment, anterior, and posterior

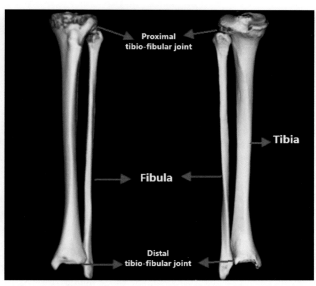

FIGURE 6.16: Volume rendering 3D image showing tibia and fibula bone anterior and posterior view showing proximal and distal tibiofibular joint.

cruciate ligaments cross each other and give extra strength to the knee joint.

Tibia (Figure 6.16)

The tibia is the next longest bone after the femur; it is located medial to the fibula. It has a proximal and a distal end along with a shaft. The proximal end is expanded, consisting of medial and lateral condyles, intercondylar area and the tibial tuberosity where the patellar tendon is attached. At the posteroinferior aspect of the lateral condyle, the fibular facet lies where the head of the fibula articulates with the tibia and forms the proximal tibiofibular joint. The shaft is triangular in cross-section, having anterolateral, anteromedial, and posterior surfaces separated by the anterior, medial, and lateral or interosseous border. The anterior border descends from the tuberosity to the anterior margin of the medial malleolus and is subcutaneous throughout. A smaller distal end projection is located medially, and it forms the medial malleolus. The distal inferior surface articulates with the talus to form a saddle-shaped ankle joint. A triangular fibular notch is present at the lateral surface of the distal end; there, the distal tibiofibular joint is formed by articulation with the distal end of the fibula.

Fibula (Figure 6.16)

The fibula is the bone of the leg which is not involved directly in the transmission of body weight and is positioned lateral to the tibia. It consists of a proximal head, a narrow neck, a shaft, and a distal lateral malleolus. The head is irregular in shape, having a round facet on the superomedial aspect which articulates with the corresponding facet on the inferolateral aspect of the condyle of the tibia and forms the proximal tibiofibular joint. Roughly, the shaft has anterior, posterior, and medial or interosseous borders. It also has lateral, anteromedial, and posteromedial surfaces; each of the surfaces is related to a specific group of muscles. The lateral surface is associated with the fibular group of muscles; the anteromedial surface is associated with the extensor group of muscles, while the posterolateral surface is associated with the flexor group of muscles. The distal end of the fibula has a projection at the posterior aspect called the lateral malleolus. The lateral surface of the lateral malleolus is subcutaneous, while the medial surface has a triangular articular facet which articulates with the lateral talar surface.

Foot bones (Figure 6.17)

The foot bones consist of tarsal bones, metatarsals, and phalanges. The ankle joint, also known as a talocrural joint, is formed by the articulation of the distal end of the tibia and fibula with the body of the talus. It is the only mortise joint present in the human body. The foot has a planter and a dorsal surface, which refers to the inferior and superior surfaces, respectively. The proximal half of the foot is occupied by the tarsal bones, which are homologous to the carpal bone in the hand but longer in size. Like carpal bones, the tarsals are also arranged into proximal and distal rows, but on the medial side, the navicular bone is articulated in between two rows, the talus and cuneiform. Talus and calcaneus form the proximal row; however, the distal row is made up of medial, intermediate, and lateral cuneiform and arranged from medial to lateral direction. These tarsal bones, along with the metatarsus, are arranged in such a manner that helps the foot make longitudinal and transverse arches which are responsible for not transmitting the thrust and weight directly from the tibia to the ground or vice versa but distributed throughout the tarsal and metatarsal bones. Similar to the phalanges of the hand, the toes also have 14 phalanges; two in the great toe and three each in the remaining four toes articulated in an almost similar manner as the hand.

Integument and soft tissue

The skin of the lower limbs is generally stronger, thicker, and hairier than that of the upper limbs. Because of its weight-bearing nature, the sole is the thickest among all of the regions of the skin. Similarly, in the sitting posture, the skin of the buttocks and posterior thigh become the weight-bearing area which consequently is relatively thick. The anteromedial region of the thigh is particularly fragile and is more prone to injury even by trivial trauma. The lower limb's deep fascia is well-defined and separates a group of muscles from others. These fascial planes prevent the spread of pathological fluids within the limb due to their attachment with bone and play a significant role in determining the degree and direction of displacement of fractured long bones. Compartment syndrome is another common condition due to this arrangement of the deep fascia in the leg, where an increase in pressure in one compartment affects the neurovascular flow and needs a fasciotomy procedure to relieve the local pressure rise. The muscle groups of the anterior and posterior aspects of the hip are responsible for flexion and extension, respectively, and the reverse is true for the thigh and leg. The muscle group in the thigh is divided into anterior, posterior, and medial compartments according to its functions which are extension, flexion, and adduction, respectively.

Injuries to the limbs

Epidemiology

Generally, males, especially those of younger age, are commonly known to suffer from limb trauma. Limb trauma can range from simple skin abrasions to complex conditions like limb amputations or conditions with complications of vascular compromise leading to advanced limb ischaemia.

Injury due to road traffic accidents

Lower limb injuries are commonly due to road traffic accidents, and the most vulnerable victims are pedestrians and motorbikers. Pedestrians sustain an injury over different parts of the lower limb or upper limb, depending on the vehicle colliding with them. The other factors which determine the primary impact region include the height of the bumper or wheel of the vehicle striking, whether the vehicle was accelerating or

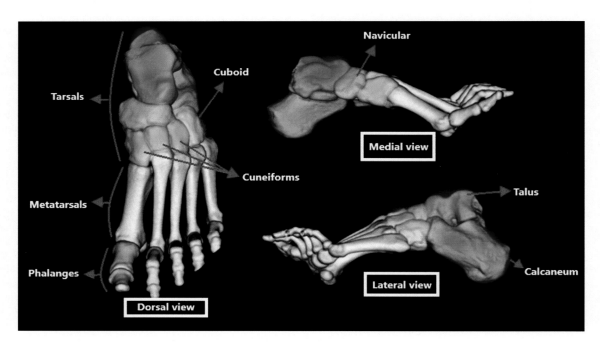

FIGURE 6.17:   Volume rendering 3D image of foot bones in dorsal view, medial view and lateral view showing tarsal bones, metatarsals and phalanges.

decelerating at the time of the accident, whether the pedestrian was in a static position or dynamic position, etc. all these determine the position and also the type of injury sustained by the pedestrian. Among vehicular accidents, bike versus car collision is a common mechanism of producing limb injuries to the victim and also by bike versus pedestrian collision. The leg is the part of the lower limb most commonly injured in an RTA, followed by the thigh and knee. In the upper limb, fractures of the humerus and clavicle are commonly seen, and this usually happens due to falls after the loss of balance. In the upper limb, wrist dislocation is also quite common and to a lesser extent, elbow and shoulder dislocations are also common; these happen mostly due to falls with an outstretched hand.

Injury due to falls from a height

Skeletal injuries due to falls from a height are potentially preventable as mostly these incidences occur in a domestic setting and due to poor construction plans. Accidental injuries from falling from a height are one of the leading causes of death, and usually, the victims are very young or very old people. Hospital admission with skeletal injuries following a fall from a height account for a significant portion of admissions. Musculoskeletal injuries due to falling from a height are also observed mostly in the first four decades of life, predominantly in males, which leads to disability and affects the most productive portions of society along with an increased burden on healthcare facilities.

As per the reports of the Council on Injury, Violence and Poison Prevention, the United States' most frequent sites of fracture in pediatric falls are the radius, ulna, and femur. Other studies also showed similar observations along with hip injuries and fractures of the tibia and fibula as common sites. Spine, pelvis, and calcaneum injuries are seen less commonly seen in children. Children are more vulnerable to head injury due to falls from a height as their heads have a larger head-to-body ratio in comparison to adults, who are more prone to limb injuries. Some authors opine that the height of the fall and the age of the individual are significant factors in the determination of the severity of the trauma, while others disapprove of them. Soft tissue injury is more frequent than fractures of the extremity in falls.

Injury due to other causes

Limb injuries differ as per the sports. The association of sports and its impact on injury is an important factor; some of the most common injuries associated with sports are:

- Marathon: Most of the injuries reported are knee injuries, ankle and foot injuries, followed by leg injuries.
- Skiing and snowboarding: Lower limb injuries are very common in skiing and snowboarding, especially among men.
- Tennis: Tennis mostly contributes to upper limb injuries involving the elbow, wrist, and shoulder joints.
- Cricket: Due to the rigorous action of bowling, upper limb injuries are common, especially the shoulder and wrist.
- Football: Being a contact sport, players are prone to lower limb injuries most commonly of the ankle and knee joints.

Types of limb injuries
Injuries produced by blunt weapons (Figure 6.18)
Abrasions

An abrasion is a type of blunt injury caused when tangential or perpendicular force is applied to the skin surface resulting in a breach of continuity of the epidermal layer of skin and dermal papillae. The tangential force produces scratch and grazed abrasions, while the perpendicular force produces pressure or impact abrasions. A combination of innumerable scratch abrasions is collectively known as a grazed abrasion, generally produced during roadside automobile accidents. In general, when a small perpendicular force is applied for a long time over the skin surface, the epithelium gets crushed and produces a pressure abrasion-like ligature mark. In cases where a relatively large force is applied for a short time period, it produces an impact or imprint abrasion-like tyre print, as in cases of heavy vehicle runover. The colour and morphology of abrasions vary with time from bright red, reddish scabs, dark brown scabs, and blackish scabs to falling scabs with no scar after a long time. Abrasions are superficial injuries and are better appreciated by naked-eye external examination compared to volume rendering 3D surface images in PMCT (Figures 6.19 and 6.20). A few abrasions which involve a larger area of skin and deeper tissue may be identified (Figures 6.21 and 6.22), but artefacts may be produced due to PMCT, which makes it difficult for identification.

Bruises/contusions

A bruise/contusion is a term for the extravasation of blood into the tissue with an intact skin layer due to blunt force trauma (Figure 6.23). Extravasation can occur due to multiple causes, many of which are non-traumatic; depending upon the

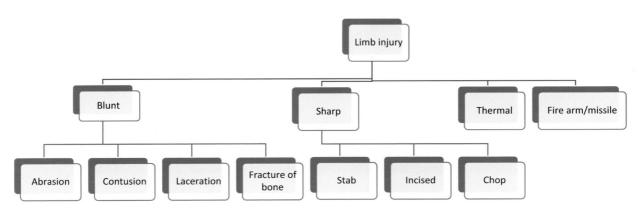

FIGURE 6.18:   Classification of the types of limb injuries based on the different types of external force

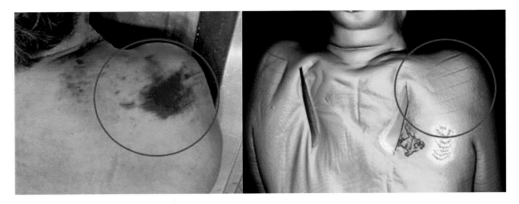

FIGURE 6.19: Abrasion over the back of right shoulder seen encircled in naked-eye external examination and volume rendering 3D image. The superficial abrasion is not well appreciated in volume rendering 3D images.

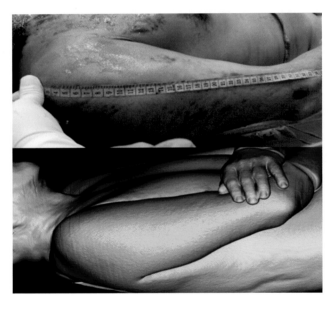

FIGURE 6.20: Superficial abrasions over the outer aspect of the right arm and elbow, which is well appreciated in naked-eye external examination and is poorly appreciated in volume rendering 3D image.

size of extravasation, its name varies like petechial haemorrhage for the size of 0.1 to 2 mm, ecchymosis for 2 to 5 mm and bruises for more than 5 mm. The term haematoma is used when a large, organized blood clot is formed. Depending upon the location of bruises, they are generally classified as intradermal, subcutaneous, or deep bruises. Soft and delicate subcutaneous tissue, less musculature, higher amounts of fat, and highly vascular and loose tissue shows more evident bruise. The colour of bruises varies with time, but it is difficult to estimate the exact age of the bruise with any degree of certainty because it varies from case to case depending on the size and depth of the bruise. Plain PMCT has a limited role in detecting bruises as it is difficult to identify without knowing the exact location of trauma because of almost similar HU for normal muscle and contused muscle; however, contrast-enhanced PMCT could be helpful to rule out any extravasations if done before decomposition starts. The significance of PMCT is to get findings of fissured or hairline fractures underlying bruises, which can be easily missed out during conventional autopsy. The PMCT is also helpful in identifying contusions in visceral organs and the brain due to the relatively higher difference of HU between blood and organs.

Lacerations

Splitting or tearing of the skin, subcutaneous tissues, muscles, or internal organs beyond its elastic strength due to

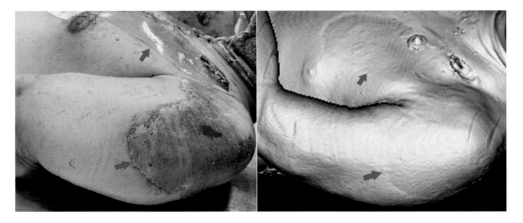

FIGURE 6.21: Grazed abrasion over the anterior aspect of the left chest, left shoulder and lateral aspect of the left arm is better appreciated in naked-eye examination; the margins of the abrasion are appreciated in the volume rendering 3D image due to the depth of the injury.

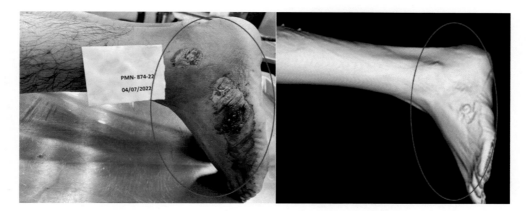

FIGURE 6.22: Grazed abrasion over the lateral aspect of the left foot is better appreciated in naked-eye examination; the margins of the abrasion are appreciated in the volume rendering 3D image at places where the depth of the injury is more.

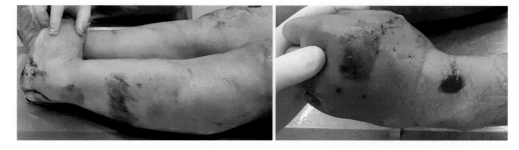

FIGURE 6.23: Contusion over the left lower limb and left dorsum of the hand.

individual or collective effects of blunt force trauma are called lacerations. Depending on the effects of blunt force over the body, lacerations are classified into tears, splits, stretches, cuts, and avulsed or shear lacerations. PMCT also helps in identifying the lacerations due to the break in the overlying skin or other structures, which can be appreciated in volume rendering 3D images and also in various sections of the CT. External examination of laceration gives clear information regarding the laceration, but PMCT, in addition, gives details of other associated injuries like fracture/dislocation of the underlying bone and rupture of the muscle (Figure 6.24) or tendon and these examinations can be done without further mutilating the surrounding structures giving a more dignified humanitarian approach for the examination.

Fractures

Fractures are a common presentation in cases of trauma to the limbs, especially in fatal cases coming for autopsy examination. Fractures can include closed fractures or open fractures; the fracture types commonly seen are fissure fractures, comminuted fractures, compound fractures, spiral fractures, wedge fractures, etc. The PMCT has a large role in identifying bone fractures, especially small or obscure sites like the scapula, facial bones, hand bones, and vertebrae which are not routinely checked in traditional autopsy and checking them would result in mutilation of the dead body. This PMCT examination also helps in the study of undisplaced fractures and in differentiating from artefact fractures caused due to the dissection procedure.

Scapula fracture

Fractures of the scapula are rare, accounting for just about 0.4 to 1% of all fractures. Among the shoulder fracture cases, scapula fractures account for only 3%. The scapula may fracture at any site if direct force is applied to it; however, if the impact is on the humeral head and is then transmitted to the glenoid cavity, the common site of fracture is the scapular neck and glenoid process. External examination of the scapular region may be deceitful due to the presence of bulky muscles, which make the identification of fracture very difficult (Figure 6.25); in such cases, PMCT is a boon where the position and type of fracture can be identified (Figures 6.26 and 6.27).

Humerus fractures

Humerus fractures are an important category encountered in routine autopsy practice. They are seen in cases of falls from a height, RTAs, assaults, firearm injuries, etc. Elderly people are more prone to proximal humeral fractures. Supra condylar fractures in the lower end are generally seen in younger individuals and are mostly due to accidental falls from a height. Fracture of the shaft of the humerus occurs due to a direct blow to the upper arm (Figure 6.28) or due to indirect trauma due to a fall (Figure 6.29) or a twisting movement, usually causing spiral or oblique fractures. Comminuted fractures may also occur if a higher impact is applied to a localized area, or fracture dislocation of the shoulder or elbow joint (Figure 6.30) may occur if higher impact happens over a larger surface. In some cases, an open fracture may also be seen also seen with bone-deep laceration caused by local blunt force or by stretch laceration

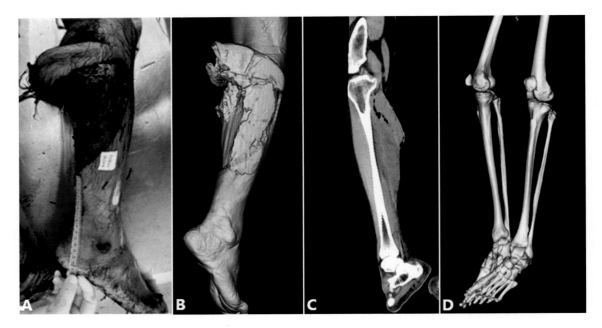

FIGURE 6.24: Laceration of the back of right leg: A: External examination showing the laceration, B: Volume rendering 3D image replicating the gross image of the laceration, C: Sagittal section of the leg showing laceration with the break in skin and muscle continuity and intact bone, D: Volume rendering 3D image of bone showing intact bones.

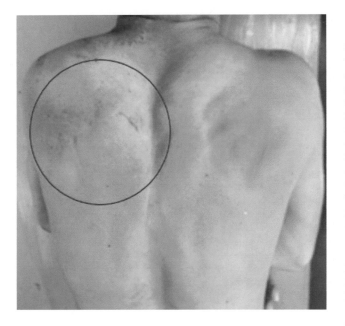

FIGURE 6.25: External examination of the scapular region in a case of scapular fracture doesn't show many external changes like contusion or any gross deformity making the detection of fracture difficult.

produced by the fractured fragment. Epicondylar fracture of the humerus is another important category which is commonly seen in children and adolescents and is among the most challenging fractures to be identified because that age period is the period of fusion of ossification centres of the lower end of the humerus, and there is a risk of misdiagnosing or over-diagnosing the fracture.

Forearm fractures

The forearm consists of two major long bones, namely the radius and ulna. Forearm fractures are routinely encountered fractures in medical practice, and the common mechanism of such fractures is by axial loading of force over the forearm bones, usually due to a fall onto an outstretched arm. Some of the most common causes of forearm bone fractures include RTAs, falls from a height, athletic/sports injuries, assaults, firearm injuries, etc. Common fractures of the radius from proximal to distal end are radial head fracture, radial neck fracture, Essex–Lopresti fracture-dislocation, Galeazzi fracture-dislocation, Barton fracture, Colles fracture, and Smith fracture. Common fractures of the ulna from proximal to distal are noted as olecranon fracture, coronoid process fracture, Monteggia fracture-dislocation, nightstick fracture, and ulnar styloid fracture. The fractures may involve an isolated radius or ulna bone or maybe a combination of fracture/dislocation of both bones, like Galeazzi and Monteggia fractures. Galeazzi fractures include the fracture of the distal third of the radius with dislocation of the distal radioulnar joint. Monteggia fractures include the fracture of the proximal ulna with dislocation of the head of the radius bone. A Colles fracture is a common type of fracture involving the distal radius bone; it is particularly common among the elderly group with osteoporosis due to falling on an outstretched hand at ground level. It involves the complete fracture of the radius bone in the lower part close to the wrist with an upward (posterior) displacement of the fractured fragment and also a classic deformity termed the 'dinner fork deformity' (Figures 6.31 and 6.32). A Smith fracture is also a fracture of the distal end of the radius where the fractured end gets displaced or gets angled in the direction of the palm, this type of injury happens when a person falls over the back of the flexed wrist of an outstretched hand resulting in the formation of a garden spade deformity.

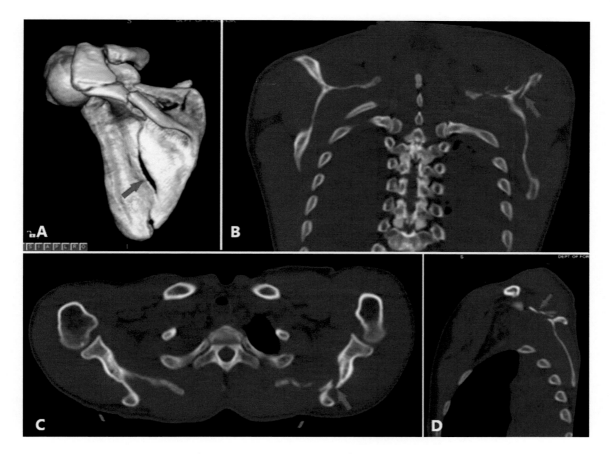

FIGURE 6.26: PMCT examination in the same case as Figure 6.25 showing: A: Volume rendering 3D image of the scapula with linear fracture extending from the superior border to the inferior angle of the scapula, including the spine. B: Bone window coronal section shows fracture of the left scapula near the spine. C: Axial section shows the fracture near the spine of the scapula. D: Sagittal section shows the fracture near the spine of the scapula.

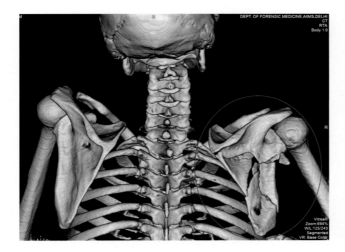

FIGURE 6.27: Volume rendering 3D image in a case road traffic accident showing comminuted fracture of right scapula.

Pelvis fracture

Pelvic fractures are commonly seen in motor vehicle accidents, falls from a height, sports injuries, and any case where high-velocity blunt force/trauma is transmitted to the pelvic bone. The type of external force, which could be local impact or compression, the energy transferred, and the integral strength of the bone are the determining factors for the resultant type of pelvic bone fracture. Young and Burgess have described four main types of fracture, namely:

1. Open book or sprung pelvis fracture (Figure 6.33) due to anteroposterior compression force.
2. Windswept pelvis due to lateral compression force.
3. Bucket handle or Malgaigne fracture due to vertical shear force.
4. Complex fracture pattern if a combined mechanical force is applied from two different directions.

Isolated fractures of the pelvic bone, like acetabular fracture, pubic ramus fracture (Figure 6.34), iliac bone fracture (Figure 6.34), avulsion fractures of ASIS, iliac crest, ischial tuberosity, etc., can also be seen in cases of local impact. Major vessels that can be damaged in cases of fracture pelvis are the internal iliac, superior gluteal, obturator, and internal pudendal vessels leading to haemorrhagic complication and death. PMCT scan is the investigation of choice to identify pelvic fractures as autopsy examination of them is difficult, and any dissection to examine the entire pelvic bone will lead to mutilation of the body and also causes difficulty in suturing back the pelvic region in proper shape. PMCT is a great help in screening for pelvic fractures, which could be missed by conventional autopsy.

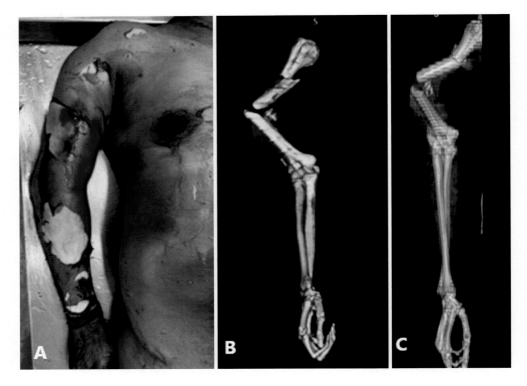

FIGURE 6.28: Examination of the right arm: A: External examination showing gross deformity of the arm with contusions over the mid-arm; B: Volume rendering 3D image of bone comminuted fracture of shaft of right humerus bone; C: Volume rendering 3D image in bone implant view.

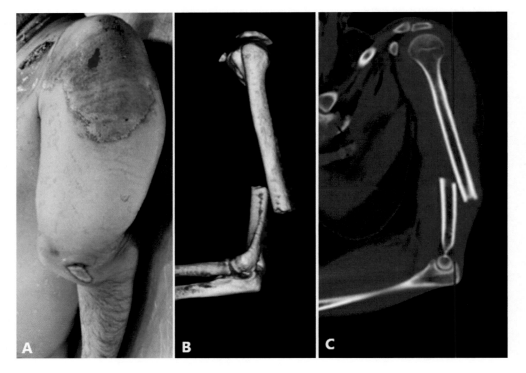

FIGURE 6.29: Examination of the left arm: A: External examination showing grazed abrasion over left shoulder and chest with disfigurement of arm; B: Volume rendering 3D image of humerus bone showing fracture-dislocation of shaft of humerus; C: PMCT image of the left arm in the bone window showing fracture-dislocation of shaft of the humerus.

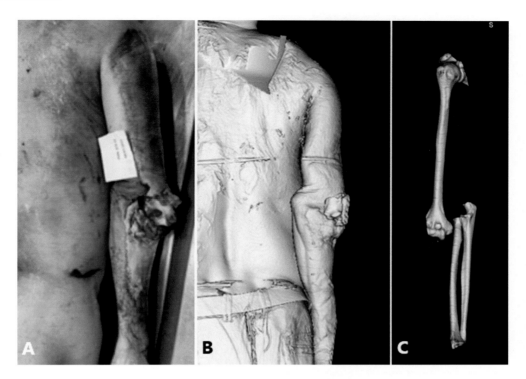

FIGURE 6.30: A: External examination showing grazed abrasion over right arm and forearm with open fracture-dislocation of elbow joint also seen in volume rendering 3D image of PMCT (B); C: Anterior view of volume rendering 3D image of bones of upper limb showing dislocation of the elbow.

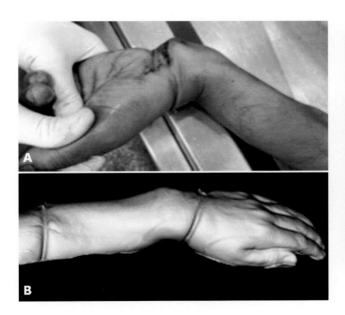

FIGURE 6.31: A case of Colles fracture of the left hand seen in autopsy: A: External examination showing the deformity; B: Volume rendering 3D image of the same case showing classic 'dinner fork deformity' due to colles fracture.

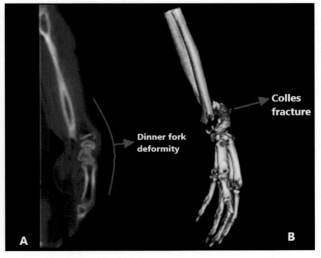

FIGURE 6.32: A case of Colles fracture in autopsy same as in Figure 6.31: A- Dinner fork deformity identified in coronal section bone window; B- Fracture-dislocation of the distal end of the radius along with dislocation of the wrist joint.

Femur fracture

The femur is the longest bone of the human body, and it is one of the most common bones to be fractured, especially in the elderly. Fractures of the femur can be classified into proximal end fractures, which include femoral head, neck, and trochanteric fractures; then shaft fractures; and finally, distal end fractures, which include the condylar, inter-condylar fracture, etc. The proximal femur fracture is more common in the elderly age group due to the fact that the femur neck is the weakest part of the femur bone, and osteoporosis makes it more vulnerable. Femoral head blood supply is disrupted when neck fractures cause avascular necrosis. Mechanisms of injury causing femur fracture in elderly and younger people are different; in the elderly, falls are the common cause and in younger patients,

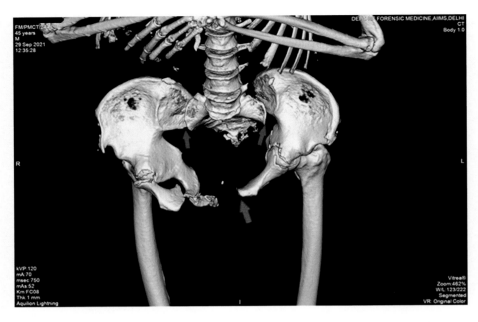

FIGURE 6.33: Sprung fracture with separation of the symphysis pubis (red arrow) and both sacroiliac joints (blue arrow).

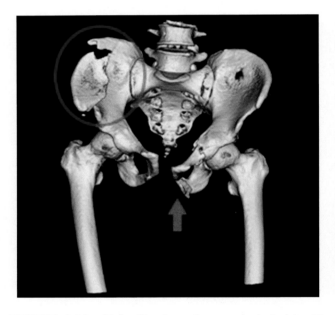

FIGURE 6.34: Right iliac bone fracture (red circle) with separation of the symphysis pubis (red arrow).

the common cause is motor vehicle collision. The fractured neck of the femur can be detected by plain radiograph with high sensitivity; PMCT, on the other hand, is much more sensitive and has the additional advantage of 3D viewing and understanding the overall fracture pattern. The distal femur fracture is a relatively rare type of femoral fracture; at autopsy, this type of injury can be seen as swelling, bruising, or deformity just above the knee joint (Figures 6.35–6.38). Since some of the distal femoral fractures are intra-articular, a PMCT scan is very helpful in these cases. In cases with a fracture, a femur previously treated for some duration, or old femur fractures, common complications of the fractured femur like osteoarthritis, aseptic fracture, mal-union, non-union, and infection in the form of localized pus collection may be appreciated.

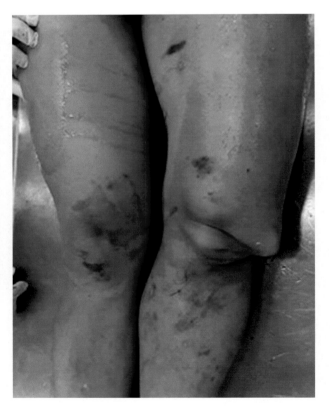

FIGURE 6.35: Fracture-dislocation of the femur with associated fracture of the tibia at the knee joint, external examination of leg showing deformity.

Pathologic lesion in femur resembling fracture

Focal lesions in bone are common and can be frequently seen in post-mortem imaging. These focal bone lesions can range from normal variants to neoplastic lesions. Commonly encountered lesions include congenital abnormalities in bone, old traumatic/iatrogenic lesions, bone deformities due to

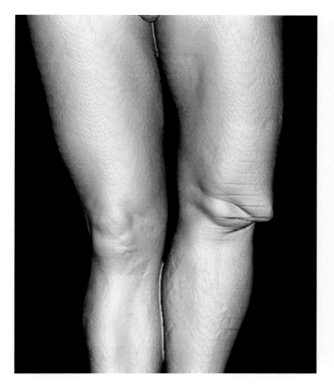

FIGURE 6.36: Fracture-dislocation of the femur with associated fracture of the tibia at the knee joint, Volume rendering 3D image showing deformity.

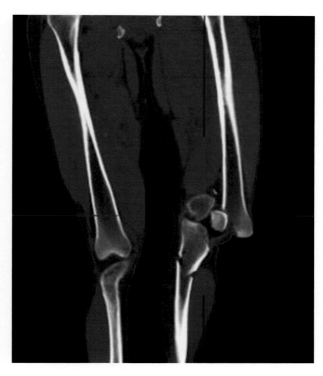

FIGURE 6.38: Coronal section PMCT image in the bone window showing fracture-dislocation of the distal end of the left femur and the proximal end of the left tibia.

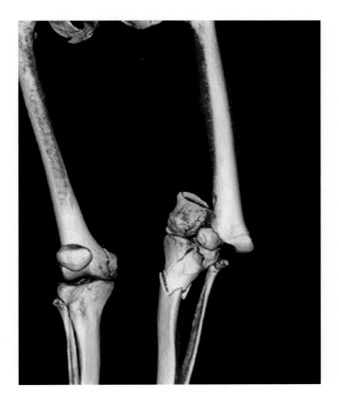

FIGURE 6.37: Volume rendering 3D image showing left lower femur fracture-dislocation with fracture of upper left tibia and fibula.

metabolic or arthritic changes, local bone infection and, many times, artefacts of post-mortem imaging. It is important to differentiate between them as, in certain cases, an incidental minor injury may be seen in the region with underlying bone deformity; this may be confused with trauma or fracture in the bone. In the case mentioned in Figure 6.40, a superficial minor abrasion was found over the left knee joint, and incidentally, the left femur showed a deformity along with a lytic lesion (Figures 6.39–6.42). It is essential to differentiate these lesions and avoid misinterpretation of the findings of post-mortem imaging.

Injury to the knee joint

Trauma to the knee is frequently encountered in cases of RTAs, falls from a height, sports injuries, and, rarely, in an assault. A patellar fracture is a common fracture associated with knee injuries, which may be appreciated as a swelling or bruise in the knee region. Patellar fractures occur due to a direct blow to the patella, severe force applied by the extensor mechanism of quadriceps muscles, and complications post-surgery to the knee or total knee reconstruction. Morphologically among the fractures of the patella, a transverse fracture is the most common type, followed by comminuted fracture and vertical fracture of the patella. Examination of the knee joint, including the patella, by traditional autopsy involving the dissection of the joint could disfigure the cadaver.

Another type of fracture in the knee joint is associated with the disruption of the anterior cruciate ligament (ACL) and is termed a Segond fracture, where there is an avulsion fracture of the knee involving the tibial plateau at the lateral aspect because of internal rotation and varus stress. Post-mortem

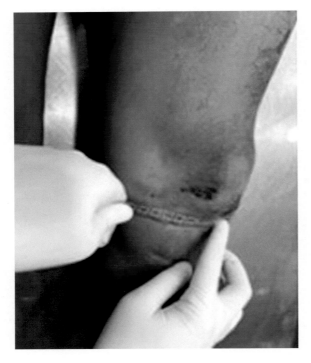

FIGURE 6.39: The lytic lesion in the shaft of the left femur has incidental small abrasion on the same leg.

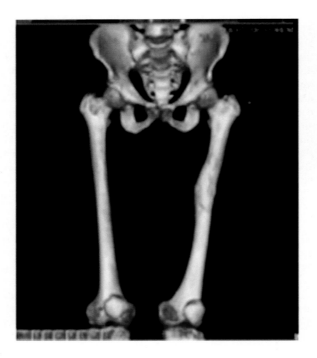

FIGURE 6.40: Volume rendering 3D PMCT image showing the lesion in left femur.

radiograph or PMCT show a curvilinear or elliptical bone fragment parallelly projecting to the lateral aspect of the tibial plateau, but a post-mortem MRI is essential to identify the tear in ligaments which is difficult to identify in a PMCT. The role of PMCT in cases of knee injury is limited because death is less

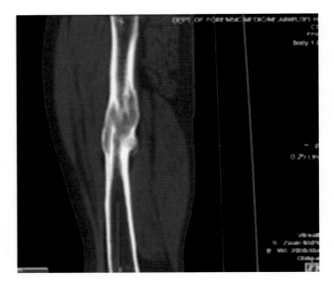

FIGURE 6.41: PMCT coronal section showing the lytic lesion in the shaft of the left femur.

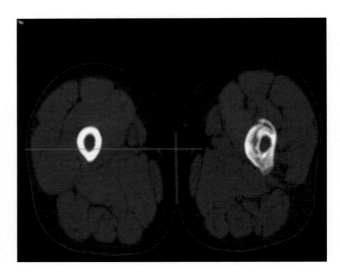

FIGURE 6.42: PMCT axial section showing the lytic lesion in the shaft of the left femur.

likely in case of isolated knee injury unless there is an associated injury to a major vessel.

Tibia and fibula fractures

Fractures of the leg bones are a common finding; the deformity is very obvious in cases where there is a fracture of both bones. Tibia fractures are common in all age groups and are divided into proximal, shaft, and distal fractures according to the Orthopedic Trauma Association classification system. The proximal tibial fracture is mostly seen in elderly females, while in young males fracture of the shaft is common with distal tibial fracture is frequently seen in middle-aged persons. The proximal tibial fracture is encountered in RTAs where there is direct impact near the knee or tibial tuberosity. The proximal tibiofibular fracture can be commonly associated with the injury of the knee joint and also the lower femur (Figure 6.43).

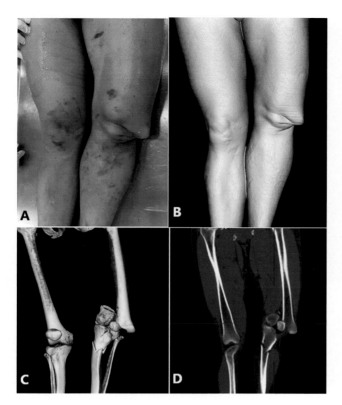

FIGURE 6.43: Fracture-dislocation of proximal tibia-fibula along with lower femur. A: External examination of leg showing deformity, B: Volume rendering 3D image showing deformity, C: Volume rendering 3D image showing fracture of the upper left tibia and fibula with left lower femur fracture-dislocation, and D: PMCT image in the bone window showing fracture of the proximal end of left tibia with fracture-dislocation of the distal end of the left femur.

Mid-shaft tibial/fibular fractures usually have a bimodal distribution in occurrence, and among young patients, the cause is due to high-energy mechanisms like RTAs, falls from a height, sports injuries, etc., and in older patients, the cause is lower energy mechanisms like falls from a standing position, tripping while walking, twisting of the legs, etc. The lower energy mechanisms like twisting may cause an indirect torsional injury resulting in spiral fractures of the mid-shaft of the tibia or fibula along with minor soft tissue injury. In cases of high-velocity injuries to the leg, the resultant fractures could be a wedge fracture, oblique fracture, or a comminuted fracture at the point of impact, and it depends on the dynamics of the injury and if the leg was supported or not the associated soft tissue injury is also severe and in certain cases can even lead to the development of compartment syndrome (Figure 6.44).

Fractures of the distal leg involve both bones in the majority of cases. Distal leg fractures can occur either by low-energy mechanisms like rotational strain due to twists or due to high-energy mechanisms like RTAs, falls from a height or sports injuries (Figure 6.45).

Compartment syndrome

Groups of muscles in the limbs are organized into defined areas based on their function called compartments. This division into compartments is done by connective tissues called the fascia, which along with the bones of the limbs, form the walls of these compartments. Injuries occurring in these tightly confined compartments that result in bleeding or oedema increase the intra-compartment pressure acutely, and the non-elastic nature of the walls tends to make the compartment tense and affect the tissues. Acute compartment syndrome can occur following injuries without any bone fractures like crush injuries, burns (Figure 6.46), tight bandaging of the limb, post-limb surgery, etc. However, in the majority of cases, compartment syndrome occurs due to closed fractures of the limb bone (Figure 6.47), which leads to bleeding and an increase in

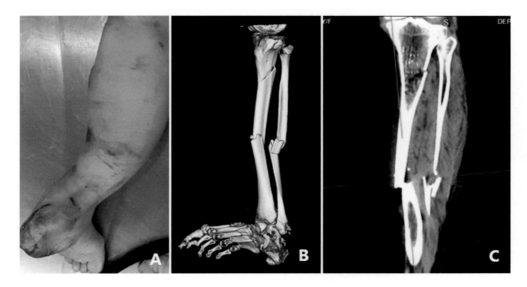

FIGURE 6.44: Fracture-dislocation of middle tibia-fibula along with upper tibial fracture in a case of a road traffic accident resulting from high-energy mechanism. A: External examination of left leg showing deformity in the middle of the leg, B: Volume rendering 3D image of the skeleton showing fracture-dislocation of the mid-third of tibia and fibula along with a fracture of the upper third of the tibia, C: PMCT image in the bone window showing fracture-dislocation of middle third of left tibia and fibula with fracture of the proximal end of the left tibia.

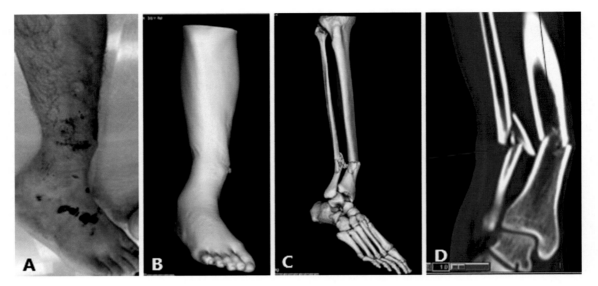

FIGURE 6.45: Fracture-dislocation of lower tibia-fibula in a case of a road traffic accident resulting from high-energy mechanism. A: External examination of right leg showing deformity; B: Volume rendering 3D image showing the deformity; C: Volume rendering 3D image of skeleton showing the comminuted fracture of the distal tibia and fibula; D: PMCT image in the bone window showing comminuted fracture of distal tibia and fibula

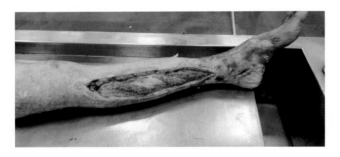

FIGURE 6.46: Fasciotomy was done to relieve compartment syndrome in a case of burns to the left leg.

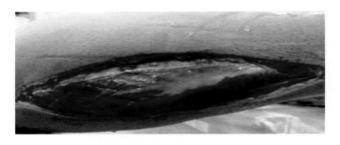

FIGURE 6.47: Fasciotomy in a case of trauma to the lower limb with closed fracture.

intra-compartment pressure. A fracture of the pelvic bone can lead to blood loss of around 3–5 litres; a femur fracture can cause around 1.5–2 litres of blood loss; a tibia/fibula fracture can cause a loss of around 1 litre, a humerus fracture can lead to around 800 ml of blood loss and radius/ulna fracture can cause a loss of about 400 ml. During an autopsy, the tense swollen feeling of limbs can point towards compartment syndrome

and underlying trauma; however, it needs to be differentiated from cases of limb cellulitis which may mimic the appearance. The presence of fasciotomy during examination is clear-cut evidence of the underlying compartment syndrome and directs us to identify the nature of the injury which caused the compartment syndrome (Figure 6.46 and 6.47).

Injuries produced by sharp force/weapon

A sharp-force injury can be due to any of the sharp-edged weapons resulting from an accidental, self-inflicted, or homicidal manner. Common weapons used are knives, blades, razors, scalpels, broken glass, or daggers. Mostly sharp-force injuries are homicidal, but other means are not uncommon. Injuries due to broken glass are usually accidental, and due to homicidal means are rare. A sharp-force injury to the limbs is more obvious as a defensive or accidental injury rather than a self-inflicted or homicidal injury. Various types of sharp-force injury to the limbs are encountered in forensic practice; common injuries are incised wounds, chop wounds, stab wounds, animal bites, surgical incisions, venipuncture, etc.

Incised wounds

An incised wound is a sharp-cutting wound produced by a sharp-edged weapon. On the limbs, it could be present as a hesitation cut over the upper limbs commonly seen in suicidal cases (Figure 6.48), accidental injury by a sharp weapon, or, rarely in homicidal cases, as a defensive wound. Characteristically the incised wound is greater in length than depth, with sharp and clean-cut margins, usually spindly in shape, deeper at the beginning, and shallower towards the tailing end. The length could be any size and with no correlation between the length of the weapon because a cutting weapon may be drawn across the body to any distance. The width of the wound can correspond to the thickness of the

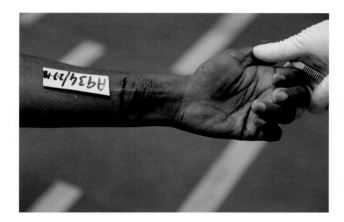

FIGURE 6.48: Hesitation cuts present over the wrist region of the left forearm in a suicidal death case.

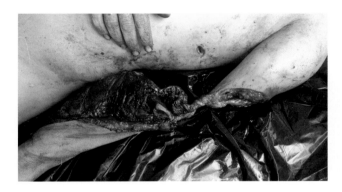

FIGURE 6.49: Chop wound involving the lower arm with near total amputation of the left upper limb with only skin attachment. The underlying humerus bone is fractured, corresponding to the chop wound.

weapon, but factors like skin elasticity, gaping, and movement of the weapon also should be considered. Beveling of the cut surface may be seen if the weapon enters the skin surface at an angle and not perpendicularly. The external examination of these wounds would give a more exact idea to correlate with the nature of the weapon than PMCT, but it can be more useful in cases where a broken piece of weapon is retained inside the body, which can be located and collected.

Chop wounds

A chop wound is produced when a sharp heavy weapon causes an injury; it appears like a cut laceration. The characteristic feature of this wound involves a mixture of sharp and blunt injury with contusion and laceration of the margins of the wound. The length of the injury is generally more or less the same as the length of the blade. There is usually a fracture of the underlying bone, which corresponds to the injury and also the edge of the blade (Figure 6.49).

Stab wounds

A stab wound is an injury caused by a sharp weapon which has a greater depth than the length and width of the skin injury (Figure 6.50). It occurs due to thrusting motion along the long axis of a pointed object into the depth of the body either by an overhand or underhand method. Any object that has a pointed end can cause a stab wound. An object/instrument that has a sharp edge but lacks a point can produce incise but not a stab. Similarly, a pointed but edgeless instrument can stab but not incise, and an instrument which has both a point as well as an edge (like a kitchen knife), can produce stab and incision injuries. Stab wounds could be in the form of a puncture, penetrating, or perforating wound. The punctured wound is superficial and may go up to muscle or bone deep but does not enter a body cavity. If the stab wound enters any body cavity (like the chest, abdomen, skull, knee joint, orbit, scrotum, etc.), it is termed a penetrating wound with respect to the body; however, it is a perforating wound to a particular structure or body part when the entry and exit wounds exist in a single track. The depth of a stab wound is determined by multiple factors like sharpness,

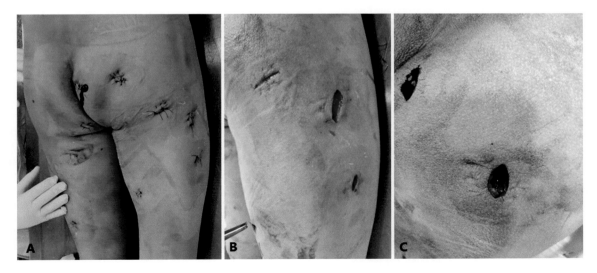

FIGURE 6.50: Stab wound at gluteal region and back and lateral aspect of thigh. A: in sutured condition; B: after opening of sutures; C: close view at gluteal region.

width, thickness and shape of the weapon, resistance offered by tissue, nature of clothing, relative momentum between body and weapon, degree of skin stretching, and angle of the strike. The depth is not always the same as the length of the weapon; it may be greater than the actual length of the weapon because of the laxity of the surface and thrusting of the weapon or lesser when the weapon is thrust partially and when a bony hindrance is present. The shape of the stab wound depends upon the cleavage line of the langer (a cut across the line produces a greater gap, and parallel to the line causes a minimum gap while an oblique cut gives an oval shape of the wound), the shape of weapon (single-edged sharp weapon produces a wedge or fishtail shaped wound while a double-edged sharp weapon produces a spindle-shaped wound and a pointed and cylindrical weapon produce a circular wound with bruised, inverted, and ragged edges).

Studies of the comparative prevalence of homicidal, suicidal, and accidental stab wounds show that homicidal stab wounds are more common and frequent while accidental stab wounds are rare. Common areas involved in stab injuries are the thorax, neck, and abdomen as the assailant's intention is to cause a fatal injury to the person, preferably in a single stab or sometimes more than one stab wound for assurance of lethality. Stab wounds in the limbs are very rare and could be possible as defensive wounds or can be produced during the dynamics of the situation and relative movements of the victim and assailant. The shape of a stab wound is better appreciated by external examination rather than volume rendering a 3D image in PMCT; however, the depth and track of the wound and collection of blood inside the body due to the stab can be easily assessed by PMCT.

Animal bites

Animal bites found on a dead body could be due to antemortem or post-mortem animal activity. Animal bites, though they can be found in any part of the body, it is common in the limbs due to the proximity to the animal and also, limbs being the peripheral part, are more exposed and accessible to the animal than the central trunk. Ante-mortem animal bites are one of the major problems which result in higher morbidity and mortality. Though most of the time, animal bites are mild, they require medical attention to prevent the spread of any infection. Common animal bites encountered in routine medical practice include those made by snakes, dogs, cats, and monkeys. Snakes have a typical fang mark on biting, whereas animals like dogs, cats, and monkeys have teeth marks. The carnivore bites usually have a pattern which shows pits, punctures, and furrows on the skin and bones, while patterns like scalloping, disarticulation, and fracture are seen over the bones (Figure 6.51). There is evidence of vitality at the edge of the wounds which helps in differentiating them from post-mortem animal scavenging.

Post-mortem animal activity on corpses is a common phenomenon which is part of the natural food chain/cycle for the recycling of the nutrients like proteins, carbohydrates, fats, etc., back to the source. The type of animal causing scavenging activity depends on the place where the cadaver is found. It could be indoor corpses which can be scavenged by animals like rodents (Figure 6.52), cockroaches, ants, pet cats or dogs, etc. Outdoor corpses again depend on the varying geography; it could be urban, rural, forests, shallow/deep water, etc. Outdoor

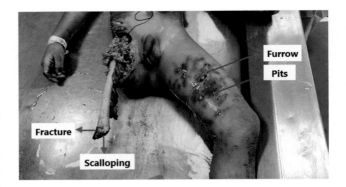

FIGURE 6.51: A case of a young boy attacked by dogs which caused major injuries to the lower limbs, including disarticulation of the right leg below the level of the lower third of the right thigh and also exposing the underlying bone, muscles and soft tissue. The vital reaction can be seen at the edges of the wound.

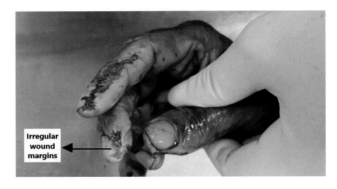

FIGURE 6.52: A case where the deceased was found dead inside a house, the fingertips show wounds with irregular margins. The edges and margins of the wound show no vital reaction.

scavenging animals could be rodents, dogs, cats, ants, wild carnivores, eagles, vultures, or aquatic animals like fish, crabs, etc. All these post-mortem injuries lack vital reactions along the edges unless in peri-mortem animal scavenging, where it happens immediately after death; here, the gross appearance could be deceiving.

Firearm/missile injury

The injury pattern due to firearms depends upon the type of weapon used, the nature of the bullet/pellets and the distance between the firing point and the target. The entry and exit wounds can be examined better by inspecting the external surface of the body during the external examination/visual autopsy (Figures 6.53 and 6.54). PMCT has a role in the determination of the path of the traversing missile into the body. PMCT has a greater role in ruling out any retained bullet/pellets or foreign particles inside the body. The identification and retrieval of such bullets/pellets or foreign particles is an important part of the autopsy. Precaution should be taken while removing the retained material so that no

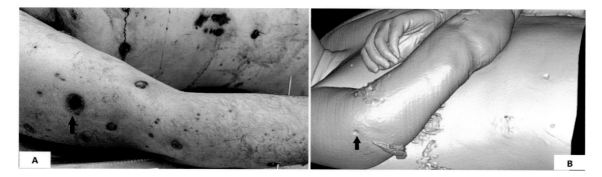

FIGURE 6.53: Firearm wound marked with black arrows in A: External examination; B: Volume rendering 3D image showing the firearm wound.

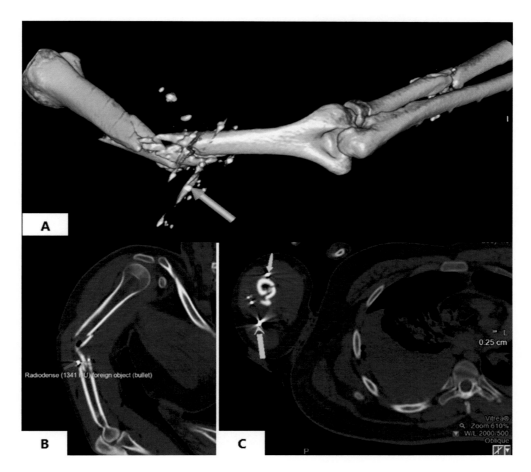

FIGURE 6.54: In the same case as Fig. 6.53: A: Volume rendering 3D image of the skeleton showing comminuted fracture-dislocation of the humerus bone and fracture of the radius bone. The foreign particle/projectile fragments are present, which are marked with an arrow. B: Coronal section of PMCT showing comminuted fracture-dislocation of the humerus bone and projectile fragment. C: Axial section of PMCT showing comminuted fracture-dislocation of the humerus bone and projectile fragment.

extra mark should be made over the surface for determination and identification of the nature and type of firearm. With the help of PMCT exact location of the bullet/foreign material can be accessed, and retrieval can be done by a minimally invasive procedure (Figures 6.55 and 6.56). The assessment of the underlying bone to identify the presence of any fracture/dislocation is also possible with PMCT in a better way. Firearm injuries involving the limbs could be fatal if any major vessel is injured or a bone fracture causes a haemorrhagic shock.

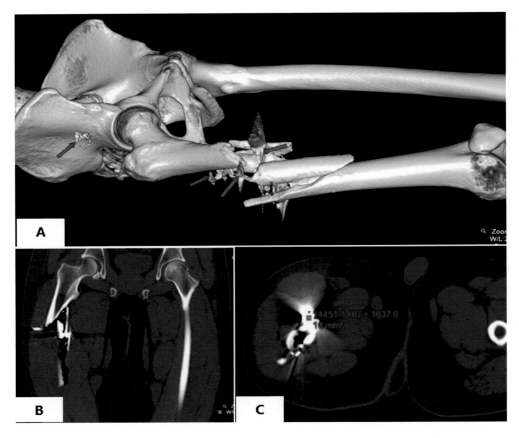

FIGURE 6.55: In a case of firearm injury to the lower limb, A: Volume rendering 3D image showing comminuted fracture of the right femur bone and right iliac bone. B: Coronal section of PMCT showing comminuted fracture of the right femur and presence of metallic projectile. C: Axial section of the right thigh showing comminuted fracture of the right femur and presence of metallic projectile.

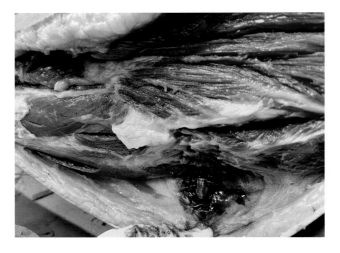

FIGURE 6.56: In the same case as Fig. 6.55 of firearm injury to the right thigh, a traditional autopsy showing the presence of a bullet corresponding to the position of the metallic foreign body identified in PMCT.

Bibliography

Benoudina S, Weerakkody Y. Winquist classification of femoral shaft fractures. Reference article, *Radiopaedia.org.* (accessed on 13 October 2022) https://doi.org/10.53347/rID-48180

Committee on Injury and Poison Prevention. American Academy of Pediatrics: Falls from heights: Windows, roofs, and balconies. *Pediatrics* 2001;107:1188–1191.

Datir A, Hacking C. Supracondylar humeral fracture. Reference article, *Radiopaedia.org.* (accessed on 13 October 2022) https://doi.org/10.53347/rID-2130

Datir A, Qureshi P. Patellar fracture. Reference article, *Radiopaedia .org.* (accessed on 13 October 2022) https://doi.org/10.53347/rID-1357

Feger J. Distal femoral fracture. Reference article, *Radiopaedia.org.* (accessed on 13 October 2022) https://doi.org/10.53347/rID-77861

Francis P, Whatman C, Sheerin K, Hume P, Johnson MI. The proportion of lower limb running injuries by gender, anatomical location and specific pathology: A systematic review. *J Sports Sci Med.* 2019 February 11;18(1):21–31. PMID: 30787648; PMCID: PMC6370968.

Gaillard F, Knipe H. Humeral shaft fracture. Reference article, *Radiopaedia.org.* (accessed on 13 October 2022) https://doi.org/10.53347/rID-18154

Gaillard F, Weerakkody Y. Proximal humeral fracture. Reference article, *Radiopaedia.org.* (accessed on 13 October 2022) https://doi.org/10.53347/rID-18277

Gulati D, Aggarwal AN, Kumar S, Agarwal A. Skeletal injuries following unintentional fall from height. *Ulus Travma Acil Cerrahi Derg.* 2012;18(2):141–146.

Harvey H, Shaggah M. Pelvic fractures. Reference article, *Radiopaedia.org.* (accessed on 13 October 2022) https://doi.org/10.53347/rID-15002.

Jones J, Lustosa L. Proximal femoral fractures. Reference article, *Radiopaedia.org.* (accessed on 13 October 2022) https://doi.org/10.53347/rID-28267

Knipe H, Yap J. Atypical femoral fracture. Reference article, *Radiopaedia.org.* (accessed on 13 October 2022) https://doi.org/10.53347/rID-28969

Kumar N. Pattern of fractures and dislocations in road traffic accident victims in a Tertiary Care Institute of Central India. *Int J Sci Stud* 2016;4(4):147–149.

Lapostolle F, Borron SW, Gere C, Dallemagne F, Beruben A, Lapandry C, et al. Victims of fall from height. Study of 287 patients and determination of clinical prognostic factors [Article in French] *Ann Fr Anesth Reanim.* 2004;23:689–693.

Libby C, Frane N, Bentley TP. Scapula fracture [Updated 2022 Jul 18]. In: *StatPearls [Internet].* Treasure Island (FL): StatPearls Publishing, 2022 January.

Ngunde PJ, Akongnwi ACN, Mefire CA, Puis F, Gounou E, Nkfusai NC, Nwarie UG, Cumber SN. Prevalence and pattern of lower extremity injuries due to road traffic crashes in Fako Division, Cameroon. *Pan Afr Med J.* 2019 January 30;32:53. https://doi.org/10.11604/pamj.2019.32.53.17514. PMID: 31143358; PMCID: PMC6522147.

Pan RH, Chang NT, Chu D, Hsu KF, Hsu YN, Hsu JC, Tseng LY, Yang NP. Epidemiology of orthopedic fractures and other injuries among inpatients admitted due to traffic accidents: A 10-year nationwide survey in Taiwan. *Sci World J.* 2014 February 5;2014:637872. https://doi.org/10.1155/2014/637872. PMID: 24672344; PMCID: PMC3932229.

Radswiki T, Fortin F. Tibial tuberosity avulsion fracture. Reference article, *Radiopaedia.org.* (accessed on 13 October 2022) https://doi.org/10.53347/rID-15612

Radswiki T, Lustosa L. Tibial plateau fracture. Reference article, *Radiopaedia.org.* (accessed on 13 October 2022) https://doi.org/10.53347/rID-15615

Shkrum MJ, Ramsay DA. *Forensic pathology of trauma, common problems for the pathologist.* Chapter 6, 7, and 8. Totowa, NJ: Humana Press, 2007.

Sip M, Serniak B, Rogozinski D, Kosec R, Zajo A, Vokaty S, Bräutigam T, Krawczuk P, Zawada B, Dabrowski M. Tactical medicine inspiring civilian rescue medicine in the management of haemorrhage. *Disaster Emerg Med J.* 2018;3(1):15–21.

Sonbol AM, Almulla AA, Hetaimish BM, Taha WS, Mohmmedthani TS, Alfraid TA, Alrashidi YA. Prevalence of femoral shaft fractures and associated injuries among adults after road traffic accidents in a Saudi Arabian trauma center. *J Musculoskelet Surg Res.* 2018;2:62–65.

Torlincasi AM, Lopez RA, Waseem M. Acute compartment syndrome. *StatPearls [Internet].* 2022 January.

7 SUDDEN DEATH

Sudden death is commonly defined as (i) a natural death that occurs within 6 hours of the beginning of symptoms in an apparently healthy subject, (ii) one whose disease was not so severe that a fatal outcome would have been expected, or (iii) In cases of unwitnessed death, which is a common situation in forensic practice, this definition requires that the deceased was last seen alive and functioning normally 24 hours before being found dead.

Sudden death (SD), also known as sudden and unexpected natural death, refers to deaths not preceded by significant symptoms. Thus, it excludes violent or traumatic deaths. The World Health Organization (WHO) defines sudden natural death as being within 24 hours from the onset of symptoms. However, this is too long clinically and pathologically, so conventionally accepted is death within 1 hour from the onset of illness. The description of 'unexplained' death may be an equally common reason for medico-legal investigation as the terms 'sudden' or 'unexpected' are not always accurate in explaining the cause of death. Death may appear sudden or unexpected, but it is the outcome of the pathological processes culminating in a terminal event. As defined by Madea, sudden death is 'any rapid (without prodrome), unexpected or unforeseen, that occurs in apparently healthy people or ill patients during a benign phase of their disease'. Pre-autopsy information is crucial for the forensic pathologist and requires the statements of witnesses, family members of the deceased, and, lastly, treating physicians or the rescue team that attempted resuscitation. Medical history among the family, the drugs consumed, and the type of activities performed by the deceased in the moments before death can be important in assessing the whole scenario associated with the death. Traditional autopsy helps in histopathological and toxicological analysis of the samples to find the cause of death; however, post-mortem computed tomography (PMCT) offers the potential to avoid open autopsy in many cases due to its evolving role in the investigation of non-suspicious adult death. Imaging has had a role in autopsy investigations for many decades revolving around plain radiograph identification of foreign objects (e.g., bullets) and fractures. With the advent of computed tomography (CT) and magnetic resonance imaging (MRI), diagnostic imaging has become extremely important in routine cases. For many reasons, the demand for non-invasive or minimally invasive post-mortem imaging has increased in recent years. Public concern about open autopsy has been on an uprise due to ethical and religious objections, possibly furthered by organ retention scandals

The most prevalent cause, in any case of SD, is related to cardiovascular diseases, which are also known as sudden cardiac death (SCD). SCD is defined as an unexpected death from cardiac complications occurring in a previously healthy individual or unwitnessed natural death of a person observed to be well within 24 hours of being found dead. When a post-mortem examination is not able to identify any cardiac abnormalities, then it is referred to as non-cardiac sudden death. The main organs involved in non-cardiac sudden deaths are the central nervous system (CNS) and respiratory systems (RS). The common causes of death in RS are fatal pulmonary emboli, severe pneumonia, anaphylaxis, and sudden airway obstruction. In CNS, intracerebral haemorrhage, brain infarct, subarachnoid haemorrhage, and status epilepticus are the cause of SD.

Cardiac causes

According to the literature, SCD affects more than 3 million people annually worldwide. SCD in young is a tragic event, with an incidence of 1–2 per 100,000 per year; the burden of SCD in young is disproportionately large because of their greater life expectancy and the burden on their families. The most common cause of SCD in people above 50 years is coronary artery disease and associated myocardial ischaemia/infarction. But SCD in individuals less than 45 years of age is mainly due to genetic, congenital, or structural anomalies. The most common ones documented are genetic cardiomyopathies like hypertrophic, dilated and restrictive cardiomyopathies, congenital anomalies of the coronaries, and specific genetic mutations causing electrophysiological abnormalities. Mak et al. showed that sudden arrhythmia death syndrome accounts for about 30% of sudden cardiac death in young people. Their study revealed that coronary artery disease was the major cause of death, followed by structural heart diseases (35–40%), and the remaining 25% of the deaths were unexplained. Genetic analysis showed the presence of positive heterozygous genetic variants in 29% of them. Hence, they concluded by emphasizing the importance of next-generation sequencing molecular autopsy adjunctive to conventional forensic investigations in diagnosing young SCD victims. Another study done by Thiene reported that around 50% of sudden cardiac death cases are genetic in origin, and the genetic approach should be part of the routine post-mortem study of SCD cases.

A study by Eckart et al. revealed that the incidence of SCD was 6.7 per 100,000 in males and 1.4 per 100,000 in females. The overall incidence of SCD was 1.2 per 100,000 persons per year for persons below 35 years of age. The incidence of fatal atherosclerotic coronary artery disease was 0.7 per 100,000 in ages less than 35 years of age, and it was 13.7 per 100,000 for those above 35 years of age. Identifiable structural heart diseases causing SCD were found in 79% of the cases, and normal heart morphology was seen in 21%.

Doolan et al., in their study, mentioned that they could not be able to identify the exact cause of death in 31% of the cases and most of which were presumed to be primary arrhythmogenic cardiac disorders. Coronary artery diseases were encountered in 24%, HCM/unexplained left ventricular hypertrophy was encountered in 15%, and clear evidence of myocarditis was noted in 12% of the cases.

Dressler's syndrome

Dressler's syndrome is also known as post-myocardial infarction syndrome or post-cardiac injury syndrome. It is a form of pericarditis that is seen in cases of myocardial infarction or injury to the myocardium, which results in an autoimmune inflammatory reaction to myocardial neo-antigens. It commonly occurs about 2 to 10 weeks after the myocardial injury. Dressler's syndrome is more common in cases where there is transmural infarction of the myocardium. It is common in the younger age group with MI and has no gender or racial predilection.

Case of sudden death due to complications of MI

A 30-year-old male was brought to the hospital with a history of sudden onset of chest pain; the person was unconscious

DOI: 10.1201/9781003383703-7

on arrival, and examination in the casualty revealed he was brought dead. The person had no history of any medical illness or was not on any medications. A medico-legal case was registered as he was declared dead on arrival, and the cause of death was not known. The body of the deceased was shifted to the mortuary for post-mortem examination. Externally there was no injury or any other signs of trauma or disease. PMCT examination of the deceased revealed features of pulmonary oedema. Autopsy internal examination of the chest revealed a pericardium adherent to the myocardium over the anterior surface of the left ventricle with features of fibrin-haemorrhagic pericarditis (Figure 7.1). Explant coronary angiography was done in the case which showed areas of the myocardium of the anterior wall and anteroseptal area near the apex with perfusion deficits (Figure 7.2) and occlusion of the left anterior descending artery in the lower one-third (Figures 7.3 and 7.4). The area of perfusion deficits corresponded to the transmural myocardial infarct and necrosis region (Figure 7.5).

Haemopericardium/cardiac tamponade

Haemopericardium/cardiac tamponade is another important cause of sudden cardiac death. Haemopericardium is the condition where blood accumulates in the pericardial sac, which could be due to heart wall rupture consequent upon necrosis/trauma or due to an intrapericardial rupture of the ascending aorta, usually following an aneurysm. In both these case varieties, death commonly occurs due to an obstructive type of cardiac shock following the accumulation of blood in the pericardium leading to increased intrapericardial pressure, which compresses the heart chambers. This, in turn, increases the intracardiac pressure and causes impaired venous return and an increase in venous pressure culminating in diastolic ventricular

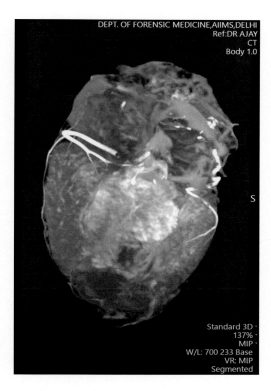

FIGURE 7.2: Explant coronary angiography was done in the case, which on 3D volume rendering MIP showed areas of the myocardium of the anterior wall and anteroseptal area near the apex with perfusion deficits.

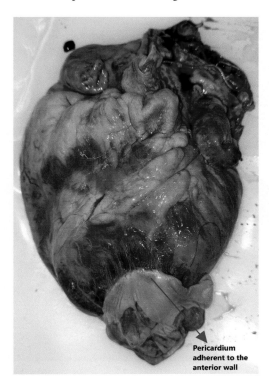

FIGURE 7.1: The pericardial sac is adherent to the left ventricle on the anterior, the ventricle wall showing roughened and reddened epicardial surface suggestive of fibrin-haemorrhagic pericarditis above the place of the transmural infarct.

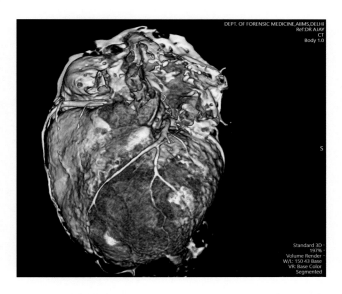

FIGURE 7.3: Explant coronary angiography was done in the case, which on 3D volume rendering with a base colour, showed narrowing and occlusion of the left anterior descending artery in the lower third.

collapse and cardiac arrest. The normal pericardial fluid volume is 30–50 ml, and a rapidly collecting haemopericardium even up to the volume of 200–300 ml is likely more fatal due to cardiac tamponade rather than a slowly accumulating pericardial fluid even up to the volume of 500–2000 ml as in the latter situation there is time for the accommodation of greater volumes

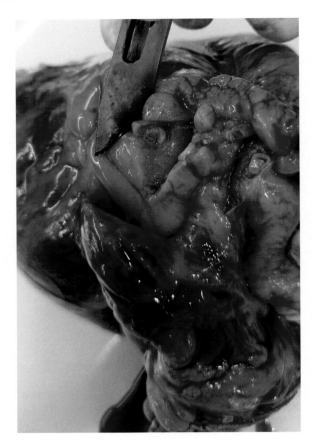

FIGURE 7.4: Occlusion of the left anterior coronary artery seen in the lower third region corresponding to the occlusion seen in the explant angiography.

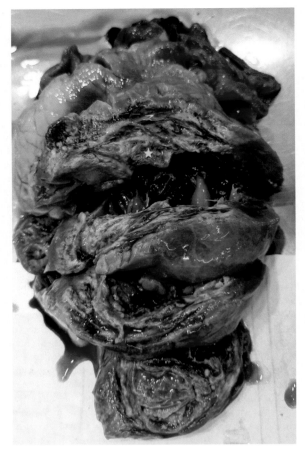

FIGURE 7.5: The case showing transmural infarct involving the anterior wall of the left ventricle (green star) with necrosis (yellow star) and infarct involving the anteroseptal region (red star).

due to gradual distension of the pericardial sac. Ascending aortic dissection is also a common cause of cardiac tamponade, and it is usually due to the dissection of the ascending aorta occurring as a result of medial cystic necrosis, chronic hypertension, Marfan's syndrome, aortic coarctation, or bicuspid aortic valve. Hemopericardium can be present with or without sedimentation and with or without forming a so-called 'target' or 'armoured heart' sign in the post-mortem setting.

Case of cardiac rupture due to MI

A 49-year-old suddenly collapsed while walking; he was taken to the hospital, where he was declared dead on arrival. The body was shifted to the Department of Forensic Medicine & Toxicology, AIIMS, New Delhi, to determine the cause of death. The deceased had no significant medical history, and on external autopsy examination, two small abrasions were appreciable over the forehead and left knee due to the sudden collapse while walking. PMCT examination revealed a pericardial hyperdense ring and flattening of the anterior surface of the right chamber of the heart, referred to as the flattening heart sign; both of these are suggestive of a possible cardiac tamponade (Figures 7.6 and 7.7). An internal autopsy revealed a blood clot in the pericardial sac surrounding the heart (Figure 7.8). The examination of the heart revealed that there was a ventricular rupture on the posterior wall of the left ventricle (Figure 7.9). Short-axis dissection of the heart showed features of old myocardial infarction on the posterior wall and rupture of the posterior wall near the junction with the inter-ventricular septum (Figure 7.10).

Case of sudden death with previous MI and coronary stents

A 58-year-old male was running on a treadmill in the gym when he suddenly became unconscious. He was brought to AIIMS, New Delhi's, emergency room, where resuscitation was

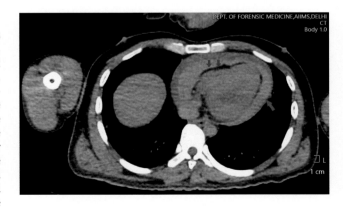

FIGURE 7.6: Axial section of PMCT chest in soft tissue window showing pericardial hyperdense ring (red arrow) and flattening of the anterior surface of right heart chamber called flattened heart sign; both findings are suggestive of cardiac tamponade in the case.

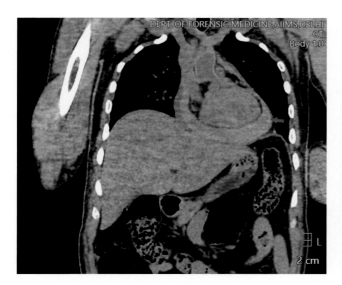

FIGURE 7.7: Coronal section of PMCT chest in soft tissue window showing pericardial hyperdense ring suggestive of cardiac tamponade in the case.

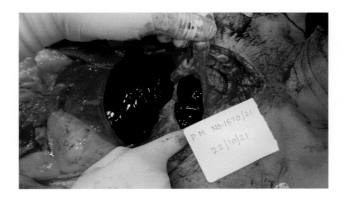

FIGURE 7.8: Autopsy internal examination of the thoracic cavity showing a blood clot surrounding the heart present within the pericardial sac.

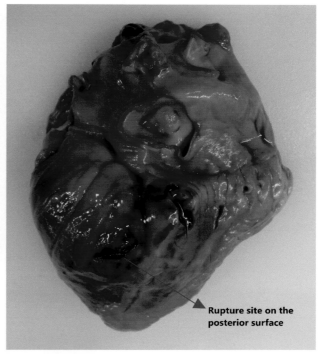

FIGURE 7.9: Examination of the heart shows a rupture on the posterior wall of the left ventricle with haemorrhagic infiltration in the surrounding epicardial surface.

PMCT were recorded in this case. There were diffuse ground glass opacities and septal thickening in both lungs (Figures 7.11 and 7.12). The examination of the heart showed the presence of the previous three PCI stents in the three vessels: left anterior descending artery, left circumflex artery, and right coronary artery (Figures 7.13–7.16). The cause of death in the case was concluded as myocardial infarction and its subsequent medical complications. Cases like these do not require an autopsy, but due to the legal binding of an MLC case, it becomes compulsory to conduct an autopsy. In these cases, Virtual autopsy is of immense use as it helps to reconfirm the treatment records

immediately done, and the person was revived. The deceased, on revival, was diagnosed with acute coronary syndrome with lateral wall myocardial infarction. He didn't regain consciousness and was admitted to the cardiac intensive care unit for close monitoring. The deceased had a medical history of diabetes mellitus, hypertension, and three previous PCI procedures. The patient was taken to the hospital by bystanders who gave an unclear history. The person was unconscious, and the reason for becoming unconscious was not clear at the time of admission; a medico-legal case (MLC) was registered. During the course of treatment, he died. Since a medico-legal case was registered, the police requested an autopsy as a standard protocol in India for legal purposes. A virtual autopsy was conducted in this case, and the dead body of the deceased was not dissected. There were clear medical records of the treatment received at AIIMS, New Delhi, which showed that the deceased had suffered from a myocardial infarction of the lateral wall due to acute coronary syndrome during the course of the hospital treatment. Autopsy, in this case, was mainly to confirm the medical record findings and to rule out the presence of any unnatural means causing death. Digital X-ray and

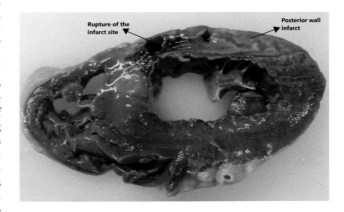

FIGURE 7.10: Short-axis dissection of the ventricles showing old infarct over the posterior wall of the left ventricle and posterior inter-ventricular septum. The rupture site is seen near the junction of the posterior wall and inter-ventricular septum with surrounding haemorrhagic infiltration.

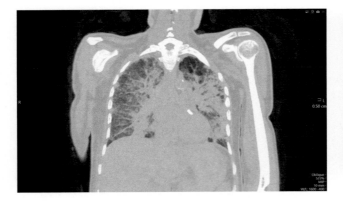

FIGURE 7.11: Chest PMCT showing diffuse GGO, septal thickening, and consolidation of multiple places of the lung.

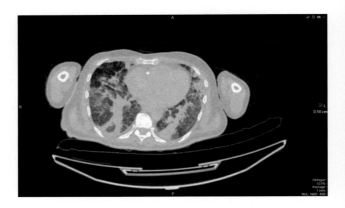

FIGURE 7.12: Chest PMCT showing diffuse GGO, septal thickening, and consolidation of multiple places of the lower lobe of both lungs.

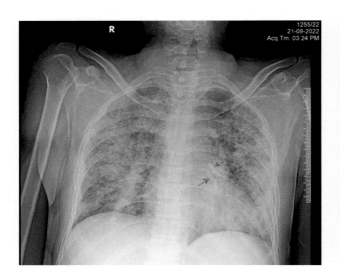

FIGURE 7.13: Chest X-ray AP view showing multiple cardiac stents of previous PCI in the case and diffuse ground glass opacity with consolidation at places.

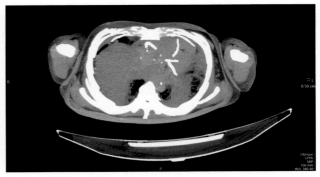

FIGURE 7.14: Chest PMCT in MIP showing multiple cardiac stents of previous PCI.

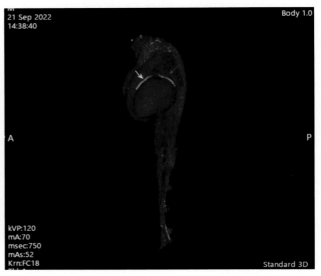

FIGURE 7.15: Volume rendering 3D image of the heart showing PCI stents of the left circumflex artery (blue arrow) and the left anterior descending artery (yellow arrow).

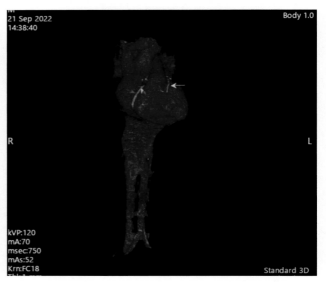

FIGURE 7.16: Volume rendering 3D image of the heart showing PCI stents of the right coronary artery (red arrow) and the left anterior descending artery (yellow arrow).

and also rule out unnatural means causing death and the same time, supports the dignified management of the dead by avoiding unnecessary invasive autopsy.

Coronary calcification

Computed tomographic scanning has the advantage of both rapid image acquisition and high contrast and spatial resolution, which helps in the quantification of coronary calcium. Post-mortem studies have shown that the extent of coronary calcification can be correlated with the severity of coronary stenosis and the frequency of myocardial infarction. Coronary artery calcification (CAC) is predictive of major cardiovascular events, and coronary calcifications measured by CT are usually expressed as an 'Agatston score'. The image analysis technique is used to calculate the degree of stenosis and the histological presence of calcification. Coronary calcium quantification by CT is an accurate, cost-effective screening method of examination for coronary heart disease since coronary artery calcification (Figures 7.17–7.19) unequivocally reflects CAD. Any region of interest with a CT density >130 HUs is used to define Agatston's score, and the PACS system requires dedicated software to calculate it. The sum of the Agatston score obtained from the evaluation of calcified lesions within each artery (LCX, LAD, and RCA) is computed as the total coronary artery calcification score (CACS). The stenosis within the lumen was divided into three categories, which include: mild (<25% occlusion), moderate (25–75% occlusion) and severe (with >75% occlusion) based on the calculation of the quotient percentage of the lumen diameter divided by the diameter of the internal elastic membrane. The degree of stenosis and calcification in PMCT calcification score versus histological evaluation shows PMCT calcification score is significantly higher in those with severe when compared to moderate or mild stenosis. PMCT calcification score (PMCT CS) showed a positive correlation with the presence of calcification, and PMCT CS increased with increasing severity of stenosis. LAD, followed by the RCA, is the most frequently and most extensively calcified artery, using both PMCT calcium score and histology due to the local haemodynamic and anatomic particularities. CT exhibits greater detection rates than conventional/digital

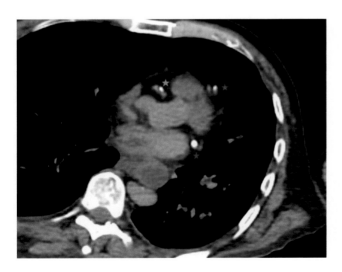

FIGURE 7.17: Axial section of chest PMCT in soft tissue window showing calcification of the left anterior descending artery (red star), left circumflex artery (blue star), and right coronary artery (green star).

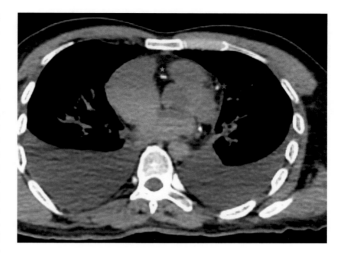

FIGURE 7.18: Axial section of the chest PMCT in soft tissue window showing calcification of the left anterior descending artery (red star), left circumflex artery (blue star), and right coronary artery (green star).

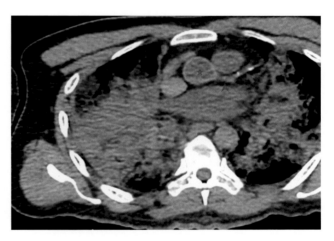

FIGURE 7.19: Axial section of the chest PMCT in soft tissue window showing calcification of the left anterior descending artery (red arrow), left coronary artery (red arrowhead), and aorta (red star).

radiography and is an extremely sensitive modality for the detection of calcium. According to the CAC score, patients/deceased may be classified into risk groups, very low risk with 0 Agatston units (AU), low risk with 1–99 AU, moderate risk with 100–299 AU and high risk with ≥300 AU. Asymptomatic patients have a sevenfold increase in the risk of myocardial infarction or coronary heart disease with an Agatston score >300 AU compared to patients with no CAC score. A high likelihood of a coronary event or at least one significant coronary stenosis is indicated by a CAC score of >400 and is a predictor of death or myocardial infarction (MI) in both symptomatic as well as asymptomatic patients. CAC is not a method to identify the severity of coronary artery stenosis, a significant CAC may be present in the absence of flow-limiting coronary artery stenosis and also coronary artery disease may be present in the absence of CAC. In patients classified as 'low risk' by traditional risk factor scoring systems, a high burden of CAC may be present and conversely absent in patients classified as 'high risk'. Coronary artery disease risk stratification is improved by combining CAC with traditional risk factors.

Valve calcification

The most common cardiac valve disease in developed countries is aortic valve disease, with moderate or severe aortic stenosis reported in ~5% of patients aged >75 years. The leading cause of aortic stenosis is calcific valvular degeneration. The presence of aortic valve calcification (Figure 7.20) should be identified, and quantification is described as None, Mild, Moderate, or Severe. To identify severe stenosis the cut-off values for the aortic valve Agatston calcium score is ≥2065 AU for males and ≥1274 AU for females. Moderate/Severe aortic valve calcification may indicate the presence of aortic valve stenosis. In cases with aortic valve calcification, the diameter of the root of the aorta and ascending aorta should also be reviewed on multiplanar reformats where possible. Coronary CT calcium scoring can be quantified, and calcification is the predominant driver of aortic stenosis.

Calcification of the mitral leaflets or mitral annulus is a common incidental finding. Mitral leaflet calcification (Figure 7.21) may be associated with rheumatic heart disease or advanced

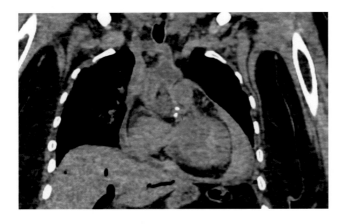

FIGURE 7.20: Coronal section of the chest PMCT in soft tissue window showing calcification of the aortic valve in a case with haemopericardium.

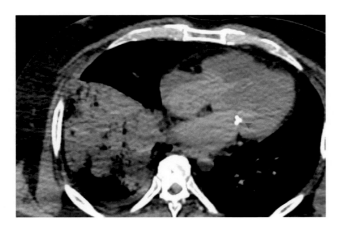

FIGURE 7.21: Axial section of chest PMCT in soft tissue window showing calcification of the mitral valve.

renal impairment. Mitral annular calcification can be extensive and usually demonstrates a curvilinear morphology in the posterior and outer rings of the valve. Mitral annular calcification is commonly mistaken as calcification in the left circumflex coronary artery. Mitral calcification can be graded by CT using a simple visual grading of None, Mild, Moderate, or Severe.

Myocardial calcification

Myocardial calcification usually occurs secondary to myocardial infarction or also in conditions like trauma, inflammation, neoplastic infiltration, hypertrophic cardiomyopathy, or infection. A thin curvilinear appearance with associated myocardial thinning or fatty infiltration is associated with dystrophic myocardial calcification. Chronic rheumatic mitral stenosis may also demonstrate left atrial wall calcification. Pericardial calcification is usually present at sites of previous fibrosis or pericardial inflammation. Infection (especially viral and tuberculosis), cardiac surgery, trauma, radiotherapy, rheumatic heart disease, collagen vascular disease, uraemic pericarditis, and hemopericardium are conditions associated with pericardial calcification.

Coronary artery disease (CAD) is a common cause of death, and diagnosis can be made using PMCT augmented by angiography (PMCTA). However, the cost and invasiveness of the procedure increase with the addition of angiography to PMCT. A clinical risk ratio assigned with the Agatston score, the volume and density of calcification in the coronary arteries can be measured. A cause of death can not be diagnosed by a high CAC score. If there is significant CAC, as demonstrated by a CAC (Agatston) score of >400, the subsequent targeted coronary PMCTA will demonstrate significant CAD in 97.4% of cases.

Cardiothoracic ratio (CTR)

Cardiomegaly is defined as greater heart weight or ventricular thickness, known as hypertrophy of the heart or enlarged chamber size, known as dilation. Increased heart weight is indicative of underlying cardiovascular disease and is significant in the medico-legal context. Studies have shown that the discriminative power of the CTR was 73–79% on using a 0.5 cut-off value for differentiating normal heart weight from cardiomegaly. Increasing the CTR cut-off value to 0.57 shows an improved ability to diagnose cardiomegaly by increasing specificity. The number of false positives is significantly restricted by setting a cut-off value of 0.57 for the PMCT CTR, and a diagnosis of cardiomegaly on PMCT will also be found at autopsy (Figure 7.22). The main limitation of the score includes the change in the size of the heart due to decomposition.

The CTR is frequently used in clinical practice as a radiographic index of the heart, and CTR >0.50 is generally defined as cardiomegaly. The threshold CTR to detect cardiomegaly on PMCT may differ from the CTR on ante-mortem CT because of radiological cardiomegaly on pPMCT in patients with a normal heart. The cardiac diameter is bordered by the outer borders of the heart, and the thoracic diameter is delineated by the inner borders of the thoracic cavity. The two measurements are made parallel to each other and are not necessarily made at the same level. CTR generally increases post-mortem; therefore, it is important to avoid overestimating cardiomegaly by using 0.5 as the cut-off value. Discrimination between normal heart weight and overweighed heart at PMCT cannot be done alone by CTR and also include parameters that influence the CTR, such as means BMI, age, and gender.

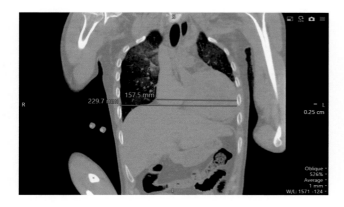

FIGURE 7.22: Chest PMCT coronal section, measurement of the heart and the thoracic diameter for calculating cardiothoracic ratio (CTR). In this case, CTR is 0.68, which clearly shows cardiomegaly.

Studies have shown that the heart wall was significantly thicker on PMCT than on AMCT (p < 0.0001). AMCT with and without contrast medium at any site of the ventricle shows no significant differences. When measured without papillary muscles or epicardial fat according to conventional methods, the heart wall was significantly thicker on PMCT than on pathology specimens.

The relationship between actual heart weight and left ventricular circumferential area (LVCA) is important as LVCA has been proposed as a simple and effective measure of heart weight. The mean measured LVCA, and actual heart weight (p < 0.0001, correlation coefficient 0.707) has a significant and strong positive correlation. LVCA and calculated heart weight reflect actual heart weight, which is found as almost the same as autopsy, according to studies.

Negative autopsy cases

The most common cause of SCD in the elderly above 50 years of age is coronary artery disease and associated myocardial ischaemia/infarction. But SCD in young individuals <45 years of age can occur due to genetic, congenital, or structural cardiac anomalies. The most common ones documented are genetic cardiomyopathies like hypertrophic, dilated and restrictive cardiomyopathies, congenital anomalies of the coronaries, and specific genetic mutations causing electrophysiological abnormalities. Examining the heart thoroughly by an expert can help identify all the structural heart abnormalities causing SCD, but in the majority of cases, heart examination for SCD in a young will be normal; hence, these cases are considered negative autopsy cases, where the exact aetiology cannot be determined. A thorough literature search on SCD in young says that the majority of these cases are due to cardiac channelopathies and ventricular tachyarrhythmias of a genetic cause, like short QT and long QT syndromes, Brugada syndrome, Wolff–Parkinson–White syndrome, and other genetic electrophysiological syndromes. Regular autopsy in these patients will usually not be informative and does not yield any gross structural abnormality. Hence, all these cases are referred to as negative autopsy cases. The exact cause and diagnosis in these cases can only be made by doing proper genetic work to identify the cause of death. Hence, a molecular autopsy can give an explanation for all these cases of negative autopsy SCD.

Sudden death and COVID-19

Recent literature reviews based on a PubMed search of 'autopsy', 'lung', and 'COVID-19' report more than 500 cases in about 45 publications from North and South America, Europe, and Asia. Out of these, histopathology of post-mortem samples was described in over 450 cases. A high incidence of deep vein thrombosis and pulmonary embolism was reported among COVID-19 decedents, suggesting vascular injury, inflammation, and vascular remodelling in COVID-19-infected endothelial cells. Capillary microthrombi were seen frequently in acute lung injury patients of COVID-19 along with thrombosis of all sized vessels at extra-pulmonary sites.

Mukerji et al. reviewed 24 autopsy studies published in January 2020 for neuropathological findings of COVID-19. In most of the studies, gross brain examinations reported either no significant findings or no acute abnormalities. In rest, haemorrhage was the most common abnormality reported, ranging from petechial bleedings and punctate subarachnoid haemorrhages to large cerebral/cerebellar haemorrhages and haemorrhagic middle cerebral artery stroke. Large acute and/or subacute infarcts as well as lacunar infarcts/microinfarcts and watershed infarcts, were identified in several cases. Severe oedema resulting in herniation as well as mild to moderate oedema without herniation was also present. Mild focal perivascular, parenchymal, and leptomeningeal T-cell predominant lymphocytic infiltrates were identified in a large number of cases without clear evidence of vasculitis or meningoencephalitis. Moderate to intense microglial activation was also noted.

There are also reports of COVID-19-infected asymptomatic patients who died suddenly due to acute pulmonary embolism, which was discovered on post-mortem examination. These types of cases imply that sudden, unexpected deaths outside of the hospital may also be associated with COVID-19 infection during the pandemic period and now in the post-COVID-19 era where we witness an increase in sudden (cardiac) deaths in healthy people during physical activity due to acute catastrophic thromboembolic events. The long-term cardiovascular outcomes in COVID-19 survivors remain largely unclear. There has been significant interest in the impacts of COVID-19 infection on patients after they have recovered. At present, the data on the real incidence and relative risk of cardiovascular disease (CVD) after COVID-19 infection are limited. A nationwide cohort study from Estonia using electronic health care data on SARS-CoV-2 RNA-positive cases (n = 66,287) and reference group subjects (n = 254,969) with linkage to SARS-CoV-2 testing and death records documented that people infected with SARS-COV-2 had more than three times the risk of dying over the following year compared with those who remained uninfected. Mainous et al. performed an analysis of electronic health records (EHR) for a cohort of 13,638 patients, including COVID-19-positive and a comparison group of COVID-19-negative patients, who were followed for 12 months. The 12-month adjusted all-cause mortality risk was significantly higher for patients with severe COVID-19 compared to both COVID-19-negative patients (HR 2.50; 95% CI 2.02, 3.09) and mild COVID-19 patients (HR 1.87; 95% CI 1.28, 2.74).

Evidence of the factors related to and the total mortality impact of COVID-19 is needed to inform preventive measures and the clinical management of COVID-19 patients. However, information on causes of sudden death and the contribution of pre-existing health conditions to post-COVID-19 mortality is scarce.

Yadav et al. (2020), mention that SCD has emerged as a disturbing concern with COVID-19 infections. There is compelling evidence of an association between influenza epidemics and major cardiovascular events like myocarditis, stroke, and SCD. Although the direct causal association between SCD and COVID-19 remains unproven, data analysis suggests a plausible association. An increased incidence of SCD has been reported both in community and hospital settings. The mechanism of SCD in COVID-19 is considered to be multifactorial as there is a lack of data to support the exact causal relationship.

Baldi et al. (2020), from Italy, also observed that there is a significant positive association between the spread of COVID-19 and an increased number of out-of-hospital cardiac arrest. There is a 58% rise in cardiac arrest as compared to the previous years.

Guo et al. (2020), studied hospital data from China, which revealed that 27.8% of the admitted COVID-19 patients had evidence of myocardial injury with elevated troponin levels and also had more frequent malignant arrhythmias. The overall mortality was much higher in elevated troponin levels.

Gopimathannair et al. (2020), reviewed global surveys by the Heart Rhythm Society. Atrial fibrillation showed that tachyarrhythmia was most commonly reported than bradyarrhythmias in all the COVID-19 hospitalized patients.

Najaf et al.'s (2022) review on sudden cardiac death in COVID-19 patients mentions that the most commonly observed cardiovascular findings in COVID-19 infections are myocarditis, arrhythmias, acute coronary syndrome, atherosclerosis, DCM, myocardial infarction, and congestive heart failure. This was commonly observed in elderly individuals with a history of comorbidities like hypertension, diabetes, and dyslipidemias COVID-19 has led to the early development of COVID-19 vaccines primarily to help the healthcare workers and to prevent the severity of infection in the general population. Observational studies indicate that fever, myalgia, fatigue, and headache are the most common symptoms after vaccinations. However, meta-analysis data also reveals thrombosis, cerebral venous thrombosis, thrombocytopenia, myocarditis, pulmonary emboli, and hepatic portal vein thrombosis after the second dose of COVID-19 mRNA vaccination.

Myocarditis is a rare complication of COVID-19 mRNA vaccination, especially rare in young and adolescent males. According to the US Centers for Disease Control and Prevention, myopericarditis rates are 12.6 cases per million doses of second-dose mRNA vaccine that usually presents 2–3 days after the second dose of mRNA vaccination. Increasing evidence of myocarditis and pericarditis is reported as a complication of vaccination.

Sudden and unexpected death and conclusion in a legal autopsy report

In India, as per the Code of Criminal Procedure, 1973, when the **cause** and **manner of death** requires to be established by the police or magistrate in an investigation and the case of sudden unnatural death is sent for post-mortem examination, it is called a medico-legal case. The cases of sudden death due to natural causes which are explained completely and are due to evident documented natural causes, beyond any reasonable doubt and suspicion or when the death has been certified by a registered medical practitioner are non-medico-legal cases and not subjected to post-mortem examination. In some cases when there is reasonable doubt or suspicion, a complaint to the police or contradiction into the cause of death or the case is

dead on arrival without a clear medical history and circumstances of death, such cases are marked by a doctor as a medico-legal case.

There are various cases seen where death occurred suddenly during strenuous physical work or even during daily pursuits like in a toilet or while sleeping. Some cases are also seen where there is death in police custody due to mental stress as a precipitating factor of death. These deaths are unexplained and sometimes deemed suspicious by the relatives of the deceased, police, or the public although the death is due to a compromised diseased condition of the heart, coronary vessels, or other previously established diseases. There are certain cases examined where death was precipitated as a result of a simple blow, fall, or during heated arguments in a person of compromised cardiac condition. The purpose of post-mortem examination in these cases is to rule out or clarify the involvement of a criminal angle into the cause of death as autopsy plays an important role in determining the exact cause and manner of death. The possible causes of sudden and unexpected death keeping in legal view are:

1. Unnatural causes
2. Natural causes
    i)   Explained natural causes and diseases
    ii) Unexplained or suspicious death due to natural causes
3. Coexistence of unnatural and natural causes
    i)   Coexistence of evident certified natural cause with an unnatural cause
    ii) Coexistence of uncertified natural causes with an unnatural cause

1. **Unnatural causes**

   Unnatural causes are one of the most common causes of sudden and unexpected deaths. The manner may vary from accidental, suicidal, or homicidal. Accidental deaths include RTAs, railway accidents, natural calamities, aircraft accidents, traumatic asphyxia due to getting buried under a falling wall, earthquakes, etc. Suicidal causes are seen in cases of hanging, drowning, poisoning, firearm injury, cut wounds, etc., and homicidal varies from strangulation, firearms, stabbing, physical assault, poisoning, etc. Unnatural deaths may appear suspicious in most cases, but the post-mortem examination plays an important role to differentiate the manner of death. The details of unnatural death have been covered in the chapter on regional injury, mechanical injuries, and medico-legal aspects of injuries.

2. **Natural causes**

   Sudden deaths due to natural causes, with a history of illness or pre-existing disease of heart or other systemic diseases, are subjected to post-mortem examination. When there is a police complaint of foul play into the cause of death or the deceased is brought to the hospital as brought dead or dead on arrival and the doctor labels the case as medico-legal case due to the unawareness of cause and circumstances of death. In cases of dead on arrival where there is a fully explained medical document suggestive of death due to natural causes available and there is no injury or suspicion, the doctor can give a cause of death and death certificate and hand over the body to the legal heirs as a non-MLC case and there is no need of post-mortem examination. However, there are certain situations when the explanation is non-satisfactory or there is a criminal complaint, the post-mortem becomes mandatory to clarify and authenticate the cause of death by post-mortem examination and eliminate any foul play. It has been further classified into two types:

i) **Explained natural causes and diseases:** In such cases, the history of ailment or pathology is already present but not known to be in the advanced stage or grave enough to produce death. The abnormalities establish beyond any doubt the identity of the disease which causes death, e.g., coronary arteriosclerosis, chronic heart disease, or pneumonia. Post-mortem examination does not reveal any other reasonable cause of death, and the location, nature, severity and extent of the anatomical changes are sufficient to cause death but are not conclusive proof. As per *Gradowohl's Legal Medicine*, in many cases, the autopsy revealed that a case clinically recorded as coronary thrombosis has been one of a fatal condition in a completely different organ such as a cerebral haemorrhage or a mesenteric thrombosis. Such inaccuracy naturally gives rise to concern about unsuspected cases of homicide. 'Double pathology in death is not a rarity'. This aspect is explained in various causes of natural death.

ii) **Unexplained or suspicious death due to natural causes:** There is no history of any illness in an apparently healthy person who dies suddenly raising the suspicion in the minds of relatives and friends and a police complaint is made for any suspecting foul play. The police in such type of cases carry out an investigation to establish a cause of death – whether it is natural or unnatural or if there is any criminal intent/force behind the sudden and unexplained death. In cases of spontaneous intracerebral haemorrhage, ruptured myocardial infarction, and massive pulmonary thromboembolism such types of situations arise and during the autopsy the cause is established. This aspect is explained in various causes of natural death. We are citing below a case of such a category.

Case report of elevator accident injury with death due to heart attack

An elderly person was found crushed under an elevator and the police brought the body for post-mortem examination. On post-mortem examination, the presence of a contused abrasion over an area of 22 × 6 cm on the back and multiple abrasions and contusions over both upper and lower arms were analyzed and found to be post-mortem in nature. Hence the heart of the deceased was examined and was found to weigh 401 gm with an 80% blockage of the left coronary artery, a 40% blockage of the circumflex branch, and a 60% blockage of the right coronary artery. The injury over the back was caused due to the fall of the lift and the rest of the injuries were caused in an attempt to drag him out. All the injuries were post-mortem in nature having no contribution to death. The cause of death was due to massive myocardial infarction which occurred prior to being hit by the elevator. It was a case of unexplained suspicious death due to natural causes.

3. **Coexistence of unnatural and natural causes:** A number of cases are seen when there is a natural disease which may convert into death; however, sustaining some trauma – mental or physical resulting in death – such type of cases require a very meticulous autopsy for making an opinion for legal purposes. The victims of sudden natural death may sustain non-contributory injury incidents to agonal episodes where they collapse and fall without being able to protect themselves and may sustain injuries, which may suggest that trauma is somehow involved in these deaths. The correlation of terminal circumstances is essential to disclose the role, if any, played by trauma in these deaths. Again, natural diseases can create situations that may lead to fatal injuries, e.g., an epileptic patient may drown due to a seizure or a cardiac patient may sustain injuries from an automobile accident that occurs from his losing consciousness during a myocardial infarction as he drives along the highway. This probable interplay of trauma and natural disease in causing or contributing to death may give rise to very complex and challenging situations. If a victim dies of injury shortly after being hurt or at some considerable time interval in a continuous chain of complicated events, there is no doubt as to the manner of death. However, the situation becomes challenging when there is a symptom-free interval between apparent recovery from trauma and death from a known natural disease. In medicine, absolute diagnostic opinions, like mathematical calculations, are rare. In criminal cases, medical conclusions are based on a **reasonable degree of certainty** and it is beyond any reasonable doubt expected from a doctor as witness/expert witness in a court of law. The autopsy surgeon's opinion is based on the highest level of probability. A medical opinion is based on the facts and findings as they are available at the time of making a medico-legal opinion and the same may be revised in cases of the facts which form the basis for the opinion change. The following cases help to elaborate on this.

Case report of alleged poisoning with fatal pathological findings in the heart

An autopsy was conducted in AIIMS, New Delhi on a 48-year-old person, who was found unconscious in the bathroom of his house which was bolted from the inside. He was declared dead on arrival at the hospital. There was a strong allegation from the various family members that he has been killed by poisoning and should be treated as murder. The deceased was a known case of coronary artery disease and his angiogram was showing blockage of the coronary artery up to a level of 70%. During the post-mortem examination, the heart was soft and flabby weighing about 315 gm. The left anterior descending artery was 70% blocked and the left circumflex artery was 20% blocked. The right coronary artery was 70% blocked. The viscera was analyzed and showed no common poison. After thorough investigation and post-mortem examination, the final cause of death given by the medical board, in this case, was 'cardiac disease and coronary insufficiency cannot be ruled out'. The deceased family again filed a case in the Delhi High Court and asked for further viscera analysis from abroad. The High Court allowed the viscera to be sent to a foreign laboratory. The case is still not concluded as final. Hence our opinion may get a revision in case any significant finding of viscera test report from abroad.

i) **Coexistence of a certified natural cause with an unnatural cause:** The deceased may be suffering from some systemic disease which was under control with medication, and was not expected to die. However, he/she dies and the death is not properly explained, also foul play cannot be ruled out by the investigating agency as there is a complaint of foul play or there may be unexplained injuries. During autopsy, injuries may be found which may not appear to be sufficient to cause death in a healthy person, but these injuries may be the cause of death due to complications arising directly from the injury, but which is not demonstrable at autopsy. In such cases, it enables the doctor to attribute death to the injury with reasonable certainty.

Example: An elderly person known to be a cardiac patient subjected to minor trauma by local criminals dies within hours of the incident. During autopsy, evident findings of heart pathology are noted and opined to be the cause of death, but trauma, though minor, cannot be ruled out to be the triggering factor. So the cause of death would be heart pathology triggered by the traumatic incident.

Case report of pushing and shoving incident, Chandigarh, India

An 80-year-old male was allegedly pushed and shoved by some police officials while raiding his house and the person died in hospital after about 6–12 hours after the incident. As local police officials were involved, the case was handed over to CBI by the Hon'ble High Court, which requested AIIMS to provide an expert opinion to rule out natural or unnatural causes of death. During the post-mortem examination, no external or internal injuries were present. Grossly, the heart weighed about 415 gm and the right atrium contained a thrombus with clotted blood, the root of the aorta showed atherosclerotic changes and both the coronary arteries were thickened. The microscopic examination of the heart showed complicated lesions of atherosclerosis with calcification in the walls of both the coronary arteries and the myocardium showing focal areas of recent infarction. Viscera were negative for the presence of any poisonous substance. After due deliberations and consideration of all the facts, the AIIMS Medical Board opined that the cause of death, in this case, was myocardial infarction (heart attack) which is a natural cause in a person suffering from heart ailments and is responsible for his death. A person suffering from heart ailments may die after a lag of about 6–12 hours after being subjected to various precipitating factors of stress including pushing and shoving.

Case report of a police officer's death, Maharashtra, India

A 55-year-old male police officer was forcefully made to drink liquor and was physically assaulted by a group of people while he was on duty. He was later admitted to hospital for 4 days. A day after he got discharged from the hospital, his condition became critical and he was declared dead on arrival at the hospital. Family members alleged that he was physically assaulted and given some poison, which ultimately caused his death. A post-mortem examination was conducted at local government hospital, which mentioned multiple abrasions over the left elbow, left knee, and left leg; and also several contusions over the left lower chest, upper lumbar region, right

thigh, and right deltoid region. Internal examination revealed that the heart showed a hard clot, which could be palpated in the left descending artery with a haemorrhagic soft area at the tip of the left ventricle; a clot was also seen in the left ventricle. Histopathology of the heart showed atheromatous plaque in the right coronary artery and left ventricular hypertrophy. The chemical analysis of the preserved viscera was negative for common poisons. The autopsy surgeons opined that death was due to coronary artery disease, a natural heart disease and his death was not due to the multiple injuries on the body. The family members were not satisfied with this and demanded further investigation. The case was handed over to CID, who sought opinions from the medical board of an eminent college, which opined that the cause of death was due to natural diseases involving the heart and not due to injuries. Later on, CID requested AIIMS to opine about the cause of death of the deceased. AIIMS Medical Board perused all relevant documents and observed that the deceased had a pre-existing coronary artery disease of the heart, i.e., atheromatous plaque and calcification with left ventricular hypertrophy leading to partial blockage of blood flow in the arteries of the heart. This condition, by itself, was not fatal unless a person is exposed to stressful conditions leading to an increased workload on the heart resulting in coronary insufficiency and heart failure, as evident in this case. The deceased was a police officer and was humiliated and beaten in a public place which caused a great impact on his mental and physical condition. The AIIMS Medical Board opined that the deceased died due to heart failure as sequelae of coronary artery insufficiency which was precipitated as a consequence of physical, emotional, and mental stress due to being beaten in a public place prior to his death.

ii) **Uncertified natural cause and coexistence of unnatural cause:** When death occurs in an apparently healthy person with no knowledge of an aliment but with a history of physical assault either grave enough or even minor to produce death. During the autopsy and histopathological examination, the pathological condition of the organ is diagnosed but the precipitating factor by the unnatural physical assault, though minor, could not be ruled out.

Example: A person with no history of any disease was found to be dead in a car accident after colliding with a tree, but during the autopsy, both gross and microscopic changes of myocardial infarction are noted. So it is up to the autopsy surgeon to determine the cause of death after considering all the factors and opine whether myocardial infarction led to the road traffic accident or vice versa.

Case report of an uncertified natural cause death and coexistence of unnatural cause – custodial death, Hoogly, West Bengal, India

In January 2013, a 38-year-old male had a heated altercation with police officers over parking his vehicle and was arrested by the police. At the police station, there was a huge hue and cry by the public disturbing the law and order situation on the arrest of the man along with the allegation that he has been subjected to physical torture. The person started feeling uneasy and complained of chest discomfort and suddenly collapsed on the floor. He was rushed immediately to the local hospital, where he was declared dead on arrival. A post-mortem examination was conducted at the local government hospital and minor abrasions and bruises were observed over the face and trunk. The heart weighed 375 gm with the left ventricular wall hypertrophied, measuring 1.5 cm and the aorta showed atheromatous streaks; the right coronary artery showed evidence of atherosclerotic changes, causing partial occlusion of the artery and the cause of death was suggested as natural. However, the family members alleged that he was subjected to custodial torture by the police and demanded a CBI investigation in the Kolkata High Court. CBI requested AIIMS to opine about the cause and manner of death of the deceased and provided the relevant documents and post-mortem videograph. After due deliberation and consideration of the entire facts, AIIMS Medical Board observed that the injuries found on the deceased were simple non-fatal in nature and the histopathological findings established that the deceased was suffering from coronary atherosclerotic disease, and hypertensive left ventricular hypertrophy, which are known common causes of acute coronary insufficiency that can result in SCD. Finally, the board concluded that the cause of death was a cardiac failure as a result of coronary insufficiency which was clearly seen in CCTV footage of the police station, which showed that the person was sweating and later fell down from the bench.

In the current practice of medico-legal autopsy, when we receive a case of sudden death where the history is not clear or dead on arrival at the hospital, there is an examination done at various levels, like verbal autopsy, visual autopsy, virtual autopsy, or traditional autopsy; and its positive findings if present along with negative autopsy will be concluded as the cause of death due to acute coronary insufficiency or the possibility of cardiac arrest cannot be ruled out after ruling out any other cause of death due to unnatural reason/disease or injury. To study the actual relationship between COVID-19 and sudden death and identify the genetic causes leading to sudden death, the author as a Principal Investigator, is currently conducting a study along with ICMR to understand the actual impact of COVID-19 in sudden death cases and also to screen genetic causes of sudden death. This study involves verbal autopsy, visual autopsy, virtual autopsy, and molecular autopsy where there is screening done for the presence of any arrhythmogenic genes in an individual, which could have triggered a sudden death. The format of data collection in this study is as follows:

Proforma – Sudden Death (18–65 years)
Department of Forensic Medicine and Toxicology
All India Institute of Medical Sciences,
New Delhi – 110029

(A) **Demographic data**
    Serial No.:
    MLC/Non-MLC
    Consent (Non-MLC): YES/ NO
    MLC No./Post-Mortem Report No.
    Virtual Autopsy Number:
    Name of Doctors:
    Name of deceased:.. S/o or D/o or W/o................................
    Age/Sex...
    Address: ....

(B) **History**
- Case History:
- COVID infection history: Yes/No, if Yes: No. of times infected ......; Last date of infection:............
- COVID Vaccine status: Yes/No
  Name of vaccine ....; doses taken: .... Booster: ...... last date of vaccination: ....
- Any adverse effects of vaccine: Fever/Allergy/Malaise/Rashes/Itching/Loss of appetite/ Irritability/Headache/ Others...
- Medical History of known illness: DM/ HTN/Allergy/Asthma/Epilepsy/Others ....
- Family history of illness or sudden death:

(C) **GENERAL DESCRIPTION**
    Length of Body................................... Weight of the body: ....
    Clothes worn & their condition
        Post-Mortem Changes: Rigor Mortis, Lividity, Decomposition Changes:
    1. External appearances: Eyes, Mouth, Nostrils, Ears, Nails, Condition of orifices.
    2. External Injuries (Type, size, shape, location and direction, etc.)

(D) **HEAD AND NECK**

Sl. No	Structures Examined		Virtual Autopsy	Traditional Autopsy
1	Scalp and Sub-scalp:			
2	Skull: Obits, Nasal Orifices, Sinuses, Aural Cavities, Mouth, Tongue, Laryngeal complex, Hyoid, Other Neck Structures			
3	Brain	Parenchyma 1. Brain infarction 2. Intracerebral haemorrhage 3. Uncal herniations due to cerebral oedema 4. Cerebellar tonsil herniations due to cerebral oedema 5. Mid brain and brain stem compression due to cerebral oedema 6. Spac-occupying lesions like tumours 7. TB meningitis 8. Brain confusions 9. Brain abscess 10. Diffuse axonal injury 11. Fat embolism 12. Air embolism 13. No findings		
		Ventricles 1. Intraventricular haemorrhage 2. Pus in ventricles		
4	Meninges and Cerebral Vessels 1. Meningitis 2. Circle of Willis abnormalities 3. Aneurysmal ruptures 4. Subdural haemorrhage 5. Subarachnoid haemorrhage 6. Brain stem haemorrhage			

(E) **CHEST (THORAX)**

Sl. No	Structures Examined	Virtual Autopsy		Traditional Autopsy	
1	Ribs and Chest Wall				
2	Diaphragm				
3	Esophagus				
4	Tracheo-Bronchial Tree 1. Choking due to foreign bodies 2. Aspiration 3. Mucous plugging 4. No findings				
	Pleural Cavities	**Right**		**Left**	**Right**	**Left**
5	1. Pleural effusion 2. Haemothorax 3. Adherent lungs 4. Spontaneous pneumothorax 5. No findings				
6	Lungs 1. Bronchopneumonia 2. Lobar pneumonia 3. Lung infarction 4. Pulmonary embolism 5. Granulomatous inflammation due to pulmonary TB, sarcoidosis, etc 6. Pulmonary fibrosis 7. Pulmonary oedema 8. Pulmonary asbestosis 9. Mesothelioma of the lung (following chronic exposure to asbestos seen as severe black pigmentations) 10. Lung abscess 11. Emphysema of lung 12. Atelectasis of lung 13. Bronchiectasis 14. Bronchial asthma 15. No findings				

7	Heart and Pericardial Sac		
	1. Pericardial effusion		
	2. Hemopericardium		
	3. Pericarditis		
	4. Congenital anomalies of the heart		
	• Transposition of great arteries		
	• Ventricular septal defect		
	• Atrial septal defect		
	• Coarctation of aorta		
	• Bicuspid aortic valve		
	• Hypoplastic left heart syndrome		
	5. Spontaneous cardiac rupture.		
	6. Cardiomyopathy		
	• Left atrial		
	• Left ventricular		
	• Right ventricular		
	• Right atrial		
	7. Coronary artery dissection		
	8. Coronary artery thrombus		
	9. Valve calcifications		
	• Mitral		
	• Tricuspid		
	• Aortic		
	• Pulmonary		
	10. Valve abnormalities		
	• Mitral stenosis		
	• Mitral regurgitations		
	• Tricuspid stenosis		
	• Tricuspid regurgitations		
	• Aortic stenosis		
	• Aortic regurgitations		
	• Pulmonary stenosis		
	• Pulmonary regurgitations		
	11. Sudden death due to valve leaflet escape in a previous valve replaced patient		
	12. Sudden death due to stent displacement in a previous valve replaced patient		
	13. Congenital anomalies of coronary artery		
	• Origin (High origin, multiple ostia, single coronary artery, anomalous origin of coronary artery from pulmonary trunk, origin of coronary artery from opposite or non-coronary sinus)		
	• Course of coronary artery (myocardial bridging, duplication of arteries)		
	• Anomalous right coronary artery		
	14. Myocarditis		
	15. Myocardial infarction		
	16. Acute coronary atherosclerosis.		
	17. Acute coronary thrombosis		
	18. Cardiomegaly		
	19. No findings		
8	Large Blood Vessels		
	1. Aortic dissection		
	2. Aortic aneurysm		
	3. Aortic rupture/transection		
9	Other structures		

(F) **ABDOMEN**

Sl. No	Structures Examined	Virtual Autopsy	Traditional Autopsy
1	Abdominal Wall		

2	Peritoneal Cavity
	  1. Biliary peritonitis
	  2. Haemorrhagic peritonitis
	  3. Ectopic pregnancy
	  4. No findings		

3	Stomach
	  1. Perforation
	  2. Ulcer bleeding		

4	Small Intestine and Mesentery
	  1. Pus over the intestines
	  2. Intestinal infarction and necrosis
	  3. Intestinal perforation
	  4. Intestine obstruction
	  5. Intestinal tuberculosis
	  6. Inflammatory bowel disease
	  7. No findings		

5	Large Intestine, Appendix, and Mesocolon
	  1. Intestinal infarction and necrosis
	  2. Intestinal perforation
	  3. Acute appendicitis
	  4. Appendix rupture
	  5. Appendix mass
	  6. Appendix obstruction
	  7. No findings		

6	Pancreas
	  1. Acute pancreatitis
	  2. Acute haemorrhagic necrotizing pancreatitis
	  3. Chronic pancreatitis
	  4. Pancreas rupture
	  5. No findings		

7	Liver and Gallbladder
	  1. Hepatomegaly
	  2. Cirrhosis of liver
	  3. Fatty change
	  4. Macro-vesicular fatty change
	  5. Micro-vesicular fatty change
	  6. Liver abscess
	  7. Tumour in liver
	  8. Laceration
	  9. Haematoma
	  10. Rupture of liver
	  11. Gall stones
	  12. Gallbladder perforation
	  13. No findings		

8	Spleen
	  1. Splenomegaly
	  2. Accessory spleen
	  3. Rupture
	  4. Haemorrhage
	  5. Calcification
	  6. Spleen abscess
	  7. Pus coated
	  8. No findings		

9	Adrenal Glands
	  1. Haemorrhage
	  2. No findings		

10	Kidney, renal pelvis, and ureter
	  1. Renomegaly
	  2. Acute tubular necrosis
	  3. Acute/chronic pyelonephritis
	  4. Acute glomerular nephritis
	  5. Micro abscess in the kidney
	  6. Malignant hypertension
	  7. Renal infarction
	  8. Renal abscess
	  9. Hydronephrosis
	  10. Calculi
	  11. Rupture
	  12. Haemorrhage
	  13. Anomaly of kidney
	  14. No findings		

11	Urinary Bladder and Urethra
	  1. Bladder rupture
	  2. No findings		

12	Genital Organs		

13	Uterus (Females)
	  1. Rupture
	  2. Haemorrhage
	  3. Pregnancy
	  4. Retained products
	  5. Placenta previa
	  6. Placenta accreta		

(G) VERTEBRAL COLUMN AND SPINAL CORD

Sl. No	Structures Examined	Virtual Autopsy	Traditional Autopsy
1	Cervical		
	Thoracic		
	Lumbar		
	Sacral		

(F) EXTREMITIES

Sl. No	Structures Examined	Virtual Autopsy	Traditional Autopsy
	Right Upper Limb		
2	Left Upper Limb		
3	Right Lower Limb		
4	Left Lower Limb		

(H) SPECIMEN PRESERVED
(I) TIME SINCE DEATH
(J) OPINION

Pulmonary causes

Recognition of pulmonary pathology in medico-legal cases of sudden death is of paramount importance as it usually contributes to the immediate or underlying cause of death. In general, a wide range of pulmonary anomalies is associated with sudden death, like pulmonary thrombo-embolism, spontaneous pneumothorax, aspiration, etc. Additionally, acute exacerbations of obstructive (emphysema and bronchial asthma) and restrictive interstitial lung diseases can cause sudden death. Cumulative evidence considers chronic obstructive pulmonary disease (COPD) a risk factor for sudden cardiac deaths both in cardiovascular patients and other patients independent from the cardiovascular risk profile.

Acute occlusive pulmonary arterial thromboembolism is one of the commonest causes of sudden and unexpected death. In approximately a quarter of pulmonary embolism patients, the first manifestation is sudden unexpected death. Overall, pulmonary embolism is responsible for approximately 4–5% of sudden deaths, and it is recognized in 8–70% of cases seen at autopsy. Unfortunately, clinical diagnosis of pulmonary embolism is missed in most pulmonary embolism patients due to either no symptoms or fairly non-specific presentation. The pulmonary embolism is revealed only after post-mortem examination. Therefore, an autopsy is essential in sudden-death patients to know the exact cause of death; otherwise, there will be considered underdiagnosis of pulmonary embolism in these cases. Computed tomography pulmonary angiogram (CTPA) is currently considered the gold standard for pulmonary embolism, while the existing post-mortem gold standard for the diagnosis of this pathologic entity is autopsy. The differentiation between true PTE and post-mortem clotting is challenging, while PMCT angiography (PMCTA) provides an opportunity of diagnosing contrast medium filling defects of the pulmonary arteries. Irregularly shaped filling defects present in pulmonary arteries allowed for a good assessment of PTE. The identification of possible PTE is possible through the identifying characteristic signs of PTE on unenhanced PMCT. A reliable diagnosis of pulmonary thromboembolism between PTE and myocardial infarction is made through the combination of the focal perivascular soft tissue oedema of the lower legs. Sufficient differentiation between pulmonary thromboembolism and post-mortem clotting is not provided by PMCTA. The definite diagnosis of PTE in a minimally invasive manner is facilitated by a post-mortem biopsy. Pulmonary thrombosis is distinguishable from hypostasis and varies in density and appearance. A non-fluid–fluid level and hyperdense cast formation are the key features suggesting pulmonary thrombus occluding the pulmonary artery. Therefore, post-mortem diagnosis of pulmonary thromboembolism is based on the combination of the radiologic findings and histopathologic examination of the potentially thromboembolic material (41). If the embolus is large, it can entirely obstruct both pulmonary arteries resulting in right heart failure; with such embolic burden, signs of right heart strain are usually present, and signs can be:

- Right ventricle (RV) dilatation causes the RV width to be more than the left ventricle width
- Inter-ventricular septum becoming straight or bulging towards the left
- Pulmonary trunk enlargement (Figure 7.23)

Case report of sudden death due to pulmonary thrombo-embolism

A 36-year-old male suddenly developed respiratory distress and breathlessness and was taken to a nearby hospital. His respiratory symptoms worsened, and he was immediately transferred to a specialist centre, but unfortunately, he died before reaching the hospital and was declared dead on arrival. As he was dead on arrival and the definitive cause of death was not known a medico-legal case was registered, and the dead body was shifted to the Department of Forensic Medicine for autopsy. There was no significant medical history in the case, and the autopsy was conducted the next day. The external examination by autopsy revealed congested conjunctivae and bluish discolouration of lips and nail beds. PMCT showed a distended pulmonary trunk, pulmonary arteries and its branches. PMCT lungs showed some ground glass opacities with features of pulmonary oedema (Figure 7.23). The internal examination by autopsy revealed a thrombus lodged in the pulmonary trunk and branching, causing a saddle-shaped thrombus and also the thrombus extending into the right and left pulmonary arteries and its branches (Figure 7.24).

Pneumothorax

Pneumothorax is a condition where there is a collection of air within the pleural cavity outside the lung. Air accumulates in these cases in the potential space between the parietal and visceral pleura. As the air accumulates in the pleural cavity, it can apply pressure on the lung and leads to its collapse. Pneumothorax can be classified as simple pneumothorax, tension pneumothorax, and open pneumothorax. A simple pneumothorax is a condition where the air in the pleural cavity does not cause any shift of the mediastinal structures or cause any severe respiratory distress. Tension pneumothorax, on the other hand, is a condition where the air is accumulated in the pleural cavity, which causes a shift of the mediastinal structures, and the pressure created results in the collapse of the lungs and also results in fatal respiratory distress. They require immediate management, or they can be fatal. An open pneumothorax is also known as a 'sucking' chest wound where the break in continuity over the skin/chest wall and visceral pleura by injury like a stab, gunshot, etc., causes a direct connection with the atmospheric air leads to the entry of air into the pleural cavity. Detection of pneumothorax in traditional autopsy is

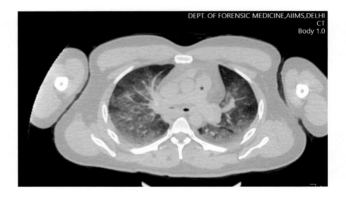

FIGURE 7.23: Axial section of chest PMCT in the lung window shows the distended pulmonary trunk and artery (red star) and the branches of the pulmonary artery (red arrow).

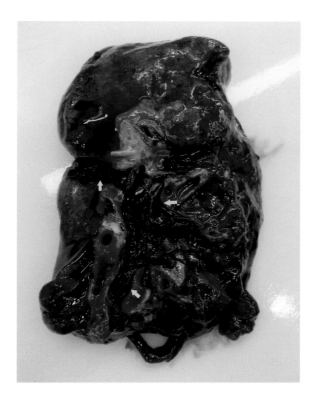

FIGURE 7.24: Pulmonary thrombus lodged in the pulmonary artery and its branches in the case (yellow arrows).

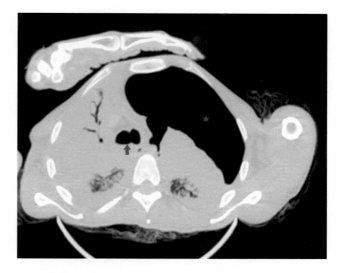

FIGURE 7.25: Axial section of chest PMCT in the lung window showing pneumothorax (red star) with the adjoining collapse of the left lung and trachea-bronchial junction shifted to the right (red arrow) along with other mediastinal structures confirming tension pneumothorax.

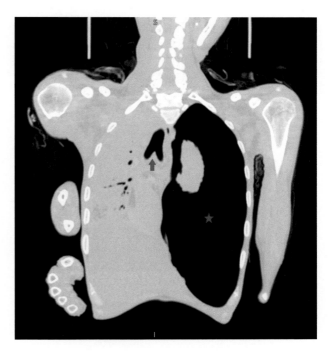

FIGURE 7.26: Coronal section of chest PMCT in the lung window showing pneumothorax (red star) with the adjoining collapse of the left lung and trachea-bronchial junction shifted to the right (red arrow) along with other mediastinal structures confirming tension pneumothorax.

quite tricky as an underwater opening of the cavity is required to appreciate the air bubbles. It is easier to appreciate the tension pneumothorax in this technique, but in cases of simple pneumothorax, it is sometimes difficult to identify pneumothorax as air is not trapped in pressure and possible local accumulation of air pockets is there away from the dissection site.

Another pattern of classification of the pneumothorax is primary spontaneous pneumothorax and secondary spontaneous pneumothorax. Primary spontaneous pneumothorax occurs in cases without any underlying lung pathology; males are more prone, and smoking nicotine or cannabis increases the risk of primary spontaneous pneumothorax. Secondary spontaneous pneumothorax occurs in cases with some underlying lung pathology like COPD, asthma, cystic fibrosis, lung cancer, or infective causes like tuberculosis, pneumocystis pneumonia, etc.

Case report of sudden death due to an acute complication of tuberculosis

A 35-year-old male was found in an unresponsive state on the footpath; he was brought to AIIMS hospital, where he was declared dead on arrival. The dead body was shifted to the mortuary for an autopsy to determine the cause of death in the case. On autopsy, external examination revealed that the deceased was thinly built and had a scaphoid abdomen. No external injuries were detected over the body. PMCT was done in the case, which showed that the deceased had tension pneumothorax with the collapse of the left lung and the trachea and mediastinal structures were shifted to the right. The lung showed some underlying pathology with ground glass opacities and consolidation at places (Figures 7.25–7.27). Though the case had a long-term lung pathology in place, an acute event deviated from the normal expected course in the case merited it to come

under the category of sudden natural death. The other possible reasons for pneumothorax were completely ruled out by the examination. All these features make the case of a secondary spontaneous pneumothorax following a lung pathology resulting in fatal tension pneumothorax, which caused the death in this case. On traditional autopsy done in the case left lung showed collapse, and both lungs showed diffuse distribution of

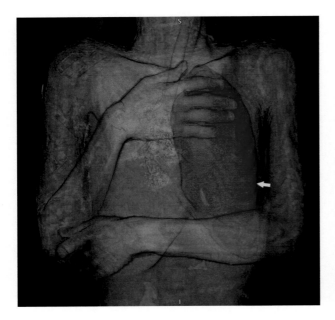

FIGURE 7.27: Volume-rendered reconstruction (VRT) with selective accentuation of air in cavities which is seen as the red colour space (yellow arrow), and it is seen shifting the trachea and mediastinal structures to the right.

miliary nodules associated with purulent secretions and areas of consolidation of the lung parenchyma. Multiple pus pockets in the parenchyma were seen more towards the periphery of the lungs (Figures 7.28 and 7.29). Histopathology examination with

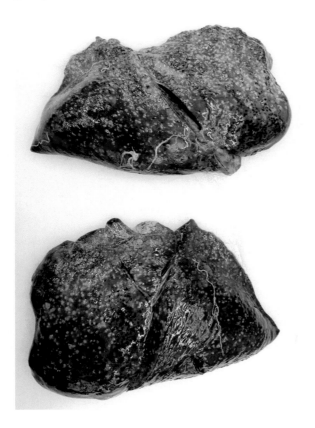

FIGURE 7.28: Gross autopsy examination of both lungs showing diffuse miliary nodularity.

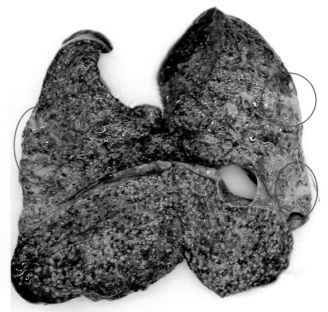

FIGURE 7.29: Gross autopsy examination of cut-section of the lung showing diffuse miliary nodularity with multiple pus pockets (red circles).

haematoxylin and eosin (H and E) stain shows the abundant sub-pleural distribution of granulomas with neutrophil infiltration, and on higher magnification (40×), multiple Langhans giant cells are seen along with palisading of giant cells around the focal area of necrosis confirming miliary tuberculosis (Figure 7.30). These lung pathologies confirm the pneumothorax to be related to the pathology and being secondary spontaneous pneumothorax.

Aspiration

Aspiration can be caused by food entering the lungs while eating, or it can be caused by stomach contents moving back up the food tube (oesophagus) and spilling over into the person's airway. Most people cough out violently when they aspirate, but some people do not; their cough reflex may have been weakened. When a person aspirates but does not cough, this is called a silent aspiration. Choking refers to an obstruction or blockage of the airway of a person, which interferes with breathing. This is an emergency if the person is unable to clear their airway on their own by coughing. The aspiration of food fragments into the distal airways/alveolar ducts is another cause of sudden death. Notably, aspiration is either not suspected before autopsy or misdiagnosed clinically as acute myocardial infarction or cardiac arrest. Aspiration, at times, may not cause sudden death but may lead to pulmonary pathologies such as partial airway obstruction, pneumonia, chemical pneumonitis, or acute respiratory distress syndrome, which causes morbidity or mortality. The final outcome after aspiration of stomach contents depends on multiple factors like volume of content aspirated, chemical composition of the aspirant, particle size, presence of infectious agents in the aspirated material, health condition of the individual, conscious state of the person to evoke a protective cough reflex, presence of any intoxicating agents, under the influence of drug or anaesthesia, etc. These foreign particles can be clearly seen on PMCT as a foreign body

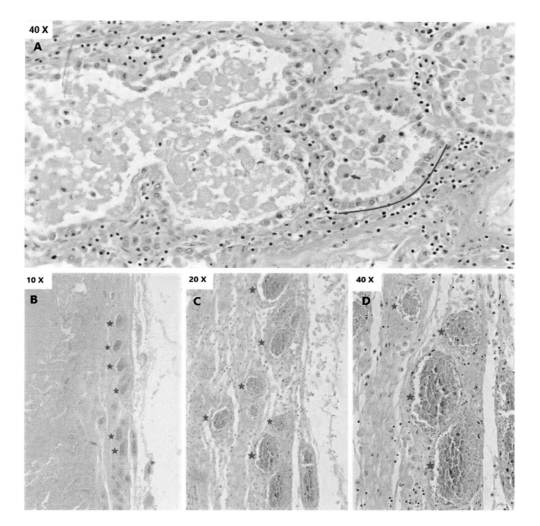

FIGURE 7.30: Haematoxylin and eosin staining of the lung tissue in the case showed A: Palisading of giant cells around the area of necrosis (red line) and Langhans giant cells (red arrow). B, C, and D: multiple subepithelial granulomas in 10×, 20×, and 40× magnification.

obstructing the airway; the same can be confirmed on traditional autopsy (Figures 7.31 and 7.32), but there is a high chance of foreign particles getting dislodged or moved or leaking out due to the process of handling and dissection.

Risk factors for aspiration:

1. **Age:** All age groups are susceptible, but young children and elderly people are at higher risk.
2. **Gender:** It equally affects both genders.
3. **Cognitive impairment:** Due to intoxication, developmental delay, or any other cognitive impairment disorders.
4. **Central neurologic impairment:** Due to stroke, seizure, raised intracranial pressure, intracranial haemorrhages, tumours, etc.
5. **Focal neurologic impairment:** Due to injury of nerves involved in deglutition, pharyngeal muscle injury, neuromuscular disorders, oesophagal dysmotility, muscular dystrophies, etc.
6. **Pulmonary diseases:** Those requiring mechanical ventilation, diseases causing poor cough reflex or poor expiratory effort.

7. **Mechanical causes:** Trauma to the neck, base of the skull or due to the presence of an NG tube, tracheostomy, iatrogenic procedures like endoscopy, bronchoscopy, etc.
8. **Miscellaneous causes:** Poisoning by CNS depressants, overuse of proton pump inhibitors, high volume of vomiting, poisoning by hydrocarbons, and position changes can cause aspiration even in healthy people.

Toxicokinetics of aspiration

A litmus test can be performed to differentiate whether the aspirate is from the stomach or from swallowing; gastric contents are acidic in nature. Aspiration of gastric contents, which are acidic in nature, into the respiratory tract can lead to chemical pneumonitis. Commonly due to the position of the right bronchus, which is less acutely angled at the carina, aspirate enters it and affects the right lower lobe. When the volume of aspirate is large, it can involve one or both sides. The position of the person at the time of aspiration also can determine the lobe that gets affected. In cases where the aspirate is large enough to block the airway completely, it can cause immediate death. Such cases need immediate clearance of the airway; even then, the acidic nature of the aspirate results in immediate damage

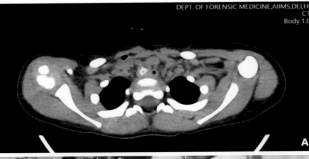

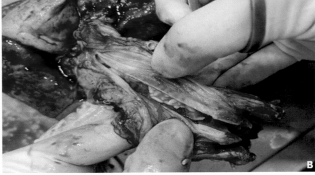

FIGURE 7.31: A case of sudden death due to aspiration; A: PMCT showing obstruction of the trachea with foreign particles; B: Autopsy showing rice particles in the trachea.

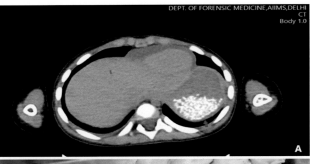

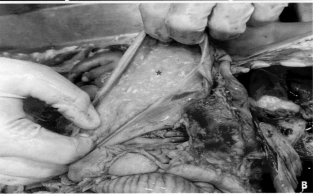

FIGURE 7.32: In the same case of aspiration as Figure 7.31, A: PMCT examination of the stomach shows particles similar to the one obstruction trachea showing the possible source of origin of the aspirate, HU can also be compared; B: Autopsy showing stomach with rice particles which are similar to the content obstructing the trachea.

to the mucosa of the respiratory tract. The pH of the aspirate is also an important determinant of the outcome, and any pH below 2.5 is highly fatal.

COVID-19 causing sudden death

Severe acute respiratory syndrome coronavirus-2 (SARS-CoV-2) is a pathogen which has been threatening the world recently. It is a new strain of coronavirus and was first reported in Wuhan, China, in December 2019. COVID-19 is a viral infection which caused a global pandemic, and it primarily affects the respiratory system. Apart from the respiratory system, it also affects other systems like the cardiovascular system, central nervous system, etc. The infection commonly spreads by droplets of nasal discharge or saliva. Though most cases progress through the common respiratory symptoms before culminating in the fatal acute respiratory distress syndrome, few cases culminate in sudden death due to the involvement of different systems and may not even have any symptoms. The common symptoms of presentation were fever, dry cough, sore throat, body pain, headache, tiredness, diarrhoea, conjunctivitis, and loss of taste and smell. A few of the proposed or witnessed causes of sudden death in cases of COVID-19 include:

- Acute massive pulmonary thromboembolism
- Acute myocarditis
- Stress-induced cardiomyopathy
- Post myocarditis sequel
- Acute coronary syndrome and coronary thrombosis
- Cardiac tamponade
- Myocardial hypoxia
- Arrhythmias
- Stroke
- Encephalitis
- Coagulopathy
- Electrolyte imbalance
- Triggering of genetic channelopathies
- Intracerebral haemorrhages
- Cytokine storm

Pulmonary thromboembolism was one commonly seen cause of sudden death in COVID-19 cases where deaths happened among cases treated in hospitals, intensive care units, and also in cases who were asymptomatic. Deep vein thrombosis and pulmonary embolism were seen in many cases of sudden death among COVID-19-infected individuals, and the possible explanation was underlying inflammation and injury to the vessels and also vascular remodelling of the endothelial cells. Capillary microthrombi were also seen commonly in acute lung injury cases infected with COVID-19, along with thrombosis of vessels of all sizes of the pulmonary and extra-pulmonary regions.

Cardiovascular changes which have been observed in COVID-19 cases include myocarditis, arrhythmias, acute coronary syndrome, myocardial infarction, congestive heart failure, etc. These were commonly seen in elderly patients who had other comorbidities like hypertension, diabetes, dyslipidemias, etc. Arrhythmias were noted in many cases, and atrial fibrillation and other patterns of arrhythmias among hospitalized COVID-19 patients showed that tachyarrhythmias were more common than bradyarrhythmias.

Radiological examination of the cases of COVID-19 by X-ray or CT scan shows the involvement of the lungs, which are seen as consolidation or ground glass opacities of lungs (Figure 7.33) with the often involvement of bilateral, peripheral, and lower

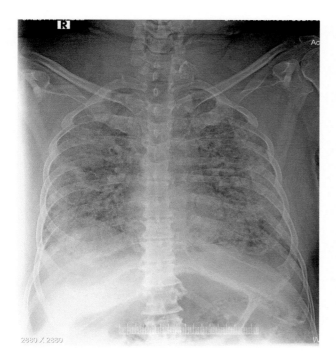

FIGURE 7.33: A case of COVID-19 digital X-ray AP showing bilateral diffuse ground glass opacities and consolidation at places with right-sided pleural effusion.

zone predominance. Pleural effusion in these cases may be seen but are rare. PMCT may also show features like crazy paving appearance (GGOs and inter-/intra-lobular septal thickening), air space consolidation, and broncho-vascular thickening in the lesion or traction bronchiectasis.

Central nervous system causes of sudden death

Sudden death by the central nervous system (CNS) related pathologies though far less common than cardiac causes, still accounts for a substantial proportion of sudden deaths. The majority of sudden deaths occur outside hospitals, and because neuropathology autopsies are uncommonly performed, a cardiac cause of death is most often assumed, and neurologic causes could be easily missed. The CNS-related pathologies causing sudden death commonly encountered in forensic autopsy practice include cerebral venous thrombosis and vascular malformations, aneurysmal subarachnoid haemorrhage, epilepsy, brain tumours, and infectious causes like meningitis and cerebral abscess, etc. In addition to history and examination, a neuroimaging and detailed autopsy is beneficial for the autopsy surgeon to conclude the cause of death in cases of sudden death due to CNS causes.

Causes of sudden death related to CNS include:

- **Vascular abnormalities:** Aneurysmal SAH, spontaneous intracerebral/parenchymal haemorrhage, arteriovenous malformations (AVM), developmental venous anomalies, etc.
- **Strokes:** Haemorrhagic or ischaemic
- Cerebral venous thrombosis
- Epilepsy
- **Brain tumours:** Primary brain tumours and metastatic tumours

- **Infectious causes:** meningitis and abscess.
- Bleeding disorders

Vascular abnormalities

Vascular abnormalities or malformations are an important cause of intracerebral/ intraparenchymal haemorrhage and sudden death. Subarachnoid haemorrhage is a frequently encountered intracranial haemorrhage, and its common non-traumatic cause is aneurysm rupture. An intracranial aneurysm is a pathological dilatation of a section or part of the artery in the cranial cavity, and the usual location of these aneurysms includes the circle of Willis. The anterior communicating artery along with the anterior cerebral artery are the common locations of these aneurysms. History, as taken before an autopsy in these cases, typically shows a presentation with a sudden severe headache due to the SAH, which is followed by features like loss of consciousness, focal neurological deficit, nausea, vomiting, etc. These aneurysmal SAH result in secondary vascular complications like rebleed or vasospasm, both of which affect the blood supply to the brain and result in stroke or death. In a minority of cases with SAH, angiography also may not be able to detect any aneurysm or vascular abnormalities; these are cases where the source of bleeding is peri-mesencephalic veins or capillaries.

Arteriovenous malformations (AVM) are another group of vascular abnormalities which leads to sudden death by intracranial haemorrhage. Arteriovenous malformations of the brain have an abnormal connection between the arteries and the veins by a bridging abnormal capillary bed known as a central nidus. The AVM of the brain may remain completely asymptomatic and may result in sudden intracranial haemorrhage, which causes fatal consequences. Among AVMs, only 12% of cases become symptomatic, of which the common presentation is intracerebral haemorrhage. Apart from the intracerebral haemorrhage, AVMs can also present as seizures, chronic headaches, and focal deficits not related to haemorrhage. In the pediatric age group, sudden unexpected death due to ruptured AVMs is considered a rare cause. However, cases of ruptured AVM of the choroid plexus of the fourth ventricle and intracerebral haemorrhages are reported. AVMs are commonly sporadic in aetiology, but a familial inheritance of the condition is also noted. The AVM abnormality can be very small, which could go unnoticed by radiological imaging or normal autopsy and may need histopathological examination for identification.

Vascular abnormalities in the cerebral vessels, especially the arteries, can occur due to hypertension and hypercholesterolemia. Both these conditions result in vessels developing atherosclerotic problems, which can cause sudden death by intracranial haemorrhage (Figure 7.34). Hypertension can lead to the following pathological changes in the vessels:

- Microaneurysms of perforating arteries (Charcot–Bouchard aneurysms) cause haemorrhages in the lenticulostriate region, pons, or cerebellum
- Thrombosis may be accelerated
- Atherosclerosis may be accelerated
- Hyaline arteriosclerosis
- Hyperplastic arteriosclerosis

Spontaneous intracranial haemorrhage

Sudden death due to spontaneous non-traumatic intr—cranial haemorrhage can occur in any one or more of the intracranial compartments, which include extradural space, subdural space, subarachnoid space, intraventricular space

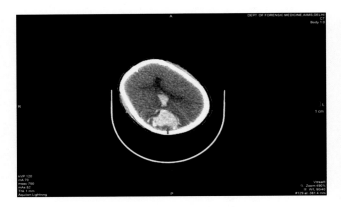

FIGURE 7.34: Spontaneous intraparenchymal bleed (red arrow) with ventricular extension (red star) in a case of an adult with chronic hypertension resulting from the vascular complications of hypertension.

or intraparenchymal. The common causes for these include aneurysm rupture and arteriovenous malformations, as discussed above. The other possible causes include alcohol consumption, anticoagulant treatment, or use like thrombolytic therapy and aspirin use. Abuse of certain drugs like amphetamines, cocaine, ecstasy, etc., can also result in fatal spontaneous intracranial haemorrhage. Spontaneous haemorrhages are also known to happen in pre-existing tumours of the brain due to their vascular nature. Spontaneous intracranial haemorrhages may also occur in cases where there is a role of physical and emotional stress involved; medico-legal scenarios like these are commonly encountered where sudden death happens in people who were involved in a verbal argument or minor assault. Deaths in such cases most frequently occur due to subarachnoid or intracerebral haemorrhage or cardiac diseases, with death possibly arising as a consequence of a sharp rise in blood pressure due to stress. There must be a clear temporal association between the stressful event and death to establish a causal link.

Intracerebral haematoma/haemorrhage of a massive type happening in the brain substance is usually of abrupt onset and also of rapid evolution. Most commonly, these large intracerebral haematomas are known to occur in middle-aged men with hypertension or in the elderly category. Intracerebral haematomas can occur in the basal ganglia (Figures 7.35 and 7.36), pons, thalamus, cerebellum (Figure 7.37), and cerebral white matter.

Cerebral venous thrombosis

Cerebral venous thrombosis (CVT) is a rare cerebrovascular condition. The condition is characterized by intracranial veins and sinuses developing thrombosis, as the name indicates. The history in such cases is of non-specific symptoms like headache, nausea, and vomiting, and these symptoms are present for a considerable duration of time. The usual symptom is a headache, which has an insidious onset and gradually increases over time. Risk factors for developing CVT include pregnancy, oral contraceptive pills, hypercoagulable conditions like factor V Leiden, deficiency of protein C, protein S or antithrombin, or related problems, nephrotic syndrome, obesity, dehydration, inflammatory bowel disease, lupus, Behçet's disease, homocysteinemia, homocystinuria, etc. In ante-mortem cases, non-contrast CT may suggest the diagnosis of CVT, but magnetic resonance angiography (MRA) or digital angiography are the most effective techniques for

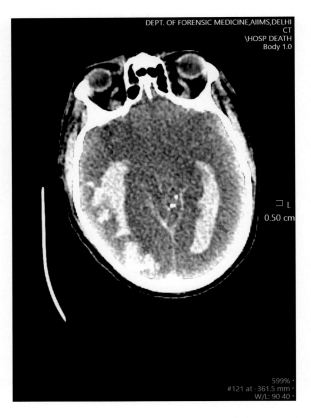

FIGURE 7.35: A spontaneous intracranial haemorrhage in the basal ganglia region and right temporal, parietal, and occipital regions with bilateral ventricular extension. The deceased was a known case of chronic liver disease and suddenly developed a headache and diminution of vision prior to collapse.

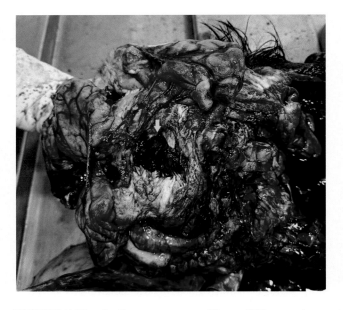

FIGURE 7.36: In the same case as Figure 7.35, an autopsy examination of the brain revealed the brain parenchyma to be softened and haemorrhaged in the basal ganglia region and right temporal, parietal, and occipital regions with bilateral ventricular extension.

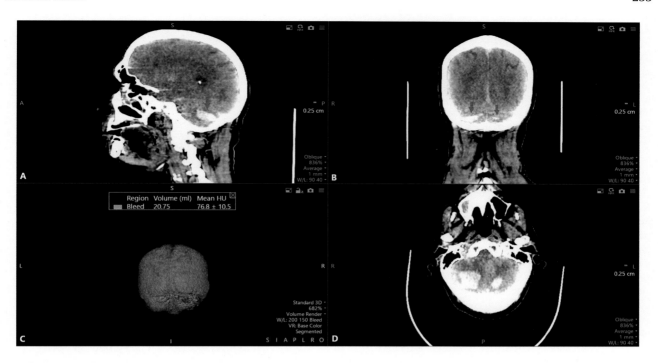

FIGURE 7.37: A case of a 72-year-old male who suddenly collapsed in the toilet and was declared dead on arrival. Spontaneous intracranial haemorrhage was seen in both lobes of the cerebellum seen on PMCT A: sagittal section, B: coronal section, C: Volume rendering 3D, and D: Axial section.

diagnosis. Cerebral angiography may show the presence of smaller clots than appreciable in CT or MRI, and when there are obstructed veins, it may give a 'corkscrew appearance'. Cerebral venous thrombosis is also an important cause of stroke due to the disruption of blood supply.

Stroke

It is a medical condition where the blood supply to the brain is disrupted, and it is possible by a blockage in the vessel or leakage of blood from the vessel. It is commonly classified into:

1. Ischaemic stroke
2. Haemorrhagic stroke

The risk factors of stroke include high blood cholesterol, tobacco smoking, obesity, diabetes mellitus, history of transient ischaemic attacks, end-stage kidney disease, etc. Stroke is the fourth most common cause of sudden death in the world. Haemorrhagic stroke, in comparison to ischaemic stroke, is a more common cause of stroke. Prior to the onset of stroke or sudden death due to stroke, some people may experience neurological symptoms, of which headache is the commonest symptom. The other common symptoms before a stroke could be weakness, numbness of the extremities or certain parts of the body, decreased level of consciousness, or other neurological symptoms. Virtual autopsy helps in identifying the stroke, especially the haemorrhagic cause; in cases of ischaemic stroke, the site of ischaemia is difficult to identify in acute cases but is helpful in identifying old ischaemic foci or regions.

Epilepsy

Sudden unexpected death in epilepsy (SUDEP) is used to define a 'sudden, unexpected, non-traumatic, non-drowning, witnessed, or unwitnessed death occurring in an otherwise healthy individual with epilepsy with or without evidence of seizure in which post-mortem examination is unrevealing'. People diagnosed with epilepsy have 24 times higher risk of sudden unexpected death compared to the normal population. People with generalized tonic-clonic seizures (GTCS) are at even higher risk. SUDEP is classified into:

- **Definite SUDEP:** An autopsy has confirmed the absence of anatomical or toxicological cause of death
- **Probable SUDEP:** An autopsy has not been done, but the circumstances of death are strongly suggestive of SUDEP
- **Possible SUDEP:** Describes a situation in which SUDEP cannot be excluded and should be considered among the explanations for death

The pathophysiology of SUDEP is unclear, and it is considered possibly due to more than one mechanism causing death, which includes peri-ictal impairment of respiratory function, post-ictal impairment of brain function, possible cardiac arrhythmias, and autonomic dysfunction.

Virtual autopsy with PMCT is an essential tool in suspected deaths due to epilepsy or seizures or SUDEP as it helps in identifying or ruling out any structural abnormalities in the brain.

Brain tumours

The global incidence rate of CNS tumours is around 4.63 per 100,000 persons. In medico-legal autopsy cases, primary undiagnosed CNS tumours causing sudden unexpected death account for about 0.02% to 2.1% of cases. Among these, the most common type histologically are neuroepithelial tissue tumours comprising about 28.2% of all primary CNS tumours. The other category of brain tumours is secondary metastasis which is commonly seen. Brain metastasis is seen in about 20% to 25% of all cancer patients, and autopsy findings report intracranial metastasis to be the cause of death in up to 25% of cases. The patients, prior to death, may present with symptoms like headache, confusion, vomiting, focal neurological deficits, symptoms of increased intracranial pressure, seizures/epilepsy, impaired level of consciousness, and cognitive dysfunction are prominent symptoms. Furthermore, fatigue, mood disturbances, tinnitus, and anxiety are also reported. The mechanisms of death in these cases of brain tumours include seizures (Figures 7.38 and 7.39), acute haemorrhage (Figures 7.40 and 7.41) and herniation due to mass effect.

Sudden death caused by intracranial infection

Intracranial infections occur most commonly in children, it is also seen in adults, and they are an important cause of sudden death. The important among these are cases of sudden unexplained deaths by either acute bacterial meningitis or a large cerebral abscess. Acute bacterial meningitis, commonly caused by pneumococci and meningococci, occurs secondary to bacteraemia in adults. Autopsy of the brain in these cases shows swollen brain along with the sulci filled by a cloudy, pale yellow/green exudate (Figure 7.42). In cases of meningococcal meningitis, the exudate can be minimal and difficult to identify. Acute bacterial meningitis is seen in cases where the individual has a poor living condition, has a history of drug abuse or alcohol abuse, is commonly associated with pneumonia, is an immune-compromised individual or even after splenectomy. PMCT though it may not show any specific features, can sometimes show sulcal effacement or slight hyper-attentuation. Further, PMCT can help identify a few of the complications related to meningitis, like hydrocephalus, abscess, infarcts, extra-axial collection, etc.

Cerebral abscess

A brain abscess is a localized area of necrosis in the brain with a surrounding membrane; it usually results from an infectious

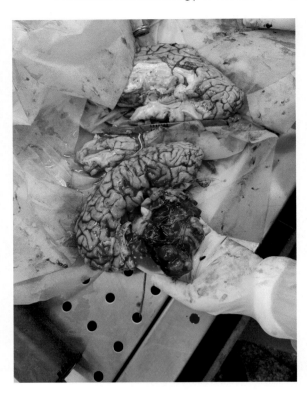

FIGURE 7.39: Autopsy examination in the same case as Figure 7.35 revealed a well-defined mass originating from the vascular structures in the brain.

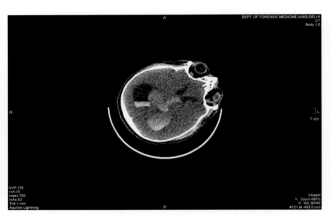

FIGURE 7.40: A case of a diagnosed pineal gland tumour who suddenly collapsed and was declared dead, PMCT in the case revealed acute haemorrhage surrounding the tumour, which had caused the sudden death.

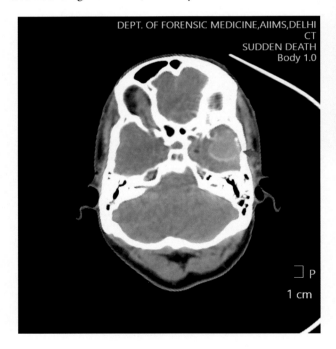

FIGURE 7.38: A case of a 32-year-old male with a history of headaches followed by seizures and sudden death. PMCT showed a well-defined mass in the left temporal region with a haemorrhage surrounding the mass.

cause or traumatic process. The most frequent microbial pathogens causing cerebral abscesses include staphylococcus and streptococcus. Brain abscesses constitute around 8% of the intracranial masses encountered in developing countries. The source of brain abscess infection could be from a direct local spread of infection or spread from a distant source.

Local sources of spread for cerebral abscess include:

- Infections of the head and neck region, like otitis media, mastoiditis, and paranasal sinus infection, especially frontal or ethmoid sinuses, spreads to the frontal lobes, and dental infection causes frontal lobe abscess.

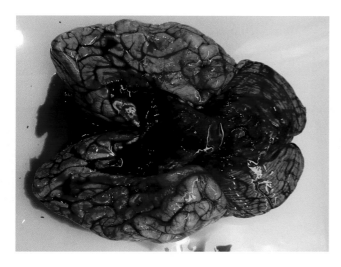

FIGURE 7.41: In the case of the pineal gland tumour, the same as Figure 7.37 traditional autopsy revealed a tumour surrounded by acute subdural haemorrhage, which caused death.

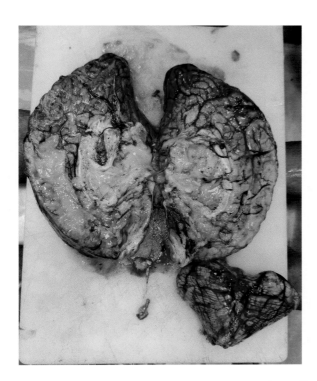

FIGURE 7.42: A case of pyogenic meningitis with swollen brain and pale yellow exudate over the cerebral hemispheres with ventricular extension. The deceased had a ventriculoperitoneal shunt.

- Generalized septicemia or haematogenous spread causes cerebral abscesses like haematogenous seeding of the brain by pulmonary infections like lung abscess, empyema, bronchiectasis, cystic fibrosis, etc., as the lung is the most common organ for the spread of infection. Congenital heart diseases causing bacterial endocarditis can act as a source. Skin infections, pelvic infections, and intra-abdominal infections are also considered high-risk

factors for haematogenous spread. Brain abscesses associated with bacteraemia commonly cause multiple abscesses, and it occurs mostly in the area of distribution by the middle cerebral artery and commonly at the grey-white matter junction.

PMCT in these cases show a brain abscess wall which is commonly smooth and regular, having a thickness of about 1 mm to 3 mm. It is also associated with oedema of the surrounding brain parenchyma. A multi-location abscess may also be seen with subjacent daughter abscesses or satellite lesions. Gas present in the abscess is suggestive of gas-forming organisms.

Bibliography

Alotaibi AS, Mahroos RA, Al Yateem SS, Menezes RG . Central nervous system causes of sudden unexpected death: A comprehensive review. *Cureus* 2022;14:e20944.

Baldi E, Sechi GM, Mare C, Canevari F, Brancagilone A. Out-of-hospital cardiac arrest during the Covid-19 outbreak in Italy. *N Engl J Med.* 2020;383:496–498.

Camps FE, Robinson AE, Lucas, BGB. *Unexpected death due to natural disease: Gradwohl's legal medicine.* Third edition. Bristol: John Wright and Sons Ltd, 1976, pp. 220–254.

De-Giorgio F, Peschillo S, Vetrugno G, d'Aloja E, Spagnolo AG, Miscusi M. Cerebral venous sinus thrombosis due to spontaneous, progressive, and retrograde jugular vein thrombosis causing sudden death in a young woman. *Forensic Sci Med Pathol.* 2015;11:88–91.

Doolan A, Langlois N, Semsartan C. Causes of sudden cardiac death in young Australians. *MJA* 2004;180:110–112.

Eckart RE, Shy EA, Burke AP, McNear JA, Appel DA, et al. Sudden death in young adults: An autopsy-based series of a population undergoing active surveillance. *JACC* 2011;58:1254–1261.

Freiman DG, Suyemoto J, Wessler S. Frequency of pulmonary thromboembolism in man. *N Engl J Med.* 1965;272:1278–1280.

Gopinathannair R, Merchant FM, Lakkireddy DR. COVID-19 and cardiac arrhythmias: A global perspective on arrhythmia characteristics and management strategies. *J Intervent Card Electrophysiol.* 2020:1–8.

Guo T, Fan Y, Chen M. Cardiovascular implications of fatal outcomes of patients with Coronavirus disease 2019 (COVID-19) *JAMA Cardiol.* 2020;5:811–818.

Hu X, Yi ES, Ryu JH. Aspiration-related deaths in 57 consecutive patients: Autopsy study. *PLOS ONE.* 2014;9:e103795.

Irwin RS, Ashba JK, Braman SS, Lee HY, Corrao WM. Food asphyxiation in hospitalized patients. *JAMA.* 1977;237:2744–2745.

Karhunen PJ, Penttilä A, Erkinjuntti T. Arteriovenous malformation of the brain: Imaging by postmortem angiography. *Forensic Sci Int.* 1990;48:9–19.

Karwinski B, Svendsen E. Comparison of clinical and postmortem diagnosis of pulmonary embolism. *J Clin Pathol.* 1989;42:135–139.

Kim AS, Moffatt E, Ursell PC, Devinsky O, Olgin J, Tseng ZH. Sudden neurologic death masquerading as out-of-hospital sudden cardiac death. *Neurology.* 2016;87:1669–1673.

Lahousse L, Niemeijer MN, van den Berg ME, Rijnbeek PR, Joos GF, Hofman A, Franco OH, Deckers JW, Eijgelsheim M, Stricker BH, Brusselle GG. Chronic obstructive pulmonary disease and sudden cardiac death: The Rotterdam study. *Eur Heart J.* 2015;36:1754–1761.

Lucena J, Rico A, Vázquez R, Marín R, Martínez C, Salguero M, Miguel L. Pulmonary embolism and sudden unexpected death: Prospective study on 2477 forensic autopsies performed at the Institute of Legal Medicine in Seville. *J Forensic Leg Med.* 2009;16:196–201.

Lucena JS. Sudden cardiac death. *Forensic Sci Res.* 2019;4:199–201.

Mainous AG 3rd, Rooks BJ, Wu V, Orlando FA. COVID-19 post-acute sequelae among adults: 12 month mortality risk. *Front Med (Lausanne).* 2021;8:778434.

Mak CM, Mok NS, Shum BC, Siu WK, Chong YK, Lee KKC, et al. Sudden arrhythmia death syndrome in young victims: A five-year retrospective review and two-year prospective molecular autopsy study by next-generation sequencing and clinical evaluation of their first-degree relatives. *Hong Kong Med J.* 2019;25:21–29.

McIntyre KM, Belko JS, Sasahara AA. Pulmonary embolism. *Arch Surg.* 1969;98:671–673.

Mukerji SS, Solomon IH. What can we learn from brain autopsies in COVID-19? *Neurosci Lett.* 2021 January 18;742:135528.

Mukhopadhyay S, Katzenstein AL. Pulmonary disease due to aspiration of food and other particulate matter: A clinicopathologic study of 59 cases diagnosed on biopsy or resection specimens. *Am J Surg Pathol.* 2007;31:752–9.

Najaf D, Tahir R, Ahmad S. Sudden cardiac death in COVID-19 Patients. *Interv Cardiol.* 2022;14:197–204.

Thiene G. Sudden cardiac death in the young: A genetic destiny? *Clin Med.* 2018;18 Supplement 2:17–23.

Van Den Berg ME, Stricker BH, Brusselle GG, Lahousse L. Chronic obstructive pulmonary disease and sudden cardiac death: A systematic review. *Trends Cardiovasc Med.* 2016;26:606–613.

Yadav R, Bansal R, Budakoty S, Barwad P. COVID-19 and sudden cardiac death: A new potential risk. *Indian Heart J.* 2020;72: 333–336.

8 IDENTIFICATION

Introduction: The problem of the unidentified

Forensic anthropology aims to achieve a unique humanitarian service owing to the prevalence of severe violent deaths. Identification is essential due to the result of the intolerable criminal and political nature of mankind. The distorted peace in the affected family can be corrected by small steps taken towards identifying the dead or missing and trying to understand their fate. Forensic anthropologists take a lead role in undertaking the methods to identify an unknown individual or an unidentified bone. However, not all the methodologies available will exactly identify the individual. The features of partial identification like stature, sex, age, etc., can help in narrowing down the pool of searches and will be a significant help to the investigative agencies. In this chapter, the author first tried to study the length of almost all the bones of the body both in males and females and calculated the regression equations from the north Indian population. However, the calculated equations will serve the purpose of identifying the stature of any abandoned unidentified bone. Second, aspects related to age, like the appearance of teeth in various ages, fusion, and the appearance of ossification centres of bone are studied. Finally, the morphological differences between gender are compared and studied using post-mortem computed tomography (PMCT).

Bones classification and description

Bones are categorized based on size and shape, location, origin, and structure.

A. **Size and shape**

Bones are classified as long bones or flat bones, while some are classified as short or irregular. Long and flat bones are easier to recognize while short and irregular bones are highly difficult to interpret in both man-made and natural disasters.

1. **Long bones:** These are much longer and not as wide. The bones of the arms, legs, fingers, and toes are long bones. Even though the bones of the fingers and toes appear short, they are longer than the width. Hence, they are considered long bones.
2. **Flat bones:** Denotes a flat appearance of bones. Bones of the skull, pelvis, and shoulder blade (scapula) are flat bones.
3. **Short bones:** These are small, rounded bones, e.g., carpal bones of the wrist, tarsal bones of the ankle, and sesamoid bones.
4. **Irregular bones:** These are the bones of the spine and the hyoid.

B. **Location**

1. **Axial skeleton:** The bones of the axial skeleton are not paired except for the ribs.
   The axial skeleton constitutes the skull, hyoid, backbone, sternum, and ribs.
2. **Appendicular skeleton:** All the appendicular bones are paired. The appendicular skeleton constitutes the pectoral girdle, arms, hands, pelvic girdle, legs, and feet.

Stature

Implications of post-mortem computed tomography in stature estimation

Post-mortem computed tomography (PMCT) is a highly useful and evolving technique. The measurements of the bones can be accurate to the nearest millimetre (mm). The main advantage of the PMCT is that it can reach all the bones which are difficult to access in traditional autopsy (TA). This aspect led to the author exploring the anthropological aspects related to stature which ultimately helps forensic pathologists to conclude the stature from the retrieved unidentified bones more scientifically.

Bones of interest

A. Long bones:
- Skull
- Sagittal suture
- Femur

B. Flat bones:
- Sternum
- Clavicle
- Scapula

C. Miscellaneous bones:
- Foot

Implications of linear regression equations in forensic anthropology

The linear regression is the linear equation that best fits the points. Linear regression describes the relationship between the dependent variable (stature) and the independent variables (various parameters).

The linear regression model calculates the stature based on the different lengths of the bones (IV, predictors). The linear regression equations, $y = (a+b)x$; where "y" is stature, "a" is the intercept where the line crosses the y-axis, "b" is regression coefficient, i.e., the slope which describes the line's direction and incline, and "x" is a predictor variable (various measurements of the bone). The linear regression equations can be used in to:

- Predict the dependent variable (stature)
- Estimate the effect of each independent variable (various bone lengths) on the dependent variable (stature)
- Calculate the correlation between the dependent variable and the independent variables
- Test the linear model significance level

In the scenario of abandoned skeletal remains, estimating the stature is a pivotal role of the forensic anthropologist. The conclusion based on these various equations can be applied to calculate the stature of the abandoned skeletal remains. This helps the investigating officer to narrow down the search of the victims in the estimated stature range. Thus the derived equations are of higher significance.

Do's and don'ts for the forensic anthropologist

- The forensic anthropologist should ensure the presence of the complete bone

DOI: 10.1201/9781003383703-8

- They should arrange all the available bones anatomically
- A PMCT of the anatomically arranged bones can be taken for the interpretation of findings
- An electronic cursor is used to measure various lengths of the bone from the landmarks as discussed below
- The calculated lengths of the bone are substituted in the calculated formula to estimate the probable stature of the bone
- The stature should always be mentioned in a range based on the standard error of the estimate

Stature measurement in PMCT

The lengths of the bones or parts of the bones can be measured using the electronic cursor (distance tool) available in the respective software. The starting point on the head end was from the most distal part of the vertex and the ending part in the lower limb was the distal-most part of the calcaneum (Figure 8.1).

Measurements of parameters of the skull in PMCT

- **Nasal breadth:** Maximum width between the left and right nasions of the nasal aperture.
- **Nasal height:** Height of the nose measured from the nasion to the nasal spine.
- **Left orbital breadth:** Width from the left mediofrontal to the left ectoconchion.
- **Right orbital breadth:** Width from the right mediofrontal to the right ectoconchion.
- **Left orbital height:** Maximum height from upper to lower borders of the left orbit perpendicular to the horizontal axis of the left orbit.
- **Right orbital height:** Maximum height from upper to lower borders of the right orbit perpendicular to the horizontal axis of the right orbit.

  The landmarks and the measurement of the above parameters are represented in Figure 8.2.

- **Minimum frontal breadth (MnFB):** Distance between both frontotemporals.

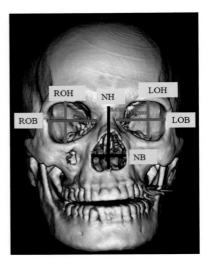

FIGURE 8.2: 3D VRT to measure the mentioned facial parameters using PMCT. (NB – nasal breadth, NH – nasal height, LOB – left orbital breadth, ROB – right orbital breadth, LOH – left orbital height, ROH – right orbital height.)

- **Interorbital breadth (IOB):** Distance between right and left dacryon.
- **Bizygomatic breadth (BZB):** Distance between most lateral points on the zygomatic arches.
- **Biorbital breadth (BB):** Distance between right and left ectoconchion.
- **Upper facial height (UFH):** Distance between nasion to prosthion (alveolare).

  The landmarks and the measurement of the above parameters are represented in Figure 8.3.

- **Palatal breadth:** The greatest breadth across the alveolar borders perpendicular to the median plane.
- **Palatal length:** Distance from the posterior palatal notch to the anterior-most border of the incisive alveoli.

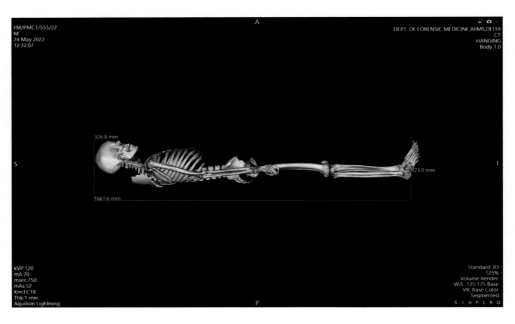

FIGURE 8.1:   3D volume-rendering technique (VRT) to measure stature using PMCT.

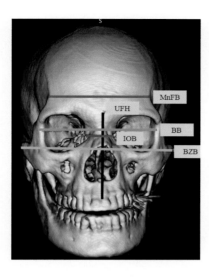

FIGURE 8.3: 3D VRT to measure the mentioned facial parameters using PMCT. (MnFB – minimum frontal breadth, IOB – interorbital breadth nasal height, BZB – bizygomatic breadth, BB – biorbital breadth, UFH – upper facial height.)

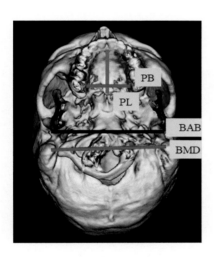

FIGURE 8.4: 3D VRT to measure the mentioned facial parameters using PMCT. (PB – palatal breadth, PL – palatal length, BAB – biauricular breadth, BMB – bimastoid breadth.)

- **Biauricular breadth (BAB):** Distance between the most lateral parts of left and right articular facets.
- **Bimastoidal diameter (BMD):** The distance between the mastoidal processes in the coronal plane.

The landmarks and the measurement of the above parameters are represented in Figure 8.4.
- **Left foramen magnum:** The leftmost lateral point of the foramen magnum.
- **Right foramen magnum:** The rightmost lateral point of the foramen magnum.
- **Maximum foramen magnum length (FML):** The anteroposterior diameter from the most anterior point of the foramen magnum to the most posterior point of the foramen magnum.

- **Maximum foramen magnum breadth (FMB):** The transverse diameter from the leftmost lateral point of the foramen magnum to the rightmost lateral point of the foramen magnum.
- **Distance between two external hypoglossal canal openings:** Distance between the right and left external hypoglossal canal openings, measured between the medial edges of the openings.

The landmarks and the measurement of the above parameters are represented in Figure 8.5. The various skull measurement in PMCT for male and female skulls are represented in Figures 8.6–8.13.

Regression equations for total population to calculate stature

Linear regression equations for estimation of stature from various skull measurements among the total population, male population and female population on both left and right sides as required are listed in Tables 8.1, 8.2, and 8.3 respectively.

Measurements of parameters of the sternum in PMCT

- **Manubrium length (ML):** It is the straight distance measured on the anterior surface of the sternum from the centre of the suprasternal notch to the centre of the manubrium-sternal junction in the midsagittal plane.
- **Manubrium width (MW):** It is measured as the distance between the midpoints of the facet for the first costal cartilage on each side.

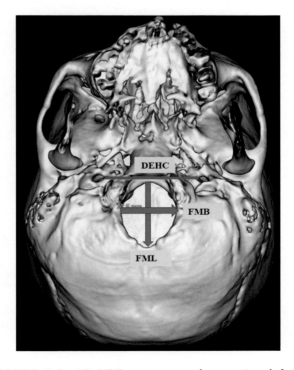

FIGURE 8.5: 3D VRT to measure the mentioned facial parameters using PMCT. (FMB – foramen magnum breadth, FML – foramen magnum length, DEHC – distance between two external hypoglossal canal openings.)

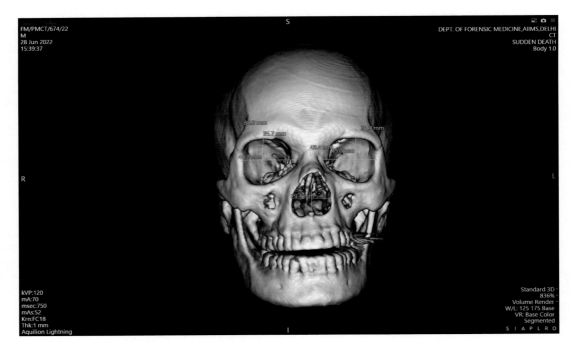

FIGURE 8.6: Measurements of skull parameters in a male skull: NB – nasal breadth, NH – nasal height, LOB – left orbital breadth, ROB – right orbital breadth, LOH – left orbital height, ROH – right orbital height.

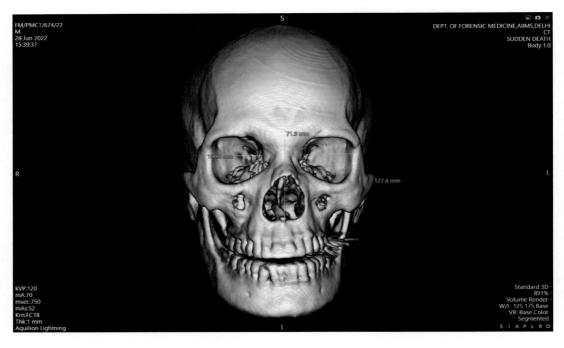

FIGURE 8.7: Measurements of skull parameters in a male skull: MnFB – minimum frontal breadth, IOB – interorbital breadth, NH – nasal height, BZB – bizygomatic breadth, BB – biorbital breadth, UFH – upper facial height.

- **Sternal body length (SBL):** It is the straight distance measured from the manubrium–sternal junction to the sternum–xiphoidal junction of the sternum in the mid-sagittal plane.

- **Total sternal length (TsTL):** Sum of the lengths of the manubrium and the sternum body.

  The landmarks and the measurement of the above parameters are represented in Figure 8.13.

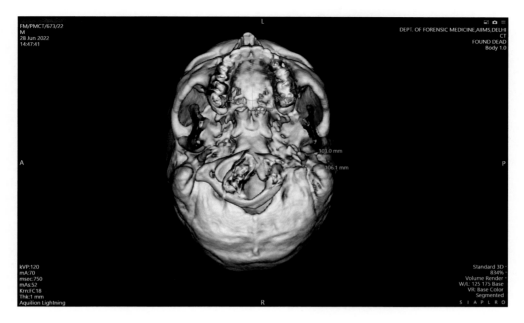

FIGURE 8.8: Measurements of skull parameters in a male skull: PB – palatal breadth, PL – palatal length, BAB – biauricular breadth, BMB – bimastoid breadth.

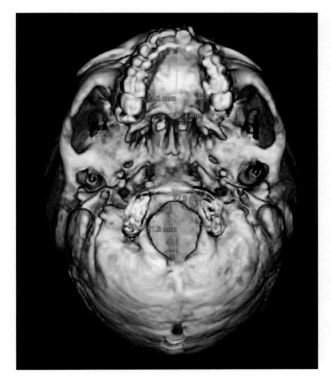

FIGURE 8.9: Measurements of skull parameters in a male skull: FMB – foramen magnum breadth, FML – foramen magnum length, DEHC – distance between two external hypoglossal canal openings.

Regression equations to calculate stature

Linear regression equations for estimation of stature from various sternum measurements among the total population, male population and female population on both left and right sides as required are listed in Table 8.4, 8.5, and 8.6 respectively.

Sexual dimorphism in lengths between gender among sternum

The various sternum measurement in PMCT for male and female skulls are represented in Figures 8.14 and 8.15.

- **Left clavicle length (LCL):** The distance between both ends of the left clavicle.
- **Right clavicle length (RCL):** The distance between both ends of the right clavicle.

The landmarks and the measurement of the above parameters are represented in Figure 8.16. The various clavicle measurement in PMCT for male and female skulls are represented in Figures 8.17 and 8.18.

Regression equations to calculate stature

Linear regression equations for estimation of stature from various clavicle measurements among the total population, male population and female population on both left and right sides as required are listed in Table 8.7, 8.8, and 8.9 respectively.

Measurements of parameters of the scapula in PMCT

- **Scapular maximum width (SMW):** The distance between the medial margin and the middle of the glenoid cavity.
- **Scapular maximum length (SML):** The distance between the end of the inferior angle and the vertex of the superior angle.
- **Longitudinal scapular length (LSL):** The distance between the end of the inferior angle and the superior margin of the coracoid process.
- **Longitudinal maximum length (LML):** The distance between the end of the inferior angle and the superior margin of the acromion process.

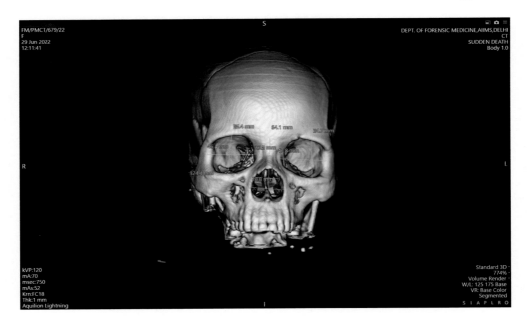

FIGURE 8.10: Measurements of skull parameters in a male skull: NB – nasal breadth, NH – nasal height, LOB – left orbital breadth, ROB – right orbital breadth, LOH – left orbital height, ROH – right orbital height, BZB – bizygomatic breadth.

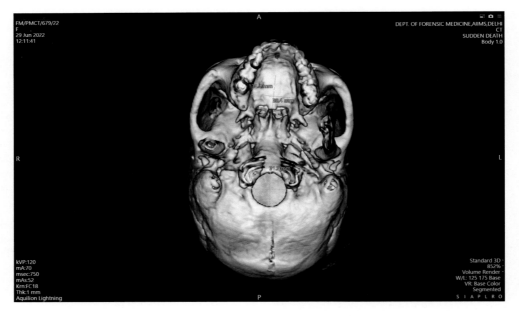

FIGURE 8.11: Measurements of skull parameters in a male skull: PB – palatal breadth, PL – palatal length, FMB – foramen magnum breadth, FML – foramen magnum length.

- **Transverse scapular length (TSL):** The distance between the medial margin and the inferior margin of the glenoid cavity.
- **Axillary margin length (AML):** The distance between the end of the inferior angle and the inferior margin of the glenoid cavity.

The landmarks and the measurement of the above parameters are represented in Figure 8.19. The various scapula measurements in PMCT for male and female skulls are represented in Figures 8.20 and 8.21.

Regression equations to calculate stature

Linear regression equations for the estimation of stature from various scapula measurements among the total population, male population and female population on both left and right sides as required are listed in Table 8.10, 8.11, and 8.12 respectively.

Measurements of parameters of the femur in PMCT

- **Right maximum femoral length (RMFL):** It is measured as the distance between a distal-most point of the superior part on the femoral head and a distal-most

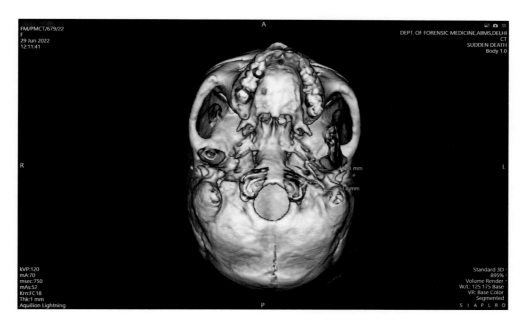

FIGURE 8.12: Measurements of skull parameters in a male skull: BAB – biauricular breadth, BMB – bimastoid breadth.

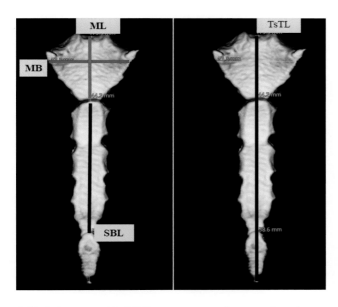

FIGURE 8.13: 3D VRT to measure the mentioned sternal parameters using PMCT: ML – manubrium length, MW – manubrium width, SBL – sternal body length, TsTL – total sternal length.

TABLE 8.1: Linear Regression equations derived from various skull measurements among total population

SKULL - Total Population	
Linear Regression Equation (y= a + b) x	**Variable**
103.48 + 4.24* (BMD)	BMD
101.39 + 5.82* (BZB)	BZB
87.31 + 5.71* (MnFB)	MnFB
66.63 + 5.70* (MxCL)	MxCL
94.78 + 6.46* (CBL)	CBL
72.80 + 6.77* (Ba-NB)	Ba-NB
119.27 + 6.30 * (BAB)	BAB
133.82 + 5.29* (NB)	NB
137.29 + 5.24* (NH)	NH
136.64 + 6.42* (ROB)	ROB
136.69 + 6.52* (LOB)	LOB
108.35+ 6.90* (BB)	BB
141.22 + 6.95* (IOB)	IOB
141.60 + 6.30* (ROH)	ROH
140.62 + 6.32* (LOH)	LOH
128.93 + 6.48* (UFH)	UFH
126.83 + 6.60* (PL)	PL
129.52+ 6.93* (PB)	PB
136.48 +6.35* (DEHC)	DEHC
130.64 + 5.81 * (FML)	FML
134.11 + 6.32* (FMB)	FMB

point of the most inferior part on the medial condyle of the right femur bone.

- **Left maximum femoral length (LMFL):** It is measured as the distance between a distal-most point of the superior part on the femoral head and a distal-most point of the most inferior part on the medial condyle of the left femur bone.
- **Right femoral bicondylar length (RFBL):** The linear distance between the distal-most point of the superior part on the femoral head and the distal-most inferior part among either condyle on the right femur.

- **Left femoral bicondylar length (LFBL):** The linear distance between a distal-most point of the superior part on the femoral head and the distal-most inferior part among either condyle on the left femur.
- **Right greater trochanter-bicondylar length (RGTBL):** The linear distance between a distal-most point of the superior part on the greater trochanter and the distal-most inferior part among either condyle on the right femur.

TABLE 8.2:   Linear Regression equations derived from various skull measurements among male population

SKULL – Male Population	
Linear Regression Equation (y= a + b) x	**Variable**
114.18 + 4.12* (BMD)	BMD
102.70 + 5.32* (BZB)	BZB
100.16 + 4.19* (MnFB)	MnFB
93.47 + 4.35* (MxCL)	MxCL
115.08 + 4.95* (CBL)	CBL
106.30 + 5.44 * (Ba-NB)	Ba-NB
136.27 + 4.77 * (BAB)	BAB
143.85 + 4.27 * (NB)	NB
145.56 + 3.79* (NH)	NH
146.97 + 4.53* (ROB)	ROB
146.95 + 4.56* (LOB)	LOB
130.74 + 5.48* (BB)	BB
150.58 + 4.30* (IOB)	IOB
150.33 + 4.65* (ROH)	ROH
150.06 + 4.63 * (LOH)	LOH
140.68 + 4.22 * (UFH)	UFH
146.57 + 4.54 * (PL)	PL
139.50 + 5.02* (PB)	PB
143.67 + 5.82* (DEHC)	DEHC
142.57 + 4.57* (FML)	FML
145.03 + 5.15* (FMB)	FMB

TABLE 8.3:   Linear Regression equations derived from various skull measurements among female population

SKULL – Female Population	
Linear Regression Equation (y= a + b)x	**Variable**
105.56 + 3.95* (BMD)	BMD
113.54 + 6.15* (BZB)	BZB
102.33 + 6.36* (MnFB)	MnFB
67.84 + 6.15* (MxCL)	MxCL
104.38. + 6.80* (CBL)	CBL
76.60 + 6.31 * (Ba-NB)	Ba-NB
105.86 + 6.02 * (BAB)	BAB
170.70 + 4.46* (NB)	NB
133.13 + 5.67* (NH)	NH
129.75 + 6.31 * (ROB)	ROB
130.23 + 6.48* (LOB)	LOB
102.29 + 5.79 * (BB)	BB
140.29 + 7.30* (IOB)	IOB
129.90 + 6.24* (ROH)	ROH
129.99 + 6.25* (LOH)	LOH
122.31 + 6.49* (UFH)	UFH
131.74 + 6.14* (PL)	PL
128.98 + 7.10* (PB)	PB
133.44 + 6.98* (DEHC)	DEHC
125.94 + 5.43* (FML)	FML
133.14 + 6.04* (FMB)	FMB

TABLE 8.4:   Linear Regression equations derived from various sternum measurements among total population

STERNUM- Total Population	
Variable	**Equation**
MW	119.72 + 7.63 * (MW)
ML	127.01 + 6.70 * (ML)
SBL	127.15 + 3.65 * (SBL)
TsTL	122.06 + 2.24 * (TsTL)

TABLE 8.5:   Linear Regression equations derived from various sternum measurements among male population

STERNUM- male	
Variable	**Equation**
MW	135.37 + 5.18* (MW)
ML	139.18 + 4.79 * (ML)
SBL	141 + 2.38 * (SBL)
TsTL	133.56 + 1.69 * (TsTL)

TABLE 8.6:   Linear Regression equations derived from various sternum measurements among female population

STERNUM- female	
Variable	**Equation**
MW	121.57 + 6.34* (MW)
ML	130.40 + 4.91* (ML)
SBL	126.90 + 3.23* (SBL)
TsTL	128.06 + 1.63* (TsTL)

- **Left greater trochanter-bicondylar length (LGTBL):** The linear distance between a distal-most point of the superior part on the greater trochanter and the distal-most inferior part among either condyle on the left femur.

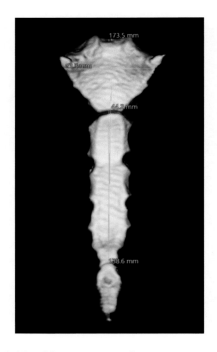

FIGURE 8.14:   Measurements of sternum parameters in a male sternum: ML – manubrium length, MW – manubrium width, SBL – sternal body length, TsTL – total sternal length.

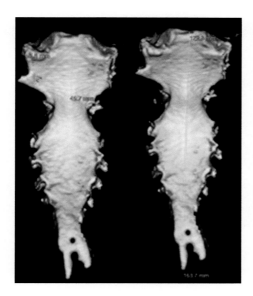

FIGURE 8.15: Measurements of sternum parameters in a female sternum: ML – manubrium length, MW – manubrium width, SBL – sternal body length, TsTL – total sternal length.

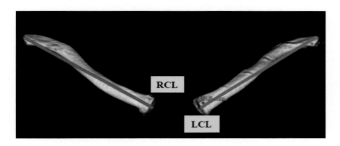

FIGURE 8.16: 3D VRT to measure the mentioned clavicle parameters using PMCT: LCL – left clavicular length, RCL – right clavicular length.

- **Right femoral epicondylar breadth (RFEB):** The linear distance between the distal-most point of the most medial and lateral points of the epicondyles on the right femur.
- **Left femoral epicondylar breadth (LFEB):** The linear distance between the distal-most point of the most medial and lateral points of the epicondyles on the left femur.
- **Maximum head diameter (RMHD):** It is measured as the maximum diameter of the femoral head on the right femur.
- **Left maximum head diameter (LMHD):** It is measured as the maximum diameter of the femoral head on the right femur.

The landmarks and the measurement of the above parameters are represented in Figure 8.22. The various femur measurements in PMCT for male and female femurs are represented in Figures 8.23 and 8.24.

Regression equations to calculate stature

Linear regression equations for the estimation of stature from various clavicle measurements among the total population, male population and female population on both left and right sides as required are listed in Tables 8.13, 8.14, and 8.15 respectively.

Sexual dimorphism in lengths between gender in the femur

Alleged history is that a human torso was found in a carry bag in an abandoned condition near the banks of a river in New Delhi. The human torso was brought by the investigating officer with queries related to the identity of the body (Figures 8.25 and 8.26).

The case was subjected to PMCT initially (Figure 8.27), along with virtual examination of important bones (Figures 8.28–8.30) and routine dissection was carried out. The sex of the individual is opined based on the external findings. The stature of the individual is opined based on the various scapula, clavicle, and sternal measurements obtained using PMCT after

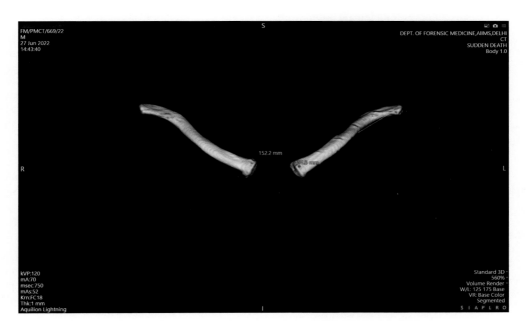

FIGURE 8.17: Measurements of clavicle parameters in a male clavicle.

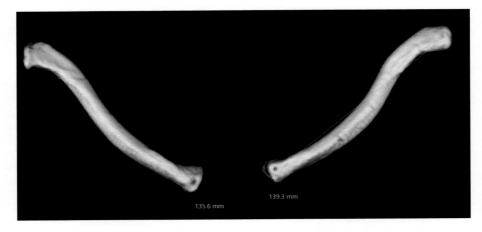

FIGURE 8.18:   Measurements of clavicle parameters in a female clavicle.

TABLE 8.7:   Linear Regression equations derived from various clavicle measurements among total population

CLAVICLE- Total Population	
Variable	Equation
RCL	83.52+ 5.46 * (RCL)
LCL	82.13 + 5.5* (LCL)

TABLE 8.8:   Linear Regression equations derived from various skull measurements among male population

STERNUM- male	
Variable	Equation
RCL	108.55+ 3.82* (RCL)
LCL	105.59 + 3.98* (LCL)

TABLE 8.9:   Linear Regression equations derived from various clavicle measurements among female population

CLAVICLE- female	
Variable	Equation
RCL	102.70 + 3.8 (RCL)
LCL	103.2 + 3.72 (LCL)

which the same was obtained on the corresponding formulae. The stature was given in a range which helped the investigating officer.

Age assessment: Possibilities and probabilities

Introduction

Estimation of age (age estimation/age assessment/age determination) is an evolving area of applied clinical research in the field of forensic medicine/science. Age can be calculated with accepted accuracy since its first appearance by around the 20th week of gestation using an X-ray-based radiological examination. It is essential to identify any individual by age, who is living (criminal culpability at court, eligibility to in any competitive sports, employment-related, permission to drive, age to get married, etc.), or in case of an unidentified person found dead (missing person found, retrieved skeletal remains). Age is an important criterion in most judicial considerations, and its absence demands assistance from a clinician to conclude their age. The principles of assessment of individuals in the healthcare setting remain uniform worldwide. The procedure is initiated by eliciting an appropriate history, performing a relevant physical examination, determining possible conclusions, and constructing a scientific plan to confirm or rule out a diagnosis. The history includes questions regarding the birth history like the date of birth in order to confirm the exact age. This is considered reliable in scenarios where the answer given by the patient is not the question in the legal sense. The answer given by the patient to the question "How old are you?" need not be challenged in a scenario where the history given by the patient is not suspicious. There are scenarios where a person masks the corpus delicti (the essence of the crime) by giving false details including preserving his/her identity. The history given differs grossly from the scientific findings that a scientific medical expert derives from his/her observations. A team of doctors from various fields of medicine is required to conduct the age estimations in the living: forensic physicians, paediatricians, and radiologists. The conclusions of the observations are always given in a range as it is highly impossible to give a specific number. This chapter outlines the scientific values and importance of age determination by using post-mortem computed tomography (PMCT) scanning to study the ossification centres of the bones.

Types of Age

There are two concepts needed for a better understanding of the processes happening in the human body. They are:

1. Chronological age
2. Bone age

1. **Chronological age:** This is the age calculated by any layman, which is the age calculated in years between the birth and the time of examination of the person.
2. **Bone age:** This is the age that is dependent on the maturation of the bones, which is modified by several physical and biological factors as discussed below.

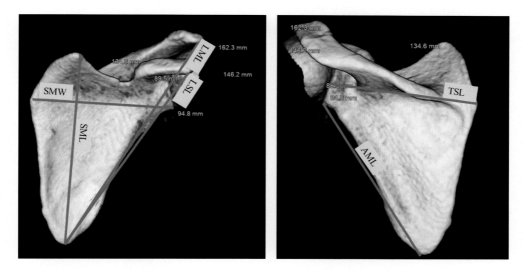

FIGURE 8.19: 3D VRT to measure the mentioned sternal parameters using PMCT: SMW – scapular maximum width, SML – scapular maximum length, LSL – longitudinal scapular length, LML – longitudinal maximum length, TSL – transverse scapular length, AML – axillary margin length.

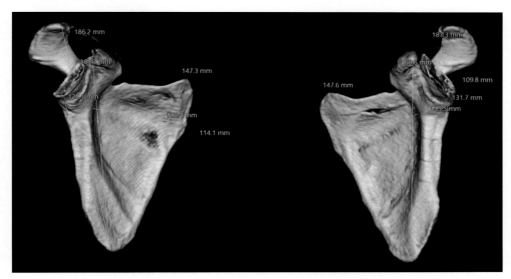

FIGURE 8.20: Measurements of sternum parameters in a male scapula.

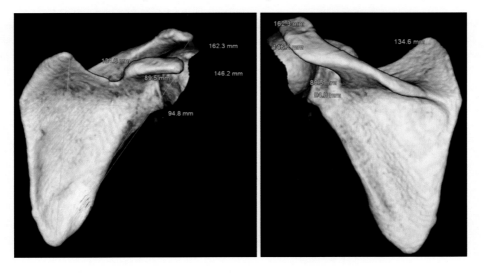

FIGURE 8.21: Measurements of sternum parameters in a female scapula.

TABLE 8.10: Linear Regression equations derived from various scapula measurements among total population

Variable	Equation
SCAPULA - Total Population	
LSMW	129.35 + 3.36* (LSMW)
LSML	102.91 + 4.11 * (LSML)
LLSL	101.07 + 3.84 * (LLSL)
LLML	86.14 + 4.28* (LLML)
LTSL	115.41 + 4.56 * (LTSL)
LAML	108.64 + 4.29 * (LAML)
RSMW	87.89 + 7.20* (RSMW)
RSML	109 + 3.67 * (RSML)
RLSL	104.42 + 3.63 * (RLSL)
RLML	86.38 + 4.25* (RLML)
RTSL	115.57 + 4.55 * (RTSL)
RAML	114.86 + 3.88 * (RAML)

TABLE 8.11: Linear Regression equations derived from various scapula measurements among male population

Variable	Equation
SCAPULA - Male	
LSMW	117.44 + 4.07* (LSMW)
LSML	98.39 + 4.24 * (LSML)
LLSL	82.66 + 4.76* (LLSL)
LLML	68.62 + 5.08* (LLML)
LTSL	99.91 + 5.62 * (LTSL)
LAML	90.79 + 5.32* (LAML)
RSMW	114.74 + 4.31* (RSMW)
RSML	101.32 + 4.01 * (RSML)
RLSL	83.75 + 4.68* (RLSL)
RLML	66.39 + 5.19* (RLML)
RTSL	96.10 + 5.99 * (RTSL)
RAML	93.49 + 5.12 * (RAML)

TABLE 8.12: Linear Regression equations derived from various scapula measurements among female population

Variable	Equation
SCAPULA - Female	
LSMW	107.52 + 4.82 * (LSMW)
LSML	106.99 + 3.48 * (LSML)
LLSL	97.11 + 3.69 * (LLSL)
LLML	81.45 + 4.23 * (LLML)
LTSL	100.52 + 5.30 * (LTSL)
LAML	110.39 + 3.43 * (LAML)
RSMW	102.06 + 5.35 * (RSMW)
RSML	112.05 + 3.09 * (RSML)
RLSL	96.50 + 3.72 * (RLSL)
RLML	78.68 + 4.39 * (RLML)
RTSL	100.85 + 5.24 * (RTSL)
RAML	111.04 + 3.39 * (RAML)

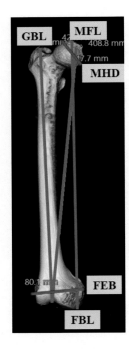

FIGURE 8.22: 3D VRT to measure the mentioned femur bone parameters using PMCT: MFLR – maximum femoral length, FBL – femoral bicondylar length, GTBL – greater trochanter-bicondylar length, FEB – femoral epicondylar breadth, MHD – maximum head diameter.

Approach for age estimation

Age estimation is a multi-factorial approach rather than a linear process. It takes into consideration history, like birth history, to rule out any developmental anomaly. Babies that are small for their gestational age appear physically and neurologically mature but their growth is less when compared to other babies due to delayed skeletal maturation. Babies diagnosed with thyroid function disorder in the form of congenital hypothyroidism during early life are shown to have delayed dental development and growth arrest. Several studies had proved the involvement of the thyroid hormone in tooth maturation in the early period of life. In addition, malnourishment associated with chronic intestinal inflammatory disease, cystic fibrosis, and celiac disease is highly prone to delayed bone age. Several children with cardiac diseases and chronic abdominal conditions affecting the liver and kidney had experienced a skeletal maturation delay. The factors associated with accelerated growth on the other hand led to overinterpretation of age. These include hyperthyroidism, weight gain (obesity), precocious puberty, and congenital adrenal hyperplasia. The major reason behind this is these conditions are associated with the production of the hormones responsible for increased maturation of the bone.

The following methodologies are considered after ruling out the mentioned conditions to conclude the age of any individuals. The history will be completely lacking in the case of a person who is found unconscious without any identity or in scenarios of retrieved skeletal remains. However, a possible age range can be given based on the history-blinded systematic approach of study which may help investigative agencies. The possible age is commented after:

- Dental development assessment
- Skeletal maturation study
- Consideration of secondary sexual characteristics

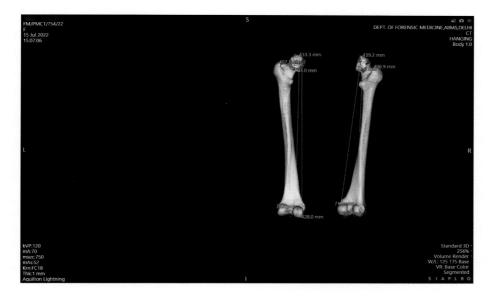

FIGURE 8.23: Measurements of various parameters in a male femur bone.

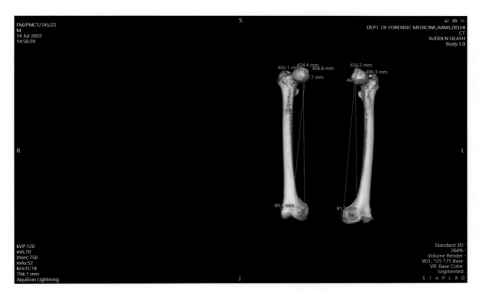

FIGURE 8.24: Measurements of various parameters in a female femur bone.

| TABLE 8.13: Linear Regression equations derived from various femur measurements among total population | | TABLE 8.14: Linear Regression equations derived from various skull measurements among male population | |

FEMUR - Total Population		FEMUR - Males	
Variable	**Equation**	**Variable**	**Equation**
MFLR	61.24 + 2.30 * (MFLR)	MFLR	107.27 + 1.33* (MFLR)
FBLR	62.66 + 2.33 * (FBLR)	FBLR	106.05 + 1.39 * (FBLR)
GBLR	64.98 + 2.35 * (GBLR)	GBLR	106.61 + 1.42 * (GBLR)
FEBR	95.6 + 8.53* (FEBR)	FEBR	122.66 + 5.47 * (FEBR)
MHDR	102.93 + 11.71 * (MHDR)	MHDR	127.99 + 7.48 * (MHDR)
MFLL	59.76 + 2.33 * (MFLL)	MFLL	120.81 + 9.97 * (MFLL)
FBLL	62.36 + 2.34* (FBLL)	FBLL	102.28 + 1.48* (FBLL)
GBLL	65.32 + 2.34 * (GBLL)	GBLL	107.55 + 1.40 * (GBLL)
FEBL	97.90 + 8.20 * (FEBL)	FEBL	122.23 + 5.51 * (FEBL)
MHDL	109.95 + 10.18*(MHDL)	MHDL	132.68 + 6.54 * (MHDL)

TABLE 8.15: Linear Regression equations derived from various skull measurements among female population

FEMUR - Females	
Variable	**Equation**
MFLR	88.53 + 1.55* (MFLR)
FBLR	92.52 + 1.50 * (FBLR)
GBLR	95.58 + 1.47 * (GBLR)
FEBR	122 + 4.34 * (FEBR)
MHDR	113.46 + 8.61 * (MHDR)
MFLL	89.22 + 1.54 * (MFLL)
FBLL	92.92 + 1.50 * (FBLL)
GBLL	94.78 + 9.70 * (GBLL)
FEBL	123.56 + 4.11* (FEBL)
MHDL	125.05 + 6.36 * (MHDL)

Tooth implications in forensic medicine (forensic odontology)

Forensic odontology is by definition, the application of dental science to the law. This speciality within the forensic sciences has been utilized for many years, principally in the area of **establishing identity.** Dental features are extremely important for age determination (see earlier in this chapter).

Identity by dentition data. Examination of the teeth may be of great value for the identification of an individual. Dental records are essential for this. These records may be of particular use in establishing identity. The identity of a body can be established from the following features:

(a) The details regarding **residual teeth** (number left behind, extracted, or missing, presence of cavities and fillings) or any other dental work and peculiarities of jaws or teeth.

(b) By **comparing artificial dentures** and their complementary jaw.

(c) **Edentulous jaw** with roots left behind after extractions.

The following case illustrates how these features helped to establish identity.

Baptist Church Cellar Case: In July 1942, some workmen, while demolishing a Baptist church in the Vauxhall district of London, found under a cellar floor a partly dismembered body which, it was thought, had lain there for about 12–18 months. Lime had been strewn over it, preserving a fracture of the larynx which suggested the death was due to strangling; parts of the arms and legs and lower jaw were missing. The premises were unoccupied but the wartime fire watcher, a man named Dobkin, was suspected since he was the only person with access to the cellar in question. About 15 months earlier his

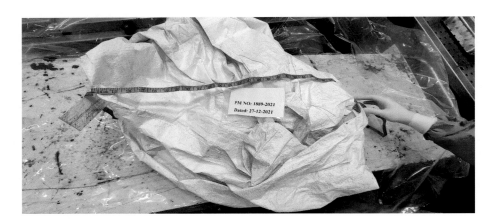

FIGURE 8.25: The body in a body bag before opening the bag.

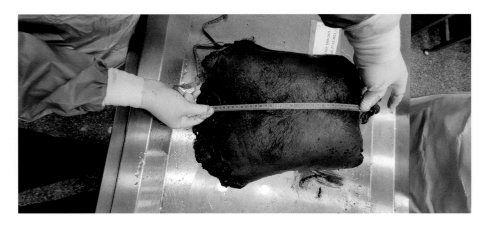

FIGURE 8.26: Autopsy examination of the torso.

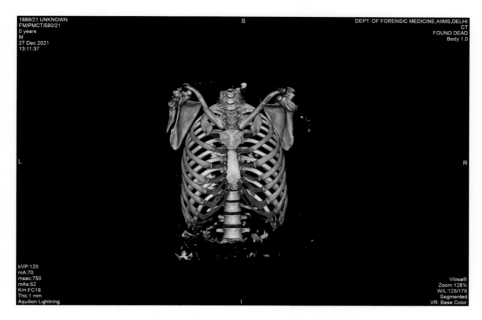

FIGURE 8.27: 3D VRT of the mentioned case.

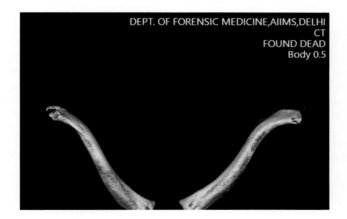

FIGURE 8.28: VRT examination of clavicles without dissection

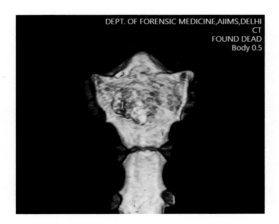

FIGURE 8.29: VRT examination of sternum without dissection

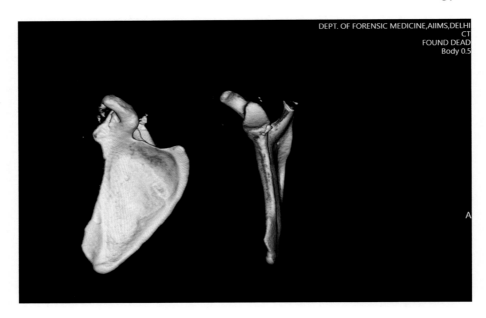

FIGURE 8.30: VRT examination of scapulae without dissection

wife had disappeared after attempting to obtain arrears of maintenance from him. Four days after her disappearance, i.e., on 15 April 1942, a fire was seen in the said place by two passing constables who drew his attention to it. Examination showed that the remains were those of a woman aged 40–50 years, 5 ft 1 in in height with dark brown hair and in whose womb, there was a fibroid. Mrs. Dobkin was 49 years old, 5 ft 1 in in height with dark brown hair going grey. The dental surgeon who had attended to her was traced and his records of the patient when last seen and features of the upper jaw collected from the cellar were compared. They were identical in number and position of teeth, the situation of fillings, marks of fittings of dentures, the remains of roots, etc. The dental surgeon later identified the skull saying 'That is Mrs. Dobkin's jaw and those are my fillings'.

Dental charting: The most widely utilized charting systems in the world today include the following:

Universal system

The universal system is widely used in the United States. According to this system, each tooth is given a number—1 through 16 for the upper, and 17 through 32 for the lower. Thus the lower right canine is designated 27 (Figure 8.31).

Palmer's notation

The system utilized the numbering system which is 8 to 1 starting with the third molars on each side and moving to the midline (Figure 8.32).

Haderup system

The Haderup system is similar to Palmer's notation except that it uses a plus sign (+) to designate upper teeth and a minus

sign (–) for the lower. The plus sign or minus sign is positioned before or after the number to designate the side of the arch. Thus the lower right canine would be designated 3– in this system (Figure 8.33).

FDI two-digit system

The FDI two-digit system advocated by the Federation Dentaine Internationale is similar to Palmer's system in that both utilize the same numbers but the FDI system substitutes a number for the quadrant sign and that number is placed before the tooth number (Figure 8.34). Therefore, the lower right canine would be number 4,3 in this system. The numbering is different for permanent and temporary teeth. Number (1,4) designates the right side and number (2,3) designates the left

Upper

8 7 65 43 2 1	1 2 3 4 5 6 7 8
8 7 65 43 2 1	1 2 3 4 5 6 7 8

Lower

FIGURE 8.32: Palmer's notation.

8 +7+ 6+ 5+ 4+3+2+ 1+	+1 +2 +3 +4 +5 +6 +7 +8
8- 7- 6- 5- 4- 3- 2- 1-	-1 -2 -3 -4 -5 -6 -7 -8

FIGURE 8.33: The Haderup system.

Permanent teeth

18 17 16 15 14 13 12 11	21 22 23 24 25 26 27 28
48 47 46 45 44 43 42 41	31 32 33 34 35 36 37 38

Temporary teeth

55 54 53 52 51	61 62 63 64 65
85 84 83 82 81	72 73 74 75

FIGURE 8.34: The FDI two-digit system for permanent and temporary teeth.

Upper

Right | 1 2 3 4 5 6 7 8 | 9 10 11 12 13 14 15 16 | Left
| 32 31 30 29 28 27 26 25 | 24 23 22 21 20 19 18 17 |

Lower

FIGURE 8.31: The universal system.

side for permanent teeth. For temporary teeth numbers (5,8) designates the right side and number (6,7) designates the left side.

Temporary teeth

Modified FDI system

There has been a modification in the FDI system that makes the even first number (2,4) designate the left side and the odd first number (1,3) designate the right. Thus the lower right canine becomes number 33 in the FDI-modified system. (Figure 8.35).

Diagrammatic or anatomical chart

Teeth are represented by diagrams or pictorial symbols of the same number of teeth, cavities, fillings, and dentures. Incisors and canines are depicted with four surfaces and molars and premolars with five surfaces.

Embryology of Tooth

The age of an individual can be stated based on dental development as the variability is low when compared to the chronological age. There are four main stages of development of the tooth (Table 8.16):

- **Stage 1 (Bud Stage):** This initial stage of development starts around the eighth intrauterine week of the development of a fetus. The enamel organs are the first part of the tooth to form in the form of swellings due to the action of the mesenchymal cells.
- **Stage 2 (Cap Stage):** Around 3 to 4 months of gestation, the enamel organ expands and leads to the formation of crown, pulp, and root partly.
- **Stage 3 (Early Bell Stage):** The disintegration of dental lamina occurs followed by the initiation of the dentine formation by the odontoblasts. Ameloblasts are columnar cells formed from the inner enamel epithelium. The secretory end of the ameloblasts is commonly called Tome's process which is responsible for the secretion of enamel matrix. This is followed by the calcification of the matrix by deposition of the calcium and phosphate ions into the enamel matrix, which forms hydroxyapatite crystallites. There occurs loss of the Tome's process in the ameloblast cells which further flattens and becomes the enamel epithelium. This enamel epithelium

protects the enamel while eruption occurs. Hence, stage 3 of development is concerned with dentine formation, enamel formation, and complete root formation.

- **Stage 4 (Late Bell Stage):** The root formation is followed by the cementum formation (cementogenesis). The cementoblasts are the cells responsible for its formation, by secreting the cementum matrix which undergoes mineralization due to deposition of hydroxyapatite crystals. Lastly, the periodontal ligament s formed from the dental follicle which differentiates into fibroblasts to secrete collagen. This collagen is responsible for the formation of the ligament, one end is connected to the cementum while the other end is embedded in the alveolar bone, which is collectively addressed as Sharpey's fibers.

Anatomy of teeth

Each tooth has four main parts, including the following:

- **Enamel:** This is the outer layer of the tooth which covers the crown completely (Table 8.17).
- **Dentin:** The inner layer and the main part of the tooth. This forms the bulk of the crown and root.
- **Pulp:** This is the soft tissue situated inside the tooth. It contains the neurovascular structures required for the tooth to maintain its vitality (Table 8.18).
- **Root:** The part of the tooth that presents inside the jaw and holds the teeth.

The anatomy of the tooth is illustrated in Figures 8.36–8.39.

Dentition

The observation of the germination and calcification of roots and eruption of deciduous and permanent dentition provides a fair guide to age from birth to 17 years of age. The temporary teeth are 20 in number and the permanent ones 32. The differences between the temporary and permanent teeth are given in Table 8.19. The gross images of the permanent dentition are depicted in Figures 8.40 and 8.41.

Methods to estimate age from teeth

1. Tooth eruption method
2. Gustafson's method
3. Boyde's method

28	27	26	25	24	23	22	21	11	12	13	14	15	16	17	18
38	37	36	35	34	33	32	31	41	42	43	44	45	46	47	48

FIGURE 8.35: The modified FDI system.

TABLE 8.16:   Stages of development of tooth

Embryology of Tooth	
Stages	**Features**
Stage 1 (Bud Stage)	Develops from 8th week of intrauterine life. Enamel develops first from mesenchymal cells
Stage 2 (Cap Stage)	Develops at 3 to 4 months of gestational age. Crown, pulp and root develop.
Stage 3 (Early Bell Stage)	Dentine formation, enamel formation and the complete root formation occurs
Stage 4 (Late Bell Stage)	Cementogenesis occurs followed by periodontal ligament formation

TABLE 8.17:   Enamel difference between temporary and permanent tooth

Enamel	
Temporary tooth	**Permanent tooth**
Thinner enamel	Thicker enamel
Colour is lighter (more whitish)	Colour is darker (more yellowish)
Broad and flat contact surface with opposing tooth	Point contact on surface with opposing tooth

TABLE 8.18:   Pulp difference between temporary and permanent tooth

Pulp	
Temporary tooth	**Permanent tooth**
Pulp chamber larger	Pulp chamber smaller
Root canal ribbon/hour glass shaped	Root canal well defined
High vascularity	Low vascularity

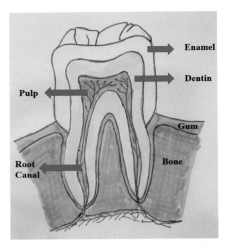

FIGURE 8.36: A diagrammatic representation depicting the gross anatomy of the tooth.

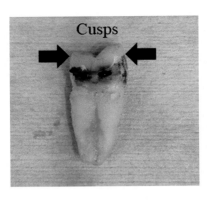

FIGURE 8.38: A premolar permanent tooth showing the cusps of a tooth.

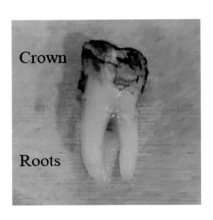

FIGURE 8.37: A molar tooth showing the roots and the crown.

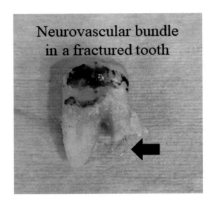

FIGURE 8.39: A fracture molar tooth showing the neuro-vascular tissue from the pulp cavity.

TABLE 8.19: Difference between temporary and permanent teeth

Features	Temporary/deciduous teeth	Permanent teeth
Size and shape	Smaller, lighter and narrower, except temporary molars which are longer than permanent premolars replacing them	Larger, heavier, and broader, except permanent premolars replacing temporary molars which are smaller.
Anterior teeth	Directed vertically	Inclined forward
Colour of crown	China white	Ivory white
Neck	More constricted	Less constricted
Roots of the molars	Smaller, more divergent	Larger and less divergent
Junction of crown and the root	Ridge is present	Ridge is not present
Radiological examination	Presence of tooth germ below tooth suggests that the tooth is deciduous	No teeth germ will be seen below tooth

4. Stack's method
5. Demirjian's method
6. Haavikko's method
7. Nolla's method

1. **Tooth eruption and calcification**

The approximate periods at which temporary (Figure 8.42 and Table 8.20) and permanent (Figure 8.42 and Table 8.21) teeth erupt and calcify are as follows:

- The **calcification of the roots of milk teeth** is usually complete by the end of 3 years of age, the incisors and the molars being the last to calcify.
- **Resorption of the roots** of the incisors starts about 4 years of age followed by molars at 6–7 years of age and the canines at 8 years of age.
- The **temporary teeth are shed** from 5 to 7 years of age.
- The **first permanent molars appear** at about 6 years of age. There is great uncertainty regarding the eruption of the third molar. In some cases, it appears very late in life.

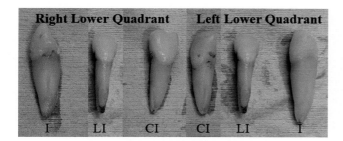

FIGURE 8.40: Gross images of the permanent dentition consisting of mandibular central incisors, lateral incisors, and canine.

Often it gets impacted and sometimes gives rise to a cyst formation called a 'dentigerous cyst'. Premolars are most erratic in eruption and are of little value in determining age.

- The **calcification of the crown** takes place 2–3 years earlier than eruption, except in the case of first molars and incisors, where calcification takes place in the intrauterine period. In general, complete calcification of roots takes place 3–4 years after eruption.

Note:

- In some cases, **temporary teeth may either appear abnormally early** or may be present even at the time of birth as in the cases of congenital syphilis and in mental retardation.
- **Eruption** of temporary as well as permanent teeth **may be delayed** for a considerable time owing to dietary deficiency of vitamins A, D, C, and calcium.
  2. **Gustafson's Method**

Gustafson (1950) studied the changes occurring in individual teeth and succeeded in estimating age with some accuracy. Longitudinal ground sections of the tooth are examined by the naked eye and microscopically for evidence of attrition, periodontosis, secondary dentin, cementum apposition, root resorption, and root transparency. **The section is prepared by grinding the tooth from two sides towards the centre until a thin film, 0.25 mm thick remains. This method is applicable only to permanent teeth**. Decalcified sections and molars are not suitable for this examination.

Attrition: Takes place with the wearing down of incisal or occlusal surfaces due to mastication and can be appreciated by macroscopic as well as microscopic examination (Figure 8.43).

Periodontosis: Loosening of the tooth or continuous eruption is characterized by changes in the attachment of the tooth. The gum margin becomes retracted. This can be seen macroscopically and microscopically.

Secondary dentin: This may form within the pulp cavity partly as a result of ageing and partly as a reaction to pathological conditions such as caries and periodontosis. The change is seen only through microscopy.

Cementum apposition: The apposition of cementum at and around the root can be seen in microscopic sections.

Root resorption: This involves both cementum and dentin and is best seen in the microscopic section.

Root transparency: The transparency of the apical parts of the root is best appreciated on the ground section but is also visible sometimes on an unprepared tooth. The transparency should be observed **before it is mounted** since the mounting medium is likely to percolate into the dentinal tubule which vitiates the root transparency (Johanson, 1971).

Ranking of age changes: Each change is ranked arbitrarily and allotted points 0, 1, 2 or 3, according to the degree of structural changes and staged as mentioned in (Table 8.22 and Figure 8.44A–D).

Point formula: The point values of each age change assessed as mentioned above are now added according to the following formula:

$$A_n + P_n + S_n + C_n + R_n + T_n = \text{Points}$$

It has been observed that an increase in age is accompanied by increasing point values. Gustafson, using the point values of teeth of known age, evolved a **regression equation** and drew a **regression line** to represent the relation between age and point value. In order to calculate the age of an individual, the point value for the tooth in question is entered on the chart, its crossing with the regression line read, and the corresponding age read off from the graph.

Subsequent workers have confirmed the utility of this method in age determination (Johanson, 1971; Pillai and Bhaskar, 1974; Ramachandran, 1974). Pillai and Bhaskar (1974) have evolved the following regression equation to calculate the age:

Age (in years) = 5.34 × point value – 4.08

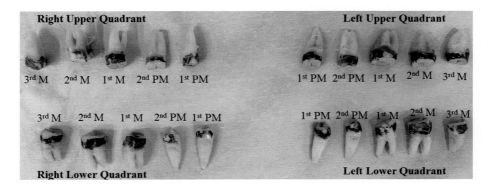

FIGURE 8.41: Gross images of the permanent dentition consisting of premolars and molars of the maxilla and mandible.

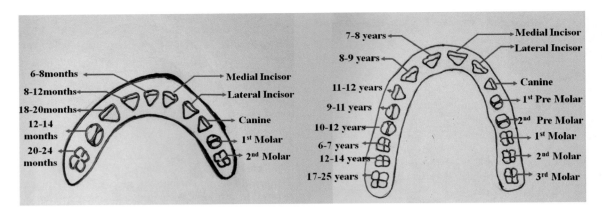

FIGURE 8.42: Line diagram showing the cusp view of temporary dentition and permanent with eruption time.

TABLE 8.20: **Time of eruption of temporary teeth**

Teeth	Time in months	Time of calicification of root in years
Lower central incisors	6–8	1½–2
Upper central incisors	8	1½–2
Upper lateral incisors	8–10	1½–2
Upper lateral incisors	10–12	1½–2
First molars	12–14	2–2½
Canines	18–20	2–2½
Second molars	20–24	2–2½

TABLE 8.21: **Time of eruption of permanent teeth**

Teeth	Time in years	Time of calcification of root in years
First molar	6–7	9
Medical incisor	7–8	10
Lateral incisor	8–9	11
First premolar	9–11	12
Second premolar	10–12	13
Canine	11–12	13
Second molar	12–14	15
Third molar (wisdom teeth)	17–25 or later or never at all.	18–25

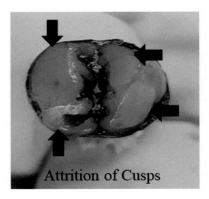

FIGURE 8.43: A molar tooth showing the attrition of the cusps.

3. **Boyde's Method**

   It is based on microscopically counting the number of cross striations or incremental lines from the **neonatal line** in the enamel of teeth. The **neonatal line** is a band of incremental growth lines seen in histologic sections of both enamel and dentine of primary and permanent teeth. It belongs to a series of growth lines in **tooth enamel** known as the **striae of Retzius**. The neonatal line is darker and larger than the rest of the striae of Retzius. It is caused by the different physiologic changes at birth and is used to identify enamel formation before and after birth. The longitudinal section of the tooth is taken and stained with iodine (2%) and collodion. It is applicable to estimate the age of infants who are dead.

4. **Stack's Method**

   It is the method to estimate the age of a fetus or infant from the weight and height of the erupting teeth. By weighing the teeth specimen, age can be obtained from 5 months in utero to postnatal age of 7 months (Tables 8.23 and 8.24).

5. **Demirjian method**

The development of the tooth is divided into eight stages (A to H) in the seven-left permanent

mandibular teeth (from the central incisor to the second molar). Each tooth is given a stage that is converted to a numerical score from a specific table. The summation of scores of the seven teeth is converted to the DA using a gender-specific table for translating the results of dental maturity.

The age-wise appearances of teeth are depicted in Figures 8.45–8.64 using PMCT.

PMCT images of tooth eruption for respective ages
   Month-old fetus
   Term fetus
   2-month female
   1.2-year male
   2-year male
   2-year female
   4.5-year female
   6-year female
   6-year male
   7-year male

TABLE 8.22:   Findings to note in different stages of eruption of permanent teeth according to Gustafson method

Stage 0	Stage 1	Stage 2	Stage 3
no attrition	attrition lying within enamel	attrition reaching the dentin	attrition reaching the pulp.
no periodontitis	periodontosis has just begun	periodontosis has passed along the first 1/3 of the root	periodontosis has passed 2/3 of the root.
no secondary dentin is visible	dentin has just begun to form in the upper part of the pulp cavity	the pulp cavity is half filled with dentin	the pulp cavity is nearly or wholly filled with secondary dentin.
Normal layer of cementum is laid down	the layer is a little greater than normal	a great layer	a heavy layer
no visible root resorption	resorption only on small, isolated spots	greater loss of substance	great areas of cementum and the dentin are affected.
transparency is not present	it is just noticeable	it extends over apical 1/3 of the root	it extends over the apical 2/3 of the root.

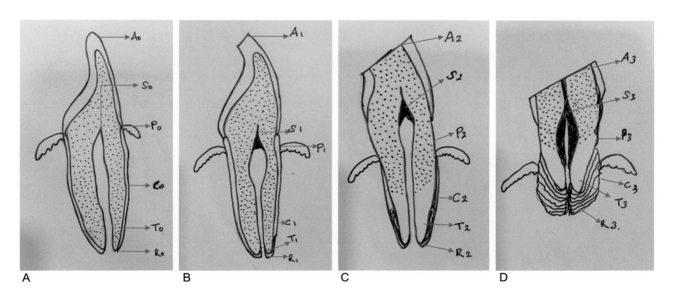

FIGURE 8.44:   A: Gustafson's analysis of age changes in teeth – Stage 0. B: Gustafson's analysis of age changes in teeth – Stage 1. C: Gustafson's analysis of age changes in teeth – Stage 2. D: Gustafson's analysis of age changes in teeth – Stage 3.

TABLE 8.23:   Estimation of pretnatal age by weight of teeth

Prenatal age (weeks)	Sum of teeth weight (mg)
28	60
40	460

TABLE 8.24:   Estimation of postnatal age by weight of teeth

Postnatal age (weeks)	Sum of teeth weight (mg)
2	530
30	1840

Age from skeletal ossification

The skeletal changes are subject to alteration depending on race, sex, nutritional status, heredity, etc. If age, based on these changes, is to be determined with confidence, one should have norms worked out by their own region. The figures given are only averages. In general, skeletal ossification changes occur earlier in girls. The age-wise appearance of various ossification centres of bone is depicted in Figures 8.65–8.78 using PMCT and listed in Table 8.25.

Findings to note in PMCT images related to age estimation

Changes in the symphysis pubis

- The irregular face of the symphysis pubis (billowing) becomes granular or smooth as age advances.
- It becomes partly granular around 25 years of age and the granularity becomes marked and involves the entire face by the age of 35 years
- Lipping of the symphyseal face commences around 35 years of age and is well marked at 45–50 years of age. The events are summarised in Table 8.26.

Closure of cranial sutures

- The metopic suture gets obliterated around 2 years of age but may persist into adult life.
- Bony replacement of the cartilage between the basisphenoid and basiocciput commences at about 17 years of age and is complete by 22–24 years of age.
- The closure of the suture of the skull's vault begins endocranially and proceeds ectocranially.
- The union in the inner aspect of the skull occurs 5–10 years earlier than externally. It occurs externally in the following order: Posterior third of the sagittal suture

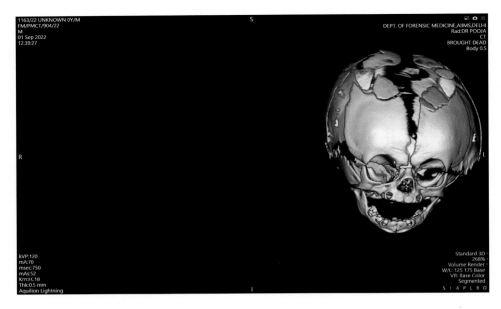

FIGURE 8.45:   3D VRT of the skull of a month-old decomposed fetus showing the absence of primary erupted teeth in both the maxilla and mandible bone.

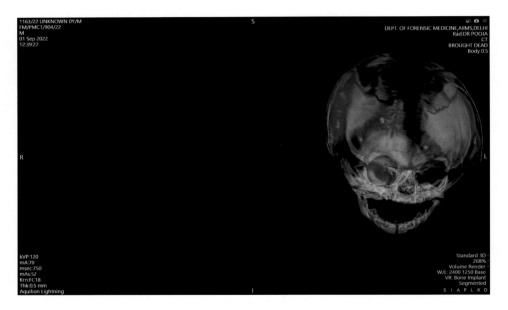

FIGURE 8.46:   3D VRT of the skull with bone-implant filter of the same fetus shows the absence of the unerupted primary tooth inside the bony margins of the maxilla and mandible.

around 30–40 years of age, anterior third of the sagittal and lower half of the coronal around 40–50 years of age, and middle sagittal and upper half of the coronal around 50–60 years of age (Table 8.27).

- The temporoparietal sutures close much later.

Frontal bone

Changes in frontal bone may be used for the determination of age (Table 8.28).

Changes in mandible and sacrum

Age estimation from the skeletal changes in the mandible and sacrum are given in Tables 8.29 and 8.30.

Other skeletal changes in advanced age (miscellaneous)

Ribs: The secondary centres for the head and tubercule of ribs appear between 16 and 20 years of age and fuse with the shaft at about 25 years of age.

Vertebrae

- The **secondary centre for each side of the arch of vertebra** appears before birth and fuses with the body and the other half of the arch at 3–6 years of age.
- Those for the **spinous, transverse, and mammillary processes** and **upper and lower surfaces of the body** appear around puberty and fuse around 25 years of age.

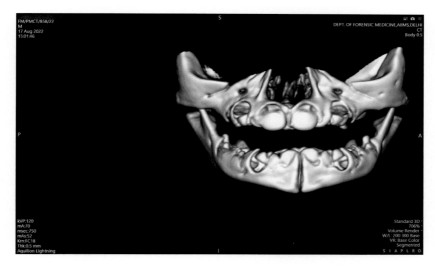

FIGURE 8.47: 3D VRT of the maxilla and mandible in the bone-white filter of a term fetus showing the absence of erupted primary teeth in both the maxilla and mandible bone.

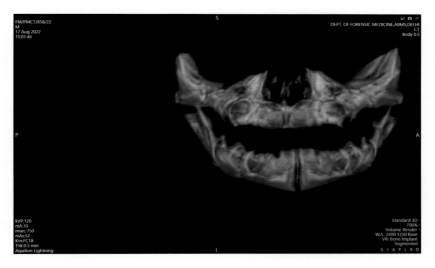

FIGURE 8.48: 3D VRT of the maxilla and mandible of the same fetus in the bone-implant filter shows the presence of the unerupted primary tooth inside the bony margins at places.

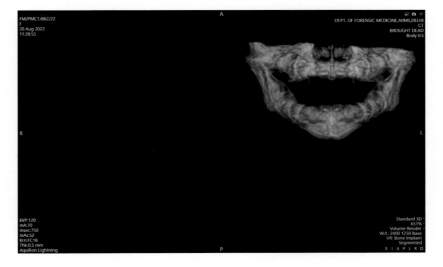

FIGURE 8.49: 3D VRT of the maxilla and mandible bone in bone-implant filter of a 2-month-old female child showing the absence of erupted primary teeth in both the maxilla and mandible bone. The blue colour denotes the presence of unerupted primary teeth inside the bone.

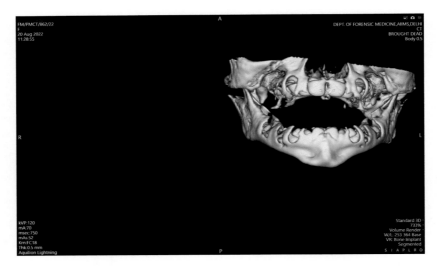

FIGURE 8.50: 3D VRT of the maxilla and mandible bone of the same fetus in the translucency filter shows the presence of the unerupted primary tooth inside the bony margins of the maxilla and mandible bone at places.

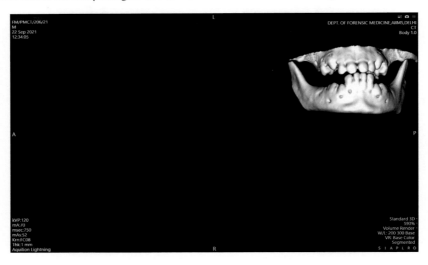

FIGURE 8.51: 3D VRT of the maxilla and mandible bone in the bone-white filter of a 1.2-year-old male child showing the presence of erupted primary teeth (14).

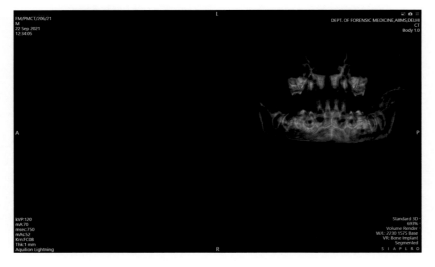

FIGURE 8.52: 3D VRT of the maxilla and mandible bone in bone-implant filter of a 1.2-year-old male child showing the presence of unerupted permanent teeth inside the bony margins (blue colour).

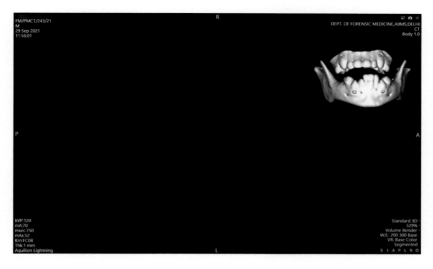

FIGURE 8.53: 3D VRT of the maxilla and mandible bone in the bone-white filter of a 2-year-old male child showing the presence of erupted primary teeth (16) in both the maxilla and mandible bone.

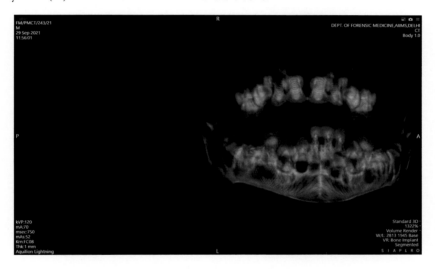

FIGURE 8.54: 3D VRT of the maxilla and mandible bone in bone-implant filter of a 2-year-old male child showing the presence of unerupted permanent teeth inside the bony margins (blue colour).

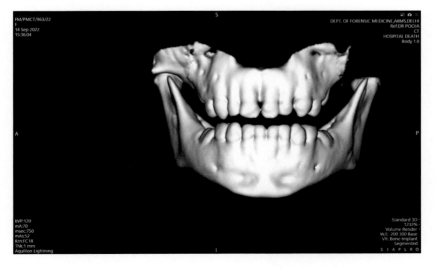

FIGURE 8.55: 3D VRT of the maxilla and mandible bone in the bone-white filter of a 2-year-old female showing the presence of erupted primary teeth (18).

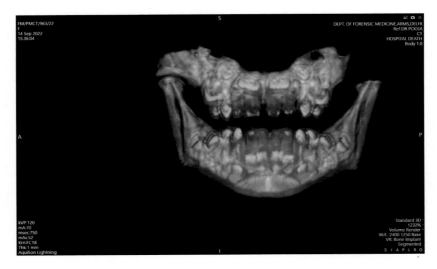

FIGURE 8.56:   3D VRT of the maxilla and mandible bone in bone-implant filter of a 2-year-old female child showing the presence of unerupted permanent teeth inside the bony margins (blue colour).

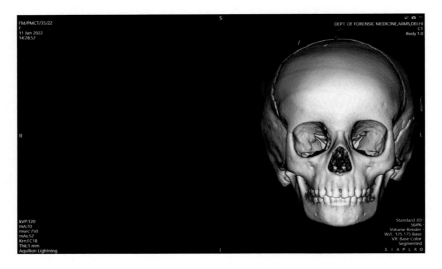

FIGURE 8.57:   3D VRT of the skull bone of a 4.5-year-old female showing the presence of erupted primary teeth (20).

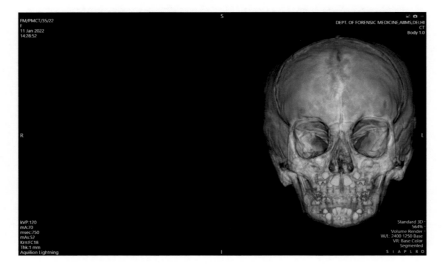

FIGURE 8.58:   3D VRT of the skull bone of a 4.5-year-old female showing the presence of unerupted permanent teeth (21).

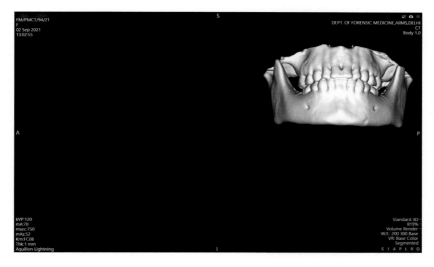

FIGURE 8.59: 3D VRT of the maxilla and mandible bone in the bone-white filter of a 6-year-old female showing the presence of erupted primary teeth (22).

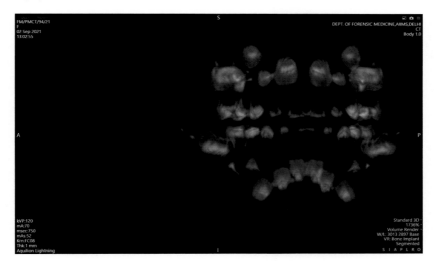

FIGURE 8.60: 3D VRT of the maxilla and mandible in bone-implant filter of a 6-year-old female showing the presence of unerupted permanent teeth (20).

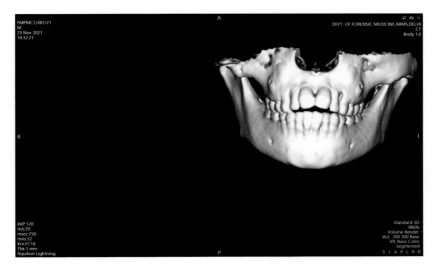

FIGURE 8.61: 3D VRT of the maxilla and mandible bone in the bone-white filter of a 6-year-old male showing the presence of erupted teeth (24).

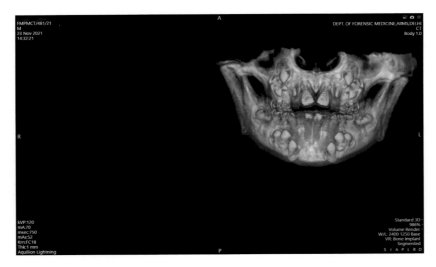

FIGURE 8.62: 3D VRT of the maxilla and mandible bone in the bone-implant filter of a 6-year-old male showing the presence of erupted central permanent incisors, and unerupted permanent teeth (20).

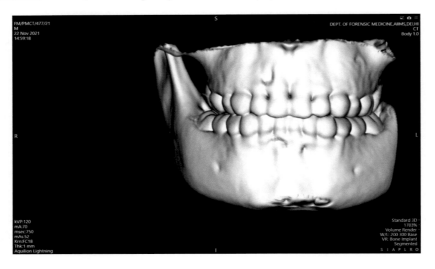

FIGURE 8.63: 3D VRT of the maxilla and mandible bone in the bone-white filter of a 7-year-old male showing the presence of erupted teeth (24).

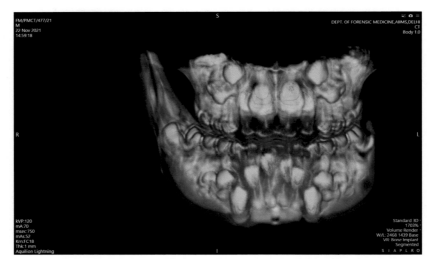

FIGURE 8.64: 3D VRT of the maxilla and mandible bone in the bone-implant filter of a 7-year-old male showing the presence of erupted central and lateral permanent incisors, and unerupted permanent teeth (20).

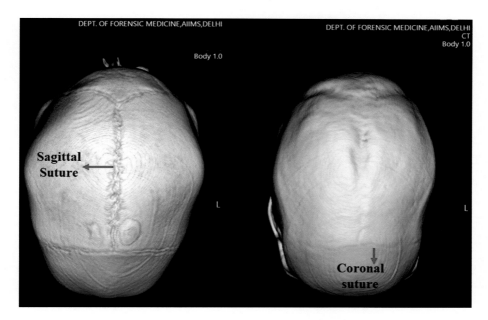

FIGURE 8.65: 3D VRT of the skull bone in the radiograph filter (left) and skeletal filter (right) showing fused (left) and unfused (right) sagittal and coronal sutures.

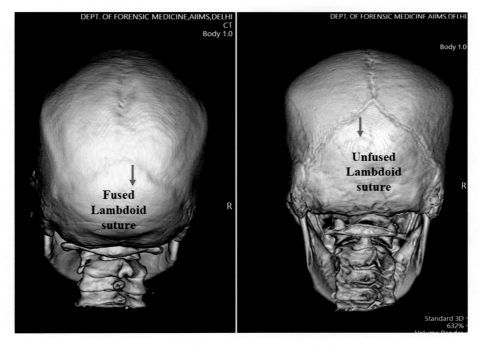

FIGURE 8.66: 3D VRT of the skull bone in the skeletal filter (left) and radiograph filter (right) showing fused (left) and unfused (right) lambdoid sutures.

- Soon after puberty, the **conjoint vertebral arches and costal elements of the sacral vertebrae** fuse with each other from below in an upwards trajectory.
- The **bodies** unite with one another at their adjacent margins by 20 years of age but the central portion may remain unossified for some more time.
- A **secondary centre for the margin of glenoid fossa** appears around 15–18 years of age and fuses around

20–23 years of age. Lipping of the margin usually commences around 30–35 years.
- Around 35–50 years of age, **lipping of vertebral bodies** can be detected.

Senile changes in the skeleton
- Beyond middle age, retrogressive changes occur in many parts of the skeleton. The thyroid and cricoid cartilages

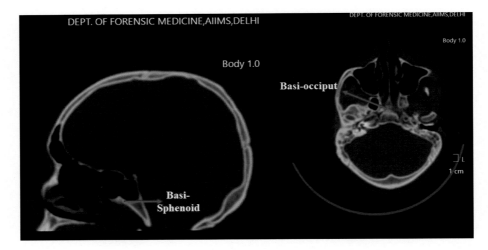

FIGURE 8.67: 3D VRT of the skull bone of 16-year-old male in the bone window of sagittal section (left) and axial section (right) showing unfused basisphenoid (left) and unfused basiocciput suture (right).

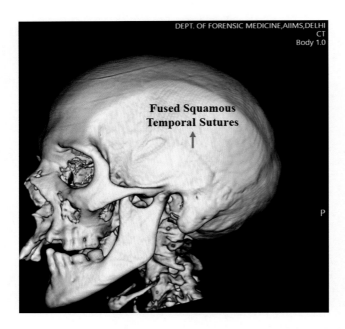

FIGURE 8.68: A 3D VRT of the lateral view of a 77-year-old female showing fused squamous temporal sutures.

of the larynx tend to calcify and the horns of the hyoid bone unite with the body.
- The costal cartilages ossify and may unite with the sternum.
- Atrophic changes occur in the intervertebral discs and osteophytes (lipping) may be seen in x-rays.
- The sutures of the skull become obliterated.
- The alveolar margins of the jaw are resorbed and the angle of the jaw is opened up.
- The manubrium sterni also unite with the mesosternum.

All the bones undergo osteoporosis
- The diploe becomes less vascular, and the venous channels are replaced by bone.
- The bone becomes more fragile.

- With the loss of cancellous tissue, the proximal end of the medullary cavity of the humerus assumes a cone shape, the tip of which gradually ascends, reaching the surgical neck during 41–50 years of age, and the epiphyseal line during the age of 61–74 years of age (Schranz, 1959).
- Similar changes involve the upper end of the femur also and can be seen on an X-ray or by longitudinal section.

Age from other factors
- The growth of hair occurs first on the pubis and then in the axilla.
- In girls, downy hair appears in the pubic region around 13 years of age and a few dark hairs around 14 years of age. The growth becomes thicker in the course of a year or two during which hair starts to grow in the axilla. In girls, breasts usually commence to develop at 12–13 years of age, but are liable to be enlarged through constant manipulation.
- In boys, the appearance of hair in the pubic region is later, by a year or two. A thick growth of hair in the pubic region, scrotum, and axilla is seen in boys around 16 or 17 years of age and hair appears on the chin and upper lip between 16 and 18 years of age. In boys, the voice becomes rather deep and hoarse, and 'breaks' at 16–18 years. The Adam's apple becomes more prominent, the testicles begin to enlarge and feel firm. The scrotum becomes pendulous and the penis enlarges.

Senile changes
- Hair on the head tends to usually become grey after 40 years of age and silvery white in old age. But grey hair is sometimes seen in young people; in some cases it is hereditary. Cases are also on record where the hair has turned grey overnight from sudden shock, fear, and grief. Patches of grey hair on the head may also be due to trophic changes. Pubic hair, chest hair, and eyebrows practically never turn grey before the age of 50.
- Atheromatous changes in arteries and cornea (arcus senilis) are rarely seen before 50 years of age. White lines around the cornea can appear even at a fairly young age

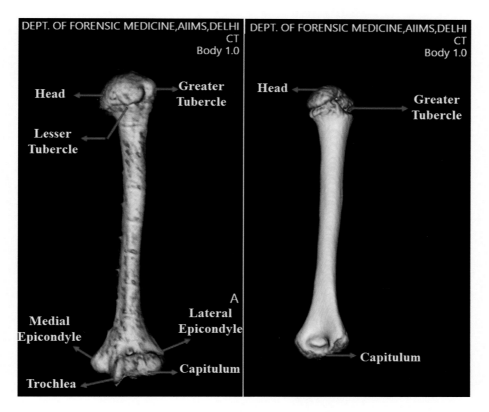

FIGURE 8.69: A comparison of 3D VRT of the left humerus bones (anterior view) of two girls aged 11 years (left) and 4.5 years old (right) showing the difference in appearance and fusion of the ossification centres according to respective ages.

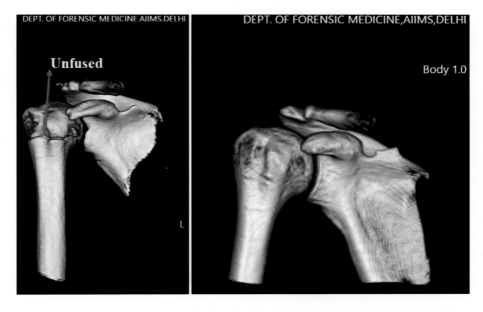

FIGURE 8.70: A comparison of 3D VRT in skeletal (left) and radiograph filter (right) of the right shoulder joint (anterior view) of two males aged 15 years (left) and 35 years (right) showing the difference in appearance and fusion of the ossification centres according to respective ages. The left image shows the unfused conjoint epiphysis on the upper part of the humerus.

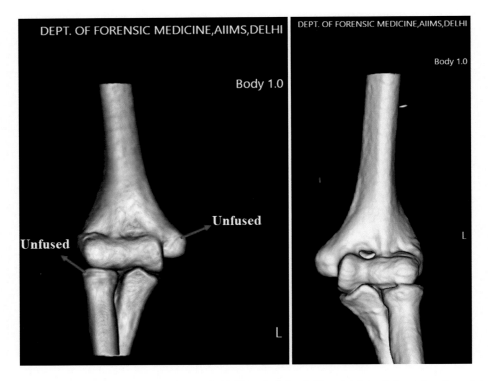

FIGURE 8.71: A comparison of 3D VRT in radiograph (left) and skeletal filter (right) of the right elbow joint and left elbow joint respectively in anterior view of two males aged 15 years (left) and 22 years (right) showing the difference in appearance and fusion of the ossification centres according to respective ages. The left image shows the unfused conjoint epiphysis on the lower part of the humerus.

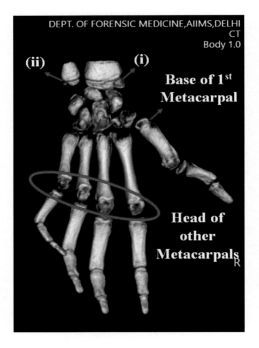

FIGURE 8.72: A 3D VRT of the left wrist joint anterior view in radiograph filter. This is a PMCT image of an 11-year-old girl where the pisiform bone has not appeared. Note the presence of (i) lower end of the radius, (ii) lower end of the unla, the base of the first metacarpal and the head of other metacarpals.

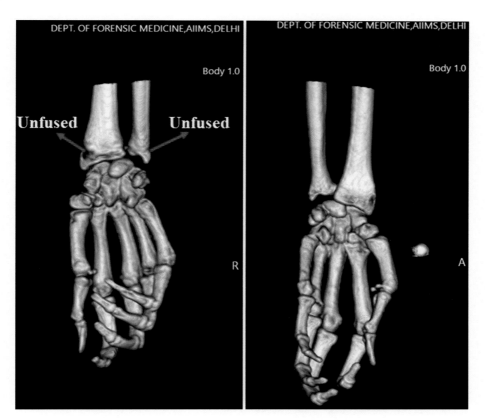

FIGURE 8.73: A comparison of 3D VRT in radiograph filter (both images) of the right and left wrist joints respectively in the anterior view of two males aged 15 years (left) and 22 years old (right) showing the difference in appearance and fusion of the ossification centres according to their respective ages. Note the presence of all eight carpal bones. The left image shows the unfused epiphysis on the lower part of the radius and ulna.

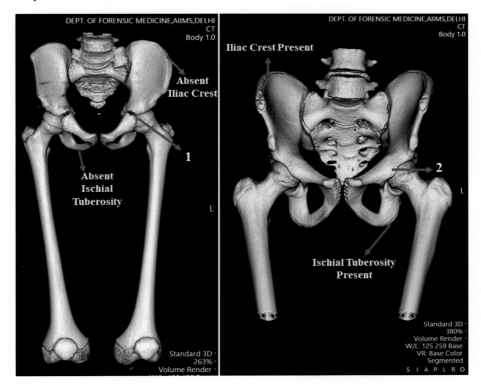

FIGURE 8.74: 3D VRT of the hip joint in the radiograph filter (left) and skeletal filter (right) showing non-fused triradiate cartilage (left) and fused triradiate cartilage (right). The presence and absence of the ischial tuberosity and iliac crest. The first image (left) is the PMCT of an 11-year-old male and the second image (right) is the PMCT of a 16-year-old male.

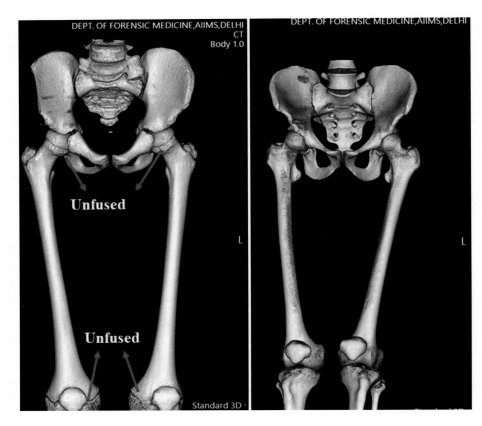

FIGURE 8.75: 3D VRT of the hip joint in the radiograph filter (left) and skeletal filter (right) showing the non-fused head of the femur and the non-fused lower end of the femur with the shaft. The first image (left) is the PMCT of an 11-year-old male and the second image (right) is the PMCT of a 16-year-old male.

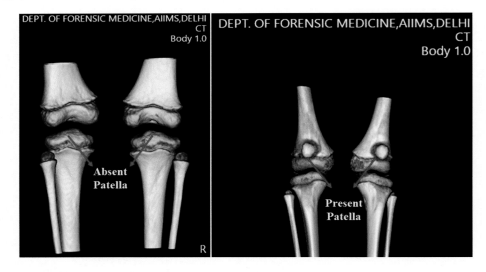

FIGURE 8.76: 3D VRT of the knee joint in the skeletal filter (left) and radiograph filter (right) showing non-appeared patella (left) and appeared patella (right). The first image (left) is the PMCT of a 4.5-year-old female and the second image (right) is the PMCT of a 6-year-old female.

(arcus juveniles) in persons suffering from disturbances of lipid metabolism such as essential hyperlipidemia.

- Around 50 years of age wrinkles begin to appear on the face, but these are variable signs.
- Atrophy of the uterus and ovary and brown atrophy of the heart, all give some indication that the body is that of an elderly person.

Age determination of human bones

When human bones are recovered following excavation and other operations, it may become necessary to decide the approximate period of burial. If the period is more than 70–100 years, the chances of the culprit being alive is almost nil. However forensic pathologists should be conversant with the methods of assessing the age of such bones.

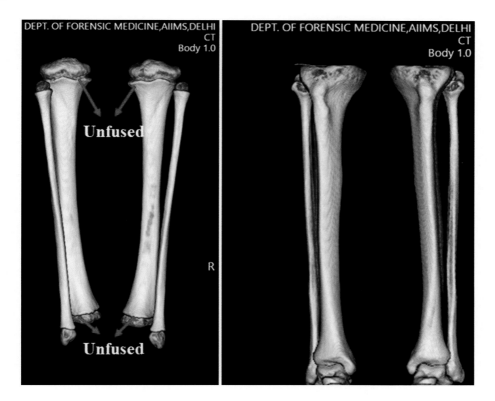

FIGURE 8.77: 3D VRT of the leg bones in the skeletal filter (left and right) showing the non-fused ends of the tibia and fibula with its shaft, on the left side which is from a 4.5-year-old female. The second image on the right is the PMCT of a 20-year-old male showing fused end both upper and lower with the respective shafts.

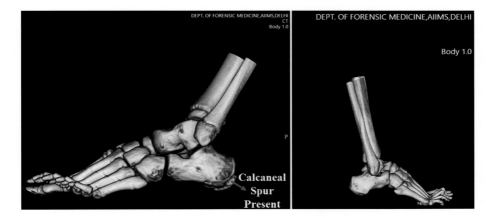

FIGURE 8.78: 3D VRT of the leg bones in the skeletal filter (left and right) showing the appearance of a calcaneal spur on a 12-year-old male. The second image on the right is the PMCT of a 20-year-old male showing a fused calcaneal spur.

Radioactive carbon C^{14} is formed in the atmosphere by the action of cosmic radiation, and it enters all living beings through various channels. After death, the C^{14} content of the remains (bones) gradually diminishes and the radioactivity weakens. The C^{14} to C^{12} ratio in the living is 1:1000 million. The half-life of C^{14} is 5750 years, which means that after this period, the C^{14} to C^{12} ratio will be 1:2000 million. Thus, by measuring the C^{14} activity of bones, and comparing it with what is known to be present in the body when alive, a reasonable estimate of the bone's age can be made. This method, however, is of little medico-legal application.

Knight and Lauder (1967) and Knight (1969) have described the following methods of dating bones:

1. **Nitrogen content** in excess of 3.5 g per cent indicates that the bone age is less than 50 years old ('modern') and nitrogen content of 2.5 g per cent or less suggests that the bone is more than 350 years old.
2. Seven or more **amino acids** can be demonstrated if the bone is less than 100 years old; proline and hydroxyproline are invariably present for up to 50 years.
3. **The entire cut surface of the freshly sawn bone will show ultraviolet fluorescence in the case of 'modern bone'.** As the age advances, the fluorescence starts disappearing from the periphery. However, traces may be detected up to 1800 years.

TABLE 8.25:   Age of appearance and union of ossification centres

Centre of ossification	Age of appearance		Age of fusion	
	Males	Females	Males	Females
Humerus				
Head	1 year	1 year	16–17 years	15–16 years
Greater tubercle	4 years	4 years	4–5 years fusion with head of humerus in both male and female	
Lower tubercle	5 years	5 years	5–7 years fusion with greater tubercle in both male and female	
Capitulum	1st year	1st year	14–15 years	13–15 years
Medial epicondyle	6–7 years	5–6 years		
Trochlea	10–11 years	9–10 years		
Lateral epicondyle	11–13 years	10–12 years		
Radius				
Shaft	Around 8 weeks of intrauterine life	Around 8 weeks of intrauterine life		
Upper end or head	5–7 years	5–6 years	15–16 years	13–14 years
Lower end	1 year	1 year	16–17 years	17–18 years
Ulna				
Upper end or olecranon	11–12 years	9–11 years	15–16 years	13–15 years
Lower end	5–7 years	5–6 years	18 years	17 years
Carpals				
Capitate	2nd month		-	
Hamate	3rd –4th month		-	
Triquetral	3 years		-	
Lunate	4 years		-	
Scaphoid	5 years		-	
Trapezium	6 years		-	
Trapezoid	6–7 years		-	
Pisiform	9 – 12 years		-	
Metacarpals (all 5 metacarpals)				
Body	8–10 weeks of intrauterine life			
Bases	2nd year		15–17 years	
Phalanges of hands				
Proximal phalanx base	2–3 years		17–18 years	15–17 years
Distal phalanx base	2–3 years		16–18 years	15–17 years
Body of both	8th- 9th week of intrauterine life		-	-
Hip bone				
Triradiate cartilage	10–13 years	12–13 years	14–15 years	14 years
Iliac crest	16 years	14 years	19–20 years	17–19 years
Ischial tuberosity	15–17 years	14–15 years	20 years	20 years
Pubis	-	-	8–9 years	8–9 years
Femur				
Shaft	8 weeks of intrauterine life	8 weeks of intrauterine life	16–17 years	14–15 years
Head	1 year	1 year	16–17 years	14–15 years
Greater trochanter	4 years	4 years	17 years	14 years
Lesser trochanter	14 years	14 years	15–17 years	14–15 years
Lower end	9th – 10th intrauterine month	9th – 10th intrauterine month	16–17 years	15–16 years
Tibia				
Upper end or olecranon	Around birth or just after birth	Around birth or just after birth	16–17 years	15–16 years
Lower end	1 year	1 year	16 years	14–14.5 years
Fibula				
Upper end	2–5 years	2–5 years	14–16 years	14–16 years
Lower end	1 year	1 year	14–16 years	13–15 years
Tarsals				
Calcaneum	5–6 months of intrauterine life		-	
Talus	6–8 months of intrauterine life		-	
Navicular	2 years		-	
Cuboid	At birth		-	
Lateral cuneiform	1–3 months of intrauterine life		-	

(Continued)

TABLE 8.25 (CONTINUED)   Age of appearance and union of ossification centres

Centre of ossification	Age of appearance		Age of fusion	
	Males	Females	Males	Females
Intermediate cuneiform	1 year		-	
Medial cuneiform	1.5 years		-	
Metatarsals (all five metatarsals)				
Shaft	9–10 weeks		18–20 years	
Base	2 years			
Head	3–4 years			
Proximal phalanges of foot				
Body	1–2 years		18 years	
Base				
Head				
Distal phalanges of foot				
Body	4 years		-	
Clavicle				
Medial end	15–17 years	14–16 years	22 years	20 years
Sternum				
Manubrium	5 months of intrauterine life	5 months of intrauterine life	Above 50 years with the body	
1st segment of body	5 months of Intrauterine life	5 months of Intrauterine life	14–25 years from below upward	
2nd segment of body	7 months of Intrauterine life	7 months of Intrauterine life		
3rd segment of body	7 months of Intrauterine life	7 months of Intrauterine life		
4th segment of body	10 months of Intrauterine life	10 months of Intrauterine life		
Xiphoid process	3 years	3 years	Above 40 years with the body	
Scapula				
Body	8 weeks of intrauterine life	8 weeks of intrauterine life	-	-
Acromian process	14–15 years	12–14 years	14–19 years	13–16 years
Glenoid cavity	Around puberty	Around puberty	17–20 years	17–20 years
Hyoid bone	From birth to 2 years		40–60 years	

TABLE 8.26:   Age related changes in pubic symphysis

Age of person*	Characteristics
< 20 years	Symphyseal surface layer of compact bone near its surface
About 20 years	Symphyseal surface is markedly irregular, the ridges run transversely across the articular surface
Between 24–36 years	The ridges gradually disappear, the surface is granular, inner and outer surfaces are well defined
During early 50s (years)	Symphyseal surface is oval, smooth with raised upper and lower
During late 50s (years)	Surface has narrow beaded rim
During 60s (years)	Surface starts to erode with breakdown of outer margin
During 70s (years)	Surface becomes irregularly eroded

When used for females, this formula underestimates age by 10 years.

TABLE 8.27:   Skull suture closure

Closure of sutures	Age of closure
Lateral and occipital fontanelles	By 2nd month
Posterior fontanelle	6–8 months
Anterior fontanelle (bregma)	1.5–2 years
Both halves of mandible	2 years
Metopic suture (between frontal bones)	3 years
Condylar portion of occipital bone with squama	3 years
Condylar portion of occipital bone with basiocciput	5 years
Basiocciput and basisphenoid	18–21 years
Sagittal suture	30–40 years
• Posterior 1/3rd	40–50 years
• Anterior 1/3rd	50–60 years
• Middle 1/3rd	
Coronal suture	40–50 years
• Lower half	50–60 years
• Upper half	
Lambdoid suture	45–50 years
Parieto temporal suture	60–70 years

4. Powdered bone gives a **positive benzidine test** up to 100–150 years. However, since false positive tests are common, only the negative test is of value.

5. **Immunological activity** with anti-human serum as demonstrated by the gel-diffusion technique ceases in five years' time. **Berg (1963)** states that the activity is continued for up to 20 years and a delayed weak reaction can be seen even up to 50 years.

6. **Aspartic acid racemization** in dentin protein during the human lifetime progresses with age. The extent of racemization of aspartic acid in the coronal dentin of normal permanent teeth can be used in forensic odontology to estimate the age of an individual at the time of death.

Sex determination

Introduction

Sex determination is a crucial aspect of forensic investigations. Sex can be easily determined with the help of external examination but the issue of sex determination mainly comes

TABLE 8.28:   **Age related changes in the frontal bone**

Centre of ossification	Age of appearance		Age of fusion	
	Males	**Females**	**Males**	**Females**
Primary	2 months of intrauterine life	2 months of intrauterine life	2–8 years	

TABLE 8.29:   **Age estimation from the skeletal changes in mandible**

Traits	Childhood	Adulthood	Old age
Body	Shallow	Longer and thicker	Shallow
Ramus	Short, oblique and forms obtuse angle with the body	Forms lesser obtuse angle with the body	Forms obtuse angle with the body
Mental foramen	Opens near the lower margin of mandible and has forward direction	Opens midway between upper and lower margins and has horizontally backwards direction	Opens near the upper/alveolar margin of mandible
Condyloid process	At a level lower than the coronoid process	Elongated and at upper level than coronoid process.	Bends backwards and is at a level lower than coronoid process

TABLE 8.30:   **Age estimation from the skeletal changes in sacrum**

Centre of ossification	Age of appearance		Age of fusion	
	Males	**Females**	**Males**	**Females**
1st segment	-	-	14 years to 25 years from lower segments towards upper	
2nd segment	3 month of intrauterine life	3 month of intrauterine life		
3rd segment	-	-		
4th segment	5–6 month of intrauterine life	5–6 month of intrauterine life		
5th segment	-	-		

when it is a case of advanced decomposition and skeletal remains. Dimorphic variation occurs during intrauterine life and afterwards, in the size, length, and weight of bones certain factors such as growth pattern and muscle attachment to the bones also play a significant role in the dimorphic features. Men's bones grow stronger and longer than women and this pattern of prolonged growth causes differences in the size of the bones.

Differences between sex and gender and intersex

Sex is an anatomical, physiological, and genetic characterization of an individual. The genetic makeup of humans is made up of 23 pairs of chromosomes, 44 autosomal chromosomes, and 2 sex chromosomes, which are either XX or XY. Females have two copies of the X chromosome, i.e., XX while males have one X and one Y chromosome, i.e., XY.

Gender is what a person identifies themself to society; it may or may not be according to his genetic makeup. It is the masculine or feminine identity of a person.

Intersex is the mixing of anatomical, physiological, and genetic characteristics of both the sex in a person.

Sex estimation in the living

The sex of an individual can easily be determined by primary sex organs (organs which are responsible for the production of male and female gamete and secretions of hormones, i.e., testicles in males and ovaries in females) and secondary sex organs (which are responsible for maturation and conduction of gametes, conduction of sperm in male and ovum in female that are responsible for the development of physical characteristics in the male and female body and change human behaviour). In the living, the presence of testicles and ovaries are strong evidence of male and female respectively. Various features of the body apart from sexual organs that help in determining the sex of the individual are mentioned in the following section (Table 8.31).

Test for sex in adults

1. **Gonadal biopsy**

   Gonadal biopsy or microscopic demonstration of ovarian, testicular, or prostatic tissues helps in distinguishing the sexes. Prostatic tissue can occur in the female also, but the amount and position distinguish it from the male.

2. **Nuclear sexing or Barr bodies**

   Nuclear sexing or demonstration of sex chromatin (Barr bodies) in the tissue cells differentiates the sexes as follows:

   - Barr and Bertram (1949) observed that the nucleus of nerve cells contained a nucleolar satellite in females. This was later identified as sex chromatin or Barr bodies. These are **inactive, condensed X chromosomes found in the nuclei of the somatic cells of females.** Barr bodies are absent in Turner's syndrome (XO), with one Barr body in genotype XX and two in genotype XXX. These can be seen during the interphase of mitosis.

   - Sex chromatin can also be demonstrated in various other cells, viz., cells of the skin, buccal mucosa, cartilage, amniotic fluid, polymorphs (drumsticks), and lymphocytes.

   - **Feulgen reactions** are the best staining technique for the demonstration of Barr bodies, though the **haematoxylin and eosin methods** can also be used. A plano-convex mass of chromatin is seen near the nuclear membrane.

TABLE 8.31:   Sexual dimorphism based on general features

Physical features	Male	Female
General built	Muscular, strong and stout	Less muscular, delicate and petite
Body hair	Thick facial hair (moustaches and beard), chest hair present	Absence of thick **facial** and chest hair
Pubic hair	Thick, coarse with apex extending towards umbilicus present	Relatively thin and horizontal covering mons veris present
Larynx	Prominent with length about 4.8 cm	Not prominent with length about 3.8 cm
Shoulders	Broader than hips	Narrower than hips
Waist	Not well-defined	Well-defined
Abdominal segment	Shorter	Longer
Thorax	Longer with more dimensions	Shorter, rounded with less dimensions
Limbs	Longer	Shorter
Arms	Flat on section	Cylindrical on section
Thighs	Cylindrical	Conical due to short femur and greater fat deposition
Gluteal region	Flatter	Fuller and rounded
Wrists and ankles	Are not delicate	Are delicate
Breasts	Not developed	Well-developed after onset of puberty
Sexual organs	Testis as gonads with penis and prostate as appendages present	Ovaries as gonads and uterus, vagina, etc. as appendages present

3. **Davidson bodies**

These are the drumstick-shaped lobes attached to the nucleus of neutrophils in females (about 3–6%) and absent in males.

The positivity percentage of various cellular level tests for males and females are shown in Table 8.32.

Classification of DSD

Disorders of sexual development (DSD) encompass a group of congenital conditions associated with the atypical development of internal and external genital structures (Table 8.33). These conditions can be associated with variations in genes, developmental programming, and hormones. Affected individuals may be recognized at birth due to the ambiguity of the external genitalia. Others may present later with postnatal virilization, delayed/absent puberty, or infertility.

TABLE 8.32:   Positivity percentage of various cellular level tests for males and females

Test	Percentage in males	Percentage in females
Barr body	0–4%	30–40%
Davidson body	0%	3%
Feulgen reaction	0–2%	50–70%
Quinacrine di-hydrochloride	45–80%	0%

Sex estimation in dead

When the **entire dead body** is available, sex can be determined in the majority of cases by **dissection.** In mutilated remains, the problem is solved when parts **bearing sex characteristics are available**, such as the uterus and its appendages, breasts, and prostate. When soft parts exhibiting sexual characteristics are not available, the determination of sex must be based on the **sexual characteristics displayed by bones.**

Identifying isolated skeletal remains and dismembered human body remains in major disasters is the most critical part of forensics. In such cases, the main focus is on establishing a person's biological profile by estimating age, sex, and race. Estimating sex is one of the most important parameters in establishing the biological profile of unknown remains. Estimation of sex is based on sexual dimorphism present in the body. It can be performed by using morphological features, morphometric measurements, and DNA analysis. The morphometric method is of higher value than the morphological method. While DNA analysis costs higher but is the confirmatory one.

Non-metric (macroscopic and visual)

Morphological study of a bone, i.e., shape, roughness, and prominences are more subjective findings varied according to the observer/examiner.

1. **Metric analysis**

As the morphological parameters are more subjective which leads to variation in diagnosis and cannot

TABLE 8.33:   Types of DSD

DSD sex chromosomes	DSD 46, XY		DSD 46, XX	
	Disorders of testicular development	Disorders of the synthesis/ action of androgens	Disorders of ovarian development	Disorders of the synthesis/ action
45, X Turner syndrome and variants	Complete gonadal dysgenesis	Defect in androgen synthesis	Ovo testicular DSD	congenital adrenal hyperplasia
47, XXY Klinefelter syndrome and variants	Partial gonadal dysgenesis	LH receptor defect	Testicular DSD	aromatase deficiency
45, X/46, XY GMD	Gonadal regression	Androgens insensitivity	Gonadal dysgenesis	maternal luteoma
Ovo testicular DSD	Ovo testicular DSD	5α reductase deficiency		

stand in a court of law. The metric analysis is more objective and eliminates the person-to-person variation. However metric analysis makes it more authentic. It can be done manually as well as virtually and could be more advanced with the help of virtual measurements. Manual measurements can be done with the help of callipers. But in today's scenario, a more advanced version could be used, i.e., PMCT, as measurements were done with it can be stored easily for further revaluation and are more accurate.

2. **Genetic analysis**

Sex chromatin, Y chromosome, amelogenin.

Bones helpful in sex determination

Recognizable differences in sex do not appear till puberty except in the pelvis in which sexual dimorphism is present since fetal life. All the mentioned bones are studied with both the aspect of morphology and the metric method. Sex determination on the basis of skull parameters alone has a degree of accuracy of up to 93% and along with pelvic measurements, it accounts for an accuracy of 95% (Krogman 1962). The accuracy of sex estimation from various bones is listed in Table 8.34.

1. Pelvis

Sexual dimorphism in the pelvic bone is established early but becomes more apparent only at puberty. The bone responds to hormonal stimuli from the pubertal ovary with active growth. The differences exhibited by the pelvis of the two sexes are more marked than in any other bone. The ilium comprises the largest component of the innominate and is the site of multiple muscle attachments, including the gluteal muscles. The ilium, positioned on each side of the sacrum, creates the sacroiliac joints. The pubis is a much smaller, comma-shaped bone anterior in the pelvis. The two pubic bones meet at the most medial and anterior portions of the pelvis and connect via a fibrocartilaginous symphysis. The ischium lies below the ilium and

TABLE 8.34: **Accuracy of sex estimation from various bones**

Portion of skeleton	Degree of accuracy
Pelvis	95%
Skull	93%
Pelvis plus skull	98%
Long bones	80–85%
Long bones plus skull	95%
Long bones plus pelvis	98%

pubis, creating a stable platform for sitting. The greater sciatic notch is recognizable early in fetal development, it is usually well preserved in archaeological and forensic remains and has shown a statistically significant level of sexual dimorphism. The parameters of sexual dimorphism are divided into two, i.e., morphological and metric analysis. Measurements obtained from 3D reconstructed images are more accurate than the manually taken measurements and it also provides a good interobserver reliability.

- **Morphological differences:** The morphological differences between males and females are depicted in Figures 8.79–8.82 and Table 8.35.
- **Metric analysis:** Metric analysis includes the measurements of different parts of bone along with the index calculated from that, which helps in a more accurate determination of sex. The various metric measurements are depicted in Figures 8.83–8.87.
  1. **Anteroposterior pelvic inlet diameter (APID):** In the midsagittal section it is the distance between the sacral promontory and superior border of the pubic symphysis (true conjugate).
  2. **Transverse pelvic inlet diameter (TPID):** On the axial oblique view it is the main determinant in defining the pelvic shape as between the widest part of the pelvic brim (maximum distance between the iliopectineal line on both sides).
  3. **Anteroposterior pelvic outlet diameter (APOD):** In the midsagittal section it is the distance between the sacro coccyx junction to the inferior pubic symphysis.
  4. **Transverse pelvic outlet diameter (TPOD):** On the axial section TPOD is the distance between the inner border of ischial tuberosities. The plane of smallest diameter is the interspinous diameter.
  5. **Greater sciatic notch width (GSW):** It is the distance between the ischial spine and piriform tubercle or posterior inferior iliac spine.
  6. **Greater sciatic notch depth (GSD):** It is the distance between the deepest point of the sciatic notch and a perpendicular line joining the ischial spine and piriform tubercle.
  7. **Sciatic notch index (SNI):** Width of the greater sciatic notch/depth of greater sciatic notch × 100.
  8. **Pubic symphysis length (PSL):** Distance between the superior and the inferior border of the pubic symphysis on the outer aspect.
  9. **Sub-pubic angle (SA):** Two lines are drawn between the inferior border of the pubic rami and a point located on the inferior midline of the pubic symphysis.

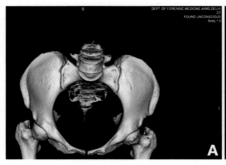
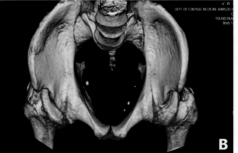

FIGURE 8.79: Craniocaudal view on a volume-rendered reconstructed image depicting (a) male heart shape pelvic inlet and (b) female oval shape pelvic inlet.

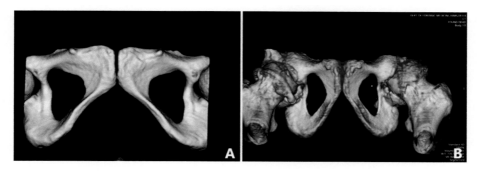

FIGURE 8.80: Anterior posterior view on a volume-rendered reconstructed image depicting female characteristics of (a) obtuse sub-pubic angle >90 and (b) male characteristic of acute sub-pubic angle<90.

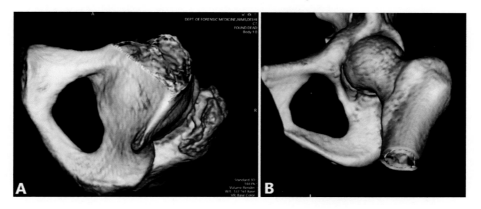

FIGURE 8.81: Oblique view on a volume-rendered reconstructed image depicting (a) male oval shape obturator foramen and (b) female triangular shape obturator foramen.

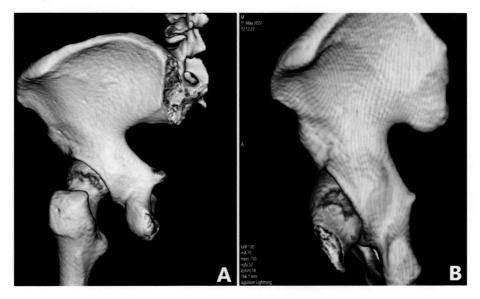

FIGURE 8.82: Posterior anterior view on a volume-rendered reconstructed image depicting (a) female characteristics such as narrow and deep greater sciatic notch and (b) male characteristics such as wide and shallow sciatic notch.

10. **Ischiopubic index (IPL):** Length of Pubis / Length of Ischium X 100.
11. **Sacrum height (SH):** In the midsagittal plane distance from the sacral promontory to the sacrococcygeal junction.
12. **Corp basal index (CBI):** Breadth of the first sacral vertebra/breadth of the base of the sacrum × 100

2. Skull

The skull is a hard structure that can be easily preserved in disasters in most cases and provides about 93% accuracy in sex determination. Basic morphological features to be analyzed on CT are depicted in Table 8.36 and Figures 8.88–8.93.

TABLE 8.35: **Sexual difference in morphological features of pelvis among males and females**

S no.	Criteria	MALE	FEMALE
1.	General	Larger, more massive, heavier	Smaller, less massive, and lighter
2.	Surfaces	Rough, rugged, thicker	Smooth, thinner
3.	Ridges	More prominent	Less prominent or absent
4.	Pelvic brim	Heart shape	Circular, elliptical (more spacious)
5.	Obturator foramen	Large, oval	Small and triangular
6.	Greater sciatic notch	Small, narrow, and deep	Large, wider, and shallow
7.	Ischial spine / tuberosity	Inverted	Everted
8.	Sub-pubic angle	V-shape	U-shape
9.	Coccyx	Less movable	More movable
10.	Sacral promontory	Well-marked	Less marked

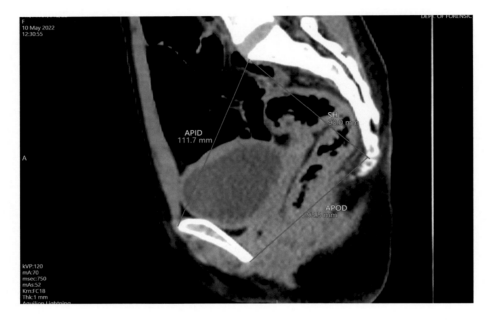

FIGURE 8.83: Midsagittal section of the female pelvic showing anteroposterior inlet diameter (APID), anteroposterior outlet diameter (APOD), and sacral height (SH).

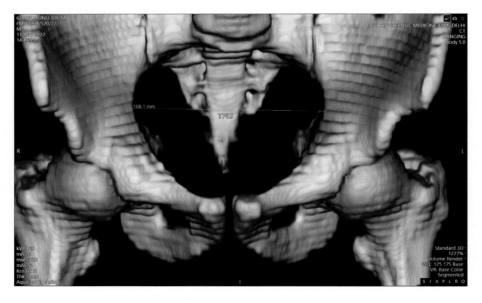

FIGURE 8.84: Craniocaudal view on a volume-rendered reconstructed image of pelvis measuring transverse pelvic inlet diameter (TPID).

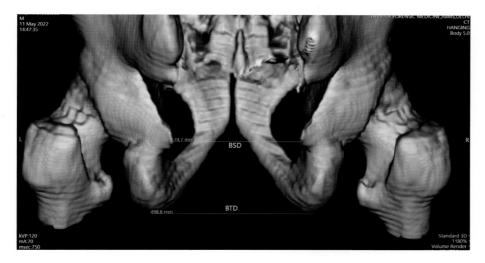

FIGURE 8.85: Posterior anterior view on a volume-rendered reconstructed image of pelvis measuring bispinous and bituberous diameter (TPOD).

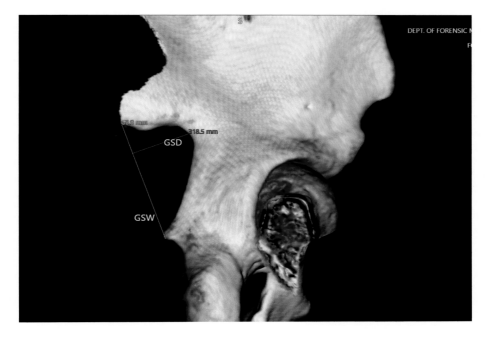

FIGURE 8.86: Posterior anterior view on a volume-rendered reconstructed image of pelvis measuring greater sciatic notch width (GSW) and greater sciatic notch depth (GSD).

Metric analysis: As morphological analysis is more subjective in nature, metric analysis provides more accuracy and less variation. Various measurement also assists in sex determination. Anatomical points should be kept in mind for measuring, which will result in higher accuracy. The various metric measurements are depicted in Figures 8.94–8.96.

1. **Maximum cranial length (MCL):** This is the distance between glabella and opisthocranion.
2. **Maximum cranial breadth (MCB):** This is the distance between the left euryon and right euryon (the meaning of **euryon** is either of the lateral points marking the ends of the greatest transverse diameter of the **skull**).
3. **Cranial index (CI):** This is the maximum cranial length/maximum cranial breadth × 100.

4. **Bimastoid diameter (BMD):** This is the distance between the most inferior part of the mastoid process. It will be discussed in detail in the section mastoid.
5. **Bizygomatic diameter (BZD):** This is the distance between the most lateral point on zygomatic arches.
6. **Bigonial diameter (BG):** This is the distance between the most lateral points in the angulus mandible.

Foramen magnum: In the base of the skull, the foramen magnum also has a favourable anatomical position as it is covered by soft tissue and the skeleton of the head that protects it from direct impact, thus preserving this area for forensic examination. Two major parameters of the foramen magnum help us in differentiation of sex to a great extent, they are as follows:

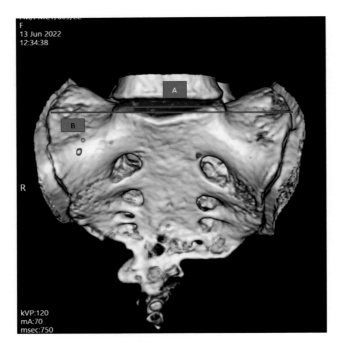

FIGURE 8.87: Anterior posterior view on a volume-rendered reconstructed image of sacrum depicting the breadth of the first sacral vertebra (A)/breadth of the base of the sacrum (B) to calculate corp basal index (CBI).

1. **Foramen magnum transverse diameter (FMTD):** The greatest width of the foramen magnum.
2. **Foramen magnum sagittal diameter (FMSD):** The greatest anteroposterior dimension of the FM (basion to opisthion). **The McRae line is a radiographic line drawn on a lateral skull radiograph or on a midsagittal section of CT that connects the anterior and posterior margins of the foramen magnum** (basion to opisthion).

Mastoid: As the mastoid process is highly resistant to physical injury its measurements are a very good method for sex determination. The mastoid process is desirable for sex determination for two reasons:

1. It is the compressed structure of the Petros section and its conserved position at the base of the skull makes the mastoid remain even if the skull is fragmented.

2. The mastoid is an area that exhibits high degrees of difference between males and females in adulthood

As far as metric analysis of the mastoid is concerned five parameters are taken into account to determine sex (Figures 8.97 and 8.98). They are as follows:

1. **Mastoid length (ML):** The distance between the porion (It is the point on the human skull located at the upper margin of each ear canal) and the incisura mastoidea in lateral view.
2. **Mastoid height (MH):** The perpendicular line of the mastoid on the line between the porion and the incisura mastoid in lateral view.
3. **Mastoid width (MW):** The distance between the most prominent point on the lateral surface of the convex mastoid triangle and the highest point on the inner surface of the mastoid triangle (within the digastric cavity) in the inferior view.
4. **Intermastoid distance (IMD):** The distance between the lowest point of the right and left mastoid triangles in the posterior view.
5. **Intermastoid lateral surface distance (IMLSD):** The distance between the most prominent convex surface points of the right and left mastoid triangles in the posterior view.

Clivus: The clivus is a denser part of bony skull that can be recovered intact from a damaged or incinerated skull. Therefore, it can alternatively be used as an anthropometric measurement for gender determination to some extent medico legally. The clivus is a bone region formed by the fusion of basisphenoid and basi-occiput. Metric analysis parameters can be considered to differentiate male from female skull to some extent as an additional or only parameter when other parameters or measures were inconclusive in medico-legal cases.

1. **Clivus length (CL):** It was measured on a reconstructed sagittal image and was defined as the longest distance superior–inferior from the upper point of dorsum sellae to the lowest point on the anterior margin of foramen magnum (Figure 8.99).

3. **Sternum**

The **sternum** completes the anterior chest wall as the ventral breastplate. It is composed of a) the manubrium, b) the

TABLE 8.36: Sexual difference in morphological features of pelvis among males and females

S no.	Criteria	MALE	FEMALE
1.	Surfaces	Rough, rugged, thicker	Smooth, thinner
2.	Ridges	More prominent	Less prominent or absent
3.	Supraorbital ridges	Prominent	Less prominent or absent
4.	Forehead	Steeper	Vertical and rounder
5.	Mastoid process	Large, blunt, M type	Small, pointed, V type
6.	Angles of mandible	Everted	Inverted
7.	Chin (Symphysis menti)	Square	Rounded
8.	Orbits	Square shape	Rounded
9.	Frontonasal angulation	Distinct angulation	Smooth
10.	Palate	Large, U-shaped and broad	Small and parabolic

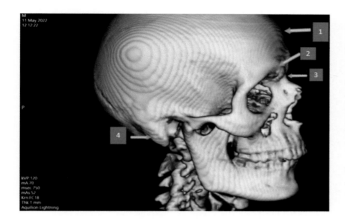

FIGURE 8.88: Volume-rendered reconstructed image of the skull of a male showing a steeper forehead (1), prominent supraciliary ridges (2), distinct angulation of frontonasal junction(3), and large and blunt shape mastoid (4).

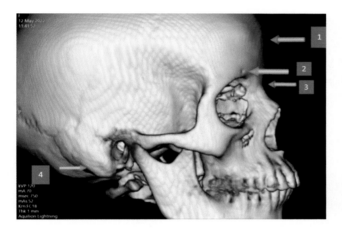

FIGURE 8.89: Volume-rendered reconstructed image of the skull of a female showing a vertical forehead (1), absent supraorbital ridges (2), frontonasal junction (3), and small mastoid (4).

body of the sternum or mesosternu, and c) the xiphoid process. Superiorly the manubrium articulates with the first rib, clavicle, and body of the sternum. The body articulates with the second rib at the stern manubrial angle (of Louis) as well as the third to seventh ribs and costal cartilages. The sternum is usually a well-preserved bone in advanced skeletal destruction making it an important candidate for sex determination in the identification process (Table 8.37). Major parameters to be evaluated for the osteometric analysis for sex determination during PMCT (Figure 8.100):

1. **Manubrium length (ML):** The longest distance from the midpoint of the manubrium (between the incisura jugularis and incisura clavicular) and the manubriosternal junction.
2. **Manubrium width (MW):** The width at the level of the line passing from the incisura costalis midpoint on the right and left.
3. **Mesosternum length (MSL)/body length:** The distance between the manubriosternal junction and mesoxiphoid junction at the midpoint.
4. **Sternebra 1 width (S1W):** The distance between the right and left first sternebra (depression between articulation notch for second and third costal cartilage.
5. **Sternebra 3 width (S3W):** The distance between the right and left third sternebra (depression between articulation notch for fourth and fifth costal cartilage.
6. **Sternal Index:** Manubrium length/mesosternum length × 100.

4. Maxillary sinus

Maxillary sinuses remain intact despite the skull and other bones getting badly disfigured in victims who are incinerated. Therefore, maxillary sinuses can be used for identification. Maxillary sinuses reach their mature sizes at about the age of 20 years. During adulthood, their shapes and sizes change, especially due to the loss of teeth. The size of the maxillary sinus can be affected due to environmental factors, genetic diseases, or post infections. Computed tomography (CT) provides

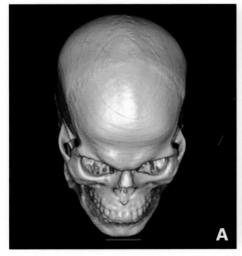
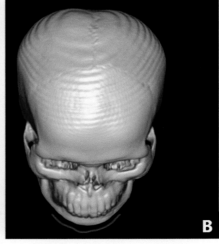

FIGURE 8.90: Craniocaudal view on a volume-rendered reconstructed image of the skull of a male showing a) Square shape symphysis menti in male with prominent supraorbital ridges and (b) rounded symphysis menti in females.

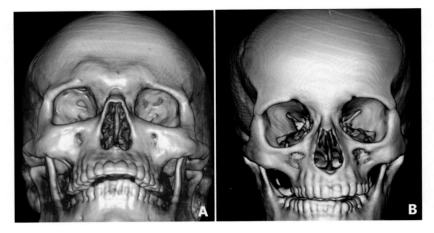

FIGURE 8.91: Antero posterior view on a volume-rendered reconstructed image of the skull of a male showing a) square shape orbit with rounded edges in males and (b) round orbit with sharp margins in females.

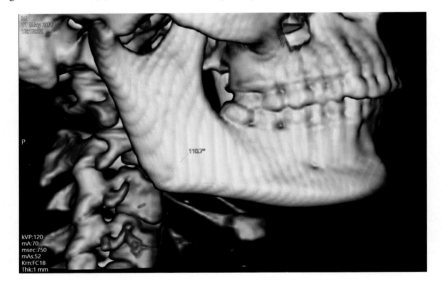

FIGURE 8.92: Volume-rendered reconstructed image of a male mandible showing the angle of body and ramus <120.

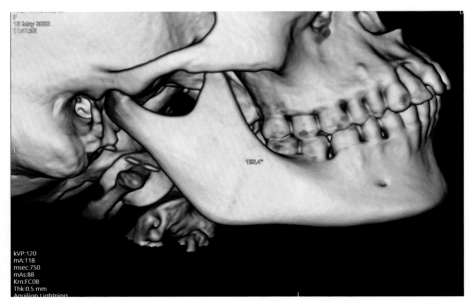

FIGURE 8.93: Volume-rendered reconstructed image of a female mandible showing the angle of body and ramus >120.

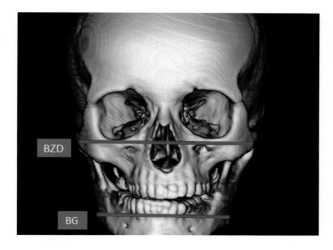

FIGURE 8.94: Volume-rendered reconstructed image showing bizygomatic diameter and bigonial diameter.

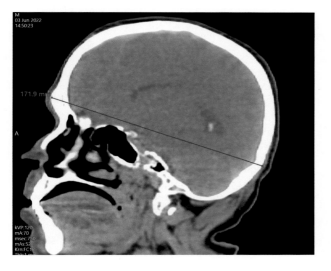

FIGURE 8.95: Midsagittal section of a skull showing maximum cranial length (MCL), i.e., the distance between glabella and opisthocranion.

an excellent method for examining maxillary sinuses. The following parameters are used for sex determination from the maxilla (Figure 8.101):

1. Mediolateral length (ML)
2. Supero-inferior length (SI)
3. Anteroposterior length (AP)
4. Volume of the maxillary sinuses

5. Vertebral column

As various disintegrated parts of the vertebral column are usually received for examination in cases of disaster. For purposes of determination of sex, it is only the extreme ends of the vertebral column, i.e., the atlas and sacrum (already mentioned above) that are of practical importance.

- In general, the male vertebral column is larger.
- There is marked lumbar lordosis in females.
- The average length of the vertebral column is 70 cm in adult males and 60 cm in females.
- The atlas is a good indicator of sex. This bone is more massive in males. The breadth (transverse diameter) of the male atlas is about 11 mm greater than the female atlas (Clavellin and Derobert 1946). It has a mean value of 83 mm in males and 72 mm in females. An adult male atlas of less than 76 mm, or a female atlas of more than 76 mm is never seen. The upper articular facets of the atlas also show sex differences.

6. Long bones

It is difficult to determine sex from a single long bone. Female long bones are shorter, slender, and smoother and the muscular markings are less prominent. The bones that are important in determining sex are the humerus and femur. Sex may be inferred from the metric analysis, i.e., lengths of these bones (Figure 8.102).

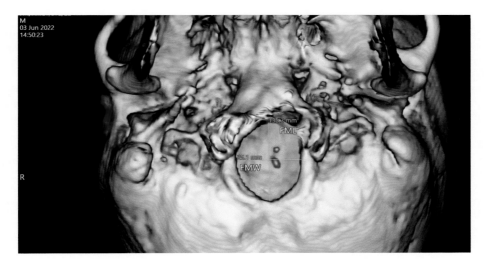

FIGURE 8.96: Volume-rendered reconstructed image of skull showing transverse diameter (FMTD) and sagittal diameter (FMSD) of the foramen magnum.

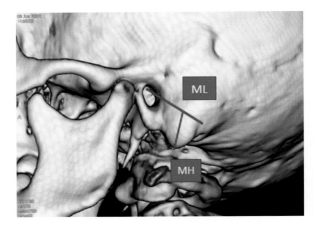

FIGURE 8.97: Volume-rendered reconstructed image of mastoid showing mastoid length (ML) and mastoid height (MH).

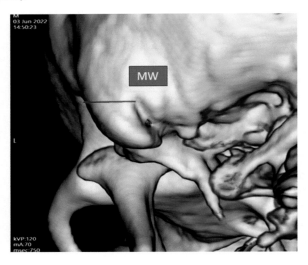

FIGURE 8.98: Volume-rendered reconstructed image of mastoid showing mastoid width (MW).

Medico-legal importance of sex

1. **Identity**

    Determination of sex is an important aspect of solving various issues related to identity. The main reasons are as follows
    - In succession to property, when the property is left to an heir of a specified sex.
    - Marriage, divorce, or the nullification of marriage.
    - Education, employment, sports, and games.

2. **Disorder of sexual development**
    - **Female pseudohermaphrodites should be always reared as females.** Most have normal internal sex organs and are capable of developing as normal

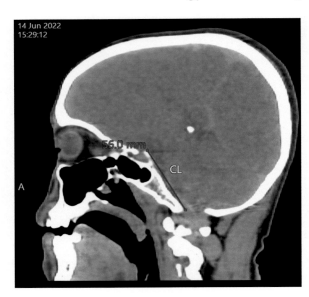

FIGURE 8.99: The sagittal reconstructed section of the skull showing clivus length.

fertile women. Labioscrotal fusion and enlarged phallus may require surgical correction.
- **Male pseudohermaphrodites with female-type genitalia should be raised as girls.** They invariably feminise at puberty. They frequently marry and lead a normal sex life even though they do not menstruate or bear children. The vagina, if too short, may require plastic surgery. Orchidectomy will be required after reaching adulthood to avoid the possible risk of malignancy.
- **Male pseudohermaphrodites with a small phallus are better raised as females.** Orchidectomy should be done in infancy to prevent masculinization, and estrogen therapy should be started at puberty to aid the development of female sex characteristics. **If the phallus is sufficiently well developed the child should be raised as male.** Appropriate correction of hypospadias and scrotal cleft and removal of uterus and tubes, if present, should be undertaken. If satisfactory masculinization does not occur at puberty, testosterone should be given in adequate doses. **Male pseudohermaphrodites with unilateral testis and contralateral gonadal aplasia are better raised as females.** Their genitalia are poorly masculinized.
- **Patients with rudimentary testis and microphallus should be brought up as females.** It is impossible for these persons to play the male sex role even after testosterone therapy.
- **True hermaphrodites** present a difficult problem in the selection of sex for rearing. If the external

TABLE 8.37:   **Sexual difference in morphometrical features of sternum among males and females**

	Male	Female
Ashley's Rule	The combined length of the manubrium and mesosternum equals or exceeds 149mm	The combined length of the manubrium and mesosternum is less than 149mm
Hyrtl's law	The body of the sternum is longer and more than the twice the length of the manubrium	The body is shorter and less than twice the length of the manubrium.

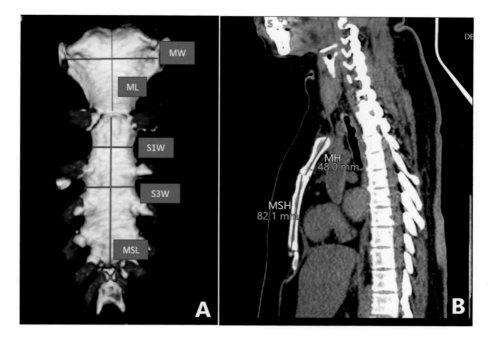

FIGURE 8.100: (a) Volume-reconstructed image of female sternum showing metric parameters, i.e., manubrium length (ML), manubrium width (MW), mesosternum length (MSL)/body length, sternebra 1 width (S1W), and sternebra 3 width (S3W). (b) Sagittal section of sternum showing manubrium length (MH or ML) and mesosternum height (MSH).

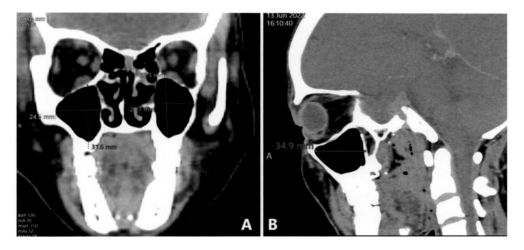

FIGURE 8.101: (a) Coronal section of maxilla measuring mediolateral length and superior–inferior length of both sides. (b) Sagittal section of maxilla showing anteroposterior length.

genitalia is inadequate for the male role, the patient should be raised as female and the testis removed. If a vagina is present and the external genitalia is well masculinized, the selection of sex is based on the nature of gonads and appropriate surgical correction should be done. If an ovary is present on one side and an ovotestis on the other side, the ovotestis should be removed and genitalia corrected to female type. Such patients mature spontaneously after puberty into fertile women, if a normal uterus and tubes are present.

3. **What is the right sex?** This question may be raised sometimes. From the practical point of view, the correct sex is that which the individual desires and to which

there is orientation (Hamblen et al. 1951). This usually conforms to that certified at birth.

Paraphilias: Homosexuality, transvestism, fetishism, voyeurism, exhibitionism, sadism, and masochism are often associated with anomalies of sex differentiation.

Laws in relation to sex

- **Section 375 IPC & Section 497 IPC:** As per this law only males are charged for rape and adultery respectively. Females are never charged under these sections.
- **Section 46(4) CrPC:** A female can be only arrested before sunset. Otherwise, permission from Judicial Magistrate has to be obtained.

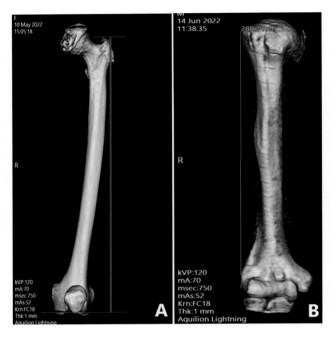

FIGURE 8.102: (a) Volume-reconstructed image of the femur showing length from the greater trochanter to the line joining both condyles. (b) Volume-reconstructed image of humerus showing length from greater tubercler to the line joining both the epicondyles.

- **Section 46(1) CrPC).** A female can be arrested preferably by a female police officer. She should not be touched by any male police officer unless the circumstances demand.
- **Section 47(1) CrPC).:** Police officers can only enter the house of a female to be arrested with proper permission and in case she is cohabitating with another female, a notice should be issued to others before entering the premises.
- **Section 53(2), 54(1) CrPC:** An arrested woman can be forced to undergo a medical examination, but only by a female medical officer.
- **Section 51 (2) CrPC:** When it is necessary to search the female body, the search shall be by another female with strict regard to decency.

Bibliography

Adebisi S Forensic anthropology in perspective: The current trend. *Internet J Forensic Sci.* 2008;4:1.

Ahmed AA. Estimation of stature using lower limb measurements in Sudanese Arabs. *J Forensic Leg Med.* 2013;20:483–488. https://doi.org/10.1016/j.jflm.2013.03.019

Asadujjaman M, Rashid MHO, Rana MS. Stature estimation from footprint measurements in Bangladeshi adults. *Forensic Sci Res.* 2020:1–8. https://doi.org/10.1080/20961790.2020.1776469

Babu YPR, Bakkannavar SM, Manjunath S. Foramen magnum as a tool of estimating stature in a male population, *J South Ind Med Leg Assoc.* 2014;6:46–48.

Brough AL, Bennett J, Morgan B, et al. Anthropological measurement of the juvenile clavicle using multi-detector computed tomography-affirming reliability. *J Forensic Sci.* 2013;58(4):946–951. https://doi.org/10.1111/1556-4029.12126

Celbis O, Agritmis H. Estimation of stature and determination of sex from radial and ulnar bone lengths in a Turkish corpse sample. *Forensic Sci Int.* 2006;158:135–139. https://doi.org/10.1016/j.forsciint.2

Cui Y, Zhang J. Stature estimation from foramen magnum region in Chinese population, *J Forensic Sci.* 2013;58:1127–1135. https://doi.org/10.1111/1556-4029.12192

De Mendonça MC. Estimation of height from the length of long bones in a Portuguese adult population. *Am J Phys Anthropol.* 2000;112(1):39–48. https://doi.org/10.1002/(SICI)1096-8644(200005)112:1<39::AID-AJPA5>3.0.CO;2

Dikshit PC. Identification. In: PC Dikshit (ed,), *Textbook of forensic medicine and toxicology*, 2nd ed. New Delhi: PeePee Publishers, 2011, pp. 86–90.

Fernandes T, Adamczyk J, Poleti ML, Henriques J, Friedland B, Garib D. Comparison between 3D volumetric rendering and multiplanar slices on the reliability of linear measurements on CBCT images: An in vitro study. *J Appl Oral Sci.* 2015;23(1):56–63. https://doi.org/10.1590/1678-775720130445

Gilbe PS, Parchake SB, Tumram NK, Dixit PG. Estimation of height from the foramen magnum in the adult population–a preliminary study, A Forensic Med Criminol. 2020;70:124–135. https://doi.org/https://doi.org/10.5114/amsik.2020.104172

Giurazza F, Del Vescovo R, Schena E, Cazzato RL, D'Agostino F, Grasso RF. Stature estimation from scapular measurements by CT scan evaluation in an Italian population. *Leg Med.* 2013;15:202–208. https://doi.org/10.1016/j.legalmed.2013.01.002

Giurazza F, Schena E, Del Vescovo R, Cazzato R, Mortato L, Saccomandi P, et al. Sex determination from scapular length measurements by CT scans images in a Caucasian population. *Conf Proc IEEE Eng Med Biol Soc.* 2013;2013:1632–1635. https://doi.org/10.1109/EMBC.2013.6609829

Giurazza F, Vescovo RD, Schena E, Battisti S, Cazzato RL, Grasso FR, et al. Determination of stature from skeletal and skull measurements by CT scan evaluation. *Forensic Sci Int.* 2012;222(1–3):398.e1–398.e9. https://doi.org/10.1016/j.forsciint.2012.06.008

Giurazza F, Vescovo RD, Schena E, Cazzato RL, D'Agostino F, Grasso RF, et al. Stature estimation from scapular measurements by CT scan evaluation in an Italian population. *Leg Med.* 2013;15:202–208.

Guhuraj PV, Gupta SK. Introduction and history. In: Guhuraj PV, Gupta SK (eds.), *Forensic medicine and toxicology*, 3rd ed., Hyderabad, India, Universities Press, 2019, pp. 1–2.

Guharaj PV, Gupta SK. Personal identity. In: Guhuraj PV Gupta SK (eds.), *Forensic medicine and toxicology*, 3rd ed. Hyderabad, India: Universities Press, 2019, p. 77.

Gustafson G. Age determinations on teeth. *J Am Dent Assoc.* 1950;41:45.

Haines DH. Racial characteristics in forensic dentistry. *Med Sci Law.* 1972;12:131.

Hamblen EC, Carter FB, Wortham JT, Zanartu J. Male pseudohermaphroditism: Some endocrinological and psychosexual aspects. *Am J Obstet Gynaec.* 1951;61:1.

Hapworth SM. On the determination of age in Indians from a study of the ossification of the epiphyses of the long bones. *Ind Med Gaz.* 1929;64:128.

Hishmat AM, Michiue T, Sogawa N, et al. Virtual CT morphometry of lower limb long bones for estimation of the sex and stature using postmortem Japanese adult data in forensic identification. *Int J Leg Med.* 2015;129(5):1173–1182. https://doi.org/10.1007/s00414-015-1228-9

Hishmat AM, Michiue T, Sogawa N, Oritani S, Ishikawa T, Fawzy IA, Hashem MA, Maeda H. Virtual CT morphometry of lower limb long bones for estimation of the sex and stature using postmortem Japanese adult data in forensic identification. *Int J Legal Med.* 2015;129(5):1173–1182. https://doi.org/10.1007/s00414-015-1228-9

Holland TD. Estimation of adult stature from the calcaneus and talus. *Am J Phys Anthropol.* 1995;96:315–320. https://doi.org/10.1002/ajpa.1330960308

Hoyte D. The cranial base in normal and abnormal skull growth. *Neurosurg Clin N Am.* 1991;2:515–537. PMID: 1821300

Ishak NI, Hemy N, Franklin D. Estimation of stature from hand and handprint dimensions in a Western Australian population. *Forensic Sci Int.* 2012;216:1–3. https://doi.org/10.1016/j.forsciint.2011.09.010

Ismail NA, Abd Khupur NH, Osman K, Mansar AH, Shafie MS, Mohd FN. Stature estimation in Malaysian population from radiographic measurements of upper limbs. *Egypt J Forensic Sci.* 2018;8:22. https://doi.org/10.1186/s41935-018-0055-9

Jit I. A Radiological study of the time effusion of certain epiphysis in Punjabis. *J Anat Soc Ind.* 1971;20:1.

Johanson G. Age determination from human teeth. *Odont Rev.* 1971;22 (suppl.):21.

Kanchan T, Gupta A, Krishan K. Craniometric analysis of foramen magnum for estimation of sex. *Int J Med Health Biomed Pharm Eng.* 2013;7:111–113.

Kanodia G, Parihar V, Yadav YR, Bhatele PR, Sharma D. Morphometric analysis of posterior fossa and foramen magnum. *J Neurosci Rural Pract.* 2012;3:261–266. https://doi.org/10.4103/0976-3147.102602

Karakas HM, Celbis O, Harma A, Alicioglu B. Total body height estimation using sacrum height in Anatolian Caucasians: Multidetector computed tomography-based virtual anthropometry. *Skeletal Radiol.* 2011;40(5):623–630. https://doi.org/10.1007/s00256-010-0937-x.

Kasprzak J. Possibilities of Cheiloscopy. *Forensic Sci Int.* 1990;46:145.

Kim W, Kim YM, Yun MH. Estimation of stature from hand and foot dimensions in a Korean population. *J Forensic Leg Med.* 2018;55:87–92. https://doi.org/10.1016/j.jflm.2018.02.011

Kira K, Chiba F, Makino Y, et al. Stature estimation by semi-automatic measurements of 3D CT images of the femur. *Int J Legal Med.* 2022. https://doi.org/10.1007/s00414-022-02921-y

Knight B, Lauder I. Practical methods of dating skeletal remains: A preliminary study. *Med Sci Laiv.* 1967;7:205.

Knight B. Methods of dating skeletal remains. *Med Sci Law.* 1969;9:247.

Kondo S, Eto M. Physical growth studies on Japanese-American children in comparision with native Japanese. In: Horvath SM, Kondo S, Matsui H, Oshimura HY (eds.), *Human adaptability: Comparative studies on human adaptability of Japanese, Caucasians and Japanese Americans.* Tokyo: Tokyo Press, 1975. https://doi.org/10.1007/s12565-014-0235-0

Koşar M, Gençer C, Tetiker H, Yeniçeri İ, Çullu N. Sex and stature estimation based on multidetector computed tomography imaging measurements of the sternum in Turkish population. *Forensic Imaging.* 2022;28:200495. https://doi.org/10.1016/j.fri.2022.200495

Krogman WM. *The human skeleton in forensic medicine.* Illinois: Charles C Thomas, 1962, p. 149.

Kumar A, Potdar P, Singh K, Dhakar JS. A study of foramen magnum and its clinical relevance, Santosh. *Univ J Health Sci.* 2019;5:72–77. https://doi.org/https://10.18231/j.sujhs.2019.015.

Lai PS, Noor MHM, Abdullah N. Stature estimation study based on pelvic and sacral morphometric among Malaysian population. *Bull Nat Res Centre.* 2021;45:142. https://doi.org/10.1186/s42269-021-00601-2

Lall R, Nat BS. Age of epiphyseal union at the elbow and wrist joints amongst Indians. *Ind J Med Res.* 1934;21:683.

Lee PA, Houk CP, Ahmed SF, Hughes IA. Consensus statement on management of intersex disorders. International Consensus Conference on Intersex. *Pediatrics* 2006;118:E488–E500.

Lee S, Gong HH, Hyun JY, Koo HN, Lee HY, Chung NE, Choi YS, Yang KM, Ha Choi BH. Estimation of stature from femur length measured using computed tomography after the analysis of three-dimensional characteristics of femur bone in Korean cadavers. *Int J Legal Med.* 2017;131(5):1355–1362. https://doi.org/10.1007/s00414-017-1556-z

Li CZ, Wu W, Zhu B, Liu XF, Huang P, Wang YZ. Multiple regression analysis of the craniofacial region of Chinese Han people using linear and angular measurements based on MRI, *Forensic Sci Res.* 2017;2:34–39. https://doi.org/10.1080/20961790.2016.1276120

Mahakkanukrauh P, Khanpetch P, Prasitwattanseree S, Vichairat K, Troy Case D. Stature estimation from long bone lengths in a Thai population. *Forensic Sci Int.* 2011;210:279.e1279.e7. https://doi.org/10.1016/j.forsciint.2011.04.025

Manoel C, Prado FB, Caria PHF, Groppo FC. Morphometric analysis of the foramen magnum in human skulls of Brazilian individuals: Its relation to gender. *Braz J Morphol Sci.* 2009;26:104–108. https://doi.org/131801091

Meadows I, Jantz RL. Allometric secular change in the long bones from the 1800's to the present. *J. Forensic. Sci.* 1995;40:762–767. PMID: 7595319

Moodley M, Rennie C, Lazarus L, Satyapal K. The morphometry and morphology of the Foramen Magnum in age and sex determination within the South African Black population utilizing Computer Tomography (CT) scans. *Int J Morphol.* 2019;37. https://doi.org/10.4067/S0717-95022019000100251

Parson FG. 1913. Cited in WM Krogman's *The human skeleton in forensic medicine.* Springfield, IL: Charles C Thomas, 1962.

Pearson K. 1898. Cited in *Medical jurisprudence in toxicology,* 16th edition. Modi NJ (ed). Bombay: Tripathi Pvt Ltd, 1967, 82.

Pearson K. 1917. Cited in WM Krogman's *The human skeleton in forensic medicine.* Springfield, IL: Charles C Thomas, 1962.

Pickering RR, Bachman DC. Introduction In: Pickering RR (ed.), *The use of forensic anthropology,* 2nd ed. New York: CRC Press Group, 2009, pp. 4–30.

Pillai MJS. The study of epiphyseal union for determining the age of South Indians. *Ind J Med Res.* 1936;23:1016.

Pillai PS, Bhaskar GR. Age estimation from teeth using Gustafson's method: A study in India. *Forensic Sci.* 1974;3:135.

Ramachandran A. *Age Determination from teeth based on structural changes.* M.D. dissertation (Forensic medicine including forensic pathology), Kerala University, 1974.

Robbins LM. The individuality of human foot prints. *Forensic Sci.* 1978;23:778.

Saco-Ledo G, Porta J, Duyar I, Mateos A. Stature estimation based on tibial length in different stature groups of Spanish males. *Forensic Sci Int.* 2019;304. https://doi.org/10.1016/j.forsciint.2019.109973

Sakuma A, Ishii M, Yamamoto S, Shimofusa R, Kobayashi K, Motani H, Hayakawa M, Yajima D, Takeichi H, Iwase H. Application of postmortem 3D-CT facial reconstruction for personal identification. *J Forensic Sci.* 2010;55(6):1624–1629. https://doi.org/10.1111/j.1556-4029.2010.01526.x

Scheuer L, Black S. *Developmental juvenile osteology,* London: Academic Press, 2000.

Schranz D. 1959. *Cited by Stewart TD in modern trends in forensic medicine.* Mant AK (ed) vol. 2. London: Butterworths, 1973, p. 206.

Shepur PM, Magi M, Nanjundappa B, Havaldar PP, Premalathai G, Saheb SH. Morphometric analysis of foramen magnum. *Int J Anat Res.* 2014;2:249–255. ISSN 2321-428.

Smith S, Fiddes FS. *Forensic medicine.* Tenth edition. London: Churchill, 1955, p. 82.

Stevens PJ. Identification of a body by unusual means. *Med Sci Law.* 1966;6:160.

Steward TD. Modern *trends in forensic medicine.* Mant AK (ed). vol. 3. London: Butterworths, 1973, p. 201.

Suzuki K, Tsuchihashi Y. Personal identification by means of lip-prints. *J For Med.* 1970;17:52.

Telkka A. On the prediction of human stature from the long bones. *Acta Anat (Basel).* 1950;9:103–117. PMID: 15403864

Torimitsu S, Makino Y, Saitoh H, Sakuma A, Ishii N, Hayakawa M, et al. Stature estimation based on radial and ulnar lengths using three-dimensional images from multidetector computed tomography in a Japanese population. *Leg Med.* 2014;16(4):181–186. https://doi.org/10.1016/j.legalmed.2014.03.001

Torimitsu S, Makino Y, Saitoh H, Sakuma A, Ishii N, Hayakawa M, et al. Stature estimation in Japanese cadavers based on scapular measurements using multidetector computed tomography. *Int J Legal Med.* 2015;129(1):211–218. https://doi.org/10.1007/s00414-014-1054-5

Trotter M, Gleser GC. Cited by Camps, FE and WB Purchase. 1956. *Practical Forensic Medicine.* First edition. London: Hutchinson, 1952, p. 187.

Trotter M, Gleser GC. Estimation of stature from long bones of American Whites and Negroes. *Am J Phys Anthropol.* 1952;10(4):463–514. https://doi.org/10.1002/ajpa.1330100407 PMID:13007782

Villarreal M. Academia. https://www.academia.edu/35905604/ Estimation_of_Stature_from_the_Foramen_Magnum_Region _in_an_American_Population_A_Validation_Study, 2015 (accessed on 8 June 2022)

Wilkins L. *The Diagnosis and Treatment of Endocrine Disorders in Childhood and Adolescence.* Third edition. Springfield, IL: Charles C Thomas, 1966, p. 309.

Wilkins L, Grumback MM, Van Wyk JJ, Shepard TH, Papdatos C. Hermaphroditism classification and diagnosis, selection of sex and treatment. *Pediat.* 1955;16:287.

Yonguc GN, Kurtulus A, Bayazit O, Adiguzel E, Unal I, Demir S. Estimation of stature and sex from sternal lengths: An autopsy study. *Anat Sci Int.* 2015;90:89–96. https://doi.org/10.1007/s12565-014-0235-0

Zhang K, Cui JH, Luo YZ, Fan F, Yang M, Li XH, Zhang W, Deng ZH. Estimation of stature and sex from scapular measurements by three-dimensional volume-rendering technique using in Chinese. *Leg Med.* 2016;21:58–63. https://doi.org/10.1016/j.legalmed.2016.06.004

Zhang K, Luo YZ, Fan F, Zheng JQ, Yang M, Li T, et al. Stature estimation from sternum length using computed tomography-volume rendering technique images of western Chinese. *J. Forensic Leg Med.* 2015;35:40–44. https://doi.org/10.1016/j.jflm.2015.07.003

Zhan MJ, Cui JH, Zhang K, Chen YJ, Deng ZH. Estimation of stature and sex from skull measurements by multidetector computed tomography in Chinese. *Leg Med.* 2019;41:101625. https://doi.org/10.1016/j.legalmed.2019.101625

9 POST-MORTEM CHANGES

Legal medicine is the branch of medicine where the most debate over how to define death takes place. In simple words, death is just the conclusion of life though it might contradict various religious beliefs. Defining death had many uncertainties in the previous century, and it was becoming more complex due to advances in resuscitation, which could potentially prolong respiratory and cardiac functioning forever.

According to section 46 of the Indian penal code, the word 'death' denotes the permanent disappearance of all evidence of life at any time. Shapiro defines death as 'the irreversible loss of properties of living matter'. *Black's Law Dictionary* defines death as 'the cessation of life'. It is better to refer to death as a process rather than an event. The dying process involves loss of function of the cardiovascular system, respiratory system, and nervous system. The blood flow, breathing, and brain functions are called the 'three feet of life' or 'Bishop's tripod of life'. Failure of one foot of the tripod will eventually cause the failure of the others, resulting in death.

The length of the dying process, called the 'agonal period', varies from case to case. It can be very short in cases like explosions, where the body is fragmented within seconds. Most of the cases in practice will have a slightly longer agonal period. This includes cases like strangulation, hanging, drowning, acute myocardial infarction, pulmonary embolism, and stab injuries causing death where the body gets time to react to trauma or disease that causes death.

The process of dying in legal medicine is further divided into two types: Somatic and cellular death. Somatic death occurs when vital centres in the brain stem cease to function, resulting in the cessation of respiration and circulation, and resulting anoxia causes the death of cells of the central nervous system. Molecular death is the death of cells and tissues that occurs after somatic death. The availability of ATP and metabolic activities determines the life span of each cell. Muscles have a longer lifespan than nervous tissue, which is the first to die from molecular death. As a result, the body dies in parts and at various stages of time. In the initial post-mortem period, the body will have both live and dead cells and tissues.

After death, the homeostatic equilibrium of the body is lost as various physiological and biochemical processes which maintain the body equilibrium cease to function. This causes the development of various post-mortem changes externally and internally. *Forensic taphonomy* is the study of the changes associated with the decomposition of organisms over a period after death. Multiple factors influence the onset, rate, and types of post-mortem changes developing in the body.

The knowledge about the semiology of normal post-mortem changes and decomposition in a particular situation will be useful in a forensic investigation as it will give insight into the time since death, the position of the body at the time of death and most importantly, prevent misinterpretations. The post-mortem changes are traditionally classified as: Immediate, early, and late.

I. **Immediate changes after death:** The immediate changes which are seen after death include loss of voluntary power, cessation of respiration and cessation of circulation. These changes are also described as signs of death. It should be kept in mind that these signs can also be seen in conditions like electrocution, syncope and catalepsy where the person is not clinically dead. The person in such cases can be brought back to life by resuscitation efforts.

II. **Early changes after death:** Early changes include pallor with loss of elasticity of the skin, contact flattening, eye changes, algor mortis, livor mortis, and rigor mortis.

III. **Late changes after death:** Late changes include decomposition, mummification and adipocere formation.

General post-mortem changes

1. Pallor mortis

In the early post-mortem period, blood present in the capillaries and venules drain, leading to paleness of skin throughout the body. This is one of the earliest changes following somatic death. The paleness observed externally over the body is known as pallor mortis. PMCT cannot detect pallor mortis.

2. Algor mortis

After death, the body stops producing heat and the body will start losing temperature till the body attains room temperature. This incremental cooling of the body is known as algor mortis. The body temperature will ultimately equilibrate with the room temperature. The rate of cooling depends on factors like the difference between body temperature and room temperature, physique, position of the body, and presence of any covering on the body. Using algor mortis to estimate the post-mortem interval is inexact because of its multifactorial dependency. Though assessment of algor mortis is not possible with the help of PMCT, PMMRI is useful in assessing temperature change.

3. Livor mortis

Livor mortis is a post-mortem change which is a sign of death. The cessation of circulation causes stagnation of blood throughout the body. Due to gravity, the blood starts to sediment. Livor mortis can be appreciated internally and externally on autopsy and imaging as it affects all the fluid compartments. The settling of blood in the vessels, internal organs, and skin leads to homogenous, hyperdense areas in the dependent areas in PMCT. Over time, the RBCs and plasma separate, and eventually the RBCs lyse and release haemoglobin. The haemoglobin and plasma move out of the vessels. The colour of the livor mortis depends on the oxygenation and quantity of haemoglobin. Normally, the livor mortis is purplish-red or bluish in colour. The colour of livor can also point to the type of poisoning. In areas that are in contact with the floor or surface on which the body is kept, the weight of the body exerts pressure, which will lead to compression of blood vessels displacing the plasma and haemoglobin, thereby producing areas of contact pallor or contact blanching. Tight clothing may also produce a similar effect, producing blanched areas. The position of the body determines where the internal and external livor develop. In a body kept in a supine position, livor will be present over the posterior aspect except over the upper back, buttocks and calves of a body. Livor can extend up to the lateral aspect of the

DOI: 10.1201/9781003383703-9

torso, neck, and upper part of the anterior aspect of the chest. In the early stages, applying light pressure with the thumb on the area of the livor mortis causes it to disappear. The amount of pressure needed to produce contact pallor increases with the post-mortem interval. Also, if the body is repositioned during the early stages, the lividity shifts to areas that are dependent on the new position. Externally, fixation of the livor mortis occurs due to progressive intravascular haemoconcentration due to leakage of plasma from the thin capillaries. In the late stages, haemoglobin released due to haemolysis of RBCs will stain the tissues adjacent to capillaries, adding to fixation. Livor mortis, a sign of death, is also the earliest visible post-mortem change. On PMCT, livor mortis is easily discernible, especially in the skin and lungs. Livor mortis can be seen in axial sections of PMCT as a gravity-dependent gradient of increasing relatively homogeneous hyperdensity.

4. Changes in muscles

Contact flattening

In the early post-mortem period, loss of muscular tone causes the body to flatten in areas which are in contact with the surface on which the body rests.

The muscles in the body after death pass through three distinct stages: Primary flaccidity, rigor mortis, and secondary relaxation.

Primary flaccidity

It is the relaxation of the muscles due to loss of tone occurring immediately after somatic death making muscles flaccid. The laxity of muscles causes limbs to fall, and relaxation of sphincters leading to involuntary urination and defecation. During this stage, as the molecular death has not happened, electrical and chemical stimuli can produce a response.

Rigor mortis

ATP plays a major role in the proper functioning of voluntary and involuntary muscles of the body during life. Though the synthesis of ATP is compromised after death, ATP consumption continues. The circulatory and respiratory arrest after death leads to the stoppage of ATP production by the aerobic system. The balance between the production and consumption of ATP is lost after death. In the initial period, the phosphagen system and anaerobic glycogen lactic acid system, to an extent does the resynthesis of ATP. It has been reported that the fall of ATP level below 85% of the normal leads to the development of rigidity. The rigidity peaks when the ATP level drops to 15%.

On gross examination, it has been observed that the rigor mortis appears first in the involuntary muscles of the heart. In the body, muscle mass determines the rapidity of development of rigor mortis. Those muscles having low muscle mass have faster depletion rates of ATPs and thus develop rigor faster than those muscles with higher muscle mass. Since children and old age people have low muscle mass, they develop rigor rapidly. Also, a top-to-bottom progression pattern may also be appreciated as the upper body muscles are smaller than those of the lower limbs.

Secondary relaxation

The rigidity/stiffness in the muscle passes off subsequently and the muscle again becomes loose and lax as decomposition starts. Though the exact mechanism which causes relaxation is not known, denaturation leading to autodigestion of myosin due to enzymatic activity and change in pH due to acid produced due to continuous rigidity have been suggested as causes. Secondary relaxation begins in roughly 36 hours. In bodies that are refrigerated after rigor mortis has fully developed, the rigor mortis can persist longer.

5. Decomposition

The process of decomposition involving autolysis, putrefaction, and/or insect and animal predation will ultimately result in the breakdown of organic material into simpler forms of matter. Within minutes after death, cells that are deprived of oxygen start to accumulate acidic by-products of metabolic reactions in the body. The enzymes present also start to digest the cell membranes, thereby commencing the process of autolysis. Autolysis is an aseptic process caused by tissue enzymes which digest tissue causing disintegration under optimum temperature and humidity.

The interaction of the body with the microbiome present inside and outside the body will ultimately lead to the putrefaction of the body. Usually, the extent to which each body may putrefy will depend on several variables, like geographical location, season, ambient temperature, body fat content, sepsis/injuries, intoxication, and clothing/insulation. Putrefaction leads to the production of gas, which can be detected in PMCT intravascularly in the early stages of decomposition and in soft tissues and organ parenchyma in later stages. Putrefactive gas will cause bloating of the body. Decomposition may significantly change the external and internal appearance of the body, rendering it more difficult to determine the cause and manner of death. Bodies which are relatively fresh or have a short post-mortem interval (Figure 9.1) have very minimal decomposition changes.

The decomposition changes can be graded from grades I–IV based on the amount of decomposition in the body. Grade I (Figure 9.2) will have features of early decomposition. Grade II will have moderate decomposition. Grades III and IV will show advanced decomposition changes. It is important to note that it is not necessary that a body at a certain period of time will have only a single grade of decomposition. Different parts of the body can thus have different rates of decomposition.

1. Grade I decomposition

Externally, Grade I decomposition includes greenish discolouration of the abdomen. The discolouration starts in the right iliac fossa due to the close proximity of the caecum to the abdominal wall. The greenish discolouration then spreads to the whole abdomen. The internal examination will reveal a dark reddish to greenish intestinal loop with dilation (Figure 9.3). The underside of the liver will show greenish discolouration. Examination of the thorax will show lungs with lividity in the dependent region. Bodies kept in a supine position will have dark reddish discolouration in the posterior aspect of the lung (Figure 9.4). On PMCT various arteries and veins including the cerebral venous sinuses are hyperdense which can be attributed to gravity-dependent blood sedimentation (Figure 9.5). PMCT will show a complete loss of grey-white differentiation in the brain. The sulci and ventricles of the brain will also show effacement. PMCT of the lung will have hyperdensity in

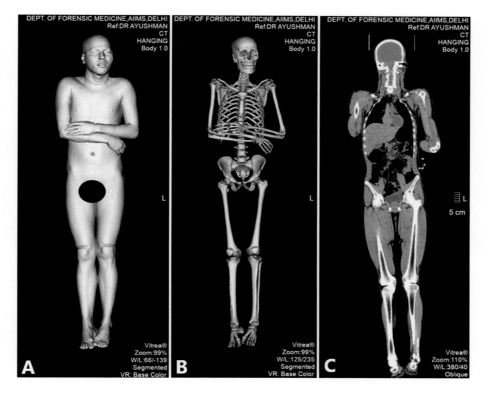

FIGURE 9.1: 3D VR (A), skeletal reconstruction (B), and the coronal section (C) of a PMCT of a body with minimal decomposition.

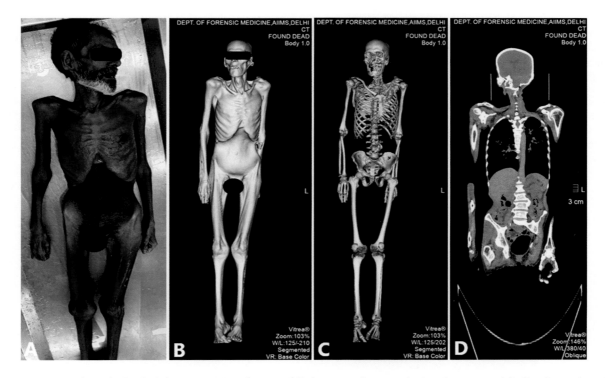

FIGURE 9.2: Body with Grade I decomposition changes. (A) Autopsy photograph showing a greenish discolouration of the abdomen. (B) and (C) 3D VR of PMCT showing good quality musculoskeletal reconstruction. (D) Coronal section of PMCT showing dilated intestinal loop.

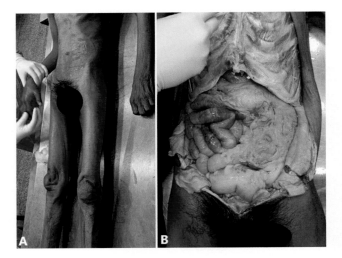

FIGURE 9.3: (A) Autopsy photograph showing a greenish discolouration of the anterior abdominal wall (B) On dissection, underlying intestinal loops show a greenish discolouration and dilation.

the dependent region of both lungs. The PMCT of the liver at this stage will have a few gas bubbles in the hepatic vasculature.

2. **Grade II decomposition** (Figure 9.6)

The bacterial propagation along the superficial veins of the body causes haemolysis and the release of haemoglobin from RBCs present in the vessels. The released haemoglobin can reach the skin due to the increased porosity of superficial veins producing a reticulated pattern on the skin known as marbling. Initially, the pattern will be purplish/reddish brown and later when acted upon by hydrogen sulphide gas produced due to putrefaction causes the colour to change to greenish (Figure 9.7). The greenish colour is due to the conversion of haemoglobin to sulfhaemoglobin. PMCT cannot identify marbling as there is minimal difference in density. A pattern similar to marbling is seen on PMCT possibly due to decomposition gas in the superficial veins.

On internal examination, the vessel walls show dark red discolouration due to the haemolysis of blood. The brain will start to soften. The bile from the gall bladder stains the adjacent liver

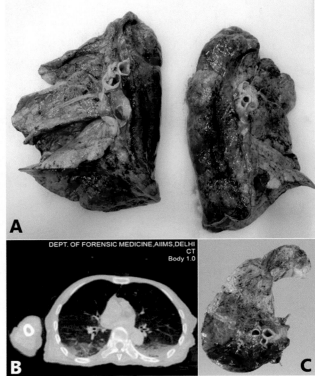

FIGURE 9.4: Lividity in the lungs in a person found in a supine position. (A) Autopsy photographs of both lungs show a darker posterior aspect. (B) Axial section of PMCT in lung window showing hyperdensity in the posterior aspect of both lungs. (C) Autopsy section of left lung showing pale anterior aspect and darker posterior aspect due to lividity in the posterior dependent area of the lungs.

parenchyma and patchy greenish discolouration appears on the surface of the liver (Figure 9.8). The liver surface may sometimes show the presence of gas just below the hepatic capsule.

On PMCT there will be minimal to moderate putrefactive gas in cerebral vasculature (Figure 9.9), arteries and veins of the body, and both chambers of the heart (Figure 9.10).

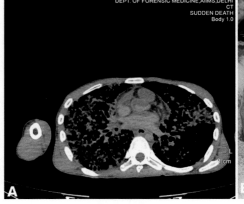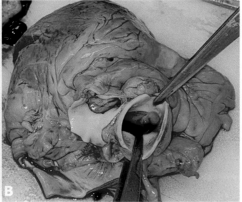

FIGURE 9.5: (A) Axial section of PMCT showing hyperdensity in the dependent portion of the aorta and pulmonary artery due to settling of blood components due to gravity. (B) Autopsy photograph showing settling of blood in the aorta.

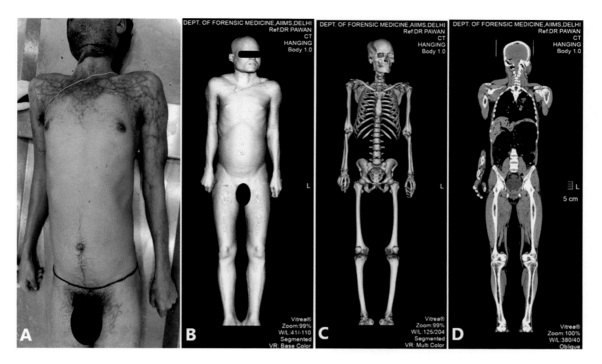

FIGURE 9.6: Body with Grade II decomposition changes. (A) Autopsy photograph showing a greenish discolouration of the abdomen and marbling in the anterior aspect of the upper chest, neck, and upper thigh. (B) 3D VR of PMCT showing skin with branching pattern in the neck, upper chest, face, and scalp due to gas produced in the superficial vessels due to decomposition. (C) 3D VR of PMCT showing good skeletal reconstruction. (D) Coronal section of PMCT showing gas in the cerebral vasculature, in the liver. There is gas in the soft tissues of the neck and upper chest. Intestinal loops also can be seen dilated.

3. **Grade III decomposition** (Figure 9.11)

During this stage, the body will be bloated with swelled face, scrotum, and penis. Due to decomposition, the joints will have gas stiffening. The brain softens and becomes papescent. The lungs collapse and will show blebs on the surface (Figure 9.12). Liver parenchyma softens and darkens.

On PMCT, the soft tissues throughout the body will have extensive gas. The brain further liquefies and settles in the cranial cavity (Figure 9.13). The paranasal sinuses, trachea and bronchi will show the presence of fluid due to decomposition caused by cell wall leakage. (Figures 9.14 and 9.15) The cranial, thoracic, and abdominal cavities will contain gas.

4. **Grade IV decomposition** (Figure 9.16)

This stage includes advanced decomposition changes. In a normal environment, the body goes through skeletonization. But due to certain environmental conditions, modification of putrefaction, like adipocere formation and mummification, can also happen. Partial skeletonization can also happen.

Bodies found in the open can have bone and soft tissue loss due to animal activity. The cranial cavity will be empty or may contain a small portion of liquefied brain settled in the dependent part of the cranial cavity. The liver and lungs will have blackish discolouration.

Asymmetric decomposition

The pace of decomposition seen on various body parts can vary since decomposition depends on multiple variables and occasionally, the full body may not be subjected to the same environmental conditions, which may develop owing to posture (Figure 9.17), clothing, injury, distance of the body part from the intestine, or even due to disease conditions. This leads to the development of asymmetric or differential decomposition.

Effect of refrigeration

The rate of decomposition will slow down significantly if the body is refrigerated as autolysis is restricted by refrigeration. It is generally accepted that PMCT imaging is unaffected by

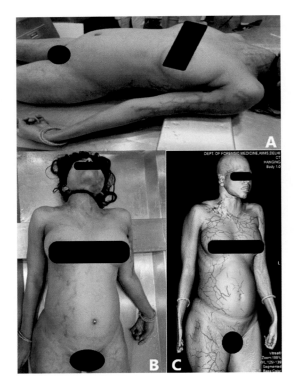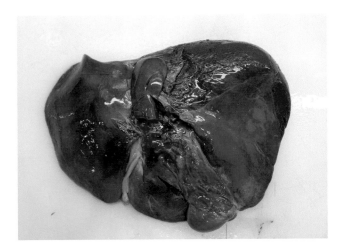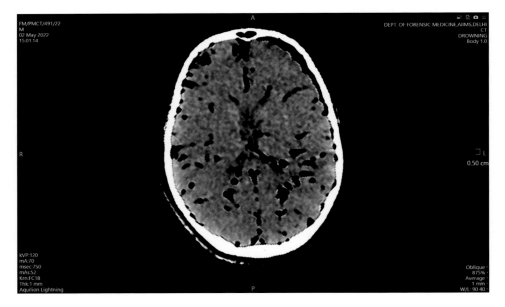

FIGURE 9.8: Autopsy photograph showing a patchy greenish discolouration of the underside of the liver. The area adjacent to the gall bladder is bile stained.

FIGURE 9.7: (A) Autopsy photograph showing purplish marbling over left upper limb and thighs. (B) Autopsy photograph showing greenish marbling over the anterior and left lateral chest in a case of hanging. (C) 3D VR of PMCT showing the reticular pattern on the skin due to decomposition gas in the superficial veins.

FIGURE 9.9 Axial section of PMCT showing air in the cerebral vasculature.

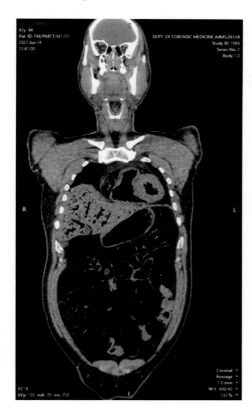

FIGURE 9.10: Coronal section of PMCT showing air in both cardiac chambers. Liver showing gas in hepatic vasculature.

refrigeration since the density of water does not significantly change between the temperatures of 0°C and the temperature of the human body.

Various organ systems in the body develop post-mortem changes which have discrete appearances in PMCT. Post-mortem radiology is distinct from clinical imaging due to post-mortem changes like decomposition changes, resuscitation, and other treatment artefacts in the body. These changes can be mistaken for pathologic findings or even injury to untrained eyes during the interpretation of PMCT.

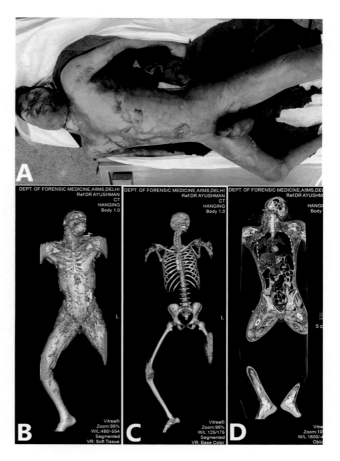

FIGURE 9.11: Body with Grade III decomposition. Both the upper limbs and portion of the left lower limb are out of scan field due to gas stiffening due to decomposition. (A) Autopsy photograph showing marbling, bullae with dark-coloured fluid, greenish discolouration of the body, and bloating of the body. (B) 3D VR of PMCT showing poor quality skin and muscle reconstruction. (C) 3D VR of PMCT showing poor quality skeletal reconstruction due to gas in the bone. (D) Coronal section of PMCT showing gas in all body cavities and soft tissues. The liver has a honeycomb-like pattern. Intestinal loops are dilated with intramural gas.

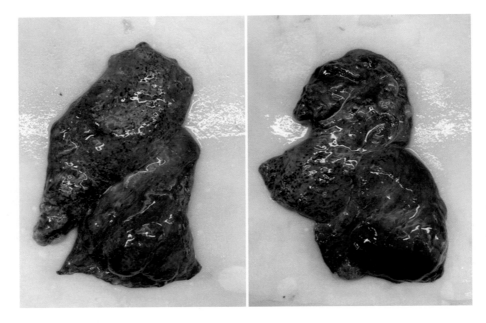

FIGURE 9.12:   Autopsy picture showing a collapsed lung with blebs on the surface due to decomposition.

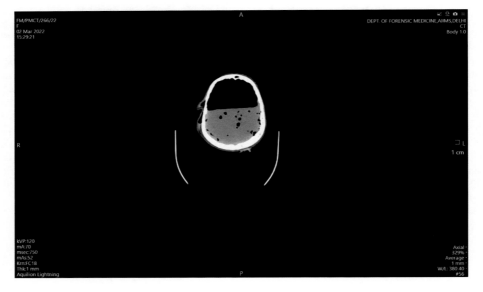

FIGURE 9.13:   Axial section of PMCT showing gas in the ante-dependent part of the cranial cavity. The brain matter shows fluid level and gas brain matter.

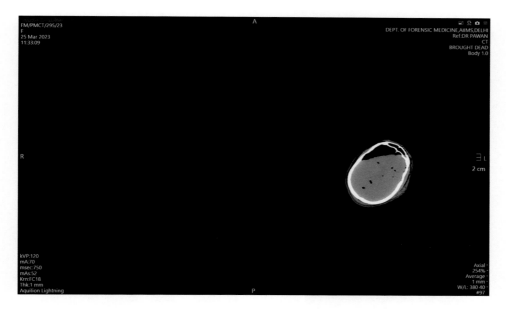

FIGURE 9.14: Axial section of PMCT showing decomposition fluid in frontal sinus in the dependent region with head resting on the left occipital area. The scalp in contact with the table is thinned out in the posterior aspect. The brain is also seen settled in the dependent region with decomposition gas in the ante-dependent region.

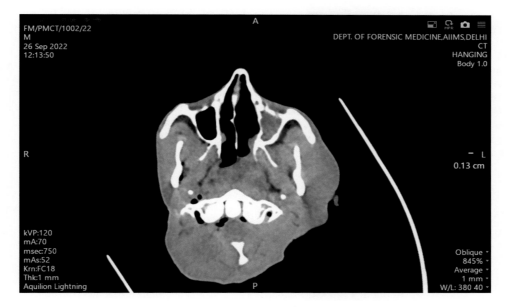

FIGURE 9.15: Axial section of PMCT showing fluid in the left maxillary sinus in a case of hanging.

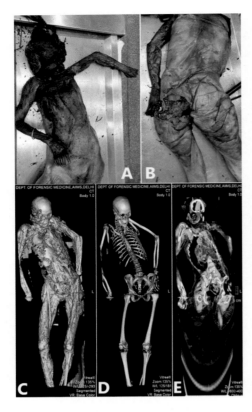

FIGURE 9.16: Body with Grade IV decomposition. (A) Autopsy photograph showing partial skeletonization of head. There are features of mummification in the body. (B) Autopsy photograph showing soft tissue loss due to animal activity in the left gluteal region. (C) 3D VR of PMCT showing poor quality skin and muscle reconstruction. (D) 3D VR of PMCT showing poor quality skeletal reconstruction. (E) Coronal section of PMCT showing gas in all body cavities and soft tissues

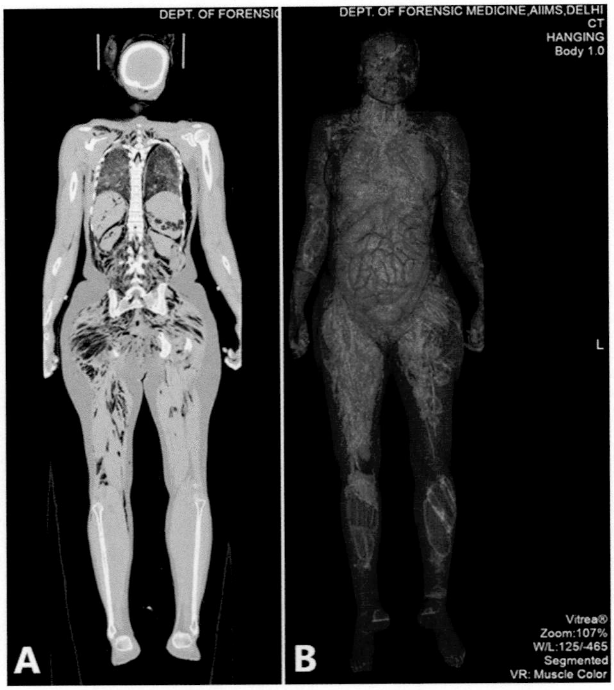

FIGURE 9.17: (A) Coronal view of the whole body shows an accelerated decomposition of the right lower limb compared to the left lower limb and upper limb in a hanging case suspended for long duration. A ligature has a knot on the right lateral aspect of the neck. (B) 3D VR of PMCT shows the pattern of gas distribution in the body. There is increased gas in the right side of the cranial cavity due to a knot on the right side. The upper limbs have minimal decomposition gas as it is farther from the intestine compared to lower limbs.

Bibliography

Dictionary BL. *Black's Law Dictionary*. 1990. 488.

Guharaj PV, Sudhir KG. *Forensic medicine and toxicology*. Universities Press, Chennai, 2019, pp. 102–120.

Ishida M, Gonoi W, Okuma H, Shirota G, Shintani Y, Abe H, Takazawa Y, Fukayama M, Ohtomo K. Common postmortem computed tomography findings following atraumatic death: Differentiation between normal postmortem changes and pathologic lesions. *Korean J Radiol.* 2015 August 1;16(4):798–809.

Jackowski C, Thali M, Aghayev E, Yen K, Sonnenschein M, Zwygart K, et al. Postmortem imaging of blood and its characteristics using MSCT and MRI. *Int J Legal Med.* 2006 July;120(4):233–240.

Madea B. History of forensic medicine. *Handbook of forensic medicine*. John Wiley. 2014 Mar 31:1–4.

Saukko P, Knight B. *Knight's forensic pathology*. CRC Press, Boca Raton. 2016, pp. 55–90.

Shapiro HA. 1950. Rigor Mortis. *Br Med J.* 2:304.

Shapiro HA. 1954. Medicolegal Mythology: Some popular Forensic Fallacies. *J Forens Med.* 1:144.

Shenton A, Kralt P, Suvarna SK. *Post mortem CT for non-suspicious adult deaths: An introduction.* Springer Nature, Switzerland. 2021 May 17, pp. 34–64.

Shirota G, Gonoi W, Ishida M, Okuma H, Shintani Y, Abe H, Takazawa Y, Ikemura M, Fukayama M, Ohtomo K. Brain swelling and loss of gray and white matter differentiation in human postmortem cases by computed tomography. *PLOS ONE.* 2015 November 30;10(11):e0143848.

Wagensveld IM, Blokker BM, Wielopolski PA, Renken NS, Krestin GP, Hunink MG, Oosterhuis JW, Weustink AC. Total-body CT and MR features of postmortem change in in-hospital deaths. *PLoS ONE.* 2017 September 27;12(9):e0185115.

10   CT ARTEFACTS AND THEIR POST-MORTEM ASPECTS

Introduction

Nowadays, post-mortem computed tomography (PMCT) leads an important role in evaluating the cause of death in deceased bodies. It is helpful in finding out the underlying pathology. There are a number of artefacts which we will encounter during the application of CT in deceased bodies, in which some artefacts vary from the routine artefacts encountered by clinical radiologists. In CT imaging, it is of utmost importance to know about the various imaging artefacts to prevent a misdiagnosis and to correctly identify any underlying pathology. This will help us to increase the accuracy of PMCT reports in deriving the cause of death. In this chapter, we will describe some important artefacts which are only commonly encountered during CT imaging in clinical PMCT and how to rectify these artefacts to an extent. Artefacts occur due to certain parameters that are not met with ideal conditions.

Parameters that should be in ideal conditions are as follows:
- High radiation dose
- High photon counts
- Perfect detectors
- Detector resolution
- Monochromatic X-rays

Common artefacts which are frequently encountered during CT imaging are as follows:

1. Beam hardening artefact
2. Metal streak artefact
3. Ring artefact
4. Partial volume artefact
5. Zebra artefact
6. Stair-step artefact
7. Noise artefact
8. Cone beam artefact
9. Motion artefact
10. Helical artefact

Some other post-mortem artefacts, specifically only seen in PMCT include (2):

1. Livor mortis
2. Decomposition
3. Blood
4. Artefacts due to resuscitation during the agonal period

In this chapter, we will discuss the most common artefacts which are observed in PMCT.

Some artefacts which routinely occur in live patients but are not encountered in PMCT are motion artefacts and partial volume artefacts.

Beam hardening artefact

- **Mechanism:** A beam hardening artefact is produced due to a variation in beam energy between two high attenuating materials or objects which come in between the X-ray beam during imaging.

For example, objects like any metallic piece present inside or outside the body surface or even the thick cortical bones present in the viewing field. This appears as a dark parallel streak where the object or material is present with high attenuation (bright image) outside that field. This increase in attenuation of the image adjacent to the beam hardening artefact may cause difficulty in the diagnosis of the pathology due to misinterpretations of the area of interest (Figures 10.1–10.6).

<u>**Reduction techniques:**</u>

- **Dual-energy CT:** The beam hardening Artefact can be reduced by using a **dual-energy CT**.
  Dual-energy CT will work on the principle of scanning at two different energy levels. Thus, the obtained images are reconstructed as monochromatic images with reduced beam hardening effects.
- **Filtration:** A metallic object can be used to pre-harden the X-ray beam before it passes through the body by filtering the components with low energy. For thinner parts of the body, we can utilize another filter, named a bowtie filter, to increase the hardness of the beam.
- **Machine calibration:** With the help of an imaging phantom, a CT machine can be calibrated for different ranges of beams. This will help us in the reduction of beam hardening effects of the deceased body at different parts of the body. However, if the deceased body does not match fully with the calibration of the phantom a cupping artefact can occur.
- **Correction software:** Preinstalled software for the reduction of beam hardening during the reconstruction of images will help us to reduce the blurring/dark bands in images during their interpretation.
- **Reduction by the operator's hands:** Also known as avoidance of hardening, it works by positioning the long cortical bones while doing scanning specific section. But this will help less in a PMCT study as we are scanning the whole body in a single study.

Metal streak artefact

Mechanism: A metal streak artefact can be produced due to various reasons. Any metallic object that is present inside or outside the body cavity will lead to the production of a metal streak artefact. When X-rays pass through metal, they get scattered and the resultant artefact on CT resembles streaks in an image, hence it is called a metal streak artefact. Even beam

DOI: 10.1201/9781003383703-10

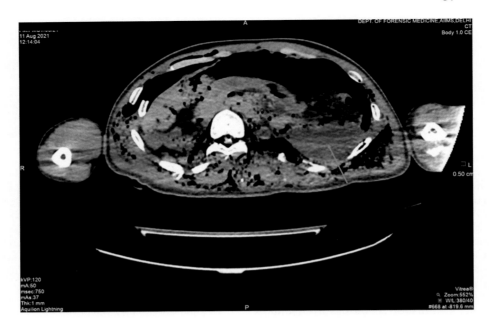

FIGURE 10.1: PMCT – axial section of the chest shows a beam hardening artefact due to cortical bone (humerus) (orange arrow).

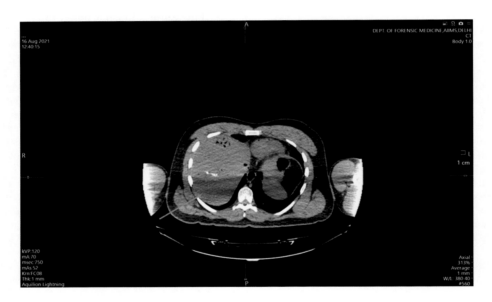

FIGURE 10.2: PMCT – axial section of the abdomen shows a beam hardening artefact due to cortical bone (ulna) (orange arrow).

hardening and noise artefacts results in a metal streak artefact (Figures 10.7–10.13).

Reduction techniques: To avoid such kinds of artefacts in PMCT we must conduct a thorough external examination body and remove metallic objects present outside the body, if any.

To reduce metal streak artefacts due to objects present inside the body, we can use the SEMAR (single energy projection-based metal artefact reduction) software. If at the time of taking a scan, we find any metal SEMAR should be activated.

Ring artefact

Mechanism: This is another type of physics-based artefact occurring due to miscalibrated detectors, which create a dark and bright streak in the shape of a ring at the centre of the image (Figures 10.14–10.16).

It can be reduced by re-calibrating the machine detectors.

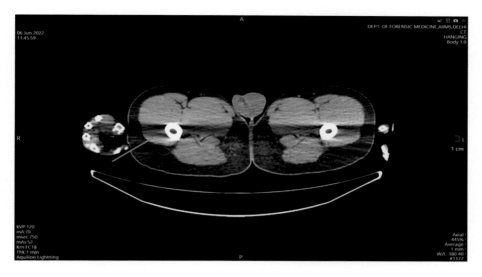

FIGURE 10.3: PMCT – axial section of the thigh shows a beam hardening artefact due to the cortical bone (femur) (orange arrow).

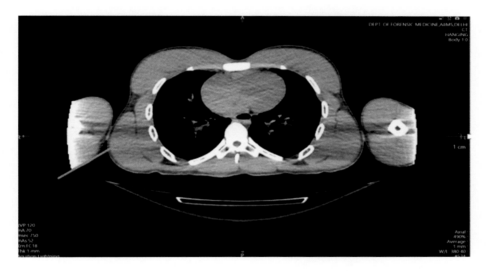

FIGURE 10.4: PMCT – axial section of chest shows a beam hardening artefact due to the cortical bone (humerus) (orange arrow).

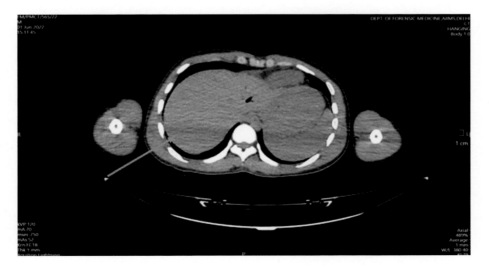

FIGURE 10.5: PMCT – axial section of abdomen shows a beam hardening artefact due to the cortical bone (ulna) (orange arrow).

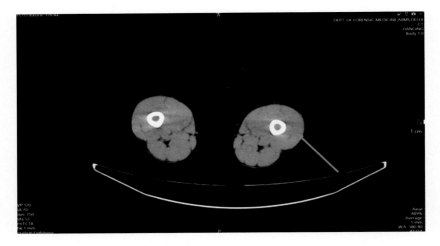

FIGURE 10.6:   PMCT – axial section of thigh shows a beam hardening artefact due to the cortical bone (femur) (orange arrow).

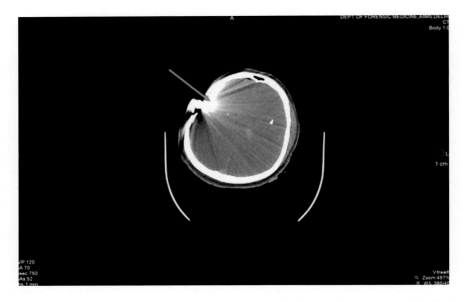

FIGURE 10.7:   PMCT – axial section of head shows a metal streak artefact due to the presence of a bullet from a firearm injury (orange arrow).

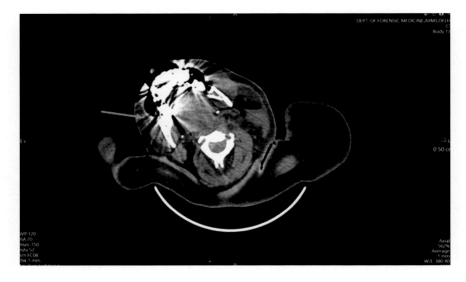

FIGURE 10.8:   PMCT – axial section of mandible shows a metal streak artefact due to the presence of dental amalgam (orange arrow).

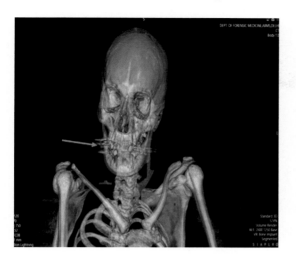

FIGURE 10.9: PMCT – MIP of mandible shows a metal streak artefact due to the presence of dental amalgam (orange arrow).

Zebra and stair-step artefacts

These types of artefacts are more common in multiplanar 3D reconstructed images. They are mostly seen at the periphery of the field of interest.

Zebra artefact

Mechanism: During the process of helical data to reconstruct 3D images a faint stripe may occur because due to helical interpolation, which gives a noise inhomogeneity (Figures 10.17 and 10.18).

This type of artefact can be overcome by reconstructing images with thin-slice data, which can be easily obtained with modern machines used nowadays.

Stair-step artefact

Mechanism: This is due to the usage of wide collimation and non-overlapping reconstruction intervals while processing the images for multiplanar 3D reconstructed images. It appears at the edges of the structures as a staircase (Figures 10.19–10.22).

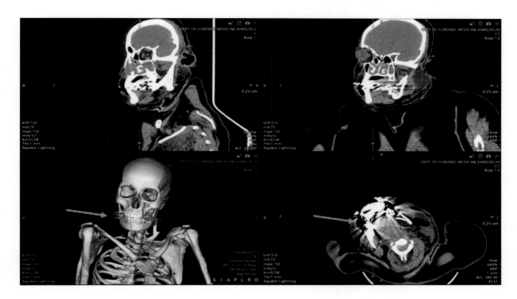

FIGURE 10.10: PMCT – MPR shows a metal streak artefact due to the presence of dental amalgam (orange arrow).

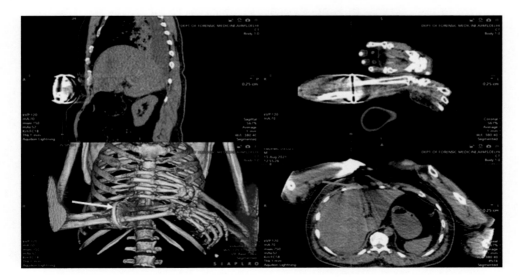

FIGURE 10.11: PMCT – MPR shows a metal streak artefact due to the presence of metal ornament over right elbow region (orange arrow).

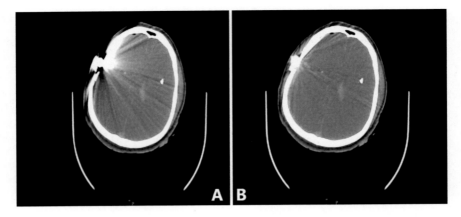

FIGURE 10.12: PMCT – axial section of the head soft tissue window shows a metal streak artefact due to the presence of a bullet from firearm injury (a: without SEMAR activation, b: with SEMAR activation).

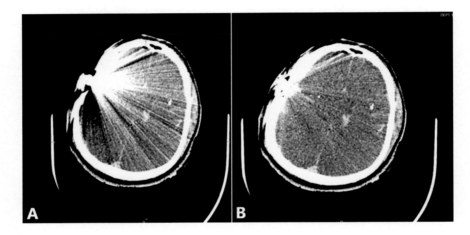

FIGURE 10.13: PMCT – axial section of brain window shows a metal streak artefact due to presence of bullet in firearm injury (a – without SEMAR activation, b – with SEMAR activation).

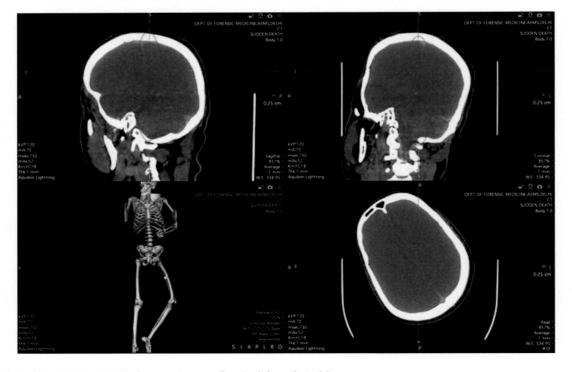

FIGURE 10.14: PMCT – MPR shows a ring artefact (red dotted circle).

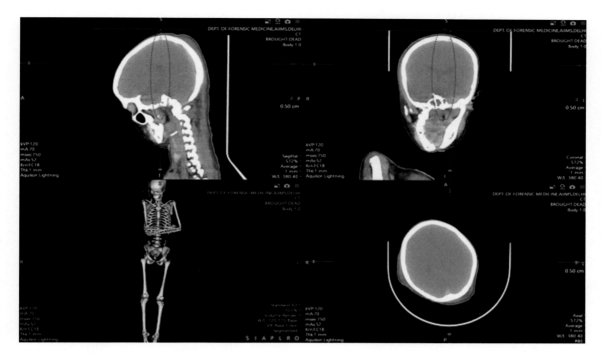

FIGURE 10.15: PMCT – MPR shows a ring artefact (red dotted circle).

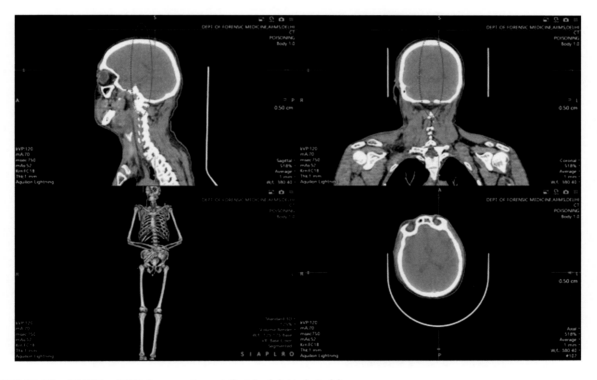

FIGURE 10.16: PMCT – MPR shows a ring artefact (red dotted circle).

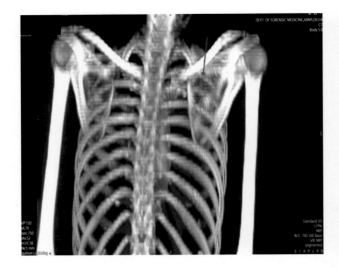

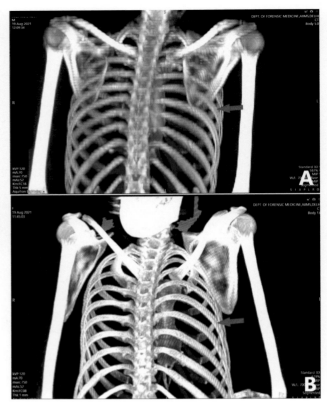

FIGURE 10.17: PMCT – MIP shows a zebra artefact (red arrow).

FIGURE 10.18: (A and B): PMCT – MIP shows a zebra arte-fact (red arrow).

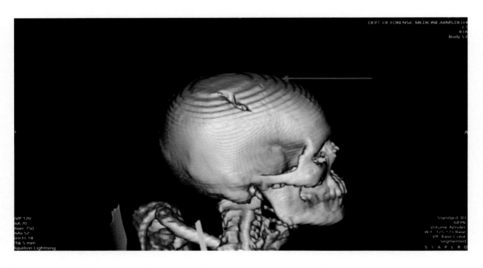

FIGURE 10.19: PMCT – VRT shows a stair-step artefact over skull (red arrow).

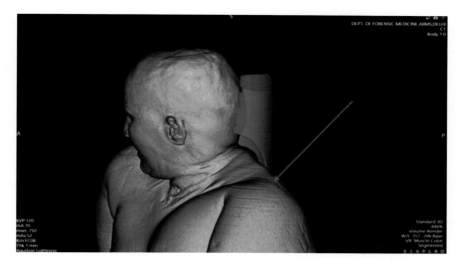

FIGURE 10.20: PMCT – VRT shows a stair-step artefact over the shoulder and arm (red arrow).

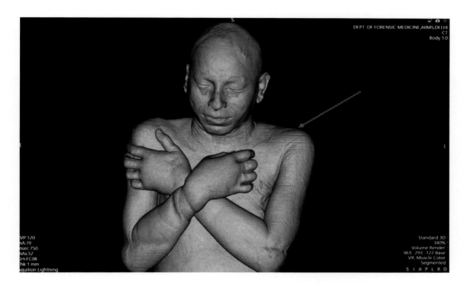

FIGURE 10.21: PMCT – VRT shows a stair-step artefact over the shoulder and arm (red arrow).

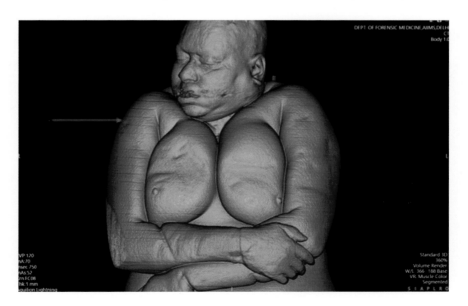

FIGURE 10.22: PMCT – VRT shows a stair-step artefact over the shoulder, arm, and forearm (red arrow).

This type of artefact can be overcome by reconstructing images with thin-slice data which can be easily obtained with modern machines used nowadays.

Noise artefact

Mechanism: This is a type of physics-based artefacts that occurs due to an error in the calculation of the photon count which results in the rays producing thin dark and bright streaks in the direction of higher attenuation (Figures 10.23–10.25).

It can be rectified by proper reconstruction techniques or by combining the data from multiple scans.

Partial volume artefact

Mechanism: When the imaging object is not fully exposed to the X-ray, a partial volume artefact is produced.

In this, the image will be darker in the fully exposed area, bright in the non-exposed area and partially dark and partially bright in the semi-exposed area (Figure 10.26).

This can be rectified by decreasing the slice thickness.

Cone beam artefact

Mechanism: This is due to multi-slice scanners where because of wider collimation, the X-ray beam becomes cone-shaped instead of fan-shaped, resulting in a cone beam artefact (Figure 10.27).

It can be rectified by appropriate reconstruction techniques of beam detectors.

Motion artefact

Mechanism: This type of artefact is mainly due to abnormal movement of the patient's body by him voluntarily or involuntarily. It is by any act such as breathing, shivering due to panic attacks, swallowing, moving of limbs or head, etc.

Reduction techniques: It can be reduced by explaining the procedure to the patient clearly prior to the CT scanning. In PMCT this artefact rarely occurs as the dead body is not moving.

Helical artefact

Mechanism: This same as motion artefact. Here, as the gantry rotates along the z-axis, any object which changes its actual position from that axis will produce a helical artefact.

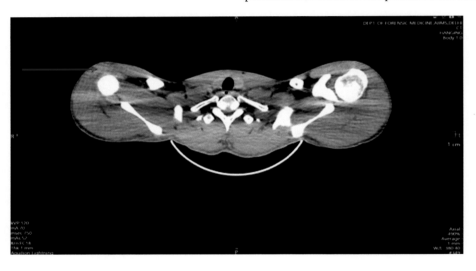

FIGURE 10.23:   PMCT – axial section of the neck shows a noise artefact (red arrow).

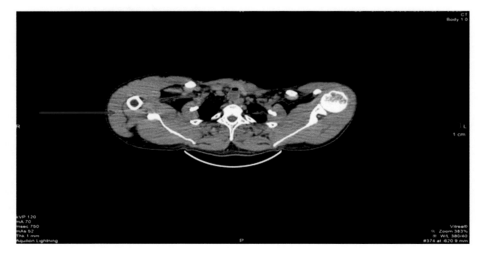

FIGURE 10.24:   PMCT – axial section of the chest shows a noise artefact (red arrow).

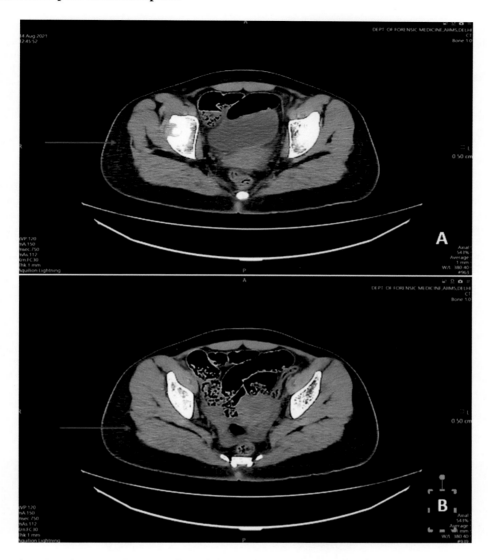

FIGURE 10.25: (A&B): PMCT – axial section of the abdomen shows a noise artefact (red arrow).

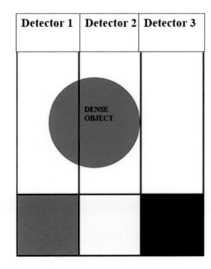

FIGURE 10.26: Picture description of a partial volume artefact.

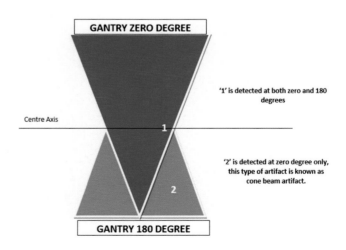

FIGURE 10.27: Picture description of a cone beam artefact.

In PMCT, motion and helical artefacts are not seen as our subjects but as dead bodies.

Post-mortem artefacts

Livor mortis

After the cessation of circulation, respiration, and brain function, the body fluids start to settle down in the dependent areas of the body. This is termed post-mortem hypostasis/lividity/livor mortis. It is observed as reddish discolouration in the dependent areas of the body as per its position at the time of death on external examination during conventional autopsy. In CT, this will appear as a thickening of the skin turgor in the dependent areas, increasing radio density in dependent aspects of the lungs, and haematocrit formation in blood vessels (Figures 10.28–10.30).

However, to conclude livor mortis in both conventional autopsy and PMCT, we must know the position of the body at the time of death.

Decomposition

Decomposition is a process of putrefaction and autolysis of the body of the deceased, occurring with the help of bacterial microorganisms. In PMCT, this may lead to various imaging artefacts which may confuse most observers.

Decomposition changes on PMCT will appear as gas inside the vessels, organs, and subcutaneous tissues, and an apparent increase in the skin density (Figures 10.31–10.44). Air (gas) will appear as black in CT.

In some areas like the peritoneal cavity, which contains more fluid, decomposition will result in fluid–fluid levels and thus, we must be more cautious as we may confuse such a finding with haemoperitoneum. Here, the role of Hounsfield units as the attenuation coefficient of the decomposition changes, in dependent area it is as low as water (0 to 10) and in the anti-dependent areas it is negative (–10 to –110), whereas blood on the other hand has a positive HU value (in a range between +30 to +65).

Blood

After death, blood inside the vessels will clot and become stagnant and it is very difficult to differentiate between ante-mortem and post-mortem clots. This is often seen in large vessels, coronaries, and heart chambers. Clotted blood is seen as hyperdense (bright) in dependent parts and hypodense (dark) in non-dependent parts, as is well demarcated by intravascular serum on PMCT (Figures 10.45–10.48).

Artefacts due to resuscitation during the agonal period

We must know about any attempted resuscitation procedures performed on the deceased. This is because many artefacts can happen during the agonal period, like a buckle rib fracture due to CPR, dislodgement of teeth during artificial respiration procedure, etc. (Figure 10.49).

These types of artefacts can be rectified and ruled out with proper history taking.

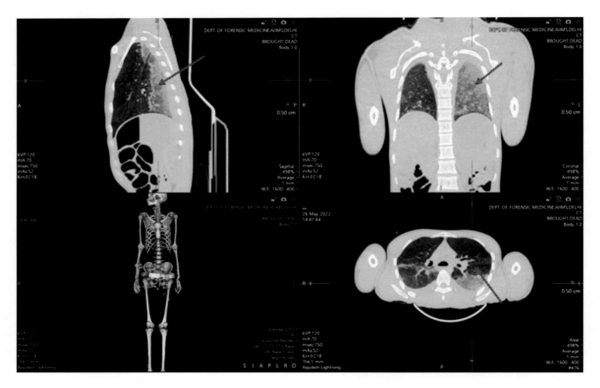

FIGURE 10.28:   PMCT – MPR shows livor mortis over the posterior aspect of the left lung (hyperdense area) (red arrow).

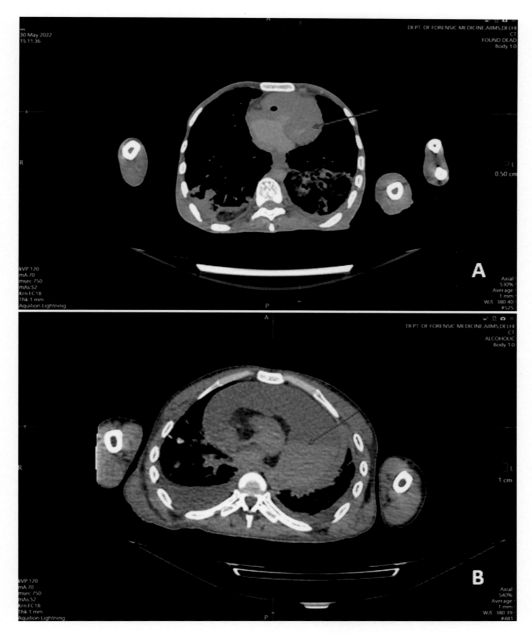

FIGURE 10.29: (A and B): PMCT – axial section of the thorax shows a clear demarcation of livor mortis over cardiac tissue (red arrow).

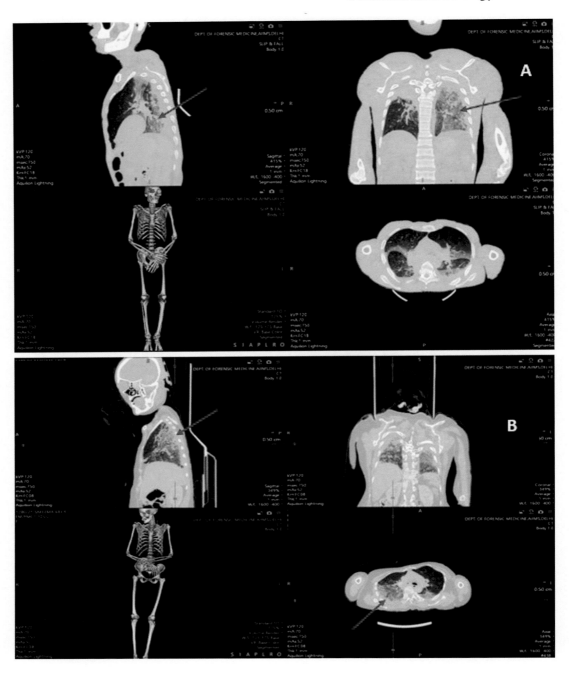

FIGURE 10.30: (A and B): PMCT – MPR shows livor mortis over the posterior aspect of the left lung (hyperdense area) (red arrow).

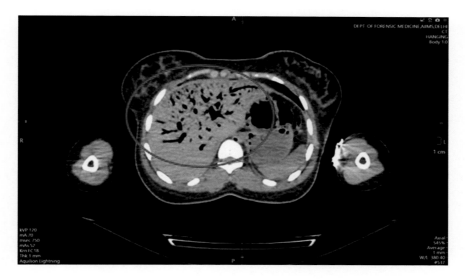

FIGURE 10.31: PMCT – axial section of the abdomen shows air (gaseous) distension of blood vessels of the liver, signs of decomposition – black in colour (red circle).

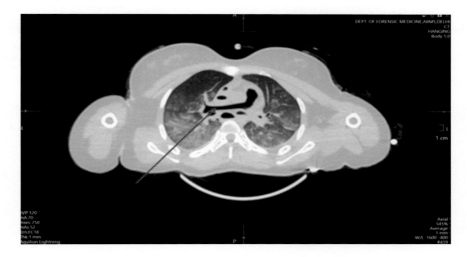

FIGURE 10.32: PMCT – axial section of the thorax shows air (gaseous) distension of pulmonary trunk and cardiac vessels, signs of decomposition – black in colour (red arrow).

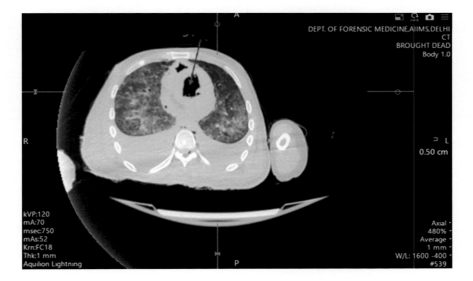

FIGURE 10.33: PMCT – axial section of the thorax shows air (black) over the cardiac region, signs of decomposition (red arrow).

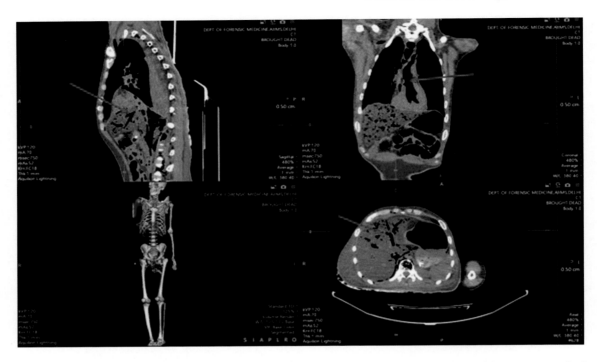

FIGURE 10.34:   PMCT – MPR shows air (black) over the cardiac region and blood vessels, signs of decomposition (red arrow).

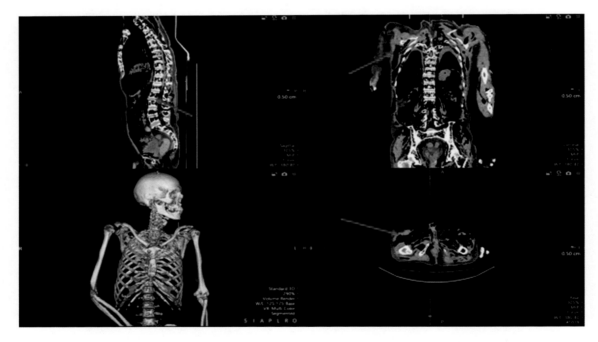

FIGURE 10.35:   PMCT – MPR shows air (black) over muscles, bone marrow, and blood vessels, signs of extensive decomposition (red arrow).

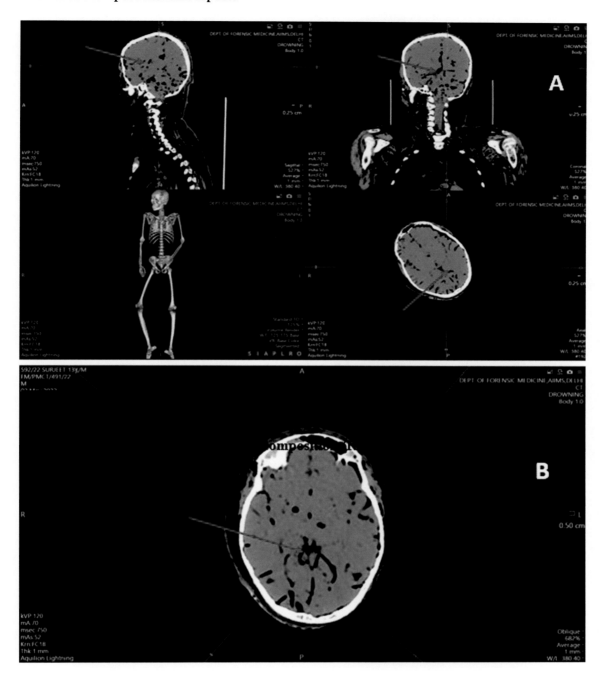

FIGURE 10.36: (A): PMCT – MPR shows air (black) over brain vessels and muscles. (B) PMCT – axial section of the brain shows pneumocephalus, signs of extensive decomposition (red arrow).

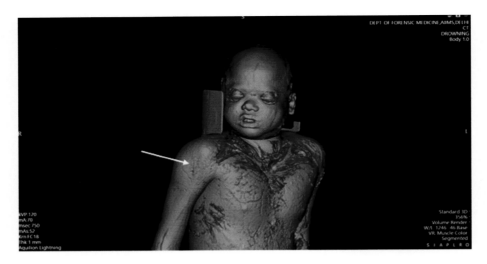

FIGURE 10.37: PMCT – VRT shows swollen face with distension of vessels (marbling), signs of decomposition (white arrow).

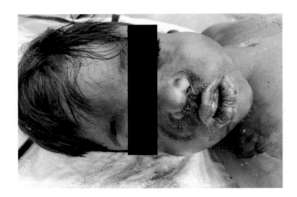

FIGURE 10.38: External examination shows swollen face with fine, blood-tinged, lathery foam is present around the nostrils due to drowning.

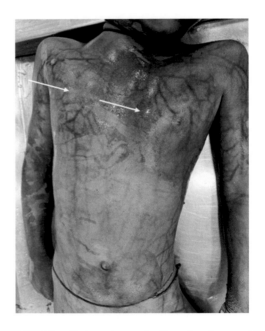

FIGURE 10.40: External examination showing marbling.

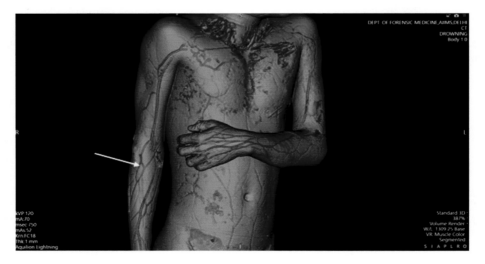

FIGURE 10.39: PMCT – VRT shows distension of vessels (marbling), signs of decomposition (white arrow).

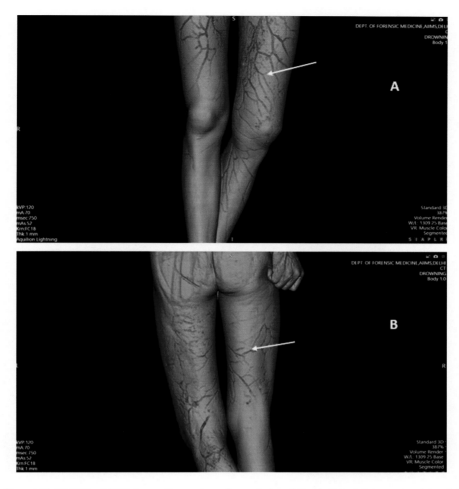

FIGURE 10.41: (A and B): PMCT – VRT shows distension of vessels (marbling), signs of decomposition (white arrow).

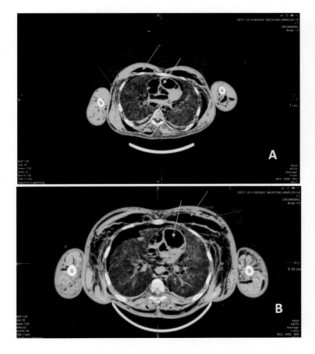

FIGURE 10.42: (A and B): PMCT – axial section of the thorax shows air (black) over cardiac vessels (yellow arrow), muscles (green arrow), and subcutaneous vessels (red arrow), signs of extensive decomposition.

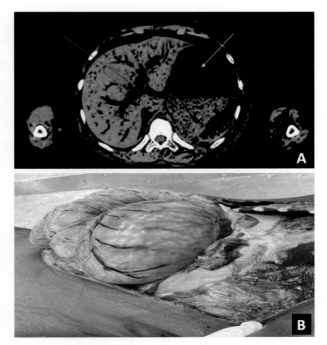

FIGURE 10.43: (A) PMCT – axial section of abdomen shows air (black) inside stomach (yellow arrow) and liver vessels (red arrow), signs of extensive decomposition. (B) PMCT – gaseous distension of stomach in conventional autopsy (yellow arrow).

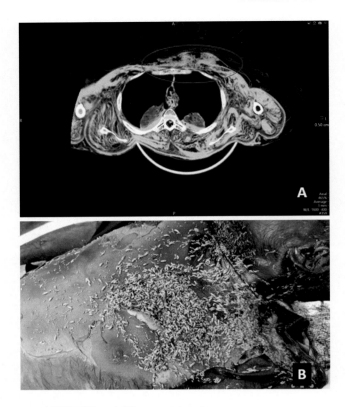

FIGURE 10.44:   Maggot activity in (A) PMCT and (B) conventional autopsy.

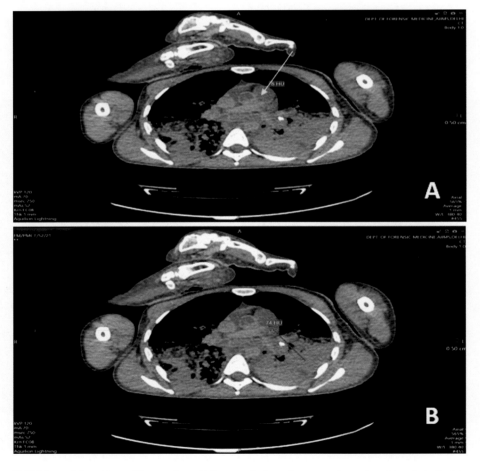

FIGURE 10.45:   PMCT – axial section of thorax in soft tissue window shows post-mortem blood clotted in pulmonary vessels with demarcation of intravascular serum. (A) Non-dependent area of vessels shows less HU and denotes serum (yellow arrow). (B) Dependent area of vessels shows higher HU and denotes blood (red arrow).

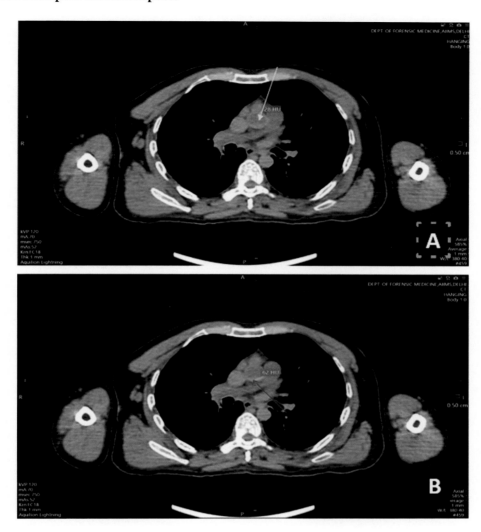

FIGURE 10.46: PMCT – axial section of thorax in soft tissue window shows post-mortem blood clotted in ascending aorta with demarcation of intravascular serum. (A) Non-dependent area of vessels shows less HU and denotes serum (yellow arrow). (B) Dependent area of vessels shows higher HU and denotes blood (red arrow).

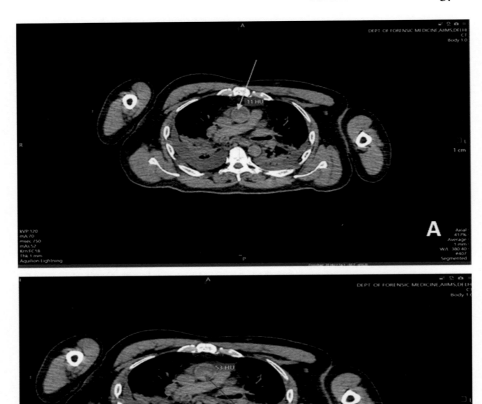

FIGURE 10.47:   PMCT – axial section of the thorax in soft tissue window shows post-mortem blood clotted in ascending aorta with demarcation of intravascular serum. (A) Non-dependent area of vessels shows less HU and denotes serum (yellow arrow). (B) Dependent area of vessels shows higher HU and denotes blood (red arrow).

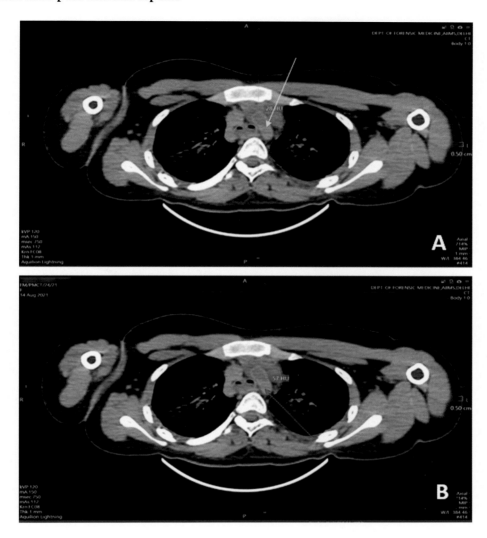

FIGURE 10.48: PMCT – axial section of the thorax in soft tissue window shows post-mortem blood clotted in aortic arch with demarcation of intravascular serum. (A) Non-dependent area of vessels shows less HU and denotes serum (yellow arrow). (B) Dependent area of vessels shows higher HU and denotes blood (red arrow).

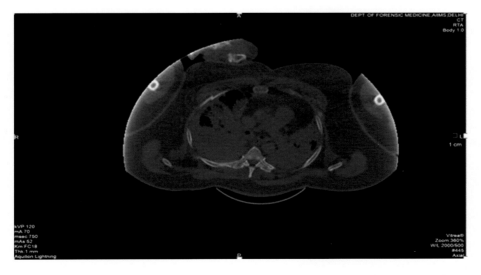

FIGURE 10.49: PMCT – axial section of the thorax in bone window shows a buckle fracture of a rib due to CPR (red circle).

Bibliography

Barrett JF, Keat N. Artefacts in CT: Recognition and avoidance. *RadioGraphics*. 2004;24:1679–1691. Available from: http://dx .doi.org/10.1148/rg.246045065

Berger F, Niemann T, Kubik-Huch RA, Richter H, Thali MJ, Gascho D. Retained bullets in the head on computed tomography – Get the most out of iterative metal Artefact reduction. *Eur J Radiol*. 2018;103:124–130. Available from: http://dx.doi.org/10.1016/j .ejrad.2018.04.019

Brook OR, Gourtsoyianni S, Brook A, Mahadevan A, Wilcox C, Raptopoulos V. Spectral CT with metal Artefacts reduction software for improvement of tumor visibility in the vicinity of gold fiducial markers. *Radiology*. 2012;263:696–705.

Di Maio VJM. An introduction to the classification of gunshot wounds. In: *Gunshot wounds: Practical aspects of firearms, bal-listics, and forensic techniques*, 2nd ed. CRC Press, Boca Raton, FL, 1998, pp. 64–121.

Douis N, Formery AS, Hossu G, Martrille L, Kolopp M, Gondim Teixeira PA, et al. Metal Artefact reduction for intracranial projectiles on postmortem computed tomography. *Diagn Interv Imaging*. 2020;101:177–185. http://dx.doi.org/10.1016/j.diii.2019 .10.009

Hsieh J. Image Artefacts: Appearances, causes and corrections. In: *Computed tomography: Principles, design, Artefacts, and recent advances*. Bellingham, Washington: SPIE Press, 2009, pp. 207–295.

Hussein MN, Heinemann A, Shokry DA, Elgebely M, Pueschel K, Hassan FM. Postmortem computed tomography differentiation between intraperitoneal decomposition gas and pneumoperitoneum. *Int J Legal Med*. 2021;136:229–235. http://dx.doi.org/10 .1007/s00414-021-02732-7

Kidoh M, Nakaura T, Nakamura S, et al. Reduction of dental metallic artefacts in CT: Value of a newly developed algorithm for metal artefact reduction (O-MAR). *Clin Radiol*. 2014;69:e11–e116.

Levy AD, Harcke HT, Mallak CT. Postmortem Imaging. *Am J Forensic Med Pathol*. 2010;31:12–17. http://dx.doi.org/10.1097/PAF .0b013e3181c65e1a

Sonoda A, Nitta N, Ushio N, Nagatani Y, Okumura N, Otani H, et al. Evaluation of the quality of CT images acquired with the single energy metal Artefact reduction (SEMAR) algorithm in patients with hip and dental prostheses and aneurysm embolization coils. *Jpn J Radiol*. 2015;33:710–716. http://dx.doi.org/10.1007/ s11604-015-0478-2

Sutherland T, O'Donnell C. The artefacts of death: CT post-mortem findings. *J Med Imaging Radiat Oncol*. 2017 December 11;62(2):203–210.

Thali MJ, Viner MD, Brogdon BG. Forensic radiology of gunshot wound, new developments in gunshot injury. In: *Brogdon's Forensic Radiology*, 2nd ed. CRC Press, Boca Raton, FL, 2014, pp. 211–252.

Thali MJ, Yen K, Vock P, Ozdoba C, Kneubuehl BP, Sonnenschein M, et al. Image-guided virtual autopsy findings of gunshot victims performed with multi-slice computed tomography (MSCT) and magnetic resonance imaging (MRI) and subsequent correlation between radiology and autopsy findings. *Forensic Sci Int*. 2003;138:8–16. http://dx.doi.org/10.1016/S0379 -0738(03)00225-1

Yang K moo, Lynch M, O'Donnell C. "Buckle" rib fracture: An Artefact following cardio-pulmonary resuscitation detected on postmortem CT. *Legal Med*. 2011;13:233–239. http://dx.doi.org/10 .1016/j.legalmed.2011.05.004

11 VIRTUAL AUTOPSY CASES

The author has, in his experience, seen many cases, a few of which are mentioned in the last chapter, indicating the potential areas that forensic radiology can be used as a substitute for dissectional autopsy in trauma deaths, foreign body discovery, mass fatality, and body identification postmortem computed tomography (PMCT). In cases of trauma like RTAs, gunshot injuries, stab injuries, fall-from-height, etc. there is a good agreement of PMCT and autopsy in detecting fractures, haemorrhages (like intracranial, intrathoracic, and intraperitoneal) and pneumo-pathologies (like pneumothorax, pneumoperitoneum, etc.). PMCT detected most injuries found at autopsy but was superior to autopsy in detecting facial skeleton and spine fractures, detecting intraventricular haemorrhages, and air-related findings. This confirms that PMCT is an important adjunct before an autopsy in cases of trauma that could also serve as an adequate alternative when a traditional autopsy is unavailable.

Road traffic accidents

In cases of roadside accidents and fall from height cases a virtual autopsy can be a very useful tool in determining the cause of death, as well as any potential contributing factors. A virtual autopsy is a detailed examination of the body, which can be conducted virtually, using digital imaging and 3D reconstruction technologies. It can provide valuable insight into the condition of the body and the events leading up to the accident. This can include analysis of the injuries, such as fractures, abrasions, and lacerations, as well as examination of the internal organs and tissues. By combining this information with other evidence, such as witness statements and physical evidence, it is possible to build a full picture of the accident and how it occurred. This can be invaluable for a legal investigation into the cause of the roadside accident.

Here a few cases are discussed in which the cause of death was solely given on the basis of a verbal autopsy, external examination, and virtual autopsy without a traditional autopsy

Case of poly-trauma following an RTA

A case of a 28-year-old male who was part of an RTA in Uttar Pradesh. He was initially treated in the local hospital, and from there referred to Banaras Hindu University's trauma centre, Varanasi, for further treatment. Later he was brought to Indraprastha Apollo Hospital, New Delhi, for further management, but unfortunately, he was declared dead after 2 days of hospital treatment. After analysis of inquest papers and hospital records, the deceased was diagnosed with polytrauma, severe traumatic brain injury, subdural haemorrhage, subarachnoid haemorrhage, diffuse axonal injury, and facial bone fractures.

On external examination, brownish-black scabbed abrasions were present over the face involving the forehead, both eyebrows, nose, both lips, and left cheek with bilateral periorbital haematoma (Figure 11.1). Apart from that, multiple brownish-black scabbed abrasions were present on both the upper and lower limbs, abdomen, chest, and back of the trunk (Figure 11.2).

On PMCT examination

Skull: A comminuted fracture of the left frontal bone with hyperdensity in the frontal sinus, the left orbital plate of the frontal bone, the roof of the left orbit, and the lateral wall of the left maxillary antrum with hyperdensity in the maxillary sinus seen. A comminuted fracture of the left zygomatic arch is also seen. A fracture of the nasal bone and nasal septum. A fracture of the sphenoid bone with hyperdensity in the sphenoid sinus. A fracture of the right mastoid. A fracture of the bilateral mandible. A fracture of the left maxillary bone is also seen. (Figures 11.3 and 11.4).

Brain and meninges: A diffuse subarachnoid haemorrhage can be seen. A ventricular haemorrhage is present. A haemorrhagic contusion is seen over the bilateral temporal and frontal lobes (Figure 11.5). A subdural haemorrhage can be seen with a midline shift. Basi-frontal and basi-temporal contusions were also seen.

Chest: The bilateral pleural cavities show hyperdense areas with attenuation ranges (50 HU–110 HU) seen suggestive of haemothorax. The bilateral lungs show diffuse ground glass opacity (Figure 11.6). The pericardial sac is intact. No pericardial effusion is seen. No calcification is noted.

Abdomen and pelvis: No abnormality was detected in the rest of the organs.

After analysis of the history, inquest papers, hospital records, external examination, and PMCT the cause of death in this case was given as shock due to polytrauma consequent upon blunt force/surface impact and all injuries were ante-mortem in nature.

Case of RTA with delayed complications

A case of a 53-year-old male who sustained injuries during an RTA was taken to Indraprastha Apollo Hospital, New Delhi. Unfortunately, after 2 months of treatment, he died. As per the submitted inquest papers and hospital records, the cause of death was given as an RTA with the following injuries sustained: chest injury, critical illness polyneuropathy, fungemia, bacterial sepsis, septic shock, disseminated intravascular coagulation, and multi-organ failure. On external examination (Figure 11.7) the deceased was noted as average build and moderately nourished. The face was congested. Yellow discolouration of the whole body with pitting oedema was present. Multiple IV cannulation needle puncture marks were present over the left side of the neck, bilateral cubital fossa and right inguinal region. An open tracheostomy wound of 2 cm × 1 cm was present on the anterior aspect of the neck. A sutured insertion wound for an intercostal drainage tube with four intact black-coloured stitches was present on the left side of the chest, 2 cm below the nipple. Multiple fluid-filled blisters were present over the posterior surface of the back of the abdomen and lower limbs. A bed sore with peeling skin with a size of 2.5 cm × 1.5 cm was present over the back of the abdomen, 2 cm left of the midline. Two injuries were present one was an old scar of 2 cm × 0.3 cm present over the forehead midline, and the other was a blackish scabbed with a size of 3 cm × 2 cm with a base containing pus, granulation tissue, and black necrotic eschar present over the lateral side of the left lower limb.

DOI: 10.1201/9781003383703-11

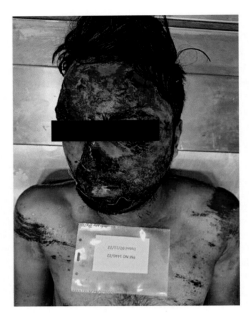

FIGURE 11.1: A gross examination of the deceased showed brownish-black scabbed abrasions over the whole face with clotted blood, and grazed brownish-black abrasions on the bilateral shoulder and chest.

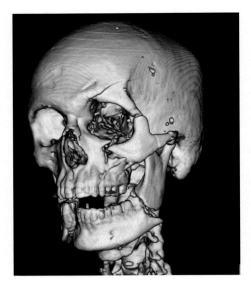

FIGURE 11.3: Volume rendered image showing fracture of the left orbital plate of the frontal bone, roof of the left orbit, lateral wall of the left maxillary antrum, comminuted fracture of the left zygomatic arch, and fracture of the mandible at two points.

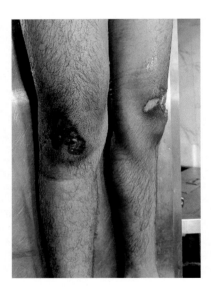

FIGURE 11.2: Gross examination of the bilateral lower limbs showing brownish-black scabbed abrasion over the knee joint.

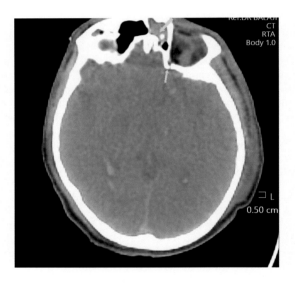

FIGURE 11.4: Axial section of PMCT showing a fracture of the left orbital plate and effusion in the frontal sinus.

On PMCT examination

Skull: The right nasal bone was fractured. The vomer bone is deviated to the left side.

Chest: The manubrium and body of the sternum along with the fourth to tenth ribs of both sides were fractured at multiple sites. Bilateral pleural cavities showed hyperdensity in dependent regions with HU in the range of 14.1 +/−15.6 to 15.6 +/−16.9 suggestive of haemorrhage in bilateral pleural cavities. The bilateral lungs were collapsed, and ground glass opacities were present over all of the lobes (Figure 11.8), which is suggestive of consolidation pericardium is intact, a hyperdense

area was present in the left ventricular wall and valves. All four chambers are intact. Multiple hyperdense areas were present in the coronary arteries at places. Hyperdensity is seen in the arch of the aorta suggestive of calcification.

Abdomen and pelvis: No abnormality detected.

Spinal Column and Spinal Cord: A fracture of the transverse process of the second, third, fourth, and fifth lumber vertebrae was noted.

After perusal of the inquest papers, treatment records, and autopsy findings the cause of death was given as septicemic shock consequent upon blunt force impact/trauma to the chest. .

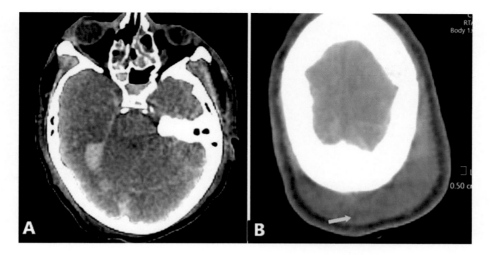

FIGURE 11.5: (A) Axial section of PMCT showing a fracture of the nasal septum and haemorrhage in the brain parenchyma with subdural haemorrhage at the periphery. (B) Diffuse subgaleal haematoma is present below the scalp (marked with a red arrow).

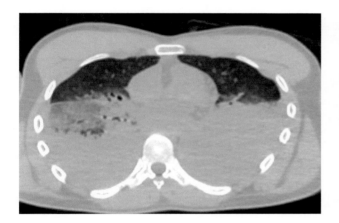

FIGURE 11.6: Axial section of PMCT showing bilateral hyperdense areas with the seen attenuation ranges (50 HU–110 HU) suggestive of haemothorax. The bilateral lungs show diffuse ground glass opacity.

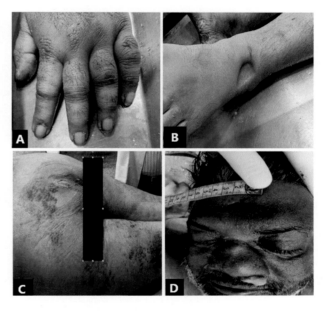

FIGURE 11.7: External examination of the deceased shows (A) diffuse swelling over the limbs, (B) pitting oedema present over the lower limbs, (C) bed sores present over the lower back, and (D) wound scar present on the forehead in the midline.

Case of poly-trauma with transection of vertebral column following an RTA

A case of a 58-year-old female who encountered an RTA after which she was taken to hospital but was declared dead on arrival. On external examination, the deceased was obese in appearance.

A periorbital haematoma was present over the right eye and the bilateral conjunctiva was pale and hazy. All fingernails were pale in appearance. Multiple grazed abrasions were present over the face, chest, abdomen, and limbs (Figure 11.9). On PMCT in volume rendered image the ribs of the right side, from fifth to ninth along the parasternal area, and the left side, from second to twelfth along the paravertebral line, and from seventh to eleventh along the midaxillary line were fractured. Complete transaction of the vertebral column is seen at the level of T12–L1 along with a fracture of the transverse process of T12 and L1 to L5 (Figure 11.10). Fracture of the left side of the sacrum, superior and inferior ramus of the right pubis, and inferior ramus of the left pubis were fractured (Figure 11.11 a, b, and c). No abnormality was detected in the head and neck

except dilated ventricles. Calcification was noted in the coronary arteries. Haemoperitoneum is present. Multiple lacerations were present over the spleen and liver parenchyma with avulsion of the left lobe of the liver (Figure 11.12). After perusal of the inquest papers, external examination, and PMCT findings the cause of death was given as polytrauma due to blunt force/surface impact.

Falls from a height

Case of poly-trauma following fall from height

A case of a 77-year-old female who sustained injuries as a result of a fall from the third floor of her residential building.

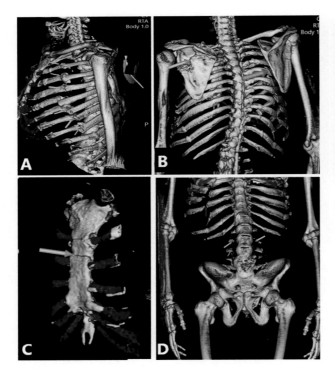

FIGURE 11.8: PMCT volume rendered image showing (A) old healed malunited fracture of the ribs on the left chest side, chest cavity. (B) Old healed malunited fracture of the left side scapula along with a non-united fracture of the right side ribs along the paravertebral area. (C) Old healed fracture of the body of the sternum. (D) Fracture of the transverse process of the lumbar vertebra.

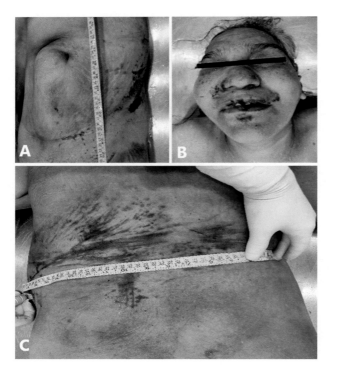

FIGURE 11.9: Gross external examination showing (A) graze abrasion and bruise over the front and lateral part of the abdomen. (B) Periorbital haematoma present over the right eye. (C) Graze abrasion and bruise present over the back of the trunk.

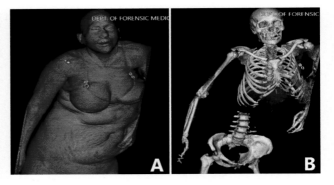

FIGURE 11.10: PMCT volume rendered image showing (A) external examination of the body and (B) skeletal examination showing the complete transaction of the body at the levels of T12–L1.

After which she was taken to hospital but was declared dead. As per the inquest papers, the deceased had a history of diabetes and hypertension. On external examination, multiple reddish abrasions were present over the posterior aspect of the chest and abdomen across the midline in an area of 36 cm × 30 cm. Along with these, multiple abrasions and lacerations were present over the upper and lower limbs (Figure 11.13). On PMCT examination the head and neck showed no abnormality. In the chest, a rib fracture from the second to the ninth was present on the right side along the midclavicular line as well as a scapula and clavicle fracture. On the left side a rib fracture from the third to ninth rib, along with the eleventh rib, was present (Figure 11.14). In the pelvic area, a fracture of the superior and inferior pubic rami was present along with disruption of the pubic symphysis (Figure 11.15). Haemopneumothorax was also present (Figure 11.16). Calcification in the left anterior descending artery and the right coronary artery were present. The abdomen shows haemoperitoneum with normal air–fluid levels in the intestines. Fractures of the C5 and C6 vertebra were noted along with fractures of the T1 to T3 vertebra. After perusal of the inquest papers, external examination and PMCT findings cause of death was given as polytrauma due to blunt force/surface impact.

A study on 100 RTA cases was conducted by the Department of Forensic Medicine, AIIMS, New Delhi, with the motive of comparing radiological (CT scan) findings vis-a-vis traditional autopsy and to detect the feasibility of virtual autopsy as an alternative method to traditional autopsy. Results of the study were divided into four sections as PMCT analysis of injuries to the head, chest, abdomen, pelvis, and limbs. The study showed that fractures (vault, base of skull and facial bones), haemorrhages (SDH, SAH, IPH, IVH, brain stem haemorrhage and sub-scalp haematoma), Pneumocephalus, brain oedema, and midline shifts are more easily appreciated on PMCT as compared to traditional autopsy (Figure 11.17).

In the results for the chest, rib and vertebral fractures, pneumothorax, haemothorax, pneumonia, pneumohaemothorax, pleural effusion, and injury to the lungs by penetrating or perforating, and surgical emphysema were more easily appreciated while the proper extent of injuries can be appreciated on PMCT as compare to traditional autopsy. Fractures in the abdomen and pelvis along with haemo and pneumoperitoneum are easily differentiated on PMCT. Similarly, on both limbs analysis concluded that fractures are detected more easily on PMCT as compared to traditional autopsy.

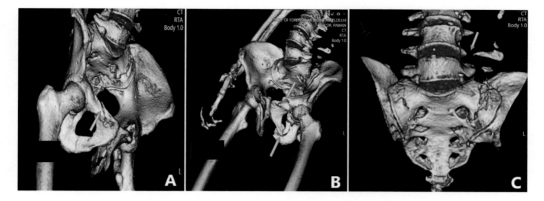

FIGURE 11.11: Volume rendered image showing (A) fracture of the right side superior pubic rami. (B) Fracture of left side superior and inferior pubic rami. (C) Fracture of the transverse process of the lumbar vertebra and left side of the body of the sacrum (fracture site marked with a yellow arrow).

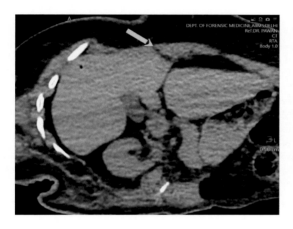

FIGURE 11.12: Axial section of PMCT showing laceration of the left lobe of the liver (marked with a yellow arrow)

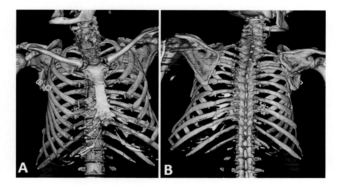

FIGURE 11.14: Volume rendered image showing (A) anterior aspect of the chest with a right side fracture of the clavicle and the second to ninth ribs along the midclavicular line. (B) Posterior aspect of the chest with a fracture of the right side scapula.

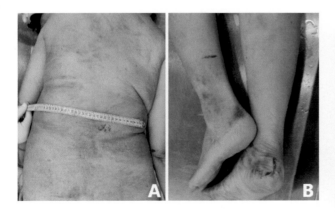

FIGURE 11.13: External examination showing (A) injury over the back of chest and abdomen (B) injury, i.e., laceration and bruise present over the lower limbs.

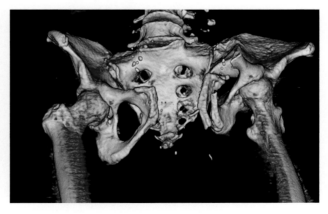

FIGURE 11.15: Volume rendered image showing dislocation of the pubic symphysis along with the fracture of superior and inferior rami of the left side of the pelvic bone.

Gunshot wounds

Identification of entry and exit wounds is important in the postmortem examination of victims of gunshot injuries. However, this is possible in the external examination itself except for the analysis of underlying fracture patterns. PMCT examination helps in this scenario by analyzing the dispersion of bone fragments and studying fracture patterns.

Foreign bodies are commonly associated findings of fatal gunshot injuries. PMCT imaging will be beneficial in identifying, localizing, and demonstrating this foreign material in 3D view. If it's retained superficially, minimally invasive procedures can be adopted for its removal.

The establishment of a bullet wound track is instrumental in the medico-legal analysis of gunshot wounds, which can be helpful in unveiling the background mechanism of causation of that fatal injury such as whether it is suicidal, homicidal, or accidental. PMCT examination can identify bullet wound tracks.

Case of suicidal gun shot

Alleged history of a 36-year-old male who shot himself with a pistol in the early morning. He was found lying on the ground

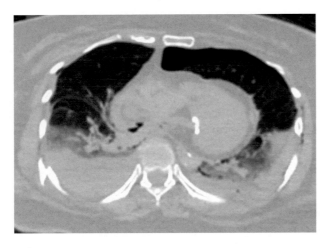

FIGURE 11.16: Axial section of PMCT showing fracture of right side ribs with pnemo and haemothorax present.

with blood oozing from his head. Near him, a pistol and an empty cartridge were found. He was taken to the Emergency Room of AIIMS Hospital where he was admitted after 1.5 days, and during the course of treatment, he died. The autopsy was conducted the next day.

External appearance: Showed the deceased was a male of moderate build and well nourished. Evidence of the ongoing treatment was seen in the form of multiple injection marks over the bilateral cubital fossa, right forearm, and endotracheal intubation. Bilateral black eyes were seen along with subconjunctival haemorrhage (Figure 11.18).

Entry wound: The gunshot entry wound with a size of 3 cm × 2 cm was present with an inverted margin. The wound exposed the brain matter over the right temporal region, associated with a cruciate laceration on the periphery. It was located 8 cm above the zygomatic process, 8 cm from the midline, and 168 cm above the right heel (Figures 11.19 and 11.20).

The entry wound tract extended into the right temporalis muscle and right temporal bone causing a defect of size 1.1 cm × 0.5 cm with a round margin in the outer table and a bevelled margin in the inner table associated with comminuted fractures over an area of size 18 cm × 16 cm present over the right half of skull vault (Figures 11.21 and 11.22).

Exit wound: The gunshot exit wound was a size of 1.5 cm × 0.7 cm with an everted margin and expulsion of soft tissue present over the left temporal region. It was located 8 cm above the left zygomatic process, 13 cm from the midline, and 168 cm above the left heel (Figures 11.23 and 11.24).

A fracture of the left temporal bone with a defect of size 1.3 cm × 1 cm with round margin in the inner table and a bevelled margin in the outer table associated with comminuted fracture over left half of the skull vault (Figures 11.25 and 11.26).

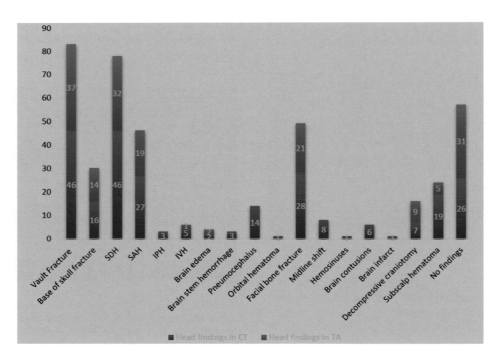

FIGURE 11.17: Chart showing analysis of the findings on PMCT and traditional autopsy. A blue bar depicts the percentage of findings on PMCT and orange bar depicts the percentage of findings in traditional autopsy.

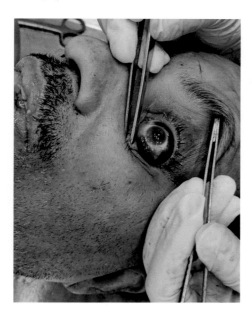

FIGURE 11.18: Left eye with a black eye seen along with subconjunctival haemorrhage.

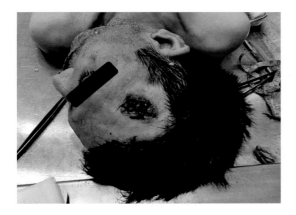

FIGURE 11.19: Gunshot entry wound present in the right temporal region.

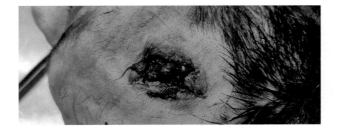

FIGURE 11.20: A closer view of the stellate-shaped gunshot entry wound showing laceration and contusion of the margins and blood clot and brain parenchyma seen in the wound.

Track of the bullet: The bullet entered the cranial cavity over the right temporal bone then perforated the dura and right frontal lobe. The tract further extended through and into the left frontal lobe and perforates the left side of the dura along

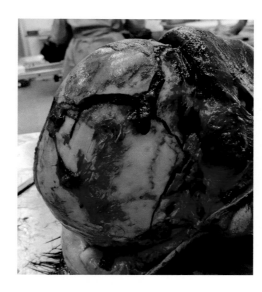

FIGURE 11.21: Gunshot entry wound causing a bony defect and surrounding comminuted fracture involving the right half of the skull vault.

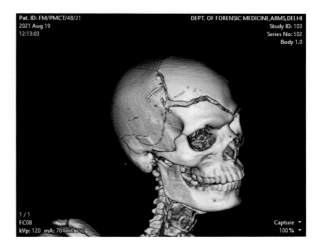

FIGURE 11.22: PMCT showing a gunshot entry wound causing a bony defect and the surrounding comminuted fracture involving the right half of the skull vault.

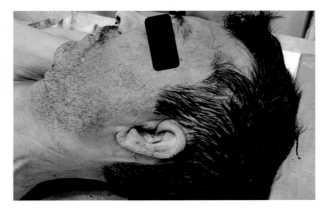

FIGURE 11.23: Exit wound present over the left temporal region.

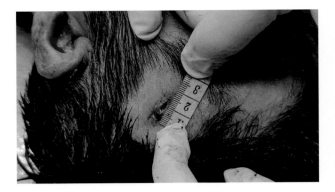

FIGURE 11.24: A closer view of the exit wound size 1.5 cm × 0.7 cm after shaving the surrounding hair showing the everted margin and expulsion of soft tissue.

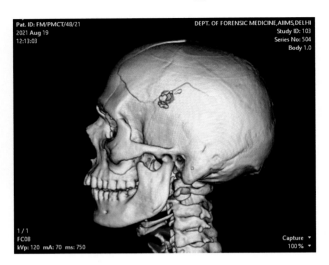

FIGURE 11.26: PMCT showing a fracture of the left temporal bone with a defect of size 1.3 cm × 1 cm and bevelled margin in the outer table associated with the surrounding of a comminuted fracture.

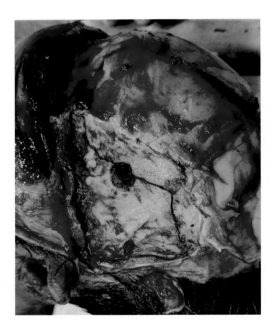

FIGURE 11.25: Fracture of the left temporal bone with defect of size 1.3 cm × 1 cm and bevelled margin in the outer table associated with comminuted fracture over the left half of the skull vault.

with haemorrhage and blackening all along the track (Figures 11.27 and 11.28).

Base of the skull: In this case, it showed a comminuted fracture involving bilateral anterior cranial and left middle cranial fossa. This can also be well appreciated in the PMCT where 3D reconstruction of the base of skull shows the fracture (Figures 11.29 and 11.30).

Case of suicidal gunshot to the head with no projectile

A case of a 30-year-old male who shot himself at an air force station and was declared dead on arrival in the hospital. External examination showed an entry wound in the left temporal scalp (Figure 11.31 a and b) and an exit wound in the parietal scalp near the midline (Figure 11.32 a and b). The external examination findings were confirmed by 3D reconstructed PMCT images. PMCT showed multiple comminuted

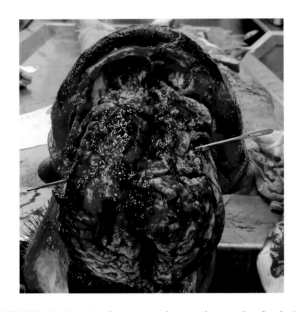

FIGURE 11.27: Probe inserted into the track of a bullet piercing the brain parenchyma running horizontally backwards from right to left.

fractures of the skull (Figure 11.33 a and b) depressed along the left side and protruding out along the right side confirming the direction of the track of the wound. Pneumocephalus is also clearly seen (Figure 11.34 a and b). No metallic fragments or bullets were detected in the body. All the PMCT findings corresponded with the traditional autopsy findings.

Case of suicidal gunshot to the head with retained projectile

A 36-year-old male was found unconscious with a gunshot wound to his head and he was declared dead on arrival in the hospital. External examination showed one gunshot entry wound at the right temporal scalp (Figure 11.35) and one exit wound at the left occipital scalp (Figure 11.36). PMCT showed

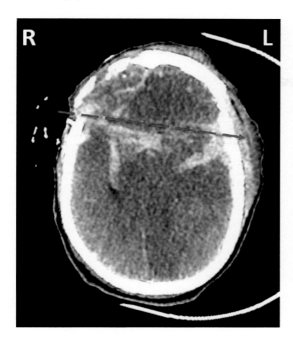

FIGURE 11.28: Red arrow showing the track of bullet piercing the brain parenchyma running horizontally backwards from right to left along with surrounding haemorrhage extending into the left lateral ventricle and surrounding parenchyma.

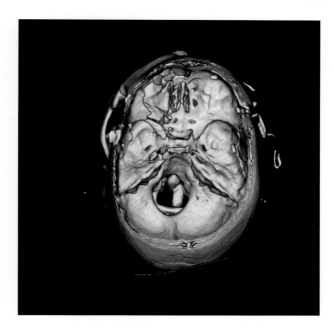

FIGURE 11.30: 3D reconstruction of the base of the skull showing the comminuted fracture.

retrieving the already fragmented bullet without any further damage. Ventricles did not show haemorrhage and mild midline shift was present. All the PMCT findings corroborated with traditional autopsy findings. The direction and the track of the gunshot wound were also clearly evident with PMCT itself. It augmented the traditional autopsy findings. Small pockets of pneumocephalus were additional PMCT findings that were not appreciable in traditional autopsy.

Stab wound deaths in PMCT

Stab wounds are one of the common types of sharp force injuries encountered in regular medico-legal practice. Postmortem X-rays can detect only the presence of a foreign body in such cases. With the advent of PMCT, the track of the stab wounds can be studied in detail without disrupting the anatomy by dissection. This helps to establish the exact cause of death and incident reconstruction can also be tried after analyzing 3D reconstructed PMCT images.

Stab wounds are caused by sharp pointed weapons. The most commonly used weapons are knives, daggers, scissors, screwdrivers and glass shards. The characteristic feature of stab wounds is that the depth of the wound is greater than its width. Traditional autopsy techniques assess depth by using probes (obsolete old technique) and by layer-by-layer removal of tissues which can cause alteration or destruction of vital findings. The use of PMCT can prevent the loss of vital information in contrast with the traditional autopsy. Documentation of stab wounds is vital for the legal process. Conventional autopsy uses photography which is generally 2D in nature. PMCT helps in 3D documentation and storage of the injury.

Some findings of stab wound injury like air embolism, pneumothorax, and pneumoperitoneum, are exclusively diagnosed by PMCT as compared to traditional autopsy. With the advent of PMCT-guided gas aspiration, air pockets can be aspirated and sent for gas composition analysis. PMCT angiography (PMCTA) can help in the detection of pseudoaneurysms of large blood vessels arising as a complication of stab wounds.

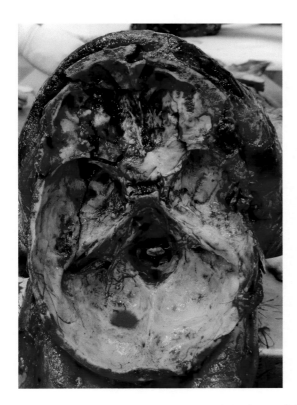

FIGURE 11.29: Comminuted fracture of the base of the skull involving bilateral anterior and left middle cranial fossa.

the entry wound and metallic fragments along with the track of the wound clearly shown (Figure 11.37). The exit wound had a fragmented bullet lodged in the left occipital bone. The detection of the bullet before a traditional autopsy helped in

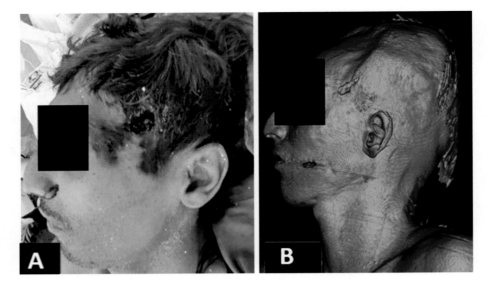

FIGURE 11.31: A and B showing External examination and 3D reconstructed PMCT image of left temporal scalp showing a gunshot entry wound.

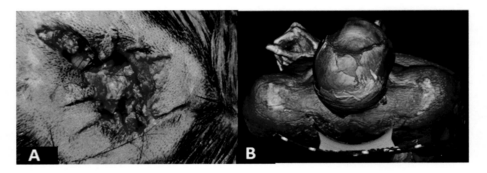

FIGURE 11.32: A and B External examination and 3D reconstructed PMCT image showing gunshot exit wound in the parietal scalp.

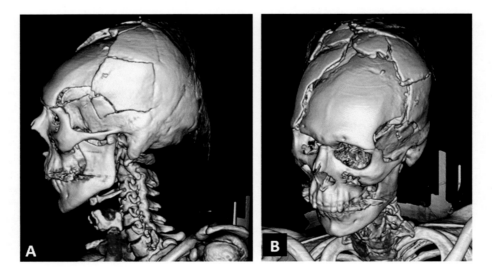

FIGURE 11.33: A and B 3D reconstructed PMCT showing comminuted fractures of the skull with outward displacement on the right side depicting the direction of the track of the wound.

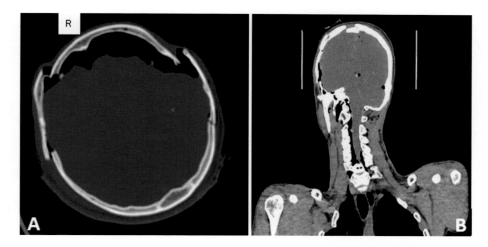

FIGURE 11.34: A and B Axial section and coronal section of PMCT showing comminuted fractures and pneumocephalus.

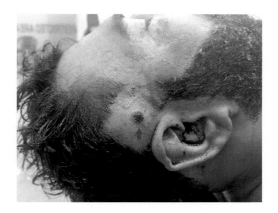

FIGURE 11.35: External examination of the deceased showing gunshot entry wound at the right temporal scalp.

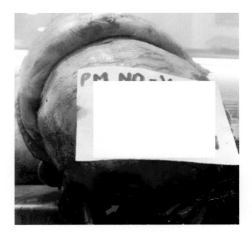

FIGURE 11.36: Traditional autopsy showing gunshot exit wound on the left occipital area of the skull with a retained bullet fragment in the left occipital bone.

Case of homicidal multiple stabs with also a gunshot wound

The case of a 20-year-old male assaulted and stabbed by two people and declared dead on arrival in the hospital. On external examination, multiple stab wounds were present in the neck and the chest (Figures 11.38 and 11.39) with one of the wounds in the neck being a grazed gunshot injury holding the bullet superficially in the neck (Figure 11.40). PMCT showed a foreign body in the neck resembling a bullet. Later, all the wounds in the external examination corroborated with PMCT findings. Internal findings in the PMCT showed pneumothorax, haemothorax, and pneumoperitoneum. The lungs and heart showed suspected stab wounds in PMCT which was confirmed by traditional autopsy. The direction and the depth of the wound were also clear, especially in the case of stab wounds which went up to the lungs or heart (Figures 11.41–11.46).

Case of multiple stab wounds in mother and child

A 28-year-old female, along with her baby, sustained multiple stab wounds and both were found lying on their bed in an unresponsive state. External examination of the female showed five stab wounds (Figure 11.47) and PMCT showed haemopericardium and left haemothorax (Figure 11.48); while external examination of the baby showed three stab wounds (Figure 11.49).

PMCT was done and all the stab wounds were corroborated well with 3D reconstructed PMCT. The axial section of the PMCT of the baby showed a breach of skin and air in subcutaneous tissue which represents the track of the stab wound (Figure 11.50). Pneumothorax and haemothorax were also present.

Case of stab with haemo-pneumothorax and pneumoperitoneum

A 24-year-old male sustained multiple stab injuries and was admitted to the hospital where he died during treatment. A stab injury in the left side of the torso is clearly seen in the PMCT below the intercostal drain site wound (Figure 11.51) The axial section of PMCT showed a breach in the skin, air in subcutaneous tissue, and pneumothorax suggestive of track of the wound (Figure 11.52). Haemothorax (Figure 11.53) and pneumoperitoneum (Figure 11.54) were also appreciated in PMCT.

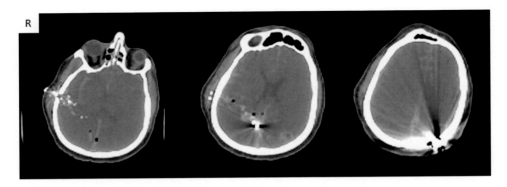

FIGURE 11.37: Axial sections of PMCT showing gunshot entry wound in the right temporal bone, metallic fragments depicting track of the wound, and the skull exit wound with retained bullet fragments in the left temporal bone.

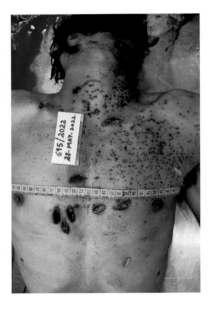

FIGURE 11.38: External examination showing multiple stab wounds on the front of the chest.

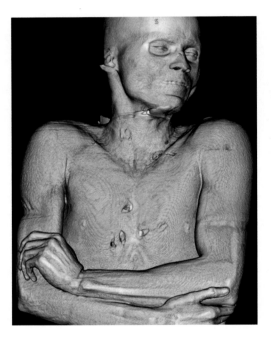

FIGURE 11.39: Volume rendered image of PMCT showing external examination with multiple stab wounds on the front of the chest.

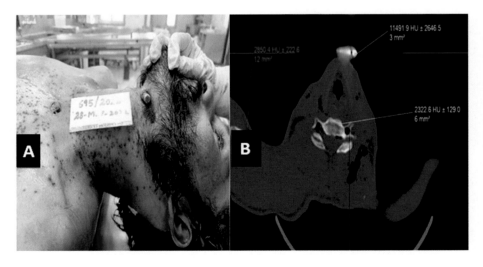

FIGURE 11.40: A and B External examination and axial section of PMCT showing a bullet in the left side of the neck.

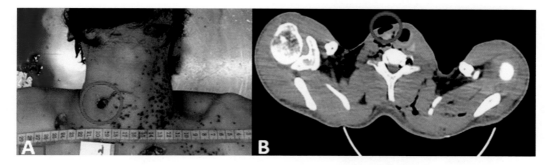

FIGURE 11.41: A and B External examination and axial section of PMCT of the neck showing corresponding stab injury (marked with a red circle).

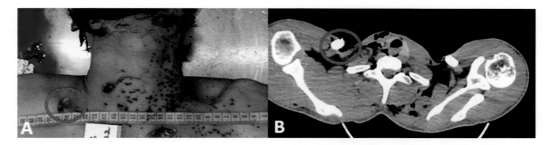

FIGURE 11.42: A and B Axial section of PMCT neck showing corresponding stab injury findings from an external examination (marked with a red circle).

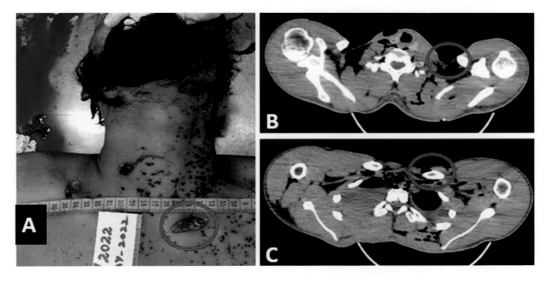

FIGURE 11.43: A, B, and C Axial section of PMCT showing the chest with a corresponding stab injury finding in external examination (marked with a red circle).

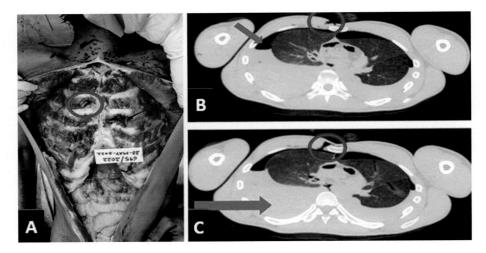

FIGURE 11.44: A, B, and C Gross examination of stab injury to chest in intercostal space (marked with a red circle). Axial section of PMCT chest showing pneumothorax (small blue arrow), haemothorax (large blue arrow), and corresponding stab injury findings from an external examination (marked with a red circle).

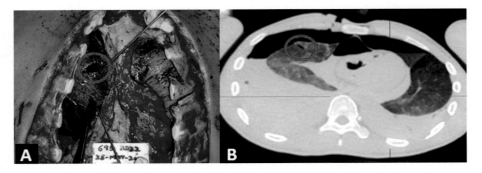

FIGURE 11.45: A and B Gross examination of an injury to the right lung in traditional autopsy and axial section of PMCT showing a chest stab injury to the right lung corresponding to the findings from an external examination (marked with a red circle).

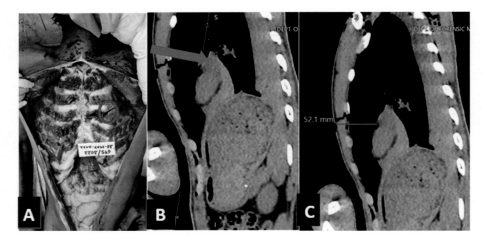

FIGURE 11.46: A, B, and C Gross examination of a stab injury to the left side of the chest (marked with a red circle). Sagittal section of PMCT showing a chest stab injury to the heart corresponding with findings from an external examination. The direction and depth of the wound can also be appreciated in the sagittal section.

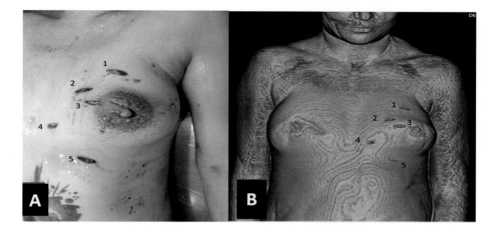

FIGURE 11.47: A and B External examination and 3D reconstructed PMCT showing corresponding stab wounds.

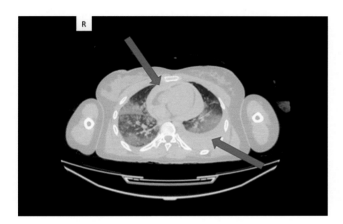

FIGURE 11.48: Axial section of PMCT showing haemopericardium and left haemothorax.

Case of stab in the back with knife in-situ

A 19-year-old male with stab wounds and a knife in situ in the back; the person was declared dead on arrival. The knife in situ was present in the back of the trunk on external examination (Figure 11.55). On PMCT examination exact the direction of the wounds along with the extent of injury can be easily appreciated (Figures 11.56 and 11.57).

Thorough knowledge of PMCT can help us to avoid the traditional autopsy in cases in which we have sufficient findings on verbal autopsy, visual autopsy, and radiological examination, i.e., PMCT. This helps not only in the dignified management of the dead but also in collecting better evidence.

Credible forensic autopsy opinion for investigators and judiciary in the interest of justice

In the realm of forensic medicine, the process of determining the manner of death, be it suicide, homicide, or accident, carries immense significance. The credibility of the opinion rendered by forensic doctors in such cases holds pivotal importance, particularly when it is presented in a court of law during cross-examination. Forensic doctors undertake a comprehensive investigation, employing various methods, including traditional, virtual, and documentary analysis, as well as examining photographic and inquest evidence. The formulation of a medical opinion that can withstand the scrutiny of the court becomes a subject of critical deliberation, necessitating necessary checks and balances to consider alternative probabilities in the case. It is noteworthy that the opinion of forensic medical experts might exhibit a certain degree of conventionality, mutability, and variance among different professionals. Nevertheless, the determination of suicide, accident, or

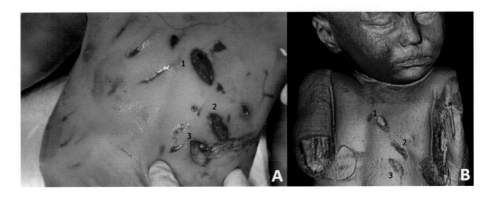

FIGURE 11.49: A and B External examination and 3D reconstructed PMCT showing corresponding stab wounds.

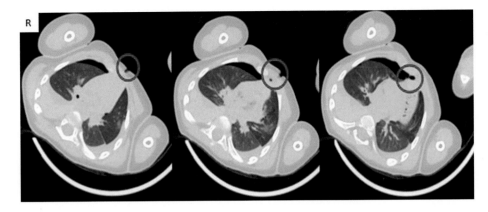

FIGURE 11.50:   Axial section of PMCT showing the track of a chest stab wound leading to the right pneumothorax.

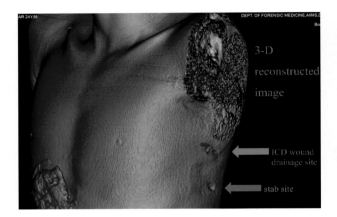

FIGURE 11.51:   Volume reconstructed image showing the external stab wound over the left side of the chest along with the ICD site.

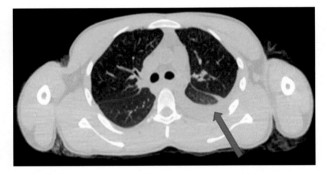

FIGURE 11.53:   Axial section of PMCT showing the left haemothorax of the chest (marked with a blue arrow).

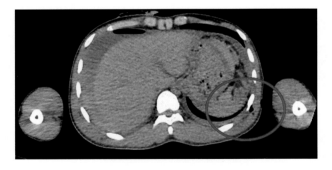

FIGURE 11.52:   Axial section of PMCT showing chest stab wound to left thorax and pneumothorax.

homicide is mandatory and is regarded as the gold standard for conducting death investigations. While forensic investigations cater to diverse audiences, the court emerges as the most crucial one. The manner in which forensic doctors gather and handle evidence and arrive at their conclusions significantly influences the outcomes of the legal proceedings, particularly during direct and cross-examination.

Drawing on experiences from various CBI cases, where the author interacted with investigative authorities, visited crime scenes, and meticulously analyzed postmortem reports, crime scene photographs, and witness and accused statements, a credible opinion with scientific justification was formed. In-depth analysis of relevant scientific documents and consultation with other forensic doctors, forensic scientists, and ballistic experts further contributed to the validity of the expert opinion.

The author underscores the vital role of credible forensic medical expert opinions in delivering justice. These opinions are instrumental in addressing the unrest that often arises at national and international levels concerning sudden and suspicious deaths, as society seeks clarity on the cause and manner of death. The credibility of the investigating agency, government, forensic laboratory, and doctors conducting postmortem examinations comes under scrutiny during such instances. Therefore, meticulous analysis and interpretation of forensic evidence in correlation with circumstantial and investigative findings become imperative.

The formulation of a credible forensic medical expert opinion hinges upon five fundamental principles, namely, the expertise and credibility of the medical experts, the basis of the expert opinion, providing a speaking opinion with justifications, eliminating alternative possibilities, and drawing upon credible references. Instances where forensic medical opinions lack adherence to these principles can lead to confusion for investigative agencies, resulting in prolonged delays in reaching logical conclusions. It becomes evident that a criminal case may sway in favour of or against the prosecution depending on the doubts cast upon the credibility of the chain of custody or at times even the expert opinion.

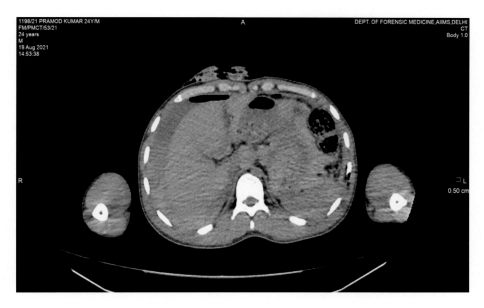

FIGURE 11.54: Axial section of PMCT of the abdomen showing pneumoperitoneum.

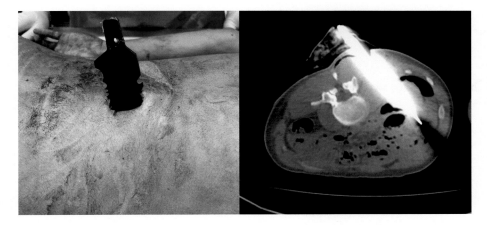

FIGURE 11.55: External examination and axial section of PMCT showing the knife in situ at the back of the trunk.

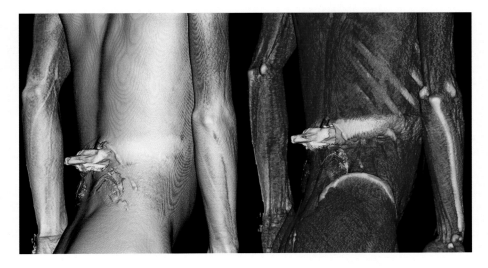

FIGURE 11.56: Volume reconstructed image showing a knife in situ in the back of the trunk in case of a stab wound.

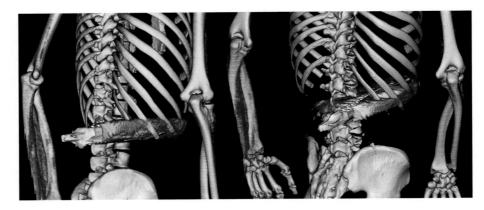

FIGURE 11.57: Extent of the injury can be appreciated on volume reconstructed PMCT showing the knife in situ in case of a stab wound.

Consequently, it is incumbent upon medically trained forensic doctors to practice their profession with utmost legal propriety, basing their opinions on sound medical justifications, supported by credible references. The section further presents three illustrative cases published in an Indian police journal by the author Dr Sudhir K. Gupta that exemplify the application of these basic principles in formulating a credible forensic medicine expert opinion, proving beneficial to both investigators and the judiciary in ensuring justice is served impartially.

A case report of death due to suicidal gunshot

A 26-year-old woman who was the wife of a Chief Judicial Magistrate was discovered dead in an open area (Figure 11.58) with multiple gunshot wounds on July 17, 2013. A revolver was found near the body, which was later identified as the licensed weapon of the deceased's husband. The family members suspected that the husband might have killed her due to alleged dowry demands. The State Police registered a First Information Report (FIR) against the husband and his parents under section 302/34 of the Indian Penal Code (IPC) and began an investigation.

Case findings

The postmortem examination conducted on July 18, 2013, at a government hospital revealed the following injuries.

1. Grazed abrasion 3.5 cm × 1.5 cm on the left side of the lower lateral abdominal wall with tapering round the edge posterior, blackening present on the wound with bright red clotted blood (Figure 11.59).
2. Entry wound with laceration of size 9 mm × 9 mm on the left side of the chest (Figure 11.60), upper one-third, 13 cm below and medial to the left shoulder tip, with inverted margins, 1 mm abrasion collar seen surrounding the wound in a circular pattern, wound seen to be continuous inside with blackening seen in the initial track up to lung tissue, piercing the subcutaneous tissue, muscles, intercostal muscles, between the 2nd and 3rd ribs, left upper lobe of lung near apex with pleura, lacerating the posterior thoracic wall correspondingly and exiting through the exit wound 1.5 cm × 1.5 cm, 17 cm below and medial to left shoulder tip with bright red clotted blood.

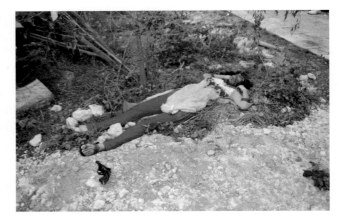

FIGURE 11.58: Body of deceased at the scene of incidence.

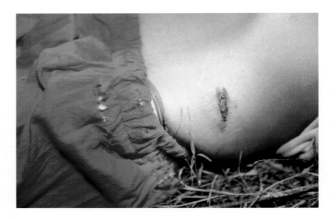

FIGURE 11.59: Grazed abrasion on lower lateral aspect of abdominal wall (injury no. 1).

3. Entry wound with laceration of size 9 mm × 9 mm, 4 cm below chin (Figure 11.61), inverted margins, 1 mm abrasion collar seen Surrounding the wound circularly, seen continuous inside with blackening seen in the initial track traversing the neck lacerating the neurovascular structures of neck, lacerating the posterior neck wall correspondingly and exiting through the exit

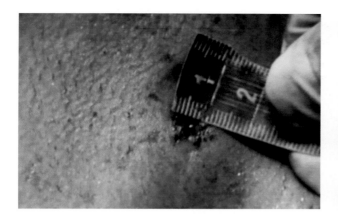

FIGURE 11.60: Lacerated wound on left side of chest (injury no. 2).

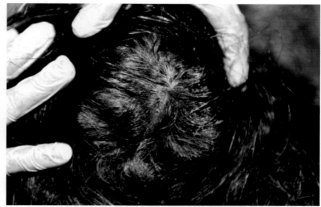

FIGURE 11.62: Lacerated wound on parietal region of right side of scalp (injury no. 4).

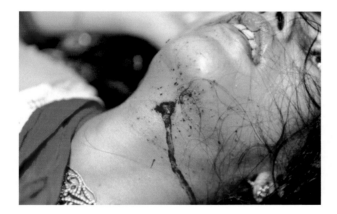

FIGURE 11.61: Entry wound below chin.

wound 1.5 cm × 1.5 cm, 12 cm posterior and below to left ear lobule with bright red clotted blood.
4. Lacerated wound 3 cm × 1 cm, right parietal region scalp, sagittal scalp deep with bright red clotted blood (Figure 11.62).

Postmortem opinion: The cause of death was opined as shock and haemorrhage following antemortem multiple firearm injury, external injuries no. 2 and 3 described above, and its consequences were sufficient to cause death in the normal course of life.

The viscera and vaginal swab of the deceased were examined, and no poison or semen was detected. The examination of clothes and articles did not reveal any struggle or drag marks. The bullets recovered from the crime scene were found to have been fired from the revolver found near the body.

CBI investigation stage I

Due to dissatisfaction with the progress of the State Police investigation, the case was transferred to the Central Bureau of Investigation (CBI) on August 7, 2013. A medical board of experts from prominent medical institutes in New Delhi was formed to give their opinion. The following observations were made by the medical board:

1. An individual firing multiple bullets over herself is a remote possibility, especially when at least two of the bullets are sufficient to cause death. Multiple firearm ammunition wounds were present on the body of the deceased.
2. The CFSL ballistic experts opined that two bullets were fired over her abdomen; it was observed that injury no. 1 was caused by a bullet fired from a distant range.
3. It has been observed usually that in suicidal/self-inflicted injuries, the weapon of suicide is found either clenched in the hand of the deceased, or if fallen, it is located very near the body of the deceased. In this case, the revolver, which is the alleged weapon of offence, was recovered at some distance from the dead body.
4. Injury no. 2 showed powder tattooing and injury no. 3 did not show any powder tattooing. Hence they were neither contact nor near contact firearm wounds.
5. Injury no. 4 mentioned as a lacerated wound in the postmortem report appears to have been caused by grazing of the projectile of a firearm weapon.
6. The direction of track of injury no. 2 was outward to inward, which would be highly unlikely to be caused by a right-handed person shooting herself.
7. Hand wash of the deceased taken at the scene of the crime and during the postmortem were negative for any gunshot residue.

The board concluded that the injuries were unlikely to be self-inflicted, and the possibility of homicide could not be ruled out.

Polygraph and Brain Electrical Oscillation Signature Profiling Test (Brain Mapping) were conducted on the husband of the deceased. The conclusions were:

1. He demanded dowry or favours from his wife/her family.
2. He was pressurizing his wife for sex determination tests but she refused to listen to him.
3. He did not find the revolver in its place, he got scared and came downstairs and went to his room after asking his wife's whereabouts from his cousin sister. Hence he was aware that the revolver may have been taken by his wife, causing his concern to increase and he started searching for his wife.
4. The subject did not have any prior knowledge about the death of his wife and her suicide or murder.

5. The subject did not do any planning with respect to the death of his wife.
6. The subject did not send his wife with his revolver to the scene of the incidence.

Psychological tests conducted on the husband indicated no prior knowledge or planning related to the death of his wife. The final opinion, based on the psychological autopsy study, was that the deceased might have committed suicide.

CBI investigation stage II

Subsequently, the investigation persisted for over two-and-a-half years, yet no breakthrough or substantial evidence emerged to suggest foul play. In light of the prolonged inquiry, the Central Bureau of Investigation (CBI) sought the expertise of the Head of Forensic Medicine at AIIMS to guide the investigative process. To this end, a medical board was convened on February 11, 2016, which conducted a thorough examination and arrived at the following observations and conclusions:

1. The body was found in a secluded place with no scuffle injuries present over the body.
2. The deceased was not under the influence of any intoxication as the viscera report is negative for poisons.
3. Injury no. 1 shows superficial grazing firearm injury showing blackening, indicating that the shot was of close/contact range. It is located in the accessible and approachable part of the body. The injury is suggestive of hesitation-type shots seen in suicidal cases.
4. Injury no. 2 and 3 are fatal injuries produced by a firearm and show blackening in the entry wound, suggestive of close contact firearm injury. Injury no. 3, present underneath the chin, is a close contact wound showing blackening inside the track of the wound. It is located in the accessible and approachable part of the body and it is one of the preferred sites for a suicidal wound.
5. Injury no. 4 (lacerated wound) present on the top of the head could be produced by grazing of bullet, anterior to posterior, and could be self-inflicted.
6. Injury no. 3 under the chin can cause instant incapacitation due to injury to the vital centre of the brain. It is likely to be the last shot before death.
7. It is not necessary in all cases to have the presence of the gun shot residue (GSR) on the hands of a deceased

in cases of suicide/self-firing. It depends upon the type of firearm. One study showed that in about 50% of cases, hand washing was positive for GSR and the value decreased to 32% for automatic pistols.[4]

8. Injury no. 3 is due to firearm missile injury associated with cranio-cerebral damage which led to concealed bleeding and clotting in the brain resulting in haemorrhagic shock and coma. So, there will not be much appreciable/visible bleeding, as it causes instantaneous death. This is a usual surgical feature in a case of fatal firearm missile injury to the brain.
9. The cause of death in this case was due to haemorrhagic shock due to firearm injuries no. 2 and 3.

It was concluded that injuries 1, 2, 3, and 4 could be suicidal/self-inflicted in nature.

Final unanimous opinion dated February 6, 2016: Death was caused by haemorrhagic shock as a result of firearm projectile injuries, which is suicidal in nature.

Current status of the case

The CBI agreed with this opinion and submitted the charge sheet for abetment of suicide, which is currently under evaluation by the Honorable Court.

A case report of suicidal ligature strangulation

On March 26, 2009, Sh Philomeenaraj and his daughter Pramila Gandhi embarked on a train journey. After arrival at the railway station, Sh Philomeenaraj went to work, while Pramila allegedly headed to her Aunt's house. However, her whereabouts became uncertain as her father could not reach her on the phone. When inquiring with her Aunt, it was revealed that Pramila had not visited them. Concerned, Sh Philomeenaraj lodged a missing complaint, and on March 27, 2009, a female body was discovered in a secluded area, identified as Pramila Gandhi (Figure 11.63). The case was registered under U/s 174 of the IPC on the complaint of her father. The neck of the deceased was found encircled by three rounds of thread (Naada) of the Chudhidaar which she was wearing. One end of the thread was tied to the finger of her right hand and the other end of the thread was found in her left hand in a loosened grip (separated from the finger). On the body of the deceased, no deep wounds were present. The two hands of the deceased and the two fists were fully tightened and she was holding hairs in both her fists.

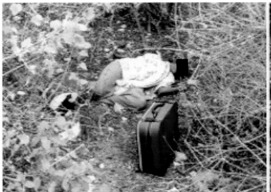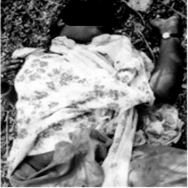

FIGURE 11.63: Body of deceased at scene of incidence.

Case findings: The postmortem examination conducted on March 28, 2009, at Bangalore Medical College revealed the following: The face and sclera were congested, tongue bitten, blood-stained fluid present at nose and mouth while the nail beds were blue in colour. The ligature material is the chudidara string, which is dirty green in colour and in two rows around the neck. Hair strands are entangled in between the ligature material and the ligature mark. There is a horizontal ligature mark in front of the neck below the thyroid cartilage, which runs on both sides of the neck and back of the neck. It measures 31 cm × 1 cm and is situated 6 cm below the right ear lobule and 6 cm below the left ear lobule, and 9 cm below the mandible. The ligature mark completely encircles the neck and is in the form of a deep groove and the skin underneath is hard and parchmentised. On dissection, there is extravasation of blood in the tissues of the neck all around. The hyoid bone and thyroid cartilage are intact. Other injuries:

1. In right little finger and right ring finger imprint abrasion of size 3 cm ×1 cm and 2 cm × 1 cm and left thumb 2 cm × 1 cm are present.
2. Crescentic shaped nail marks present on right angle of jaw, lower border of right lower jaw, and left side of neck ranging from 1.5 cm × 0.1 cm to 2 cm × 0.1 cm.
3. Abrasion on both knee caps present of size 3 cm × 2 cm each.
4. On reflection of scalp, there is extravasation of blood in left temporal and parietal regions over 6 cm × 3 cm to 4 cm × 2 cm size.

Postmortem opinion: The findings are suggestive of ligature strangulation and self strangulation is ruled out as at a stage of cerebral anoxia, ligature is loosened and death does not occur.

The *viscera and vaginal swab* of the deceased were also preserved and sent to the State Forensic Science Laboratory. Viscera report did not reveal any common poison. Semen could not be detected on vaginal swab. From the Forensic Science Laboratory findings, sexual assault has been ruled out.

CBI investigation stage I

The case was initially handled by the Bengaluru Police, but dissatisfaction with the progress led the deceased's parents to file a writ petition to the Honorable High Court of Karnataka. Consequently, the case was transferred to CBI Chennai. During their investigation, CBI probed the complainant, relatives, friends, and neighbours but failed to trace any culprits. The main challenge was distinguishing between homicidal and suicidal strangulation.

CBI investigation stage II

After more than two-and-a-half years of investigation without a breakthrough, CBI sought the expertise of the Head of Forensic Medicine at AIIMS. The medical board conducted an in-depth evaluation and arrived at the following observations:

1. Strangulation may be homicidal, accidental, or suicidal, particularly ligature strangulation. Distinction between homicidal and suicidal strangulation by ligature is often impossible on the basis of anatomical findings alone, although fractures of the larynx in suicidal strangulation are distinctly unusual. The type of noose and knot as well as the number of turns around neck and circumstances under which the body is found may suggest the manner of death.

2. Postmortem report as well as Forensic Science Laboratory is negative for any sign of biological evidence of sexual assault, which rules out any sexual assault. Also, there are no signs of struggle or any signs of defence injury over the body, which is seen in cases of self-strangulation.

3. The medical board also observed that the ligature material was tied in the right hand finger and another end was in the left hand (Figure 11.64). As per the postmortem report, it was seen that the thyro-hyoid complex was intact. In cases of strangulation by assailant, the thyro-hyoid complex is likely to be broken due to the greater force which is applied in cases of strangulation by an assailant to ensure death. However, no injury in the thyro-hyoid complex suggests light compression force in neck, which could be possible by self-inflicted ligature force.

4. The ligature material, a green-coloured cotton cloth naada with metallic safety pin attached to one end was examined by the AIIMS Medical Board. The length of the ligature material was 190 cm and its breadth was 1 cm. The use of this ligature material and the body being found in an accessible, non-remote place again suggests self-infliction, thus ruling out a homicidal angle.

5. The opinion of the autopsy surgeon mentions that "Self-strangulation is ruled out as at a stage of cerebral anoxia, ligature is loosened and death does not occur." It is inconceivable that anyone could die from compression of the neck by his own hand because loss of consciousness would cause relaxation of the constricting fingers. When a ligature is involved the matter is different, and if the ligature is found in situ suicide is unusual but a distinct possibility.

6. As per Taylor, self-strangulation involving a ligature is possible in four ways, as follows:
   i. When constriction of neck occurs due to multiple turns sufficient to maintain constriction without a knot at a point accessible to the person's own hands.
   ii. The neck may be compressed by twisting a rod inserted under a knot and by twisting it like a tourniquet, which is the most common method used.
   iii. The free end having a weight, which is attached to a running noose.
   iv. The free end being attached to the hand with a running noose, with the hand and forearm compressing the neck.

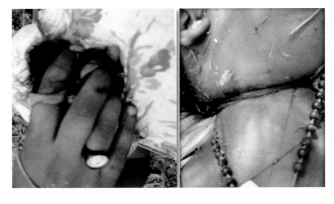

FIGURE 11.64: Ligature material tied to the right hand and in situ around the neck of deceased.

Final unanimous opinion dated April 22, 2015: The cause of death in this case is asphyxia as a result of ligature strangulation. It is a case of self-achieved strangulation, which is suicidal in manner.

Current status of the case

CBI concurred with the AIIMS medical board opinion, and based on compelling justification and references, submitted a closure report to the Honorable Court, stating that the case is a suicide without any other possibility.

A case report of suicidal partial hanging

On June 20, 2009, the police were informed of a possible suicide involving Tannu Jaswal, a 22-year-old female, in Baddi, Himachal Pradesh. The body was found lying on a bed with ligature material nearby. Photography of the ligature material and dead body was done. An injury was observed on the left side of the face, along with a ligature mark around the neck. The deceased's father raised doubts about the manner of death, leading to the registration of a case under U/S 306 of the IPC at Solan, HP. A postmortem examination was performed on 21 June, 2009, at ESI Hospital, Baddi.

Case findings

At the crime scene, photographs revealed a faint reddish-purple broad ligature mark on the left postero-lateral aspect of the neck with a small area of discontinuity below the left mandible area. Additionally, an injury with a bleeding clot was observed on the middle part of the left cheek below the zygomatic process, as well as an ovoid-shaped injury on the middle part of the lower border of the left side of the mandible (Figure 11.65).

Postmortem examination: The postmortem examination, conducted by a single doctor at ESI Nalagarh, Solan, indicated no external wounds. The ligature mark was yellowish-brown, inverted V-shaped on the left side, encircling the entire neck except below the left ear. The ligature mark was situated above the level of the thyroid cartilage, between the larynx and chin, with a width of 2.5 cm–4 cm. All internal organs appeared normal, and no external injury was observed, except for the ligature mark.

Postmortem opinion: Cause of death is asphyxia due to antemortem hanging. Probable time between injury and death is within one hour. Probable time between death and postmortem is within 24 hours.

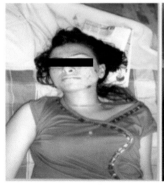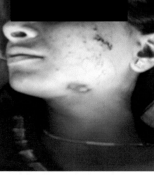

FIGURE 11.65:   Body of deceased at scene of incidence.

Viscera examination: The viscera of the deceased were sent to the State Forensic Science Laboratory, where no common poison was detected. Human blood was found on the bed sheet, but no struggle or drag marks were detected on the clothes/articles.

Initial investigation and expert opinions: The initial investigation was conducted by Shimla Police. Subsequently, the case was transferred to the Chief Investigating Authority, Himachal Pradesh. CIA submitted the documents to Indira Gandhi Medical College, Shimla Medical Board for an expert opinion. Board 1 comprising six doctors from IGMC, Shimla, perused all the relevant documents and observed that:

1. The drooling of saliva should have been present on the clothes of deceased, mainly on right side, which is not evident.
2. The haemorrhages in the conjunctivae are neither mentioned nor visible in the photographs. No bleeding is present from nose, mouth, or ear.
3. The neck does not stretch in all cases of hanging, so is not a very good criterion to ascertain the hanging and strangulation.
4. The board has examined the available record thoroughly and is of the opinion that the autopsy surgeon is the best judge to answer many of the facts in question and he may be asked to clarify the facts.

Opinion of IGMC, Shimla Board dated September 7, 2009: From the available record it is not possible to give the exact cause of death due to want of complete record and partial findings; however, there is nothing to suggest the possibility of strangulation in absence of struggle marks, poisoning, and any other factor contributing to the cause of death.

CBI investigation stage I

Due to differing opinions, the case was transferred to the Central Bureau of Investigation (CBI). Board 2, comprising experts from AIIMS, New Delhi. A board comprising three doctors from the Department of Forensic Medicine & Toxicology, AIIMS, New Delhi, perused all the relevant documents and observed that:

1. In absence of signs of struggle and Forensic Science Laboratory report being negative for common poison, the hanging in this case could be suicidal in nature.
2. Dribbling of saliva is considered to be the surest sign of antemortem hanging, whenever it is present. But it is not necessarily seen in all cases of hanging.
3. Neck is not necessarily found stretched and elongated in cases of hanging.
4. The faint ligature mark as mentioned in the postmortem report could be possible by the dupatta/chaddar as mentioned. But ligature mark is unlikely to be caused by the cable wire.
5. The photographs are showing acne vulgaris on face with slight bleeding on left side cheek as well as impression of ligature on left side chin, near angle of mandible. The bleeding from acne could have occurred during the process of hanging and is unlikely to be because of injury.

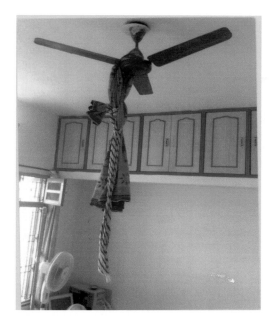

FIGURE 11.66: Ligature material at scene of incidence.

Opinion of AIIMS, New Delhi Board dated January 2, 2010: The cause of death in this case is asphyxia due to antemortem hanging by ligature.

CBI investigation stage II

On February 7, 2011, High Court Shimla rejected the LHMC opinion. The CBI investigation continued for more than 20 months and no breakthrough/evidences was found as to the manner of death. The CBI then requested Dr Sudhir K. Gupta, an expert from AIIMS, to give an opinion. Dr Gupta visited the scene of the crime and conducted a detailed analysis along with CFSL experts on June 4, 2011. It was observed that the height of the room from floor to roof level was 9 feet 8 inches. The deceased was seen in a kneeling position over the Newar cot. The height of the ligature from the floor was 5 feet 6 inches and the length of the dupatta was 3 feet 6 inches (Figure 11.66).

Final opinion: Dr Sudhir Gupta's final opinion confirmed the cause of death as a result of combined asphyxia and ischemia due to antemortem partial hanging by an alleged ligature. The case was considered a suicide without any other possibilities.

Current status of the case: The CBI concurred with the AIIMS Medical Board's opinion, and the case of abetment of suicide is currently under trial. This chapter emphasizes the importance of thorough investigation and the challenges involved in forming expert medical opinions in forensic cases.

The observation, basis of credible opinion, and the final opinion were:

1. The medicolegal inference of neck injury, specifically a ligature mark, raised questions about whether the death was due to antemortem hanging resulting in asphyxia. The focus was on determining if the hanging was suicidal or homicidal based on the characteristics of the ligature mark:
   i. The geometry of the ligature mark was crucial in interpreting the nature of the fatal event. In strangulation, the ligature mark would fully encircle the neck horizontally at a lower level, crossing just below the larynx and merging with the nape of the neck. In cases of homicide, where only one turn of the ligature is used, the ligature mark's two ends may overlap, appearing at the front, side, or back of the neck depending on the assailant's position relative to the victim.
   ii. The pressure abrasion or imprint/pattern abrasion from the ligature material in the neck can be found in both antemortem and postmortem hanging or strangulation. In cases of strangulation followed by postmortem hanging, there would be two ligature marks—one more horizontal for strangulation and another more oblique for hanging. The ligature marks might partially overlap but not fully encircle the neck, suggesting antemortem strangulation followed by postmortem hanging to simulate death by hanging.
   iii. Despite the expectation of two ligature marks due to the combination of strangulation and postmortem hanging, the examination of photographs, postmortem reports, and discussions with relevant personnel did not reveal evidence of double ligature marks, except for a single faint oblique ligature mark. Consequently, the possibility of death resulting from strangulation followed by postmortem hanging was ruled out.
   iv. The Forensic Science Laboratory report on the victim's viscera did not indicate the presence of common poisons, suggesting that the victim was not under the influence of intoxication or poisoning before death.
   v. There were no findings of injuries indicative of active struggle or resistance on the deceased's body during the autopsy examination and postmortem report. Given that homicidal hanging typically involves a more violent form of asphyxial death and is not feasible without complete physical overpower/gagging of mouth/tying of limbs and struggle leaving significant injuries in the body of a normal victim. It was concluded that the cause of death as antemortem hanging or homicidal hanging by use of force/overpower/poisoning is ruled out.

2. The medicolegal inference of an oval-shaped injury on the neck and another injury on the left side of the face was as follows:
   i. Both injuries were deemed antemortem based on their coloration as seen in photographs, and individually and collectively, they were considered simple in nature.
   ii. The injury due to the knot of ligature would be an abrasion particularly in the case of partial hanging and there would be no such colouration of injury on the skin because the pressure abrasion is appreciated by the epidermis of the skin which is devoid of blood vessels. In light of this, the oval shape injury as an imprint/pattern abrasion due to the knot of the ligature was ruled out.
   iii. The possibility of the injury being caused by hot liquid, resulting in a burn injury, could not be ruled out, as the visual assessment of a burn injury was a common practice for doctors.

iv. The injury on the left side of the face appeared to be acne vulgaris with slight bleeding, indicating an antemortem injury that occurred prior to death. This type of injury was unlikely to occur during the hanging process. Self-inflicted injury was also ruled out, as it would typically involve multiple scratch abrasions during the hanging process.

v. It was clarified that both the injury on the face and the oval-shaped injury on the neck were simple in nature and did not directly contribute to the cause of death.

Basis of credible opinion:

1. The faint ligature mark described in the postmortem report and seen by the investigating officer could have been caused by the examined dupatta found at the crime scene.
2. The position of the deceased's body was consistent with self-suspension.
3. The negative result from the Forensic Science Laboratory indicated the absence of common poisons.
4. The ligature mark encircled the entire neck, except for the left side below the left ear.
5. The ligature mark was located above the level of the thyroid cartilage, positioned between the larynx and the chin.
6. The width of the groove of the ligature mark was 2.5–4 cm, compatible with the ligature material used. The ligature was positioned high up on the neck and was incomplete.
7. All internal organs showed no abnormalities.
8. The case was considered one of partial hanging.
9. No injuries were present on the hands or other parts of the victim's body suggestive of resistance.

Final opinion of Dr Sudhir Gupta dated June 23, 2016: The cause of death was due to the combined effect of asphyxia and ischaemia as a result of antemortem partial hanging by alleged ligature. Partial hangings are generally suicidal in nature and in this case it is a suicidal death.

Current status of the case: The CBI concurred with the AIIMS medical board opinion that it is a case of suicide without any other possibility, which is speaking in nature with justification and references, totally corroborative with their investigation and a case of abetment of suicide is currently under trial.

Discussion

In the three presented cases, the postmortem findings remained consistent, but different opinions were given at different stages of the investigation. This inconsistency can lead to confusion and erode trust in both the judiciary and the investigators. A suitable analogy to illustrate this point is the interpretation of a CT scan film, where the expertise of the reader matters significantly. Just as a radiologist or neurosurgeon can analyze the film accurately, a dermatologist or microbiologist may not possess the necessary expertise to do so. Similarly, forming a medicolegal opinion requires not only experience but also scientific knowledge and credentials of the medical professional providing the opinion.

In criminal cases, medical conclusions must be based on a **reasonable degree of certainty** and be beyond any reasonable doubt, as expected from a doctor acting as a witness or expert witness in the Court of Law. The opinion given by the autopsy surgeon is based on the highest level of probability. However, it is crucial to recognize that the same postmortem findings may be present in different circumstances. Therefore, forming an opinion in such complex cases necessitates a meticulous examination of minute details, including crime scene findings, analysis of trace evidence, and investigative discoveries.

In the case report of death due to suicidal gunshot, too much emphasis was placed on the non-detection of gunshot residues on the deceased's hands. It is essential to note that non-detection does not necessarily mean the absence of gunshot residues; rather, it implies that the testing laboratory failed to detect their presence. Moreover, various fallacies and reasons can affect the detection of gunshot residues.

In the case report of suicidal ligature strangulation, the autopsy surgeon did not consider the variations that could be found in ligature strangulation cases, nor did they consider the manner in which the ligature material was positioned over the neck and tied to the fingers of the deceased. The investigation revealed that the deceased had psychiatric problems and was on medication, and the parents eventually accepted that she had committed suicide, leading to the closure of the case.

In the case report of suicidal partial hanging, it was a typical hanging case, but different medical boards were unable to scientifically guide the investigation and address the parents' concerns about certain autopsy findings.

Conclusion

Forensic doctors' opinions should be considered the "gold standard" and based on scientific findings. Each medicolegal case is unique and holds its own distinct characteristics. Forensic experts should continuously update their knowledge about the latest developments in the field through case reports and research articles.

A forensic expert must avoid forming opinions hastily, especially concerning the manner of death. Postmortem findings are objective facts that should be recorded accurately and objectively. Forensic Medicine does not offer absolute diagnostic opinions like mathematical calculations, but rather, conclusions should be based on the nearest possible option with a reasonable degree of certainty, without any reasonable doubt and without any other plausible alternatives.

In forming a medical opinion, circumstantial and direct pieces of evidence play pivotal roles. The opinion is based on the facts and findings available at the time of its formulation, and it may be revised if the underlying facts that shape the opinion change over time.

Bibliography

Di Maio VJM. *Gunshot wounds: Practical aspects of firearm, Ballistics and forensic techniques.* Second edition. London: CRC Press, 1999, pp. 327–346.

Dixit N. Shehla Masood case: Police, forensic doctors botched up probe. *India Today.* 2011 October 12. [Internet] [Cited 2018 September 14]. Available from: https://www.indiatoday.in/india/north/story/shehla-masood-case-police-forensic-doctors-botched-up-probe-143223-2011-10-12

Furukawa S, Sakaguchi I, Morita S, Nakagawa T, Takaya A, et al. suicidal ligature strangulation without an auxiliary mechanism: Reports of two cases with a cotton rope or a T shirt. *Rom J Leg Med.* 2013;21:9–14.

Gupta S, Dey A, Sharma N, Kanwar H, Tyagi S, Yadav A, et al. Credible forensic medical expert opinion for investigators and judiciary. *The Indian Police Journal* January–March 2020;67:63–72.

Gupta SK. *Forensic pathology of asphyxial deaths.* Boca Raton: CRC Press, 2022 July 5.

Mant KA. *Taylor's principles and practices of medical jurisprudence.* Thirteenth edition. Edinburgh: Churchill Livingstone, 1984, pp. 309–311.

Narayana BK, Mishra AK, Honourable Allahbad high court justice: Rajesh Talwar & Nupur Talwar vs state of Uttar Pradesh. *Criminal appeal no* 293 & 294 of 2014. 2017 October 12.

Spitz WU. *Spitz and fisher's medicolegal investigation of death.* Fourth edition. Springfield, IL: Charles C Thomas, 2006, p. 811.

INDEX

Page numbers followed by 'f,' and 't' refer to figures and tables respectively.

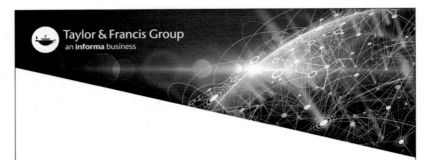